Geriatrics & Gerontology of the Dog and Cat

RICHARD T. GOLDSTON, DVM, MS, Diplomate ACVIM, Diplomate ABVP
Internist and Director
Animal Hospital of St. Petersburg
St. Petersburg, Florida

JOHNNY D. HOSKINS, DVM, PhD, Diplomate ACVIM
Professor
Department of Veterinary Clinical Sciences
School of Veterinary Medicine
Louisiana State University
Baton Rouge, Louisiana

Geriatrics & Gerontology of the Dog and Cat

W.B. SAUNDERS COMPANY
A Division of Harcourt Brace & Company
Philadelphia London Toronto Montreal Sydney Tokyo

W.B. SAUNDERS COMPANY
A Division of Harcourt Brace & Company

The Curtis Center
Independence Square West
Philadelphia, Pennsylvania 19106

Library of Congress Cataloging-in-Publication Data

Geriatrics and gerontology of the dog and cat / edited by Richard T. Goldston, Johnny D. Hoskins.—1st ed.

p. cm.

ISBN 0–7216–4584–4

1. Dogs—Aging. 2. Dogs—Diseases. 3. Cats—Aging. 4. Cats—Diseases. 5. Veterinary geriatrics. I. Goldston, Richard T. II. Hoskins, Johnny D.

SF991.G46 1995 636.7′089897—dc20

95–8334

GERIATRICS AND GERONTOLOGY OF THE DOG AND CAT ISBN 0–7216–4584–4

Printed in the United States of America.

Last digit is the print number: 9 8 7 6 5 4 3 2 1

To my wife and daughter, Sharon and Lesley Goldston,
whose love and support I need and covet very much,
and to my mother, Lucy Goldston,
whose love, strength and faith has been a constant inspiration.

RTG

To all practicing veterinarians who are caring for the older dogs
and cats of the world.

JDH

Contributors

DAVID P. AUCOIN, DVM, Diplomate ACVCP
Senior Vice President, VCA-Vet's Choice, Santa Monica, California
Drug Therapy in the Geriatric Pet

JENNIFER AUTHEMENT, DVM, Diplomate ACVIM
Internist, Animal Hospital of St. Petersburg, St. Petersburg, Florida
Drug Therapy in the Geriatric Pet

BRIAN S. BEALE, DVM, Diplomate ACVS
Surgeon, Gulf Coast Veterinary Specialists, Houston, Texas
The Skeletal System

COLIN F. BURROWS, BVetMed, PhD, MRCVS, Diplomate ACVIM
Professor of Medicine, College of Veterinary Medicine, University of Florida, Gainesville, Florida
The Digestive System

JANICE L. CAIN, DVM, Diplomate ACVIM
Staff Internist, Norris Canyon Veterinary Medical Center, San Ramon, California
The Reproductive System and Prostate Gland

BARBARA L. CHAPMAN, BVSc, MACVSc
Clinician, Victoria, Australia
Behavioral Disorders

C. B. CHASTAIN, DVM, MS, Diplomate ACVIM
Professor of Small Animal Medicine and Associate Dean for Academic Affairs, College of Veterinary Medicine, University of Missouri; Professor of Small Animal Medicine, Veterinary Medical Teaching Hospital, College of Veterinary Medicine, University of Missouri, Columbia, Missouri
The Endocrine and Metabolic Systems

AUTUMN P. DAVIDSON, DVM, Diplomate ACVIM
Staff Internist, Encina Veterinary Hospital, Walnut Creek, California
The Reproductive System and Prostate Gland

JACEK J. DeHAAN, DVM
Clinical Instructor in Orthopedic Surgery, Department of Companion Animal and Special Species Medicine, North Carolina State University, Raleigh, North Carolina
The Skeletal System

LINDA J. DeBOWES, DVM, MS, Diplomate ACVIM, Diplomate AVDC
Associate Professor, Veterinary Medical Teaching Hospital (VMTH), Kansas State University College of Veterinary Medicine, Manhattan, Kansas
The Oral Cavity and Dental Disease

SHARON M. DIAL, DVM, PhD, Diplomate ACVP
Clinical Pathologist, Southwest Veterinary Diagnostics, Phoenix, Arizona
The Hematopoietic System, Lymph Nodes, and Spleen

DONNA S. DIMSKI, DVM, MS, Diplomate ACVIM
Staff Internist, Willamette Veterinary Referral Center, Corvallis, Oregon
The Liver and Exocrine Pancreas

LISA M. FREEMAN, DVM
Clinical Instructor, Tufts University School of Veterinary Medicine, North Grafton, Massachusetts; Fellow in Clinical Nutrition, USDA Human Nutrition Research Center, Boston, Massachusetts
The Cardiovascular System

HOWARD B. GELBERG, DVM, PhD, Diplomate ACVP
Professor and Chairman, Department of Veterinary Pathology, College of Veterinary Medicine, University of Illinois, Urbana, Illinois
The Urinary System

RICHARD T. GOLDSTON, DVM, MS, Diplomate ACVIM, Diplomate ABVP
Internist and Director, Animal Hospital of St. Petersburg, St. Petersburg, Florida
Introduction and Overview of Geriatrics; Drug Therapy in the Geriatric Pet; Nutrition and Nutritional Disorders

C. GUY HANCOCK, DVM
Director of Veterinary Technology Program, St. Petersburg Junior College, St. Petersburg, Florida; Board of Directors, The Hospice of the Florida Suncoast, Largo, Florida
Client Services

COLIN E. HARVEY, BVSc, FRCVS, Diplomate ACVS, Diplomate AVDC
Professor of Surgery and Dentistry, School of Veterinary Medicine, University of Pennsylvania, Philadelphia, Pennsylvania
The Oral Cavity and Dental Disease

GISELLE HOSGOOD, BVSc, MS, Diplomate ACVS
Associate Professor of Veterinary Surgery, School of Veterinary Medicine, Louisiana State University, Baton Rouge, Louisiana
Surgical Protocol

JOHNNY D. HOSKINS, DVM, PhD, Diplomate ACVIM
Professor, Department of Veterinary Clinical Sciences, School of Veterinary Medicine, Louisiana State University, Baton Rouge, Louisiana
Health Care Program; Nutrition and Nutritional Disorders

BARBARA E. KITCHELL, DVM, PhD, Diplomate ACVIM
Associate Professor of Veterinary Medicine, Department of Veterinary Clinical Medicine, College of Veterinary Medicine, University of Illinois, Urbana, Illinois
Cancer and Its Therapy

DONALD R. KRAWIEC, DVM, MS, PhD, Diplomate ACVIM
Associate Professor of Veterinary Medicine and Chief of Small Animal Medicine Section, Department of Veterinary Clinical Medicine, College of Veterinary Medicine, University of Illinois, Urbana, Illinois
The Urinary System

DOTTIE P. LAFLAMME, DVM, Diplomate ACVN
Department of Pet Nutrition Research, Ralston Purina Company, St. Louis, Missouri
Nutrition and Nutritional Disorders

JODY P. LULICH, DVM, PhD, Diplomate ACVIM
Associate Professor, Department of Small Animal Clinical Sciences, College of Veterinary Medicine, University of Minnesota, St. Paul, Minnesota
The Urinary System

SANDRA R. MERCHANT, DVM, Diplomate ACVD
Associate Professor of Dermatology, Louisiana State University; Dermatologist, Veterinary Teaching Hospital and Clinics, Louisiana State University, Baton Rouge, Louisiana
The Skin

T. MARK NEER, DVM, Diplomate ACVIM
Professor, Department of Veterinary Clinical Sciences, School of Veterinary Medicine, Louisiana State University, Baton Rouge, Louisiana
The Nervous System

CARL A. OSBORNE, DVM, PhD, Diplomate ACVIM
Professor, Department of Small Animal Clinical Sciences, College of Veterinary Medicine, University of Minnesota, St. Paul, Minnesota
The Urinary System

ROBERT R. PADDLEFORD, DVM, Diplomate ACVA

Associate Professor and Director of Anesthesia Services, Department of Small Animal Practice, College of Veterinary Medicine, University of Tennessee, Knoxville, Tennessee

Anesthesia

JOHN E. RUSH, DVM, MS, Diplomate ACVIM (Cardiology), Diplomate ACVECC

Assistant Professor, Tufts University School of Veterinary Medicine, Co-Director, ICU and Emergency Services, and Clinical Cardiologist, Tufts University, North Grafton, Massachusetts

The Cardiovascular System

G. DIANE SHELTON, DVM, PhD, Diplomate ACVIM

Associate Clinical Professor, School of Medicine, Department of Pathology, University of California, San Diego; Director, Comparative Neuromuscular Laboratory, University of California, San Diego, La Jolla, California

Neuromuscular Disorders

JOSEPH TABOADA, DVM, Diplomate ACVIM

Associate Professor and Chief of Small Animal Internal Medicine, Department of Veterinary Clinical Sciences, School of Veterinary Medicine, Louisiana State University, Baton Rouge, Louisiana

The Respiratory System

I. VAN DER GAAG, DVM, PhD

Associate Professor, Department of Veterinary Pathology, Faculty of Veterinary Medicine, University of Utrecht, Utrecht, The Netherlands

The Ear

A. J. VENKER-VAN HAAGEN, DVM, PhD

Associate Professor, Department of Clinical Sciences of Companion Animals, Faculty of Veterinary Medicine, University of Utrecht, Utrecht, The Netherlands

The Ear

Preface

During the past few years there has been an enormous increase in interest in the geriatric health care of dogs and cats. Dogs and cats are living longer now due to better nutrition, husbandry, and veterinary care. Additionally, much more has been learned of the importance to the human of the human–animal bond that develops as more owners keep pets longer. There are only a few review papers, research articles, and case reports published over the years that contain practical information on the diagnostic, medical, and surgical management of disorders of the older dog or cat. This textbook is the first extensive accumulation of information concerning the special health needs of geriatric dogs and cats.

It is our hope and the hope of all the contributors that *Geriatrics and Gerontology of the Dog and Cat* will become a valuable and time-proved informative source for you. We hope it is a textbook that you will use often and that it will stimulate more sharing of information on the health needs of the older dog and cat.

We are indeed grateful to all of the contributors to this textbook. It has to be a caring, dedicated individual who will set aside, from an already full schedule, the time to prepare manuscripts such as those that went into this textbook. Thank you for sharing your expertise with your colleagues. We would especially like to thank our families, friends, and colleagues for their unfailing support and encouragement. It has indeed been an exciting and educational experience.

The staff at the W.B. Saunders Company deserve thanks for their extra efforts in the production of this textbook. Their desire for quality and a final product that will be of genuine benefit to the veterinary profession is representative of the high standards of the W.B. Saunders Company.

We would like to extend special acknowledgment to Mr. Ray Kersey for his excellent direction and assistance in all phases of this book's preparation. Additionally, we would like to thank the editorial and production staff of the W.B. Saunders Company for their skillful assistance, cooperation, and professionalism.

RICHARD T. GOLDSTON, DVM, MS
JOHNNY D. HOSKINS, DVM, PHD

Notice

Contents

CHAPTER 1

Introduction and Overview of Geriatrics

RICHARD T. GOLDSTON

Geriatrics is that branch of medicine and surgery that treats problems peculiar to old age. Age is defined as a complex biologic process resulting in the progressive reduction of an individual's ability to maintain homeostasis under internal physiologic and external environmental stresses, thereby decreasing the individual's viability and increasing its vulnerability to disease and eventually leading to death. Aging is not a disease itself, and there are many factors, most notably genetics, environment, and nutrition, that can influence the rate of the aging process. Table 1–1 covers these factors and the ages at which cats and dogs in different weight groups are considered to be geriatric (Goldston, 1989).

In a study of longevity and morbidity over a 10-year period for six giant breeds of dogs and seven small breeds of dogs, there was statistically significant evidence that the small breed dogs studied lived longer than the giant breed dogs studied. Only 282 of 2171 giant breed dogs (13%) lived to be 10 years of age or older, and only two (0.1%) lived to be 15 years of age or older. Conversely, 1857 of 4931 small breed dogs (38%) lived to be 10 years of age or older and 347 (7%) lived to be 15 years of age or older (Deeb and Wolf, 1994). A retrospective study by the Saint Bernard Club of America to determine the life span and morbidity for that breed revealed an average life span of 6.5 years (Saint Bernard Club of America, 1993). A similar study of the Irish wolfhound found that the average life span of that breed was also 6.5 years (Bernardi, 1988). Another survey of dogs 17 years of age or older revealed a 12:1 ratio of small to large breeds (Goldston, 1989).

An American Veterinary Medical Association pet survey in 1991 revealed that there were 52.5 million pet dogs in households in the United

TABLE 1–1. AGING FACTORS

Genetics	Smaller breeds of dogs live longer than larger breeds.
	Mixed breeds live longer than pure breeds.
Nutrition	Obese pets live shorter life spans than nonobese pets.
	High-fat and/or low-fiber diets decrease life expectancy.
Environment	"Outdoor" animals have a shorter life expectancy than "indoor" animals.
	Rural animals possibly live longer than urban animals.
	Neutered animals live longer than non-neutered animals.

Ages at which dogs and cats are considered to be "geriatric" or most likely to start having diseases associated with aging:

Small dogs	(0–20 lb):	11.48 ± 1.85 yr
Medium dogs	(21–50 lb):	10.90 ± 1.56 yr
Large dogs	(51–90 lb):	8.85 ± 1.38 yr
Giant dogs	(>90 lb):	7.46 ± 1.94 yr
Cats		11.88 ± 1.94 yr

States. Of these, 41.7 per cent (22 million) were 6 years of age or older, and 13.9 per cent (7.3 million) were 11 years of age or older. The total of 52.5 million dogs owned in 1991 indicates a stable dog population, as a similar survey done in 1987 had revealed a total dog population of 52.4 million. The same 1991 survey revealed that there were 57 million cats in households in the United States. Of these, 33.4 per cent (19 million) were 6 years of age or older, and 11 per cent (6 million) were 11 years of age or older. The cat population of 57 million in 1991 represents an approximate increase of 4.5 per cent over the cat population of 54.6 million in 1987. Thus, the estimated total dog and cat population in the United States as of 1991 was 109.5 million (Wise, 1991).

Pets provide humans with companionship, physical contact, a focus of attention, a means of safety, and a stimulus for exercise (Crow, 1986). Because of the increased problems seen in the older patient, along with the strong attachment to the pet by the average owner (human–animal bond), the percentage of practice income from geriatrics may range from 30 to 40 per cent if a complete program of geriatric medicine is offered.

THEORIES OF AGING

The underlying cause of aging has not been definitively determined, but there are many theories. Cumulative damage theories suggest that ionizing irradition of genetic material or free radical damage to subcellular organelles underlies the aging process (Allen, 1988). Waste product theories suggest that accumulation of substances such as lipofuscin and advanced glycosylation compounds in the central and peripheral nervous system affects the aging process. The effects of immunologic events as acquired cellular changes—resulting in antigenic stimulation, prolonged antigen–antibody reactions, decreases in immune surveillance, and the emergence of altered or mutated cells—may also promote the aging process.

THE CHALLENGE OF GERIATRIC MEDICINE AND SURGERY

In the geriatric patient, multiple organ systems are usually undergoing progressive and possibly irreversible change at the same time. It is rare that a geriatric patient presented for illness or surgery will have only the problem for which it is presented, with all other organ systems normal. It is a true challenge to identify and assess the multiple "hidden" organ dysfunctions or hypofunctions of the elderly patient before medical or surgical intervention for the problem for which the patient was presented. It is an even greater medical challenge to identify internal organ dysfunctions before they are externally obvious. In his 1908 book, *The Cure of Tumors by Medicines,* John H. Clarke wrote, "Anybody can diagnose an apple tree when he sees apples on it, but the skilled botanist can distinguish between an apple tree, a pear tree, and a plum tree, even when there are no leaves on them. In the same way, the skilled physician should be able to diagnose a cancer organism before any lump has appeared" (Clarke, 1908).

REWARDS OF A GERIATRIC PRACTICE

The mental challenge of diagnosing, treating, and monitoring the chronic disease processes of older pets is extremely rewarding.

The practice of geriatrics encompasses every facet of veterinary medicine. There is a continual mental challenge to stay abreast of current knowledge and understand the pathophysiology of multiple organ dysfunction. Pharmacokinetics must be understood when treating animals with cardiac, renal, and/or hepatic disease. Drug interactions must be understood when treating animals that require multiple drugs given at one time (i.e., polypharmacy). Anesthesia requires more attention to detail before, during, and immediately after surgery in the geriatric patient. Meeting the specific nutritional demands of aged patients with, for example, single or multiple organopathies, cancer, diabetes mellitus, or obesity requires continual updating of nutritional knowledge as more specific diets and "longevity" supplements are discovered.

Many veterinarians suffer early discouragement and "burnout" associated with day-to-day management of a practice and the routine of well animal care (e.g., vaccinations, dewormings, and ovariohysterectomies and orchectomies). In addition to personal gratification, however, the veterinarian will also recognize increased practice income from the detailed management of the geriatric patient.

Rewards for the owners of the geriatric patient can be both physical and emotional. Virtually every type of family unit has one or more family

TABLE 1–2. EFFECTS OF AGING

Metabolic effects	Decreased metabolic rate plus lack of activity decreases caloric needs by 30 to 40 per cent.
	Immune competence decreases, despite normal numbers of lymphocytes.
	Phagocytosis and chemotaxis decrease, and the pet is less able to ward off infections.
	Autoantibodies and autoimmune diseases develop.
Physical effects	Percentage of body weight represented by fat increases.
	Skin becomes thickened, hyperpigmented, and inelastic.
	Footpads hyperkeratinize, and claws become brittle.
	Muscle, bone, and cartilage mass are lost, with subsequent development of arthritis.
	Dental calculus results in tooth loss and gingival hyperplasia.
	Periodontitis results in gingival retraction and atrophy.
	Gastric mucosa becomes atrophic and fibrotic.
	Hepatocyte numbers decrease, and hepatic fibrosis occurs.
	Pancreatic enzyme secretion diminishes.
	Lungs lose elasticity, fibrosis occurs, and pulmonary secretions become more viscous. Vital capacity decreases.
	Cough reflex and expiratory capacity decrease.
	Kidney weight decreases, glomerular filtration rate decreases, and tubules atrophy.
	Urinary incontinence frequently develops.
	Prostate gland enlarges, testes atrophy, and prepuce becomes pendulous.
	Ovaries enlarge, and mammary glands become fibrocystic or neoplastic.
	Cardiac output decreases, and valvular fibrosis and intramural coronary arteriosclerosis develop.
	Bone marrow becomes fatty and hypoplastic, and nonregenerative anemia develops.
	The number of cells in the nervous system decreases. Senility causes loss of house training.

members with a deep bond to the geriatric pet. In families with children, the pet may be older than the eldest child; this child may have known the pet for his or her entire life and have a very deep bond with the pet (Blue, 1986). Single-person families, families without children, and families with grown children may see the pet as a child substitute (Lynch, 1977). Elderly people living alone may become dependent on the companionship of a pet (New et al, 1986). Any treatment or surgical protocol that can extend and improve the quality of life of these pets not only gives owners valuable time with their pets, but also allows them time to prepare for the pet's death.

VETERINARIAN AND OWNER COMMUNICATION AND OWNER COMPLIANCE

Successful geriatric medicine requires detailed communication between the veterinarian and the owner and exceptional owner compliance in meeting all the medical recommendations and nursing needs of the elderly patient. Most medical problems involving older patients are chronic rather than acute. Chronic diseases (e.g., renal failure, hepatic failure, cardiac insufficiency, and endocrinopathies [diabetes mellitus, Cushing's disease, and hypothyroidism]) require lifelong treatment with intermittent monitoring of the patient and modification of the treatment regimen as needed.

EFFECT OF AGING ON PETS' BODY SYSTEMS

A common characteristic of all aging systems is progressive and irreversible change. This change may be hastened by the effects of disease, stress, malnutrition, lack of exercise, genetics, and environment. Increased knowledge and improved technology increase our opportunity to effect change and improvement in the pursuit of health, longevity, and quality of life. Elderly animals seldom have a single disease, but instead have a unique combination of multiple organ disease with varying levels of dysfunction. Veterinarians should not accept that poor health and old age are synonymous. Knowledge of the common pathologic changes associated with age and their effect on function allows the veterinarian to plan and manage more effective health care programs for aged pets (Mosier, 1989). Table 1–2 outlines the common effects of aging.

The Skin

Cellular atrophy occurs in the epidermis, its appendages, and the dermis of older dogs. The skin becomes less pliable and loses its elasticity owing to pseudoelastin infiltration and calcium deposition in the skin's elastic fibers. Follicular atrophy results in hair loss, and the atrophy of pigment cells in the hair follicles may result in white hair (Muller et al, 1983). Sebum production decreases, and the sebum consistency becomes waxy so that the hair shafts are not adequately covered. This results in a haircoat that may be dry, scaly, dull, and lusterless, with patchy areas of alopecia.

The skin and haircoat of the geriatric dog and cat may be improved with external application of either oil-free humectants such as Humilac (Allerderm/Virbac) or oil-based products such as HyLyt efa bath oil coat conditioner (DVM Pharmaceuticals). Correction of any endocrinopathies, especially hypothyroidism and/or Cushing's disease, will also improve skin and haircoat in the geriatric patient.

Nasal and digital pad hyperkeratosis can also occur. These can be treated with a topical keratolytic gel such as Kera-Solv (DVM Pharmaceuticals) or with manual debridement. The median age for the development of skin neoplasia is 10.5 years in dogs and 12 years in cats (MacDonald, 1987). (See Chapter 12 for an in-depth study of geriatric disorders of the skin.)

The Digestive System

Dental calculus and tartar accompanied by either gingival hyperplasia or periodontitis with gingival retraction, atrophy, and bone loss increase with age. Loss of teeth usually results from alveolar demineralization owing to calcium deficits and/or periodontitis (Mosier, 1981). Xerostomia results from decreased salivary secretions owing to fat infiltration within the salivary glands. Proper dental hygiene includes (1) owner education on the importance of brushing the dog's teeth at least twice weekly and (2) routine dental prophylaxis when needed. Gerodontics is a vital part of a geriatric health care program and results in a decreased incidence of the internal organ disease that can occur from the postprandial bacteremia seen in dogs that have severe dental and periodontal disease.

Oral tumors are common in dogs 10 years of age and older. The most common are melanoma, fibrosarcoma, and squamous cell carcinoma (Mosier, 1987). Melanoma is the most common oral neoplasia in the dog and is also the fastest to metastasize. Squamous cell carcinomas are the most common oral neoplasm seen in cats. Benign epulides are common in geriatric dogs, especially the brachycephalic breeds. Surgical ablation by maxillectomy, mandibulectomy, or hemimandibulectomy is usually the treatment of choice for oral neoplasia when possible. Cisplatin 60 mg/m^2 once every 3 weeks for three treatments can be effective for squamous cell carcinoma in dogs but is extremely toxic in cats.

Esophageal function is decreased by loss of neurons and cellular atrophy. The incidence of atrophic gastritis and gastric polyps increases with age and can result in decreased gastric function and hypochlorhydria (Wingfield and Twedt, 1986).

Hepatic function decreases as the fat content of hepatocytes increases and the number of hepatocytes decreases. In addition, there is perilobular hepatic fibrosis and decreased bile secretion. Pancreatic enzyme secretion is diminished. Intestinal epithelial cell renewal and replacement are diminished, resulting in decreased intestinal villous height and width and, as a result, decreased intestinal mucosal surface area; this in turn causes decreased intestinal enzyme production and nutrient absorption. Colonic motility may decrease with age, predisposing the geriatric pet to constipation (Hodgkins, 1989). The addition of Viokase (½ teaspoonful per 10 kg of body weight) to a high-fiber, low-fat diet may facilitate digestion. It is not necessary to preincubate the enzyme with the food, nor is it necessary to alkalinize the stomach with sodium bicarbonate before feeding, as was previously thought. If constipation is observed, the addition of a small amount (titrated to effect) of psyllium hydrophilic mucilloid fiber (Metamucil) may be beneficial. (See Chapters 9 through 11 for an in-depth study of gerodontics and disorders of the gastrointestinal tract, liver, and pancreas.)

The Cardiovascular and Respiratory Systems

Thirty-three per cent of dogs 13 years of age or older that are examined at veterinary clinics have some form of heart disease (Mauderly, 1979). Cardiac output decreases 30 per cent in the last one third of the life span. Maximum heart rate and maximal oxygen consumption during exercise also decrease with age.

Chronic mitral valvular insufficiency is the most common cause of congestive heart failure (CHF). It occurs as a result of acid mucopolysaccharide deposition in the subendocardial layers of the valve cusps and eventually progresses to valvular fibrosis. Ascites and hepatomegaly are the most commonly seen signs secondary to right heart failure with its associated pulmonary venous hypertension. The typical murmur of mitral insufficiency is heard best at the left intercostal space. The therapeutic approach to mitral insufficiency is to reduce fluid retention (furosemide 2 mg/kg per os bid); decrease cardiac workload with the use of a low-sodium diet, restricted activity, and hypotensive drugs (enalapril 0.5 mg/kg per os bid or captopril 1 mg/kg per os tid, plus calcium channel blockers such as diltiazem 1 mg/kg per os tid); and augmentation of myocardial contraction (digoxin, dosed to maintain blood levels of 1 to 3 ng/ml, or digitoxin, dosed to maintain blood levels of 15 to 35 ng/ml.) Digoxin is excreted renally, whereas digitoxin is eliminated hepatically. Thus, digoxin is used in the presence of chronic liver disease and digitoxin in the presence of chronic renal disease.

Bronchodilation further aids tissue oxygenation in CHF. The drugs of choice are theophylline 6 mg/kg per os or aminophylline 10 mg/kg per os. Therapeutic blood levels for each are 10 to 20 μg/ml.

Common problems of the respiratory system of aged pets are increased susceptibility to infection (pneumonia) and the chronic obstructive pulmonary disease complex, which includes a number of pathologic conditions in the pulmonary airways (e.g., asthma, chronic bronchitis, bronchiectasis, and emphysema). Decreased volume and increased viscosity of pulmonary secretions along with diminished function of the mucociliary apparatus contribute to obstructive disease.

The aged lung also has reduced capability to expel air and decreased oxygen diffusing capability through enlarged coalescing alveolar membranes. In addition, there is loss of elasticity with increased pulmonary fibrosis and an increase in both surface area and fixed lung volume (Mauderly, 1979). Radiographs show a trachea dilated on both inspiration and expiration, increased pulmonary interstitial densities, and pulmonary retraction from the thoracic wall owing to fibrosis. The cough reflex is decreased as a result of decreased sensitivity of mucous membranes and atrophy and weakening of the muscles of respiration. Treatment is with bronchodilators (theophylline/aminophylline) and mucolytic/expectorants (iodinated glycerol [Organidin]) at 30 mg per os tid. (See Chapters 7 and 8 for an in-depth study of geriatric respiratory and cardiovascular disorders.)

The Urinary System

A gradual decline in kidney function is considered a normal part of aging. Renal failure is one of the top four causes of death in geriatric dogs (Polzin, 1987) and is also a major cause of mortality in cats (DiBartola et al, 1987). Of 2228 cases of feline renal failure diagnosed between 1980 and 1990 at North American veterinary colleges, 63 per cent were in cats 10 years of age or older (Veterinary Medical Data Base, Purdue University).

The process of renal failure begins with loss of functioning nephrons, decreased renal blood flow, and decreased glomerular filtration rate. A decrease in renal blood flow leads to ischemic atrophy and fibrosis of peritubular tissues, with further loss of function (Schneck, 1982). This results in progressive chronic renal failure. The progression of chronic renal failure in dogs can be slowed with the use of diets containing low amounts of highly biodegradable protein. In cats the progression of chronic renal failure can be slowed by feeding similar diets containing only 28 per cent protein. Also, dietary phosphate restriction (0.42 per cent phosphorus) in cats with severe (5/6) renal mass reduction prevents the mineralization, fibrosis, and mononuclear infiltration of the kidneys that occurs in similarly renally impaired cats receiving the usual 1.5 per cent phosphorus diets (Wingfield and Twedt, 1986). Diets for dogs with chronic renal failure should have reduced protein, salt, and phosphorus (e.g., Prescription Diet k/d or u/d [Hill's Pet Products]). Animals on protein-restricted diets should have adequate amounts of dietary fat and carbohydrates to meet 100 per cent of their daily caloric needs to ensure that dietary protein is used only for anabolism and is not catabolized to meet caloric demand.

The life span of the erythrocyte is decreased with uremia, and a concomitant decrease in erythropoietin production by the kidneys leads to a nonregenerative anemia. This can best be treated with Epogen (Amgen, Inc.), a human recombinant erythropoietin, at 100 U/kg three times weekly until the hematocrit level is 30 to 35 per cent, then as needed. Other therapies for chronic renal failure include reducing hypertension and preventing hypocalcemia and hypovitaminosis.

Urinary incontinence (UI) is a common geriatric disorder that frequently results in the owner's inability to keep the dog or cat as a pet. The most common causes of UI are urethral incompetence, urinary tract infection, and diseases that cause polydipsia/polyuria. Therefore, the treatment of UI should be directed at the specific cause. Urethral incompetence can be subjectively evaluated by interrupting the pet during urination to assess urethral tone. Also, residual urine volume (volume of urine in the urinary bladder after urination) can be measured and should not exceed 0.4 ml/kg. When a specific cause of UI cannot be determined, then nonspecific treatment of the incontinence should be implemented.

Drugs that increase contractility of the urinary bladder include bethanechol dosed at 2.5 to 7.5 mg for a small dog or cat and 10 to 25 mg for a large dog. Metoclopramide 0.5 mg/kg tid also can be used to stimulate detrusor muscle contraction in dogs. Drugs that decrease contractility of the urinary bladder include propantheline bromide (Pro-Banthine) dosed at 7.5 to 15 mg bid for dogs and 7.5 mg every 3 days for cats.

Drugs that increase urethral pressure include sex hormone replacement drugs. In bitches, diethylstilbestrol at 0.1 to 1.0 mg/day for 5 days and then twice weekly is frequently successful. In neutered males, 2.2 mg/kg of injectable testosterone propionate usually is effective. Because of rapid hepatic degradation, oral testosterone is ineffective unless dosed to levels that can cause adverse side effects. Phenylpropanolamine at 1.5 mg/kg bid or ephedrine sulfate at 25 to 50 mg bid is frequently effective.

Drugs to decrease urethral pressure are used in urethral spasm and detrusor-urethral dyssynergia. Phenoxybenzamine at 0.5 mg/kg/day orally is used to relax the smooth muscle of the urethra. Diazepam at 1 to 2 mg bid for small dogs and cats and 5 mg bid for large dogs is used to relax the striated muscles of the urethra. These may be very beneficial in feline obstructive urethropathy.

Urinary bladder tumors are the most common tumor of the urinary tract. Bladder tumors occur more commonly in dogs than in cats, supposedly because cats metabolize tryptophan differently than dogs and are less susceptible to tryptophan metabolites. Transitional cell carcinoma is the most common urinary bladder tumor. Squamous cell carcinomas and adenocarcinomas may also occur and probably develop as a result of metaplasia of transitional epithelial cells. The most effective treatment is early detection and radical surgical removal. The most successful chemotherapy is with parenteral and intravesicular cisplatin and/or doxorubicin. (See Chapter 16 for an in-depth study of geriatric disorders of the urinary system.)

Endocrine and Genital Systems

The aged animal experiences a significant decrease in the secretion of hormones by the thyroid, testes, ovaries, and pituitary glands. The testes will show flaccid atrophy and/or tumor formation. The ovaries increase in weight until approximately the age of 13 years and then atrophy. The adrenal glands may become hyperplastic, resulting in Cushing's disease. The mammary glands may become fibrocystic or develop neoplasia. Nodules or tumors are found in 60 per cent of intact females by the age of 11; mammary tumors make up 25 per cent of all neoplasms of the bitch. Fifty per cent of these tumors are malignant, and about 50 per cent of these will metastasize. Ovariohysterectomy before the first estrus eliminates virtually all mammary tumors, but this effect is lost if ovariohysterectomy is performed after 2.5 years of age.

Prostate diseases, including hyperplasia, neoplasia, cyst formation, and infection (abscessation), are the most common genital disorders of aged dogs, but prostate disease is rare in cats. Treatment for all prostatic diseases consists of castration. Other specific treatments include drainage of cysts and abscesses and antibiotic therapy. The antimicrobials that best penetrate the prostate gland include trimethroprim-sulfamethoxazole, lincomycin, erythromycin, chloramphenicol, and clindamycin. (See Chapters 15 and 20 for an in-depth study of geriatric disorders of the reproductive and endocrine and metabolic systems.)

Musculoskeletal System

Muscle and bone mass are lost in the aged animal as a result of both atrophy and decreased numbers of muscle and bone cells. Reduced muscle function is due to increasing fibrosis, muscle fiber atrophy, and reduced oxygen transport to muscles, as well as reduced use of oxygen by muscles. Reduced bone function results from fat infiltration of the bone marrow and decreased bone cortex thickness. Intestinal absorption of calcium is decreased, resulting in thinner, more dense, and more brittle bone structure. Aged cartilage has decreased tensile strength and has a tendency to split and fragment. Degenerative numbers of chondrocytes produce less mucopolysaccharide and chondroitin sulfate. Vertebral spondylosis and costochondral calcification are frequent incidental findings on radiographs of geriatric animals.

Degenerative joint disease (DJD) is the single most common problem of the musculoskeletal system; DJD is the most common form. In DJD, microfractures occur in the subchondral bone

(Muller et al, 1983), and synovial fluid becomes more viscous. In rheumatoid arthritis, the synovial fluid becomes thin and watery, and joint capsule thickening and osteophyte formation are common. Obesity, commonly seen in the aged patient, compounds the effects of arthritis.

Treatment is aimed at reducing activity, reducing fat mass, and increasing muscle mass. In DJD, a polysulfated glycosaminoglycan, Adequan I.M. (Luitpold Pharmaceuticals), given at 4 mg/kg every 4 days for six doses and then every 2 to 4 weeks as needed, has proven beneficial in long-term pain reduction in dogs. Some nonsteroidal anti-inflammatory drugs (NSAIDs) are also beneficial in treating DJD. Recommended doses of some NSAIDs are as follows:

- Aspirin (buffered), 10 mg/kg twice daily for dogs and twice weekly for cats
- Phenylbutazone, 10 mg/kg tid for dogs, not to exceed a total daily dose of 800 mg
- Meclofenamic acid, 1 mg/kg daily for 1 week, then 0.5 mg/kg daily for dogs

Ibuprofen and acetaminophen should not be used, as the therapeutic dose is very close to the toxic dose. The common side effects of NSAIDs include gastrointestinal ulcers, renal ischemia, bone marrow toxicity, and decreased platelet function. (See Chapters 17 and 18 for an in-depth study of geriatric disorders of the neuromuscular and musculoskeletal systems.)

Nervous System

The first sign of senility usually seen in animals is loss of house training. Other senile changes include cognitive dysfunction signs such as changes in the sleep/wake cycle; inattention to food; inattention to the environment, including people or other animals; and an apparent inability to recognize familiar places and people or to respond to a name or to previously learned commands. Neurotransmitters also change with age. Acetylcholinesterase and monamine oxidase b levels increase, whereas choline acetyltransferase and serotonin levels decrease. Lipofuscin, "the aging pigment," accumulates in the cytoplasm of the neurons.

Ninety-five per cent of the neurons in the brain are said to be interneurons that amplify and refine diverse signal input. In the aged brain, the effects after a stimulus are prolonged. Subsequent repetitive stimuli impede short-term memory and increase response time to external stimuli. Advanced age results in distortion of neuronal soma, loss of dendritic spines, zones of dendritic varicosities, shrinkage of dendritic spines, and neuritic plaques (Schneck, 1982).

The aged brain is chronically hypoxic as a result of arteriocapillary fibrosis and endothelial proliferation. Long-term memory, unlike short-term memory, apparently is not affected by chronic cerebral hypoxia. An abundant supply of oxygen to the brain of senile animals allows the neurons to recover from past deprivation. Mental condition improves markedly and stays improved for a time after the extra oxygen is withdrawn (Schneck, 1982).

Tremor and motor hesitancy result from impairment of the corpus stratum and corpus pallidus. Neuronophagia occurs when astrocytes surround and phagocytize neurons. Treatment of senility and cognitive dysfunction in aged dogs is currently in its infancy. Studies using L-deprenyl, a dopaminogenic, monoamine oxidase b inhibitor, are under way. (See Chapter 19 for an in-depth study of geriatric disorders of the nervous system.)

ANESTHETIC CONSIDERATIONS IN THE GERIATRIC PATIENT

Geriatric patients often have various pathophysiologic conditions and decreased organ reserve capabilities that make them more sensitive to preanesthetic and anesthetic drugs.

The use of low-dose neuroleptic/analgesic agents containing reversible opiates for preanesthetics is very effective in geriatric anesthesia. An excellent combination is acetylpromazine at 0.1 mg/kg IM or IV combined with butorphanol at 0.5 mg/kg IM or IV. Butorphanol is an excellent analgesic, with five times the analgesic potency of morphine. Its main advantage in geriatric anesthesia is its marked analgesic effect with minimal respiratory and cardiovascular depression; also, it is a noncontrolled opiate.

The inhalant anesthetics are the general anesthetics of choice for prolonged procedures in the aged patient. Methoxyflurane, halothane, or isoflurane can all be used with or without nitrous oxide. Methoxyflurane decreases cardiac output, can be hepatotoxic, and can alter renal function by decreasing renal perfusion. Halothane also decreases cardiac output, is a respiratory depressant, sensitizes the myocardium to catecholamines, and should not be used in animals with dysrhythmias. Chronic liver dysfunction should also preclude the use of halothane. Isoflurane is the least soluble of the inhalant anesthetics and as a result has the fastest induction time (3 to 5 minutes). It is the inhalant anesthetic of choice in the geriatric patient.

Regardless of the anesthetic technique used, geriatric patients should be preoxygenated for 2 to 5 minutes before induction to prevent hypoxia. The patient should be intubated to provide a patent airway, and intravenous fluids should be administered to help maintain a proper hemodynamic state. The rate of intravenous fluid administration in most cases should be in the range of 10 to 20 ml/kg/hour. (See Chapter 21 for an in-depth discussion of anesthesia in geriatric patients.)

ADVANCES IN DELAYING THE ONSET OF GERIATRIC CHANGES

Various drugs and hormones that affect the aging process are currently being studied. However, the most promising research in significantly delaying the onset of aging appears to be in genetics and gene manipulation (Kohn, 1973). Michael Jazwinski of Louisiana State University has discovered a "longevity" gene that can extend the life span of a yeast cell by 30 per cent. He has named it Longevity Assurance Gene-1 and, after sequencing and cloning it, is currently looking for a similar or identical gene in humans (Darrach, 1992).

Daniel Rudman of the Medical College of Wisconsin, experimenting with human growth hormone, found that human males who received recombinant human growth hormone in amounts equivalent to those produced by healthy young men regained 10 per cent of their muscle mass, had a 9 per cent increase in skin thickness, and lost 14 per cent of their body fat. Their liver and spleen also substantially regained mass (Darrach, 1992).

In Switzerland and at the Medical College of Virginia, Walter Peirpaoli and William Regelson induced laboratory mice to live up to 30 per cent longer than untreated mice simply by adding melatonin to their drinking water (Darrach, 1992).

Robert Flood and John Carne at Oklahoma Medical Research Foundation and the University of Kentucky have developed an active neutrino called PAN (tertiary butylphenylnitrone) that repairs brain damage in old gerbils, restoring their ability to solve mazes learned when they were younger (Darrach, 1992).

Arthur Schwartz of Temple University has reported that in laboratory animals receiving high doses of dehydroepiandrosterone (DHEA), body fat was reduced by one third. DHEA also enhances the immune system, thus reducing the risk of cancer and the development of some autoimmune diseases. The life span of mice has been increased by 20 per cent with DHEA (Darrach, 1992).

The abortifacient drug RU-486, used in France and currently being reviewed for use in the United States, could become the "wonder drug" of future geriatric medicine. Roussel Uclaf, the French company that owns the patent for RU-486, and other researchers claim RU-486 may contribute to the treatment of many disorders associated with advancing age, such as hypertension, muscle atrophy, obesity, immune deficiency, osteoporosis, and depression (Darrach, 1992).

References

Allen TA. Geriatric internal medicine. In Proceedings of the AAHA/Midwest Small Animal Association Meeting. Denver, AAHA, 1988, pp 1–4.

Bernardi G. Longevity and morbidity in the Irish wolfhound in the United States—1966–1986. Harp and Hound 1:78, 1988.

Blue G. The value of pets in children's lives. J Assoc Childhood Educ Int pp 84–90, 1986.

Clarke JH. The Cure of Tumors by Medicines. London, James Epps & Co., 1908, p. 159.

Crow SE. Psychosocial aspects of veterinary clinic oncology. Semin Vet Med Surg (Small Animal) 1:84, 1986.

Darrach B. Life. New York, Rockefeller Center, 1992.

DiBartola, SP, Rutgers Z., et al. Clinicopathologic findings associated with chronic renal disease in cats: 74 cases (1973–1984). J Am Vet Med Assoc 190:1196–1202, 1987.

Deeb BJ, Wolf NS., Studying longevity and morbidity in giant and small breeds of dogs. Vet Med 89 (Suppl 7):702–713.

Goldston RT. Preface. Vet Clin North Am 19:1, 1989.

Hodgkins EM. Geriatric nutrition. Vet Clin North Am 19:1, 1989

Kohn RR. Aging. Kalamazoo, MI, Upjohn, 1973.

Lynch, JL. The Broken Heart: The Medical Consequences of Loneliness. New York, Basic Books, 1977.

MacDonald J. Neoplastic diseases of the integument. In Proceedings of the American Animal Hospital Association, 1987, pp 17–20.

Mauderly JL. Effect of age on pulmomary structure and function of immature and adult animals and man. Fed Proc 138:173–177, 1979.

Mosier JE. How aging affects body systems in the dog. In Proceedings of the Geriatric Medicine Symposium, 1987, pp 2–5.

Mosier JE. Canine geriatrics. In Proceedings of the American Animal Hospital Association, 1981, pp 137–145.

Mosier JE. Effect of aging on body systems of the dog. Vet Clin North Am 19:1, 1989.

Muller GH, Kirk RW, Scott DW. Small Animal Dermatology. 3rd ed. Philadelphia, WB Saunders, 1983.

New JC Jr, Wilson CC, Netting FE. How community-based elderly perceive pet ownership. Calif Vet 40:22–27, 1986.

Polzin DJ. Topics in general medicine: General nutrition; The problems associated with renal failure. Vet Med 82(10):1027–1035, 1987.

Saint Bernard Club of America Research Committee. ABCA health survey. Saint Fancier March/April:59–73, 1993.

Schneck AA. Aging of the nervous system. In Schrier RW, ed. Clinical Internal Medicine in the Aged. Philadelphia, WB Saunders, 1982, pp 41–49.

Wingfield WE, Twedt DC. Medical diseases of the stomach. In Jones BD, ed. Canine and Feline Gastroenterology. Philadelphia, WB Saunders, 1986, pp 101–133.

Wise JK. The Veterinary Services Market for Companion Animals. Schaumburg, IL, American Veterinary Medical Association, 1991.

CHAPTER 2

Health Care Program

JOHNNY D. HOSKINS

Geriatric dogs and cats make up a large portion of the patients seen in most veterinary practices. The veterinarian's responsibility to older dogs and cats is to delay, or at least minimize, the progressive deterioration of the body systems from the aging process and provide an improved quality of life for the weeks or months ahead (Goldston, 1989; Mosier, 1987). Delivery of improved health care to the geriatric dog and cat through the use of state-of-the-art medical and/or surgical therapy and competent nutritional management is the primary goal for a comprehensive geriatric health care program (Hoskins, 1993).

HEALTH CARE PROGRAM

Age Guidelines. A geriatric health care program can be a natural extension of the preventive health program of the younger dog and cat. A pediatric preventive health program includes patients from birth to 1 year of age, whereas the standard annual preventive medicine program begins at 1 year of age and continues until approximately 6 to 8 years of age.

Because the aging process varies with breed and species and an animal's lifestyle, the age at which a geriatric health care program should be implemented also varies. A geriatric health care program could begin at the following ages (Goldston, 1989):

- Small dogs (less than 20 pounds): 9 to 13 years
- Medium dogs (21 to 50 pounds): 9 to 11.5 years
- Large dogs (51 to 90 pounds): 7.5 to 10.5 years
- Giant dogs (more than 90 pounds): 6 to 9 years
- Cats (most breeds): 8 to 10 years

Range of the Program. A comprehensive geriatric health care program can provide a way to target key geriatric-related health problems, to institute preventive health care measures, and to detect disorders early enough for medical and surgical management (Table 2–1). Education of

TABLE 2–1. COMMONLY ENCOUNTERED GERIATRIC DISEASES

Geriatric Dog	Geriatric Cat
Diabetes mellitus	Inflammatory bowel disease
Prostatic disease	Diabetes mellitus
Obesity	Feline hepatic lipidosis
Cardiovascular disease	Chronic renal disease
Degenerative disease	Obesity
Cataracts	Cancer
Cancer	Dental disease
Dental disease	Hyperthyroidism
Keratoconjunctivitis sicca	Urolithiasis
Hypothyroidism	Anemia
Urolithiasis	Hepatopathies
Hyperadrenocorticism	Cardiovascular disease
Anemia	
Urinary incontinence	
Hepatopathies	
Chronic renal disease	

the dog or cat owner about health risks to geriatric patients and possible preventive measures is key to the success of this program.

The acceptance of an older dog or cat into the health care program depends on its general health status, which may be determined from the case history, physical examination, and other diagnostic procedures, and not on actual age. The health care program may include different levels of health evaluation (e.g., Program 1 for the apparently healthy patient, Program 2 for the patient with minor health concerns, and Program 3 for the patient with major health concerns, as in Table 2–2).

Physical Examination. Clinical evaluation of a geriatric dog or cat initially begins with taking a complete case history and performing the physical examination. Basic information about the animal, such as breed, age, and sex, as well as owner concerns, is obtained from the case history. After the case history is obtained, the physical examination is performed in a systematic manner. Although the examination may be easier to complete by proceeding from head to tail, it is advisable to examine and record observations according to body systems. Special concerns are directed to specific age-influenced body systems (Table 2–3).

TABLE 2–2. HEALTH SCREENING LEVELS FOR GERIATRIC DOGS AND CATS

Program 1
History and physical examination, including eyes and rectum
Packed cell volume (PCV) and total protein levels
Blood urea nitrogen (BUN) and glucose levels
Complete urinalysis
Consultation regarding nutrition, teeth, ears, nails, and skin care
Weight control program
Program 2
History and physical examination, including eyes and rectum
Complete blood cell (CBC) count and blood chemistry profile
Complete urinalysis
Consultation regarding nutrition, teeth, ears, nails, and skin care
Weight control program
Program 3
History and physical examination, including eyes and rectum
CBC count and blood chemistry profile
Complete urinalysis
Electrocardiography (ECG) and thoracic radiography, possibly echocardiography
Consultation regarding nutrition, teeth, ears, nails, and skin care
Weight control program
Ancillary Diagnostic Procedures
Echocardiography
Abdominal ultrasonography
Thyroid gland function tests
Blood pressure evaluation
Liver, pancreas, and small intestinal function assays
Urine protein-to-creatinine ratio determination
Urine cortisol-to-creatinine ratio determination

TABLE 2–3. SYSTEMATIC PHYSICAL EXAMINATION OF THE GERIATRIC DOG AND CAT

Abdominal palpation
Dental examination
Ears and eyes inspection
Musculoskeletal evaluation
Rectal examination and prostate gland palpation
Skin, haircoat, and nails examination
Thoracic auscultation

Health Care. The owner of a geriatric dog or cat should be encouraged to have the animal examined by a veterinarian at least once a year. At this annual examination a checklist of health care services can be used to ensure that all the steps in the health care program are followed (Table 2–4).

Owner Education. Another important aspect in the geriatric health care program is education of the pet owner, specifically in the areas of nutrition, preventive health care, exercise, normal aging process, cancer and its effects, and bereavement (Table 2–5). Pet loss, services for the owners of geriatric dogs and cats, memorialization, and hospice concepts applicable to veterinary medicine are discussed in Chapter 24. Unabridged attention must be directed toward instructing the pet owner with regard to certain potential problems specific to geriatric dogs and cats (Table 2–6).

IMPLEMENTATION OF THE HEALTH CARE PROGRAM

A health care program for aged dogs and cats should be fashioned to meet the specific needs of the patient and pet owner. A successful program requires a team approach that includes the receptionist, technician, ward attendants, veterinarian, and pet owner. To obtain optimal results, everyone, from the hospital staff to the veterinarian to the pet owner, should completely understand the intent of the program and its benefits.

Initiation of the Program. The first step in the initiation of a geriatric health care program is for the veterinarian to understand the full scope and need for geriatric health care services in the

TABLE 2–4. A PREVENTIVE HEALTH CARE PROGRAM FOR GERIATRIC DOGS AND CATS

Geriatric Dog

A. Conduct a general physical examination and record the body weight.
B. Check for external parasites and dermatophytes and initiate appropriate therapy.
   1. Fleas, ticks, and ear mites *(Otodectes cyanotis).*
   2. Mange mites, especially *Demodex canis* and *Sarcoptes scabiei.*
   3. Dermatophytes, particularly *Microsporum* spp. and *Trichophyton mentagrophytes.*
C. Conduct fecal examination (fecal flotation test).
D. Check for heartworm disease (Knott or occult test)
E. Adjust the dosage of heartworm preventive according to body weight, especially for diethylcarbamazine (DEC) products.
F. Deworm with broad-spectrum anthelmintic product.
G. Vaccinate with DA_2PLPC* and rabies vaccine and, possibly, kennel cough and canine Lyme borreliosis vaccine.
H. Adjust the diet according to health needs and, if necessary, change grooming procedures.
I. Trim the nails and clean the ear canals.
J. Discuss age-related changes that are occurring.
K. Provide the owner with educational pamphlets on such topics as:
   1. Identification, treatment, and control of fleas, ticks, and ear mites.
   2. Dental, skin, nails, and ear care.
   3. Grooming and nutrition.
   4. Management of normal and abnormal behaviors.
   5. Exercise and its importance.
L. Fill in the health record for the owner.

Geriatric Cat

A. Conduct a general physical examination and record the body weight.
B. Check for external parasites and dermatophytes and initiate appropriate therapy.
   1. Fleas and ear mites *(O. cyanotis).*
   2. Mange mites, especially *Notoedres cati, Demodex* spp., and *Cheyletiella* spp.
   3. Dermatophytes, particularly *Microsporum* spp. and *T. mentagrophytes.*
C. Perform fecal examination (fecal flotation test).
D. Vaccinate with FVRCP,† chlamydia, feline leukemia virus, rabies, and feline infectious peritonitis (FIP) vaccines.
E. Deworm according to fecal examination results.
F. Adjust the diet and grooming procedures, as needed.
G. Discuss age-related changes that are occurring.
H. Provide the owner with educational pamphlets on such topics as:
   1. Identification, treatment, and control of fleas, ticks, and ear mites.
   2. Dental, skin, nail, and ear care.
   3. Management of normal and abnormal behaviors.
   4. Exercise and its importance.
I. Fill in the health record for the owner.

*This refers to the use of a vaccine to protect against canine distemper (D), infectious canine hepatitis (canine adenovirus type 2) (A_2), canine parainfluenza (P), leptospirosis (L), canine parvovirus type 2 (P), and canine coronavirus (C).

†This refers to the use of a vaccine to protect against feline viral rhinotracheitis (FVR), feline calicivirus infection (C), and feline panleukopenia (P).

daily routine of the veterinary hospital. The program must then be explained completely to the hospital staff, including how it fits into their daily activities. Ideas and changes should be solicited from the hospital staff, as these may improve the implementation of the program. Because the receptionist is the first person with whom the pet owner has contact, it is important that the receptionist fully understand the health care program so that he or she can explain the program in common terms to the pet owner. The technician also has an important and very visible role in this program; many in-hospital procedures in the geriatric patient, as well as laboratory procedures, radiographs, and electrocardiograms, can be done by the technician.

The daily activities of the health care program should be worked out to include appointment schedules, office and examination room procedures, maintenance of health records, provision of laboratory support, and a pet owner consultation period to review all findings, recommendations, and subsequent examinations. When geriatric patients are scheduled, appointments should be made during the slower time periods, if possible. By scheduling these patients during less busy periods during the day, week, or year and encouraging pet owners to use these time periods, additional services can be provided with minimal additional overhead.

Adequate time is set aside for pet owner consultation so that a complete case review is possible. The consultation should start with a private discussion between the hospital staff and the pet owner, without the pet, regarding various test results or other important items such as revisits or recommendations. The veterinarian should always participate in a portion of the consultation period. Specific recommendations to the pet owner should be provided in writing. Next, the pet owner makes payment for the services and schedules another appointment, if necessary. Finally, the pet is reunited with the pet owner and any final items are discussed or demonstrations using the pet are done.

TABLE 2–5. EDUCATION OF THE PET OWNER ABOUT THE GERIATRIC DOG AND CAT

Nutrition
Restrict protein, phosphorus, and sodium intake
Provide fewer calories (only in overweight dogs and cats)

Preventive Health Care
Dentistry
Health screening recommendations
Annual vaccinations
Heartworm check
Fecal examination
Feline leukemia virus (FeLV) and feline immunodeficiency virus (FIV) tests
Grooming routine

Oncology
Early cancer detection
Medical or surgical considerations

Exercise
Exercise requirements
Exercise and feeding activity

Normal Aging Process
General information on the aging process (e.g., vision and hearing loss, muscle tone, skin and haircoat changes)

Changes to Watch for at Home
Housing environment
Food and water consumption (appetite)
Abnormal urination and defecation
Body weight changes
Activity level
Abnormal odors
Skin lumps/masses/sores that do not heal
Constant coughing/sneezing
Vomiting/diarrhea

Bereavement
Support during the last few weeks of life, if needed
Final discussions and support after death of the pet
Resolution of pet loss with the owner to allow another pet to be obtained by the family

TABLE 2–6. PROBLEMS SPECIFIC TO GERIATRIC DOGS AND CATS

Weight stasis—obesity
Cancer—present or not
Halitosis—oral disease
Lusterless haircoat—skin changes
Changes in behavior
Arthritis—altered rising and/or walking
Anesthesia risk
Loss of vision and hearing
Heart murmur—heart failure
Urine production—kidney failure
Coughing—chronic bronchial disease
Urine or fecal incontinence

SUMMARY

Geriatric health care remains a virtually untapped area in spite of changing public views and scientific knowledge on aging. As pet owners live longer, healthier lives and become more aware of age-related changes in themselves, they discover that their pets also undergo age-related changes. The number of geriatric dogs and cats will continue to grow into the next century. As the senior citizen segment of society increases, the number of geriatric pets also increases. Senior citizens usually have older dogs and cats and are willing to invest in quality health care services. A geriatric health care program can expand veterinary services in a practice and is a natural extension of pediatric and adult maintenance programs.

Suggested Reading

Goldston RT. Geriatrics and gerontology. Vet Clin North Am (Small Anim Pract) 19:ix–x, 1–202, 1989.
Hoskins JD. Geriatric preventive medicine. In Geriatric Medicine. St. Louis, MO, Ralston Purina, 1993, pp 5–10.
Mosier J. How aging affects body systems in the dog. In Geriatric Medicine: Contemporary Clinical Medicine and Practice Management Approaches. Lenexa, KS, Veterinary Medicine Publishing, 1987, pp 2–6.

CHAPTER 3

Drug Therapy in the Geriatric Pet

DAVID P. AUCOIN, RICHARD T. GOLDSTON, and JENNIFER AUTHEMENT

Aging is not a disease. However, it is correlated with an increased incidence of organ dysfunction that results in the common chronic diseases of the elderly. The veterinarian is presented with a paradox in the aged patient. Age in itself is not a disorder treated with drugs, yet drug therapy is more frequently used in the elderly patient. In humans the elderly constitute 12 per cent of the population but consume a third of all prescription drugs (Sloan, 1992). As a group they account for a disproportionate number of adverse drug reactions. Since the mid-1980s much has been made about this fact, and more careful studies in elderly patients have been called for by many veterinarians who believe that the elderly have altered drug disposition and sensitivity (Williams and Lowenthal, 1992; Sloan, 1992; Tregaskis and Stevenson, 1990). Are the elderly more susceptible to drug side effects, toxicity, or change in activity? Are these effects seen in the aging dog and cat population? These questions will be explored in this chapter in more detail, as will therapeutic strategies that can be used in patients of advanced age. Drug therapy should always be individually tailored to the patient regardless of age.

The therapeutic strategies used in the elderly are identical to those used in all patients. The veterinarian must have a working diagnosis, be aware of any changes in the patient caused by existing diseases, individualize the therapy to the patient, and monitor therapy for clinical effects. Elderly patients are a very heterogeneous group in humans, and even more so in companion animals. Simply identifying a patient as "old" will not provide sufficient information for the veterinarian to maximize a drug's effect and minimize its toxicity.

This chapter will explore some of the known differences in the disposition (pharmacokinetics) and effects (pharmacodynamics) of drugs in the geriatric patient. Most of the data are from human studies in which the findings are applicable to canine and feline patients. These studies will provide guidelines for therapy for geriatric patients, for agents ranging from antimicrobials to newer agents in blood component therapy.

AGE-DEPENDENT EFFECTS ON DRUG DISPOSITION (PHARMACOKINETICS)

Pharmacokinetics is the study of a drug's tissue concentration over time and its correlation to drug efficacy and toxicity. Such information is used to quantitatively describe and predict tissue concentrations using mathematical models that calculate the concentration of a drug over time after dosing. The models recognize that the drug undergoes disposition steps after dosing, each of which is dependent on different physiologic processes. These stages of drug disposition are absorption, distribution, metabolism (biotransformation), and elimination. Alterations in the physiologic processes involved in these various functions may occur as a natural aging process. The effects these alterations have on drug disposition, however, can be overlapping and thus complex and often unpredictable.

Little information is available regarding specific aging-related alterations in the dog and cat, but information extrapolated from other mammalian species can be used as a guideline. Because altered physiology begets altered pharmacology, veterinarians should understand these processes and the potential effects they will have on their patients.

Absorption

Data regarding aging-related effects on oral absorption are conflicting. In humans an increase in gastric pH occurs with age (Castelden et al, 1977). Thus, lipophilic weak bases (i.e., trimethoprim) that depend on acidity for gastric absorption might be expected to have decreased bioavailability as a result. However, studies in humans have shown little, if any, consistent effect in the rate or amount of absorption as a result of a higher gastric pH (Green et al, 1982). Ciprofloxacin has been shown in three studies to have an increased area under the serum time concentration curve (AUC), an indicator of increased absorption. However, other quinolone antimicrobials (e.g., lomefloxacin, ofloxacin) have not shown any difference. Oral absorption is difficult to study in the clinical patient, because parameters such as AUC and peak serum concentration are also affected by the drug's distribution and its rate of elimination.

There is a loss of intestinal mucosal absorptive surface in aging animals and humans, along with a slight decline in motility. Because most drugs are absorbed by passive diffusion, a loss of absorptive surface area could decrease bioavailability, resulting in lowered plasma concentrations and a decrease in drug effects. Decreased transit time also means longer absorption time, which probably explains why a loss in intestinal drug bioavailability has been reported for some drugs in human patients.

Portal and intestinal blood flow also declines with age, potentially altering the extent of diffusion gradients on which passive absorption depends. This decline in hepatic blood flow is thought to be the major influence on decreased hepatic clearance, resulting in higher than expected serum concentrations after oral dosing (see "Biotransformation and Elimination") (Woodhouse and James, 1990). A decrease in blood supply could lower the diffusion gradient and decrease the rate of passive transfer. To date, few studies have been conducted to address this issue.

Absorption through parenteral routes in the aged has not been addressed, but it is safe to assume that the rate of subcutaneous absorption in the geriatric patient is likely to be slower owing to a general decrease with age along with an increase in fat and decreased vascularity. Studies conducted in human and veterinary medicine have shown that injection site is as likely to influence drug bioavailibility in the aged animal as in the young adult.

In summary, although aging does affect gastrointestinal (GI) function, its effect on drug disposition is of little practical concern to the veterinarian. The major parameters affecting drug distribution occur during distribution and elimination.

Distribution

Aging decreases total body muscle and body water (lean body mass) but increases the proportion of body fat (Novak, 1972). Total body water is reduced by as much as 15 per cent in humans, which affects the distribution of many drugs. The volume of distribution (V_d) is a pharmacokinetic parameter used to mathematically describe the relationship between the measured plasma concentration and the dose given:

$$V_d \text{ (ml/kg)} = \text{Dose (mg/kg)}/C_p(0) \ (\mu\text{g/ml})$$

Where V_d is the central volume of distribution and $C_p(0)$ is the concentration of the drug as estimated at time 0 if the drug was instantaneously distributed into the body. It does not necessarily relate to a real physiologic volume of fluid (i.e., in the extra- or intracellular compartments). However, from this equation one can see that, given the same dose, a lower plasma concentration is associated with a greater volume of distribution, and a higher plasma concentration with a lower volume of distribution. Lipophilic drugs (e.g., anesthetics, calcium channel blockers) leave the vascular compartment and distribute into tissue and body fat, producing lower plasma concentrations. In the geriatric patient, the percentage of total body fat is higher and lean body mass is lower, meaning that drugs with large volumes of distribution could have lower than expected plasma concentrations because of more extensive distribution. Because of this alteration in drug distribution into body fat and not necessarily to the site of action, these lower levels could decrease the efficacy of the drug.

Conversely, polar drugs (e.g., aminoglycosides) distribute poorly to body tissue and body fat, giving respectively higher serum concentrations. The loss of body water should be expected to decrease the distribution of water-loving (i.e., polar) drugs, increasing their serum concentrations. In a study of 13 elderly human patients, ciprofloxacin did have lower volumes of distribution, resulting in higher than expected drug concentrations, but pharmacokinetic studies done in 63 human patients between 65 and 79 years of age found no difference in distribution volume as long as renal function was normal (Bauer and Blouin, 1982).

There is also a decrease in protein binding as animals age, resulting in more free drug and greater volumes of distribution. However, this effect is not as clinically significant as the change in drug elimination rates, because the distribution volume is inversely related to the half-life of elimination. Distribution volume is one of two parameters of a drug's half-life ($T^{1/2}$), the other being the rate of plasma clearance.

$$T^{1/2} = 0.693 \times V_d / Cl_{plasma}$$

Where V_d is the apparent volume of distribution, the constant 0.693 is the natural logarithm of 2 (ln 2), and Cl_{plasma} is the total body clearance of the drug from plasma. The greater the volume of distribution, the longer the half-life; the smaller the V_d, the shorter the half-life. These relationships hold when comparing drugs with similar clearances and when comparing the half-life of a single drug in two different patients with different volumes of distribution. Thus, it is known that geriatric patients have a greater V_d for many benzodiazepines (i.e., diazepam) than do nongeriatric weight-matched adults, resulting in a longer half-life. However, it is the changes in drug metabolism and elimination rate that make these drugs have greater side effects in the elderly (Greenblatt et al, 1991).

A drug's half-life has an important effect on therapeutic decisions, because for many drugs the half-life determines the frequency of administration and the time it takes to reach steady-state concentrations. Steady-state concentration means simply that the changes in plasma concentrations from one dosing interval to the next are the same. A minimum of three half-lives are required to reach 90 per cent of steady state, which means that, given the same dose of a lipophilic drug (e.g., digoxin), the geriatric patient may achieve lower plasma concentrations and take longer to reach steady-state concentrations than the nongeriatric patient. For this reason digoxin is dosed as a function of lean body mass. However, it is important to remember that the thin geriatric patient still has a greater proportion of fat than the thin adult dog; this must be taken into account when formulating a dose.

Although an increase in the V_d of a drug decreases its plasma concentration, the V_d is not important in determining the amount of drug administered; this is a function of the second determinant of half-life, plasma clearance. Clearance describes a drug's elimination rate from a volume of plasma over time (ml/min) and is dependent on the rate of its metabolism (biotransformation) or renal elimination. The concentration reached at steady state is a function of drug dose and clearance rate:

$$C_{ss} = \text{Dose (mg/kg)}/Cl_{tb}$$

Where C_{ss} is the average concentration at steady state (µg/ml), dose is the amount administered per unit of time (mg/day), and Cl_{tb} is the total body clearance rate (ml/kg/min). Thus, the final concentration reached at steady state is directly dependent on how much drug is given per day and is inversely proportional to the stages of clearance.

In summary, then, the two stages of drug disposition that affect a drug's half-life are its distribution volume and its clearance rate. The volume of distribution of a drug does not affect its steady-state concentration or the dose necessary to achieve effective concentrations; these are functions of clearance and dose. However, changes in V_d in the elderly patient may change the loading dose or frequency of drug delivery. A geriatric dog receiving digoxin may have a larger than normal V_d (owing to an increase in the proportion of body fat) but a normal drug clearance rate, which would necessitate less frequent dosing but a larger than normal loading dose. This is why merely knowing a drug's half-life or a change in half-life in a given patient is insufficient to change a patient's dosage. It is important to know whether the change in half-life is a function of a change in V_d or in total body clearance. The more significant factor affecting half-life in the geriatric animal is probably the change in clearance rates, because aging has its greatest effect on this stage of drug disposition.

Biotransformation and Elimination

Once a drug has entered the systemic circulation, its ultimate fate is dependent on excretion of intact drug into the urine or bile or biotransformation into metabolite that is filtered or excreted into the urine or bile. The effect of aging on the rate of hepatic biotransformation of drugs is unclear and extremely variable (Durnas et al, 1990). The natural variation of hepatic metabolism is genetically controlled and differs widely among the normal nongeriatric population; aging does not seem to improve this heterogeneity. It is clear that hepatic metabolism decreases in the elderly, but this is probably not because of a change in enzymes (i.e., cytochrome P_{450} oxidation, conjugation) but because of a change in hepatic and portal blood flow (Woodhouse and James, 1990).

The liver has a very large capacity to metabolize exogenous compounds, including drugs, that does not appear to be overwhelmed except under severe cirrhotic conditions. However, the rate of elimination for some drugs is dependent on hepatic blood flow, which decreases with age. Such drugs are referred to as *high-clearance compounds* undergoing pathways of biotransformation that are nonsaturatable. Therefore, the rate of metabolism is dependent only on how fast the blood can get the drug through the liver. Propranolol is a high-clearance drug that is affected by aging, with geriatric patients having a slower clearance rate for this drug than young adults. In general, however, the effects of aging on any drug's metabolism appear to be minimal and, because they are unpredictable, of questionable clinical significance.

Of greater importance is the effect of aging on renal function, as most drugs use renal filtration or secretion as their major elimination pathway. Many studies have addressed the effects of aging on renal function (Kaufman, 1984). Renal mass decreases with age in the dog, as does the population of nephrons, which thereby causes a decrease in the glomerular filtration rate (GFR). Renal blood flow changes from cortical to medullar, altering distal tubular functions such as concentrating ability (Bichet and Schrier, 1982). Quantitation of this decline in GFR with simple laboratory tests is insensitive to gross changes in the young adult and even more so to such changes in the geriatric patient. Because GFR must decrease by 75 per cent before changes occur in serum creatinine level, a significant and highly important factor will be undiagnosed when this test is used alone. Moreover, aging decreases the proportion of muscle mass, sometimes profoundly, which in turn affects the production of creatinine. The creatinine level is a function of both its clearance and its production, and a "normal" range of serum creatinine values in a cachectic old dog or cat is at best misleading. A simple linear regression formula allows the veterinarian to calculate a patient's GFR. Three factors are related to GFR in humans: age, sex, and serum creatinine level. It has shown that elderly human patients with serum creatinine levels in the "normal" range may in fact have severely compromised renal function.

All the beta-lactam antimicrobials (i.e., the penicillins and cephalosporins) and aminoglycosides undergo renal elimination exclusively, meaning that changes in GFR will profoundly affect the clearance rates of these drugs. The decrease in clearance will increase steady-state concentrations, which in turn can produce toxicity. In addition, aminoglycoside toxicity is enhanced in the aged kidney owing to a decrease in nephron population and an increase filtered load per nephron (Frasier et al, 1986).

Antiarrhythmics, anti-inflammatories, and cardiotonics are some of the families of drugs that use renal pathways of elimination to some extent and for which a decrease in clearance profoundly affects their toxicity (Haass et al, 1972). Given the narrow therapeutic window of digoxin and the aged population in which it is used, it is not surprising that toxicity is sometimes an almost inevitable consequence during its use. The problem the veterinarian faces is in predicting the geriatric patient's GFR in the presence of a "normal" serum creatinine and blood urea nitrogen (BUN) level. Unlike in human medicine, there are no algorithms for determining a patient's GFR based on a few simple parameters. Therefore, the prudent veterinarian should account for the possibility of decreased renal function in the geriatric patient and assess the risk of toxicity to the patient if plasma concentrations are higher than expected. The dangers with the beta-lactam antimicrobials are negligible, and dose modification is unnecessary. However, with almost every other medication used in the aged animal (e.g., aminoglycosides, antiarrhythmics, anti-inflammatories, and cardiotonics), toxicity is a concern, and dosage modification may be prudent.

In summary, the effects of altered drug metabolism in the aged patient are at worst variable and at best probably not significant. Hepatic biotransformation is altered in the elderly, but its significance is probably slight. The real issue is alteration in renal elimination, which may occur as a function of age. The question becomes, are geriatric patients more susceptible to adverse drug effects because of "perceived" alterations in drug pharmacokinetics? A large retrospective study of all papers published from 1966 through 1990 concluded that there still are no data showing that age is responsible for adverse or unexpected drug actions in the elderly. Instead it is the individual disease state and its accompanying altered physiology that are responsible for these problems rather than age itself (Gurwitz and Avorn, 1991). As Gurwitz and Avorn stated, "Patient-specific physiological and functional characteristics are probably more important than any chronological measure in predicting both adverse and beneficial outcomes associated with specific drug therapies."

AGE-DEPENDENT EFFECTS ON DRUG EFFECTS (PHARMACODYNAMICS)

The action of any drug is dependent on its concentration at the site of effect and its actions at that site. Pharmacodynamics, or drug actions, are definitely altered in elderly human patients, and this alteration is not always due to changes in drug concentrations. The biologic systems (homeostatic mechanisms) that control blood pressure, cardiac output, cognitive functions, thermoregulation, and neuromuscular responses are also altered with age.

Changes in specific receptor density or binding affinity have been described in humans and in rodents for many beta- and alpha-adrenergic receptors (Swift, 1990). Many drug actions are manifested through receptors (benzodiazepines, calcium channel blockers, anticholinergics, adrenergics). It is this area of study that is getting a lot of attention and where further studies are needed (Abernethy, 1990).

An increase in sensitivity to hypnotics, tranquilizers, and general anesthetics may be due to altered pharmacokinetics, as well as to a change in dynamic responses to the drugs. However, propranolol has less effect in the elderly human patient than in the young adult, and thus the dynamic effects are not constant.

GUIDELINES FOR DRUG USE IN ELDERLY PATIENTS

Antimicrobials

Most antimicrobials currently used in veterinary medicine have wide safety margins, and changes in dosing schedule more often reflect an attempt to save money or make drug delivery more convenient, not an attempt to make drug delivery safer. Most antimicrobial efficacy is correlated with time during which concentration is above the minimum inhibitory concentration of the pathogen. Changes in disposition of most antimicrobials are due to a decrease in renal function, which prolongs the action of these agents and allows a decrease in dosing frequency.

Rule of Thumb. If a patient is showing significant body changes consistent with aging and renal function is unknown, it is better not to alter the dosing schedule. Having available established serum creatinine values for the geriatric patient is very important. *Veterinarians should establish baseline values for their patients before their patients are of geriatric age.* A dog or cat that had a serum creatinine level of 1.0 mg/dl at 10 years of age and currently has a level of 2.0 mg/dl at 13 years has had a 50 per cent reduction in GFR, even though a level of 2.0 mg/dl is in the normal range. I would drop one dosing interval (i.e., to bid from tid or to sid from bid).

Veterinarians should take more care when determining dosage for aminoglycosides. If unsure of renal function, use once-daily dosing at 6 to 8 mg/kg of gentamicin or 10 to 12 mg/kg of amikacin. This dosing strategy is preferable both for improved efficacy and decreased renal toxicity. Aminoglycoside efficacy is correlated with a high serum concentration and its toxicity is inversely related to frequency of dosing.

Anti-inflammatory Agents

As a group nonsteroidal anti-inflammatory drugs (NSAIDs) are used more often and for longer periods of time in the elderly than in any other age group. These drugs have a high incidence of undesirable side effects, including GI upset, ulceration, and prolonged bleeding. In humans their use in patients with decreased renal function is associated with worsening of renal function. This is due to the increased role of prostaglandins in maintaining renal blood flow in the compromised kidney. The clinical consequences of NSAID use in geriatric dogs with chronic renal disease is unclear, but caution is advised.

Rule of Thumb. Start at the lowest dose and dosing frequency for all NSAIDs. Gradually increase the frequency first and then the amount over weeks. Loss of appetite is a clinical sign of GI upset and indicates that treatment should be stopped for 1 day and resumed at one half the previous dose. An alternative is to combine the NSAID with misoprostol (Cytotec) at 2 to 4 μg/kg bid or tid as a protectorate. It does not provide any GI protection in human patients with chronic renal disease. Therefore, *reduce dosing frequency in dogs with suspected renal dysfunction.* Although many NSAIDs do not show alterations in elimination in the elderly, their dynamic effects seem more pronounced. Do not use a cytoprotectorant such as sucralfate (Carafate) in combination with NSAIDs, as absorption is greatly impaired and efficacy reduced.

Analgesics

There is an increased awareness that veterinarians have not been as concerned with the relief of pain in their patients as perhaps they should have been. Pain has been amply demonstrated to slow healing and prolong time to recovery in human patients. The use of opioid agonists-antagonists (i.e., butorphenol) or opioid agonists (i.e., morphine, oxymorphone) is becoming more common.

Rule of Thumb. The sedative effects of analgesic drugs may be enhanced in the geriatric patient as a function of age-related changes in pharmacodynamics and alteration of cognitive pathways. *It is better to use less drug more frequently than to try to prolong the action by increasing the dose.* Optimizing a dose for oxymorphone involves administering 0.01 mg/kg every 5 to 10 minutes until the patient is quiet and comfortable. The total dose used is determined, and this amount can then be given every 3 to 4 hours as needed. No drugs require as much individualization as pain relievers. There is no standard dose, only standard dose ranges. The more pronounced sedative effect of these agents in the elderly should not deter the veterinarian from using these agents; instead, they should be used with care.

Blood Component Therapy

Blood component therapy in the geriatric patient can be used for treatment of immune-mediated hemolytic anemia, acute hemorrhage from surgical blood loss, gastric ulcers, neoplasia, chronic blood loss, anemia from decreased marrow production, and acute reversible hypoalbuminemia; for platelet transfusion; and for clotting factor replacement (Cotter, 1991). Transfusions can be done most safely and efficiently by separating blood into its cellular and plasma components. This reduces unnecessary volume overload and the likelihood of transfusion reactions resulting from unnecessary cellular or plasma protein administration (Authement, 1987).

Indications for the use of fresh whole blood are hemorrhagic shock, bleeding disorders resulting from thrombocytopenia or clotting factor deficiencies, and excessive surgical hemorrhage. Packed red blood cells are indicated for replacement of all needs not requiring plasma or platelets. Indications for plasma administration include nonroutine volume expansion (i.e., in shock and burn patients), hypoproteinemia, and clotting factor deficiencies. Plasma should be separated and frozen within 6 hours of collection to be considered fresh frozen plasma (FFP). FFP may be stored for 1 year for most clotting factors or for 5 years as frozen plasma (FP) for proteins and stable factors such as vitamin K–dependent factors. Packed red cells are separated from plasma into the attached satellite bag. Red cells can be stored at 1°C to 6°C for 30 days (Cotter, 1994). Plasma should not be used for routine volume expansion; this is best accomplished by crystalloids or dextrans. Plasma is effective only for albumin replacement in cases of acute plasma loss (e.g., burn patients and protein-losing enteritis). Chronic hypoalbuminemia that occurs with liver diseases or protein-losing nephropathies is not efficiently replaced by the 3 to 4 g/dl of albumin present in a unit of plasma (Cotter, 1994).

Cryoprecipitate, a product of FFP, is rich in Factor VIII, fibrinogen, and von Willebrand's factor. It can be prepared from FFP by thawing FFP at 4°C, separating the liquid portion into a satellite bag, and saving the remaining precipitate. It is indicated in hemophilia type A, von Willebrand's disease, and hypofibrinogenemia (Authement, 1987).

Blood donors should be typed; they should be negative for dog erythrocyte antigen (DEA) 1.1 and 1.2 loci, unless the recipient is the same blood type. Cat donors are not routinely typed because of the very low prevalence of type B cats in the United States (Cotter, 1988). Collection bags with attached satellite bags can be used as a closed system for storage. A refrigerated centrifuge and −30°C freezer are needed to make and store components. Techniques for the preparation and storage of components have been described (Authement, 1987, 1991).

Clinical transfusion medicine involves consideration of several factors such as cause and severity of anemia, expectations of further blood loss, and alternative treatment options (Cotter, 1991). Immune-mediated hemolytic anemia is one of the most common clinical conditions requiring blood transfusions. Most patients have positive results on the direct antiglobulin test, which can interfere with both typing and crossmatching. Numerous transfusions and immunosuppressant therapy are necessary. Destruction of transfused cells in immune-mediated hemolytic anemia is more common with fever and hepatosplenomegaly. Rapid hemolysis of transfused red cells is detrimental to the patient, and the decision to transfuse should be made on an individual basis when signs of hypoxia (i.e., weakness and tachycardia) are present, to prevent further organ damage (Cotter, 1991).

Chronic blood loss can occur from repeated blood sampling (in small animals) and from gastrointestinal bleeding caused by parasites, ulcers, or neoplasia. Transfusion with packed red cells is indicated if the anemia is severe (Cotter, 1991). Anemia can result from decreased marrow production caused by red cell aplasia, myelodysplasia, aplastic anemia, leukemia, feline leukemia virus, feline immunodeficiency virus, chronic renal disease (i.e., lack of erythropoietin), iron deficiency, immune-mediated destruction of red cell precursors, and chronic disease (Cotter, 1991). Transfusion of packed red blood cells may be required if clinical signs of tachycardia and weakness are present. Crossmatching becomes more important in patients that receive multiple transfusions. Hematopoietic growth factors such as recombinant human erythropoietin should be used to decrease the necessity for recurrent transfusions.

Disseminated intravascular coagulation (DIC) occurs more commonly in geriatric patients with malignancies (i.e., hemangiosarcomas), immune-mediated hemolytic anemia, pancreatitis, and sepsis. DIC is classically characterized by thrombocytopenia, hypofibrinogenemia, elevated levels of fibrinogen degradation products, and prolonged prothrombin time (PT) and activated partial thromboplastin time (PTT). When a patient is actively bleeding and has a low fibrinogen level and prolonged PT or PTT, replacement of clotting factors with fresh frozen plasma (FFP) is recommended. FFP contains antithrombin III, which is a potent inhibitor of thrombin formation. In severe cases of DIC in which red cell replacement, clotting factors, and platelets are needed, fresh whole blood is indicated; individual components may be used later (Cotter, 1991). Treatment of the underlying cause of the DIC is necessary in addition to component therapy.

Thrombocytopenia can be effectively treated with platelet-rich plasma or fresh whole blood transfusions when red cell support is needed. Refrigerated platelets do not maintain function or viability as well as platelets stored at room temperature (Authement, 1987).

Appropriate filters and administration sets should be used for blood component transfusions to retain blood clots. A Y-component administration set is ideal, as 0.9 per cent saline solution can be added to packed red blood cells to reduce viscosity of packed red cells. The only fluid that can be safely added to blood components is 0.9 per cent saline solution. Lactated Ringer's solution contains calcium, which can cause clotting, and dextrose in water can cause hemolysis (Authement, 1987).

Complications of transfusion include intravascular and extravascular hemolysis, fever, urticaria, hypocalcemia, arrhythmias, volume overload, and transmission of infectious agents such as feline leukemia and immunodeficiency viruses and diseases caused by *Babesia, Ehrlichia,* Hemobartonella and Toxoplasma (Authement, 1987; Cotter 1994). Most hemolytic reactions in dogs are delayed hemolytic reactions. Nonimmunologic causes of hemolysis include overheating or freezing of blood, concurrent administration of hypotonic solutions, and mechanical trauma from infusion through a small needle (Cotter, 1994).

SUMMARY

It is clear from this discussion that the effects of aging on the disposition and effects of therapeutic agents in veterinary medicine must be studied. Theoretical concepts are important in that they may help rationalize a therapeutic regimen or help explain a drug toxicity, but they must be explored in well-controlled studies to determine which alterations in drug behavior are important and which are merely academic.

In the meantime, veterinarians are in need of guidelines in the use of these agents in the geriatric patient population. Chapters on the specific use of certain drugs are included elsewhere in this volume, but some generalizations can apply and have been given here.

References and Supplemental Reading

Abernethy DR. Altered pharmacodynamics of cardiovascular drugs and their relation to altered pharmacokinetics in elderly patients. Clin Geriatr Med 6:285–292, 1990.

Authement JM. Canine blood component therapy. J Am Anim Hosp Assoc 23:483–493, 1987.

Authement JM. Preparation of components. In Cotter S (ed). Comparative Transfusion Medicine. San Diego, Academic Press, 1991, pp 171–185.

Bauer LA, Blouin RA. Gentamicin pharmacokinetics: effect of aging in patients with normal renal function. J Am Geriatr Soc 30(5):309–311, 1982.

Bichet DG, Schrier RW. Renal function and diseases in the aged. In Schrier RW, ed. Clinical Internal Medicine in the Aged. Philadelphia, WB Saunders, 1982, p 211.

Birnbaum LS. Age-related changes in drug disposition. In Zenser TV, Coe RM, eds. Cancer and Aging: Progress in Research and Treatment. New York, Springer, 1989, pp 125–138.

Castelden CM, Volans GN Raymond K. The effect of aging on drug absorption from the gut. Age Ageing 6:138–143, 1977.

Cotter SM. Blood banking I. Collection and storage. Proc Am Coll Vet Intern Med Forum, 6:45, 1988.

Cotter SM. Clinical transfusion medicine. In Cotter S (ed). Comparative Transfusion Medicine. San Diego, Academic Press, 1991, pp 187–223.

Cotter SM. Blood component therapy. In Proceedings of the North American Veterinary Conference, Orlando, FL, 1994, pp 275–276.

Durnas C, Loi CM, Cusack BJ. Hepatic drug metabolism and aging. Clin Pharmacokinet 19(5):359–389, 1990.

Frazier DL, Dix LP, Bowman KF, et al. Increased gentamicin nephrotoxicity in normal and diseased dogs administered identical serum drug concentration profiles: Increased sensitivity in subclinical renal dysfunction. J Pharmacol Exp Ther 239:946–951, 1986.

Green DJ, Sellers EM, Shader RI. Drug disposition in old age. N Engl J Med 306:1981–1988, 1982.

Greenblatt DJ Harmatz JS Shader RI. Clinical pharmacokinetics of anxiolytics and hypnotics in the elderly. Therapeutic considerations (Part I). Clin Pharmacokinet 21(3):165–177, 1991.

Gurwitz JH, Avorn J. The ambiguous relation between aging and adverse drug reactions. Ann Intern Med 114:956–966, 1991.

Haass A, Lullmann H, Peters T. Absorption rates of some cardiac glycosides and portal blood flow. Eur J Pharmacol 19:366–370, 1972.

Kaufman GM. Renal function in the geriatric dog. Compend Contin Educ Pract Vet 6:1087–1094, 1984.

Klotz U, Avant GR, Hoyumpa A, et al. The effects of age and liver disease on the disposition and elimination of diazepam in adult man. J Clin Invest 55:347–359, 1975.

Novak LP. Ageing, total body potassium fat free mass and cell mass in males and females aged 18 and 85 years. J Gerontol 27:438–443, 1972.

Riviere JE, Carver MP, Coppoc GL, et al. Pharmacokinetics and comparative nephrotoxicity of fixed dose versus fixed interval reduction of gentamicin dosage in subtotal nephrectomized dogs. Toxicol Appl Pharmacol 75:496–509, 1984.

Shand DG. Biological determinants of altered pharmacokinetics in the elderly. Gerontology 28(suppl 1):8–17, 1982.

Sloan RW. Principles of drug therapy in geriatric patients. Am Fam Physician 45(6):2709–2718, 1992.

Swift CG. Pharmacodynamics: Changes in homeostatic mechanisms, receptor and target organ sensitivity in the elderly. Br Med Bull 46:36–52, 1990.

Tregaskis BF, Stevenson LH. Pharmacokinetics in old age. Br Med Bull 46:9–21, 1990.

Williams L, Lowenthal DT. Drug therapy in the elderly. South Med J 85:127–131, 1992.

Woodhouse KW, James OF. Hepatic drug metabolism and ageing. Br Med Bull 46:22–35, 1990.

CHAPTER 4

Nutrition and Nutritional Disorders

JOHNNY D. HOSKINS, RICHARD T. GOLDSTON, and DOTTIE P. LAFLAMME

The concept of varying nutritional needs during different life stages for dogs and cats is an accepted principle. For many years nutritional needs during these different life stages were met by either selective increases in or limitation of intake of the same diet or, alternatively, by prudent supplementation of that diet (Sheffy et al, 1985). More recently, however, the pet food industry has attempted to accommodate the recognized needs of dogs and cats, first by the introduction of puppy foods to the marketplace, followed by the presentation of lines of foods designed for a specific physiologic state; these include commercially prepared diets for aging dogs and cats (Sheffy et al, 1985).

Aging is a physiologic process that continues from birth to death. Geriatrics is an extension of the physiologic state known as adult maintenance. Veterinarians have observed a general slowing of many biologic responses in aging dogs and cats (Table 4–1) (Mosier, 1989). However, the extent to which these changes are attributable to disease or to a simple consequence of aging is not always known. Diseases associated with aging, such as cancer and cardiovascular, gastrointestinal, and renal problems, are thought to increase in frequency in aging dogs and cats (Goldston, 1989).

In addition to the differences among populations of aging dogs and cats in the age at onset of medical problems, there is great variation among individual animals within populations. Signs of aging, such as graying of the muzzle and feet, reduced activity, and/or loss of visual and auditory acuity, are the most reliable indicators of advanced age in any specific dog or cat. The presence of these signs indicates the likelihood of loss of the reserve capacity of body systems that allows young animals to adapt to changes in their environment and should raise the clinician's index of suspicion for the possibility of age-related problems (Goldston, 1989).

NORMAL FEEDING MANAGEMENT

Nutritional advice for owners of aging dogs and cats depends on the animal's usual diet and its current health status (Buffington, 1991). Owners should be asked about the specific amount and brand of food fed to their pet, what kinds of

TABLE 4–1. STRUCTURAL AND METABOLIC CHANGES ASSOCIATED WITH AGING

Oral cavity	Dental calculus, periodontal disease, loss of teeth, oral ulcers, gingival hyperplasia
Digestive system	Altered liver and pancreatic functions; altered intestinal digestion and absorption; altered esophagus, stomach, and colon motility
Endocrine system	Decreased function of thyroid glands or pancreatic islet cells, hyperplasia or tumors of pituitary or adrenal glands, neoplasia of pancreatic islet cells
Integument	Loss of elasticity; thickened skin; dry, thin haircoat; altered function of sebaceous glands; graying of muzzle; brittle nails; hypersensitivity
Cardiovascular system	Structural alterations in the heart and blood vessels
Genitourinary system	Reduced renal function, blood flow, and glomerular filtration rate; prostate gland hypertrophy; hyperplasia; squamous metaplasia; cysts; neoplasia
Musculoskeletal system	Loss of muscle mass and tone, brittle bones, degenerative joint disease, disturbed gait
Nervous system and special senses	Reduced reactivity to stimuli; altered memory; and diminished visual acuity, hearing, taste perception, and smell
Metabolism	Reduced sensitivity to thirst; reduced thermoregulation, physical activity, and rate of metabolism

"people food" are being consumed by the pet, and the type and amount of supplementation given. The quantity and brand of food provided give an indication of the dietary history of the pet. If a high-quality, commercially prepared food is being fed, there is little cause for concern for the animal's nutritional status. If the pet has existed on a diet of people food, treats, and/or a number of supplements, the possibilities of nutrient deficiencies, excesses, and imbalances are more likely. Advising the gradual introduction of a diet specifically formulated for the older dog or cat may be a way to improve the pet's diet without offending the well-meaning owner (Buffington, 1991). Young adult animals have sufficient adaptive reserves to adjust to a broad range of nutrient intakes and may tolerate seemingly bizarre diets for years, but aging dogs and cats cannot be expected to show this level of tolerance.

The veterinarian should inquire about the pet's eating habits and body weight and any recent changes in the two. Decreased food intake can be attributable to problems involving any body system, whereas increased food intake may be a time-filling activity or indicate the onset of an endocrine disease. Recent weight loss may also be attributable to a wide variety of causes in any body system, while increases in body weight are most commonly attributable to an excess of energy intake over energy expenditure or to endocrine disease (Buffington, 1991).

The examination of an aging dog or cat should include a search for signs of obesity and/or malnutrition. Obesity is a form of malnutrition that is as easy to diagnose as it is difficult to manage. Signs that result from inadequate nutrition include poor haircoat, delayed wound healing, pressure sores, edema (hypoalbuminemia), and cachexia. Laboratory evaluation of nutritional status is difficult. For example, packed cell volume and serum albumin concentration do not appear to decline with age in dogs and cats as they do in humans, so anemia or hypoalbuminemia in the absence of organ dysfunction may indicate protein-calorie malnutrition (Sheffy et al, 1985). However, packed cell volume and serum albumin concentration are insensitive indicators.

The animal's history, physical examination, and complete laboratory evaluation should allow the veterinarian to decide whether the current diet is adequate and to identify the presence of any chronic disease that may require dietary modification (Buffington, 1991). If the dog or cat is apparently healthy, the clinician should then decide if a special diet is needed for the aging animal.

RECOMMENDATIONS FOR NUTRIENT INTAKE

Owners should be told that great variability in nutrient needs exists among aging dogs and cats. They should be advised to feed sufficient quantities of food so that the animal's ribs may be felt but not seen and the abdomen is trim (Buffington, 1991; Laflamme, 1993). Dogs and cats become less active as they grow older, resulting in a need for fewer calories to maintain ideal body weight and condition. Owners should be counseled to monitor their dog's or cat's body condition and adjust food intake to avoid obesity as energy needs decline.

Dogs and cats require enough dietary protein to fill body protein reserves and maintain normal body function. Excessive intake of dietary protein may be unnecessary but is not known to be harmful. It has been suggested that at least 30 per cent of available energy be supplied by mixed protein to fill the body protein reserves for older dogs (Kronfeld, 1983). Others have suggested that at least 20 per cent of calories in the diet should consist of protein (Sheffy and Williams, 1981). Some geriatric diets contain less protein than this, and the status of protein reserves of dogs fed these diets is not known.

Fat in the diet improves palatability, provides essential fatty acids, enhances absorption of fat-soluble vitamins, and is a concentrated source of calories. Only small amounts of dietary fat are needed to meet physiologic requirements, so the trade-off is between palatability and the risk of obesity. Overweight animals should be fed low-fat diets (less than 20 per cent of calories from fat) (Buffington, 1991). Fat levels greater than 30 per cent of calories are of value for below-weight dogs or cats.

High-quality, commercially prepared pet foods contain well in excess of the requirement for any particular vitamin or mineral, so supplementation is not necessary as long as at least half the dog's or cat's food intake comes from commercially prepared pet foods and gastrointestinal function is normal.

FEEDING MANAGEMENT PROGRAM

Although it is true that the aging dog or cat has need for the same nutrients it required earlier in life (Sheffy et al, 1985), the quantities needed per unit of metabolic body size may differ, and delivery or the feeding management recommended to supply these nutrients may require change. The feeding management program for aging dogs and cats should be carried out with moderation and regularity (Buffington, 1991). The quantity of food fed should satisfy hunger but should never result in unnecessary gastric distention and discomfort. Although ad libitum feeding may be adequate for younger animals, the importance of maintaining ideal body condition and observing the animal's food intake makes at least twice-daily meal feeding advisable for older animals (Laflamme and Kuhlman, 1993).

Feeding management programs should also take into account the following (Hoskins, 1992):

- Because of reduced physical activity and a slower basal metabolic rate, most aging animals require fewer calories.
- With changes in smell, taste, oral cavity, and digestive system, the diet consumed should be highly palatable and digestible.
- Increased intake of vitamins A, B_1, B_6, B_{12}, and E is indicated because of possible changes in the digestive system and body metabolism.
- Adequate intake of unsaturated fatty acids and zinc helps to ensure proper skin health and a healthy haircoat.
- An increase in dietary fiber aids in calorie restriction and enhances intestinal function.

Because of the increased frequency of disease in aging animals, owners should be advised that any sudden, unexplained decrease in food intake should be interpreted as an early sign of disease that ought to be investigated. Overweight dogs and cats can be fed small quantities three or four times each day to reduce begging (Buffington, 1991; Laflamme and Kuhlman, 1993). Salted human snacks should not be provided, especially if heart disease is present. If the owner enjoys offering the pet snacks, low-calorie snacks or part of the daily ration should be reserved for this purpose.

SELECTION OF FOODS

All dog and cat foods fed must be complete, balanced, digestible, and palatable to provide satisfactory diets. Label guarantees of "complete and balanced for all life stages" mean that the food contains nutrients in excess of the needs of older animals. Nutrient digestibility in aging dogs and cats is usually as good as that found in young adult animals (Sheffy et al, 1985). In addition, diets need not be too palatable unless inadequate food intake is a problem, as obesity is by far the more common nutritional problem in healthy older dogs and cats.

All feeding recommendations made to owners concerning their aging dogs and cats require consideration of the individual animal. Healthy aged dogs and cats are not nutritional cripples (Sheffy et al, 1985; Buffington, 1991). Keeping them in ideal body condition, ensuring that they eat right and exercise, will go a long way toward helping them attain full quality of life.

OBESITY

Obesity is defined as an excessive accumulation of body fat due to the intake of more dietary energy than the body needs. A dog or cat is considered overweight if it weighs 15 to 20 per cent more than its ideal body weight (Hand et al,

TABLE 4–2. ASSESSMENT OF BODY CONDITION AND OBESITY IN THE DOG

ASSESSMENT	PHYSICAL FINDINGS
Emaciated	Ribs, lumbar vertebrae, pelvic bones, and all bony prominences evident from a distance; no discernible body fat; obvious loss of muscle mass
Very thin	Ribs, lumbar vertebrae, and pelvic bones easily visible; no palpable fat; some evidence of other bony prominences; minimal loss of muscle mass
Thin	Ribs easily palpated and may be visible with no palpable fat; tops of lumbar vertebrae visible; pelvic bones becoming prominent; obvious waist and abdominal tuck
Underweight	Ribs easily palpable, with minimal fat covering; waist easily noted as viewed from above; abdominal tuck evident
Ideal	Ribs palpable without excess fat covering; waist observed behind ribs when viewed from above; abdomen tucked up when viewed from side
Overweight	Ribs palpable with slight excess of fat covering; waist is discernible when viewed from above but is not prominent; abdominal tuck apparent
Heavy	Ribs palpable with difficulty, heavy fat cover; noticeable fat deposits over lumbar area and base of tail; waist absent or barely visible; abdominal tuck may be absent
Obese	Ribs not palpable under very heavy fat cover, or palpable only with significant pressure; heavy fat deposits over lumbar area and base of tail; waist absent; no abdominal tuck; obvious abdominal distention
Morbidly obese	Massive fat deposits over thorax, spine, and base of tail; waist and abdominal tuck absent; fat deposits on neck and limbs; obvious abdominal distention

1989). Obesity is often associated with an increased risk of adverse effects on health and longevity. Adverse effects that have been documented in overweight dogs or cats include increased cardiovascular and musculoskeletal disease, decreased immune competence, abnormal glucose metabolism, and increased anesthetic and surgical risk (Hand et al, 1989).

Management. An effective weight management program can be of benefit to the older dog or cat. Several programs for weight loss have been suggested for effective weight management (Hand et al, 1989; Markwell et al, 1990; Sibley, 1984). Computer software programs are also becoming available from various pet food manufacturers (Fig. 4–1) and private companies; these calculate individual maintenance energy requirements for dogs and cats and appropriate calorie restriction for weight loss and maintenance (Laflamme and Kuhlman, 1993). Points that are common to most weight management programs, and seem to be effective when completely implemented, include the following (Laflamme and Kuhlman, 1993):

- *Enlist the owner.* The owner must want the dog or cat to lose weight before he or she will be likely to adhere to a weight management program. Many owners of overweight dogs and cats do not realize their pet is obese. It may be helpful to demonstrate to owners how to assess obesity, using palpation and visual cues (Tables 4–2 and 4–3), and to educate them about the health risks associated with being overweight (Laflamme, 1993).
- *Make the owner responsible.* Overweight dogs and cats usually do not hunt for their own food, and the veterinarian does not feed the overweight dog or cat. Thus the owner is responsible for feeding and must restrict the food intake appropriately. Have the owner keep a weekly record of food intake (Fig. 4–

TABLE 4–3. ASSESSMENT OF BODY CONDITION AND OBESITY IN THE CAT

ASSESSMENT	PHYSICAL FINDINGS
Thin	Ribs visible on short-haired cats; no palpable fat; severe abdominal tuck; lumbar vertebrae and wings of ilia easily palpated
Underweight	Ribs easily palpable with minimal fat covering; lumbar vertebrae obvious; obvious waist behind ribs; minimal abdominal fat
Ideal	Well-proportioned; obvious waist behind ribs; ribs palpable with slight fat covering; abdominal fat pad minimal
Overweight	Ribs not easily palpated, with moderate fat covering; waist poorly discernible; obvious rounding of abdomen; moderate abdominal fat pad
Obese	Ribs not palpable under heavy fat cover; heavy fat deposits over lumbar area, face, and limbs; distention of abdomen, with no waist; extensive abdominal fat deposits

Welcome to the
CNM Clinical Nutrition Management®
OM-Formula® Obesity Management Program
2/22/93

Patient Directory
Clinic Information
Print Program Directions
Quit

version 1.3
Copyright 1992, All rights reserved Ralston Purina Company
Created Expressly for ABC Veterinary Hospital

®"CNM Clinical Nutrition Management" and "OM-Formula" are trademarks of Ralston Purina Company

---

A

ABC Veterinary Hospital
12345 Animal Court
Anywhere, MO 12345
123-4567
OM-Formula Obesity Management Program
Initial Diet Recommendation

For: Arnold Long

Recommended daily intake is 485.4 Kcal.
This includes 1⅝ cups of OM-Formula per day plus 49 Kcal/day in snacks or treats.
If snacks or treats are totally eliminated from the diet the recommended daily intake is 1¾ cups of OM-Formula.

Based on average caloric needs, and your dog's current body weight, this diet may result in a weight loss of 0.4 pound per week.

	Week of	Projected Weight
Start date:	2/22/93	20.0
	3/01/93	19.6
	3/08/93	19.2
	3/15/93	18.8
	3/22/93	18.4

Individual pets may have different energy requirements because of activity level, age, genetics, etc.
It is VERY important to have your dog rechecked in 4 weeks to determine its special individual energy requirements.

Your pet's next appointment is ______________

B

Figure 4–1. OM-Formula Obesity Management Program. *A*, Computer software program generated by the Ralston Purina Company (Checkerboard Square, St. Louis, MO) that will calculate individual maintenance energy requirements for dogs and cats and appropriate calorie restriction for weight loss and maintenance. CNM (Clinical Nutrition Management) and "OM-Formula" are trademarks of Ralston Purina Company. *B*, An example of a hospital–pet owner letter generated from the computer-based program on weight management.

Illustration continued on following page

OM-Formula Obesity Management Program
Patient Recheck

HELP Food List for Extra Kcal/day

Food	Approx. Kcal	Food	Approx. Kcal
Dog Biscuit (small)	20	Egg (large)	81
Dog Biscuit (medium)	40	Hot Dog (2 oz.)	170
Dog Biscuit (large)	120	Ice Cream (¼ cup)	66
Dog Vitamin	8	Ice Milk (¼ cup)	50
Apple	80	Milk 2% (½ cup)	72
Bacon (1 slice)	46	Oatmeal (¼ cup)	78
Beef, lean (1 oz.)	64	Peanuts (1 oz.)	165
Candy (1 oz.)	130	Peanut Butter (Tbs)	82
Cereal, dry (1 oz.)	105	Popcorn (½ cup)	32
Cheese (1 oz.)	106	Potato Chips (1 oz.)	162
Chicken, meat only (1 oz.)	52	Pretzels (1 oz.)	111
Cookie (1 oz.)	140	Toast (1 slice)	56
Cracker (1 oz.)	130		

To print a copy of this list press the Print Screen key
Press Enter to return to Patient Screen

C

Figure 4–1 *Continued C,* Extra kilocalories per day consumed in the form of snacks or treats. If snacks or treats are fed, they should not exceed 10 per cent of the total kilocalories per day, and the amount of pet food consumed should be reduced.

2). Encourage the owner to accurately measure and record all food given to the animal. Everyone in the household who provides food and/or treats for the dog or cat should participate in the weight management program.

- *Have regular "weigh-ins."* If the owner is able, the pet's body weight should be measured and recorded weekly in the home (Fig. 4–2) and monthly at the veterinary facility (Fig. 4–3). Weigh-ins at the veterinary facility provide an extra motivation for the owner and allow the veterinarian to adjust diet and food intake recommendations if necessary.
- *Regular exercise.* Depending on the health status of the animal and owner, various amounts of exercise should be encouraged. A 15-minute walk with the dog, twice daily, may allow both owner and pet to

PATIENT
Weekly Record

For You To Complete At Home

DATE	WEIGHT	DATE	WEIGHT	DATE	WEIGHT
....	....	....	....	....	....
....	....	....	....	....	....
....	....	....	....	....	....
....	....	....	....	....	....
....	....	....	....	....	....
....	....	....	....	....	....
....	....	....	....	....	....

Figure 4–2. An example of a patient weekly record.

CLINIC Recheck Record					
For Your Veterinarian To Complete At Office Visits					
		AMOUNT TO FEED			
DATE	WEIGHT	kcal/day	Cups/day	NEXT VISIT	COMMENTS
....	....	....	....	....	....
....	....	....	....	....	....
....	....	....	....	....	....
....	....	....	....	....	....
....	....	....	....	....	....
....	....	....	....	....	....
....	....	....	....	....	....

Figure 4–3. An example of a clinic recheck record and new feeding recommendations.

slim down. In addition, studies on human weight loss indicate that exercise aids in maintaining the weight loss.

- *Minimize treats.* Ideally, overweight dogs and cats should receive no treats or food other than their allowed ration. Some owners, however, may refuse to comply with this recommendation. Discuss the feeding of treats and associated calories directly with the owner. If the owner insists on including treats, suggest a specified quantity of low-calorie foods or commercially prepared treats and then include these calories in the dog's or cat's total daily allowance.
- *Feed several times daily.* Eating, especially eating a palatable food, causes an increase in the metabolic rate that is not dose dependent (Diamond et al, 1985; LeBlanc and Diamond, 1986). Feeding the same number of calories in four meals instead of in one or two will reduce the number of usable calories, stimulating weight loss. In addition, feeding several times daily may reduce the amount of begging done by the dog or cat. The animal should be fed by itself.
- *Individualize the program.* Be as flexible as possible in meeting the needs of the owner. For instance, some owners prefer to use a special diet for weight loss, whereas others prefer to continue with the pet's usual food.
- *Provide a support program.* In some communities weight loss clubs for dogs and cats have been organized. Support groups meet regularly to weigh their dogs or cats and discuss problems associated with weight loss (Laflamme and Kuhlman, 1993). Such a program can provide good support and motivation for the owner. The program can be coordinated by a veterinary technician or other staff member in a veterinary facility.

Feeding the Overweight Animal. Several different feeding management programs for weight reduction have been promoted for dogs and cats. Three widely accepted programs entail estimating the dog's or cat's ideal body weight (the weight at which an animal is neither too fat nor too thin), calculating the maintenance energy requirement (MER) based on ideal body weight, and then reducing that number by 25, 40, or 50 per cent to arrive at the daily caloric allowance (Laflamme and Kuhlman, 1993). Starvation is not recommended.

In one study on weight management in overweight dogs, investigators evaluated the safety and effectiveness of various levels of calorie restriction and the effect on subsequent weight maintenance (Laflamme and Kuhlman, 1993). Dogs studied were initially an average of 20 per cent overweight. Calorie allowances were based on calculated MER ($144 + 62.2 \times [\text{ideal body weight}_{kg}]$). Treatment groups were fed a commercially available diet for weight reduction (CNM CV-Formula, Ralston Purina Company, St. Louis, MO) to provide 100, 75, 60, or 50 per cent of MER for up to 16 weeks. After 16 weeks, or when each dog achieved its ideal body weight, the dogs were fed either ad libitum or sufficient quantity to maintain their reduced body weight and were monitored for an additional 6 to 9 months.

The average rate of weight loss for the four groups was 1.14, 1.56, 2.18, and 2.63 per cent per week (range, −0.32 per cent to +4.41 per cent per week). All dogs restricted to 75 per cent MER or less lost weight, as did half the dogs fed 100 per cent MER. Small breed dogs lost weight more quickly than large breeds on the same feeding program. The difference in rates of weight loss can be attributed to differences in actual MER for the individual dog. If anything, the calculation tended to overestimate MER for large dogs and underestimate MER for small dogs.

During the first week after weight loss, dogs that were allowed to eat ad libitum regained much of the lost weight. Those dogs that had lost the most weight regained the most weight. By 3 months after the weight loss program ended, there was no difference in the average per cent weight loss (3.1 to 7.7 per cent) between the four feeding groups. Dogs fed at 100 per cent MER were able to maintain their weight loss, and by 3 months after weight loss, those dogs fed throughout the study at 100 per cent MER had lost a significantly greater percentage of body weight than dogs reduced on any treatment and subsequently fed ad libitum.

This study clearly illustrates the following points about a weight management program in overweight dogs (and possibly has implications for such a program in overweight cats) (Laflamme and Kuhlman, 1993):

- Any weight loss program based on moderate calorie restriction will allow safe weight loss in otherwise healthy, overweight dogs.
- Individual dogs will respond to weight loss programs differently. This may be attributable to individual variation in MER.
- Unless food is appropriately restricted after weight loss, body weight will increase. The veterinarian should individualize every weight loss program used.

TABLE 4–4. DIETARY MANAGEMENT OF ORGAN SYSTEM DYSFUNCTION IN THE AGING DOG AND CAT

DIET TYPE	DISORDER OR CLINICAL SIGN REQUIRING FEEDING MANAGEMENT
Low protein	Uremic renal failure
	Oxalate and urate urolithiasis
	Hepatic encephalopathy
Low fat	Obesity
	Chylothorax
	Hyperlipidemia
	Hyperlipoproteinemia
	Hypothyroidism
	Small bowel disease
Low mineral	Urolithiasis
	Feline urologic syndrome
	Chronic renal failure
Restricted protein source	Food-induced allergy
	Flatulence
Low copper	Copper-associated hepatopathy
	Chronic active hepatitis
Gluten free	Gluten-induced enteropathy
Low fiber, moderate fat	Chronic liver disease
	Gastrointestinal surgery
	Gastric dilatation/volvulus
	Flatulence
	Hyperadrenocorticism
High fat, high protein	Soft tissue wounds
	Hypoglycemia
	Fractures
	Fever
	Stress, environmental or psychological
	Cachexia or starvation
	Anorexia
	Anemia
	Hepatic lipidosis
	Hyperthyroidism
Maintenance	Renal disease, nonuremic
	Steatitis
	Advanced age with reduced calorie requirements
Low fat, high fiber	Obesity
	Hyperlipoproteinemia
	Diabetes mellitus with obesity
Moderate fat, moderate fiber	Diabetes mellitus
	Large bowel disease
	Constipation
Reduced sodium	Heart failure
	Hypertension
	Chronic renal failure
	Chronic liver disease with ascites or edema

FEEDING THE SICK DOG AND CAT

Complete nutritional therapy recommendations for all diseases afflicting older dogs and cats are beyond the scope of this chapter (Table 4–4). Avoidance of sudden diet changes is particularly important. Older dogs and cats are rarely presented in such serious condition that abrupt diet modifications are necessary (Buffington, 1991).

Modifications to Diet. Modifications to the diet should be made in increments over a period of a few days to weeks, depending on the severity of the disease problem and the willingness of the animal to eat (Buffington, 1991). Dietary change is not effective if it is not instituted, and drastic changes may be resisted by the animal as well as the owner. If the owner is not convinced of the necessity of the change, it will not occur. Diet modifications will also be less likely to occur if the modification is one of many changes in owner behavior recommended simultaneously.

It is more appropriate to delay introducing the new diet or feeding program until medical therapy has succeeded in improving the dog's or cat's condition. The animal will have an improved appetite and be more likely to eat the new food.

The animal will also be less likely to associate the new diet or feeding program with the illness and to develop a learned aversion. With a learned aversion, the dog or cat may associate the food and feeding with the feeling of illness and will refuse to eat the food even though it would not result in a problem (Buffington, 1991). The animal is more likely to begin eating familiar food first and should be fed familiar food until its health condition is stabilized. The new food or feeding program should then be gradually introduced. The poor acceptance of some commercially prepared pet diets may be a consequence of trying to introduce them too early in the course of therapy.

Drug–Nutrient Interactions. Veterinarians treating older dogs and cats should also be aware of the possibility of drug–nutrient interactions (Roe, 1987). Management of such medical problems as congestive heart failure, chronic renal failure, and cancer includes drugs that may have nutritional side effects (Ogilvie, 1993). Digitalis-induced cachexia, the potassium wasting associated with diuretic use, and the depressant effects of cancer chemotherapeutic agents on food intake and nutrient absorption are examples of common drug–nutrient interactions in geriatric medicine and oncology.

ENTERAL NUTRITIONAL SUPPORT

Generally, dogs and cats with a functional gastrointestinal tract and a history of inadequate nutritional intake for 3 or more days or those that have lost at least 10 per cent of their body weight during a 1- to 2-week period are candidates for nutritional therapy (Donohue, 1989; Wheeler and McGuire, 1989). In most cases, methods to encourage food consumption should be attempted first, including uniform warming of food to just below body temperature and the use of chemical stimulants (Table 4–5). No single method or pharmacologic agent for nutritional support is best for anorexic dogs or cats. If animals do not voluntarily consume adequate food, nutritional support is warranted.

Routes of Feeding. Nasogastric tube feeding is among the most common methods used for short-term (fewer than 5 days) nutritional support (Donohue, 1989; Wheeler and McGuire, 1989). This method is especially valuable for the older animal during the initial recovery period after surgery or a short-term debilitating illness. Small, soft polyvinylchloride or polyurethane catheters will minimize complications associated with the delivery system. The distance from the nose to the last left rib is noted and marked on the feeding tube before passage. To decrease the discomfort associated with the initial placement of the feeding tube, lidocaine is instilled into the animal's nasal cavity with the nose pointing up. Occasionally, sedation of the animal may be necessary. The tube is lubricated and passed to the level of the 13th rib in dogs and the ninth rib in cats. In cats, the proximal end of the tube should be bent dorsally over the bridge of the nose and secured to the frontal region of the head or to the side of the head with a permanent adhesive. The cat's whiskers should be avoided when the feeding tube is secured. In dogs, permanent adhesive or a suture should be used to secure the tube to the side of the face ipsilateral to the intubated nostril. Most animals will tolerate the nasogastric tube, although some may require an Elizabethan collar.

Gastrostomy tubes are frequently used for an-

TABLE 4–5. MANAGEMENT OF DECREASED FOOD INTAKE

- Stay with the animal when food is offered, as petting, along with vocal reassurance, may be necessary for encouraged food intake.
- Warm the food to enhance the aroma (serve food at 78°F to 103°F [25.6°C to 39.4°C] and, if necessary, clean the animal's nasal passages to improve the ability to smell the food (especially useful in cats).
- Try different food. Cats prefer dry or canned gourmet foods, whereas most dogs prefer a good-quality canned cat food (preferably a nonacidifying diet), complete canned gourmet cat food, or meat-based dog food.
- Place highly palatable moist food on top of the regular food to increase acceptance; hand feed if the animal refuses to adequately eat from a bowl.
- Tube feed a complete and balanced semiliquid food (e.g., Prescription Diet a/d [Hill's Pet Products]; Clinical Care Liquid Diets [Pet-Ag, Inc.]) three to six times daily.
- Give 1 to 2 mEq/kg body weight daily oral potassium supplementation and 1 to 2 mg/kg oral zinc supplementation.
- Give diazepam, oxazepam, or flurazepam to stimulate food intake in animals physically able to eat; intravenous diazepam dosage is 0.05 to 0.2 mg/kg, which can be repeated once or twice a day for 2 to 3 days if effective. (Be sure to have food available when diazepam is given, as its effects last no longer than 10 min); oral oxazepam dosage is 2.5 mg in cats and can be repeated once or twice a day if effective; oral flurazepam dosage is 0.2 to 0.4 mg/kg every 4 to 7 days in dogs and cats; give debilitated animals one-half the calculated dose of diazepam, oxazepam, or flurazepam initially; if liver disease exists, these drugs should be avoided.
- Corticosteroids and anabolic steroids have helped some anorectic animals but, because of their side effects, may be contraindicated.

imals that need nutritional support for more than 7 days (Donohue, 1989; Wheeler and McGuire, 1989). These can be placed surgically or with endoscopic guidance. With surgical placement, a Pezzer mushroom-tipped catheter (No. 14 to 24 French) (Bard Urological Catheter, Bard Urological Division, Murray Hill, NJ) is used (DeBowes et al, 1993).

Percutaneous placement of a gastrostomy tube by endoscopic guidance can be quick, safe, and effective (Armstrong and Hardie, 1990; Donohue, 1989; Wheeler and McGuire, 1989). First, the stomach is distended with air from an endoscope placed into the stomach. After distention, an area just caudal to the last left rib (below the transverse processes of the lumbar vertebrae) is depressed and located by the person viewing the stomach lining via endoscopy. Be sure the spleen is located and not trapped by the inflated stomach. A polyvinylchloride over-the-needle intravenous catheter is placed through the skin and into the stomach in the area located by endoscopy. The first portion of a 5-foot length of suture material is introduced through the catheter into the stomach and grasped by a biopsy snare passed through the endoscope (Fig. 4–4).

The suture material and endoscope are pulled up the esophagus and out the oral cavity. After the stylet is removed from the catheter and discarded, the end of the gastrostomy tube opposite the mushroom tip is trimmed so that it is pointed to fit inside the polyvinylchloride catheter. The same polyvinylchloride intravenous catheter is placed over the suture material, with the narrow end pointing toward the stomach. The free end of the suture material that extends from the animal's mouth is sutured to the end of the tube. The catheter–tube combination is pulled from the end of the suture located outside the abdominal wall until the pointed end of the intravenous catheter comes down the esophagus and out the abdominal wall. The tube is grasped and pulled until the mushroom tip and attached 3- to 4-inch piece of tubing are adjacent to the stomach wall as viewed by endoscopy (Fig. 4–5).

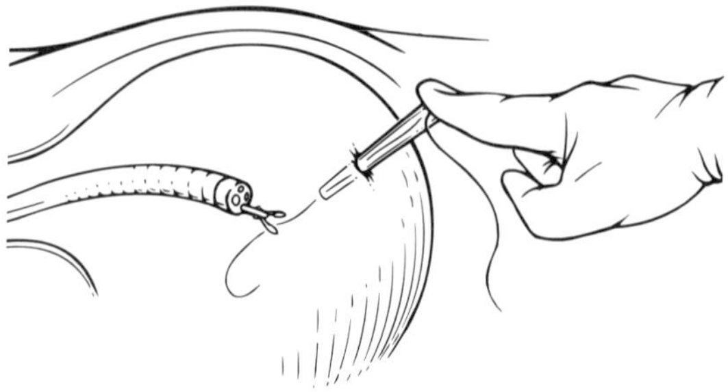

Figure 4–4. The metal stylet in the polyvinylchloride over-the-needle intravenous catheter is removed. The suture material is advanced through the catheter until it can be grasped with the endoscopic retrieval forceps. An assistant can aid the endoscopist by capping the end of the catheter with a finger to prevent air from escaping from the stomach and by keeping gentle inward pressure on the catheter.

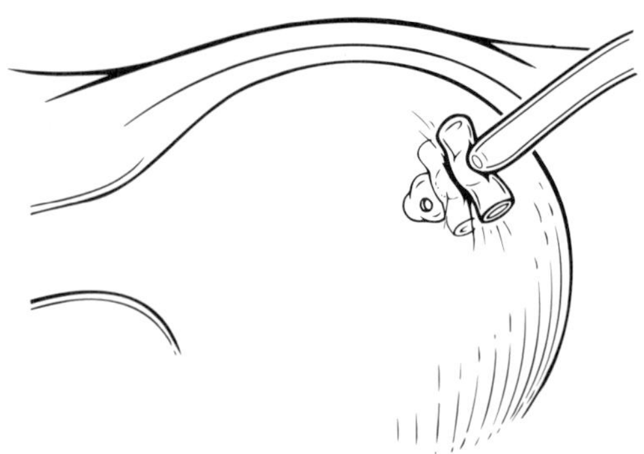

Figure 4–5. The feeding tube is snugged gently to bring the stomach and abdominal wall into loose contact. The second 3- to 4-inch piece of tubing is pierced completely through both sides, slid down the feeding tube, and brought into contact with the skin; the tubing is then sutured or taped securely in place. The feeding tube is capped after any air remaining in the stomach has been aspirated and is then bandaged in place.

To prevent slippage, the middle of a 3- to 4-inch piece of tubing is pierced completely through both sides and passed over the feeding tube to be adjacent to the body wall (see Fig. 4–5). The piece of tubing is sutured or taped securely in place, and the feeding tube is capped and bandaged in place. An Elizabethan collar is recommended.

When the gastrostomy tube has been in place for at least 7 to 10 days, it can be removed by cutting just below the bumper to allow the mushroom tip and associated tubing to fall into the stomach. Some mushroom tips can be straightened by placing a stylet into the lumen of the catheter to push the tube into a straight tube; the tube can thus be removed from the skin and stomach. The mushroom tip may need to be removed by endoscopy in small dogs and cats; otherwise, it will pass without complications in most animals.

Jejunostomy tubes should be considered for older dogs and cats that have functional lower intestinal tracts but do not tolerate nasogastric or gastrostomy tube feeding (Donohue, 1989; Wheeler and McGuire, 1989). With this method, the distal duodenum or proximal jejunum is located and isolated by surgery. A pursestring suture of 3-0 nonabsorbable material is placed in the antimesenteric border of the isolated piece of intestine. A No. 5 French polyvinylchloride nasogastric infant feeding tube or similar device is passed through a small incision in the skin and abdominal wall, through a piece of omentum (called an *omental patch*), and into the lumen of the intestine through a small stab incision in the center of the area encircled by the pursestring suture.

An ideal placement site is in the intestine 20 to 30 cm from the enterostomy site. The pursestring suture is tightened and secured around the tube. The loop of intestine with the enterostomy site is secured to the abdominal wall with four sutures, which are cut after the feeding tube is removed (in 7 to 10 days). Complications with this method are similar to those associated with gastrostomy tubes (e.g., peritonitis, diarrhea, and cramping). In addition, jejunostomy tube feeding requires constant infusion of nutrients and cannot be used as a bolus feeding method.

Enteral Feeding Methods. The type of diet selected depends largely on the type of enteral tube used and the health status of the dog or cat. Blenderized canned pet foods may be adequate for feeding by gastrostomy tubes, and human or veterinary enteral feeding products are easy to administer through nasogastric and jejunostomy tubes (Table 4–6) (Donohue, 1989; Wheeler and McGuire, 1989). In either case, feeding is usually not begun until 24 hours after tube placement. Once feeding is begun, the amount of food is gradually increased for several days; the food is administered frequently in small amounts or continuously to allow the animal to adapt to this method of feeding. The tube should be aspirated three to four times a day to prevent excessive residual volume in the gastrointestinal tract. In addition, the tube should be flushed periodically with warm water to prevent clogging. If the tubing becomes obstructed, water, cranberry juice, or cola instilled into the tube may dislodge the obstruction (Nicholson, 1987).

The following are current, simplified recommendations for determining enteral nutrient requirements. The basal energy requirement (BER, in kilocalories per day) is calculated by using one of the following formulas:

$$\text{BER} = \text{Weight}_{\text{kg}}{}^{0.75} \times 70$$

OR

$$\text{BER} = (\text{Weight}_{\text{kg}} \times 30) + 70$$

To calculate the illness energy requirement (IER, in kilocalories per day as nonprotein calories), the BER is multiplied by one of the following factors:

- For healthy dogs and cats at rest in a cage, × 1.25
- For dogs and cats that have undergone recent surgery or are recovering from trauma, × 1.2 to 1.6
- For dogs or cats that are septic or have major burns, × 1.5 to 2.0

The IER has not been determined for aging dogs and cats, and these calculations may overestimate the nutritional requirements of these animals, even without sepsis, burns, trauma, or surgery.

The protein requirement is 4 g/kg/day for healthy dogs and 6 g/kg/day for dogs with heavy protein losses. Dogs and cats with renal or hepatic failure should not be given high protein loads (recommended protein loads: ≤3 g per 100 kcal in dogs and 4 g per 100 kcal in cats).

Because most high-quality, commercially prepared canned pet foods can be put through a blender to form a gruel that will pass through a large catheter, the IER of the animal is divided by the caloric density of the pet food gruel to determine the amount to feed. The same calculation can be made with human or veterinary enteral feeding products. The volume fed may need to be increased if the enteral feeding product is diluted before administration to make it approximately iso-osmolar.

TOTAL PARENTERAL NUTRITION

Total parenteral nutrition is the delivery of a parenteral solution that provides all essential nutrient requirements of the animal (i.e., energy, protein, vitamins, and minerals). Indications for total parenteral nutrition include those situations previously discussed for enteral nutritional support in conjunction with an inability of the gastrointestinal tract to retain, digest, and/or absorb adequate nutrients to meet the animal's needs (Lippert et al, 1993). Enteral feeding has many advantages over parenteral feeding and should be used instead of total parenteral nutrition whenever possible. The use of total parenteral nutrition is becoming commonplace in many specialty veterinary facilities, but the owner should be fully informed as to the cost and potential complications of total parenteral nutrition.

Catheter Selection and Placement. Central line catheters are required for delivery of parenteral nutrition solutions; the external jugular vein is preferred. However, some lipid solutions may be given by a catheterized peripheral vein (Re-

TABLE 4–6. SELECTED CHARACTERISTICS OF SOME ENTERAL NUTRITIONAL SUPPORT PRODUCTS

PRODUCT	CALORIC CONTENT (kcal/ml)	PROTEIN CONTENT (g/100 kcal)	PROTEIN CONTENT (g/ml)	FAT CONTENT (g/100 kcal)	OSMOLARITY (mOsm/kg)
Feline p/d* (Hill's Pet Products)	0.80	9.29	0.074	6.22	—
Feline k/d† (Hill's Pet Products)	0.90	4.36	0.039	7.54	—
Feline a/d† (Hill's Pet Products)	0.62	8.87	0.055	5.96	—
Feline CNM CV-Formula‡ (Ralston Purina)	0.70	8.73	0.062	5.50	—
Canine k/d† (Hill's Pet Products)	0.62	3.06	0.019	5.29	—
Canine u/d† (Hill's Pet Products)	0.66	1.94	0.013	5.13	—
Canine i/d† (Hill's Pet Products)	0.57	5.86	0.033	3.41	—
Jevity (Ross Laboratories)	1.06	4.20	0.045	3.48	310
Osmolite (Ross Laboratories)	1.06	4.44	0.047	3.68	310
Vital HN (Ross Laboratories)	1.00	4.17	0.042	1.08	460
Vivonex HN (Sandoz Nutrition)	1.00	4.60	0.046	0.90	810
Clinical Care Feline (Pet-Ag, Inc.)	0.92	7.00	0.064	4.60	368
Clinical Care Canine (Pet-Ag, Inc.)	0.99	5.00	0.050	6.10	340

*Blenderized ½ can (224 g) + ¾ cup (170 ml) water
†Blenderized ½ can (224 g) + ⅝ cup (284 ml) water
‡Blenderized 1 can (156 g) + 1 can (156 ml) water

millard and Thatcher, 1989). Strict attention to asepsis is necessary for catheter placement, and the catheter should be used exclusively for nutritional support and not for purposes other than nutrient delivery (e.g., medication, additional fluids, or blood sampling). Alternate-day catheter care should be performed, again with strict attention to asepsis, and extension lines and connections should be changed routinely. Many catheter types are available, from expensive multiport catheters to more practical single-port varieties (Lippert et al, 1993). Catheters made of silicone (Centrasil, Baxter Healthcare Corp., Deerfield, IL) are preferred over those made of Teflon, especially for long-term placement (Remillard and Thatcher, 1989).

Parenteral Solutions. Commercially premixed parenteral nutrition solutions designed for human use are available; however, these solutions tend to be expensive, so most veterinary facilities compound their own solutions. Combination nutrition solutions are based on three primary constituents: 50 per cent dextrose (Dextrose, The Baxter Co, Columbus, OH) as an energy source; 20 per cent lipid emulsion (Liposyn II, Abbott Laboratories, Chicago, IL) as a source of energy and essential fatty acids; and 8.5 to 10 per cent amino acid solution as a protein source (10 per cent Travasol, Baxter Healthcare Corp., Deerfield, IL). Although some lipid solutions can be given alone through a peripheral vein, high-concentration dextrose and amino acid solutions require a central line (e.g., external jugular vein).

All-in-one compounding bags (Travamulsion Container, Travasol Labs Inc., Deerfield, IL) are preferred because they simplify the maintenance of asepsis and ensure that the dextrose and amino acids solutions are mixed prior to contact with the lipid emulsion, as the lipid emulsion may destabilize if combined with dextrose alone (Remillard and Thatcher, 1989). Vitamin and mineral supplementation of the base solution may be necessary as determined by the underlying disease process, electrolyte status of the animal, and the number of days parenteral nutrition is required. Multivitamins are commonly added to the total parenteral nutrition solution on a daily basis, and vitamin K_1 should be given subcutane-

TABLE 4–7. COMPLICATIONS ASSOCIATED WITH PARENTERAL NUTRITIONAL SUPPORT

COMPLICATION	SOLUTION
Infectious	
Fever, leukocytosis, unexplained glucosuria	If it persists for longer than 24 hours with no apparent clinical reason, remove catheter, culture catheter tip, and perform blood cultures. Contamination with enteric bacteria is another source of infection.
Metabolic	
Azotemia, high plasma ammonia levels	Animals with hepatic and renal insufficiency are less tolerant of protein infusion.
Hyperglycemia	Keep glucose concentration less than 200 mg/dl; animals with diabetes mellitus may require decreased glucose supplementation and increased calories from lipids.
Hyperlipemia	Visual check of hematocrit tube daily; animal may require decreased lipid supplementation.
Nonregenerative anemia, thrombocytopenia	Monitor the animal for infectious causes and treat appropriately.
Hepatocellular swelling and vacuolation	Increased alanine transaminase activity and bilirubin concentration are possible but will resolve after total parenteral nutrition is discontinued.
Mechanical	
Malpositioning or dislodgement of catheter	Monitor catheter placement and maintenance.
Thrombosis of catheter	Monitor for disseminated intravascular coagulopathy and maintain patency of catheter by frequent flushing of the catheter.

ously on a weekly basis at a dose of 0.5 mg/kg. Other fat-soluble vitamins are not usually required unless long-term (more than 10 days) total parenteral nutrition is required. Some amino acid solutions come premixed with adequate electrolytes; otherwise, it may be necessary to add potassium chloride or potassium phosphate to the parenteral solution.

Special attention to serum phosphate should be given to animals receiving total parenteral nutrition, because hypophosphatemia may develop (Thompson and Hodges, 1984). Although calcium and trace minerals are not commonly supplemented, they may be necessary for long-term maintenance. Importantly, arachidonic acid and taurine are not present in total parenteral nutrition solutions, and supplementation should be considered for total parenteral nutrition of more than 1 week's duration (Remillard and Thatcher, 1989). Delivery of total parenteral nutrition solutions can be performed either by gravity or fluid infusion pump in a continuous fashion or as an intermittent, cyclic, 6- to 15-hour delivery of daily needs.

Total Parenteral Nutrition Needs. Total parenteral nutrition is based on the animal's energy and protein needs. The first step, therefore, is to determine the dog's or cat's caloric needs; the second step is to determine the animal's protein needs. Protein requirements should be based on the calculated energy requirement, because sufficient energy must be available for protein to be used appropriately for tissue maintenance and repair (Remillard and Thatcher, 1989). If energy is inadequate in the presence of adequate protein, appropriate protein anabolism cannot occur; conversely, if excessive protein is used, extravagant energy demands are required to handle the excess nitrogen. The protein requirement is 1.5 to 4.0 g/kg/day for healthy dogs (Dudrick et al, 1968), 6.0 g/kg/day for dogs with heavy protein losses, and 3.5 to 6.0 g/kg/day for healthy cats (National Research Council, 1978). Modified protein supplementation levels should be considered in special cases (e.g., increased protein if excess protein loss; decreased protein with concurrent hepatic and renal disease [low end of the protein range is selected]). The third step is to determine the contribution of each of the three basic elements of the solution: namely, 50 per cent dextrose, lipid emulsion, and amino acid solutions.

Some authors believe that the calculated energy needs should be provided only by the dextrose and lipid solutions, and calories provided by amino acid solutions should not be taken into account (Remillard and Thatcher, 1989). This approach, however, results in the animal's receiving energy in excess of the calculated IER, resulting in nutritional support in excess of real needs. The consequences of calorie overload in animals undergoing total parenteral nutrition have been noted (Lippert et al, 1989; Mashuma, 1979). Although calorie overloads typically do not result in clinical problems until the degree of excess approaches 25 per cent, a study in 33 healthy cats receiving total parenteral nutrition reported the development of clinical disease (i.e., vomiting, depression, and oral ulceration) and excess weight gain (Lippert et al, 1989). Animals receiving identical nutritional support, with the exception of factoring in the calories present in the amino acid solution such that they were not hyperalimented, appeared to perform better clinically and maintained stable weights. However, it may be prudent to include calories derived from amino acid solutions in the total parenteral nutrition calculations for aging dogs and cats and then divide the remaining required calories between 50 per cent dextrose and 20 per cent lipid emulsion.

Beginning delivery of total parenteral nutrition should be done slowly, using a half-strength solution initially and increasing to full strength by the second day. It also may be necessary to taper the total parenteral nutrition delivery over 12 hours prior to discontinuation to avoid hypoglycemia (Remillard and Thatcher, 1989). Oral or enteral supplementation should be instituted as soon as is practical.

Complications associated with total parenteral nutrition fall into three broad categories: infectious, metabolic, and mechanical; a summary of these is presented in Table 4–7 (Lippert et al, 1993). These complications and the animal's ongoing disease process dictate that rigid clinical follow-up be maintained while the animal is on total parenteral nutrition to ensure that metabolic needs are met and electrolyte concentrations are appropriate. Vital signs, body weight, blood and urine glucose levels, serum electrolyte levels, and renal parameters should be evaluated serially, more frequently at the initiation of total parenteral nutrition and as required once the animal's condition stabilizes (Remillard and Thatcher, 1989).

In the appropriate situation, the benefits of total parenteral nutrition include maintenance of normal weight, increased response and tolerance to therapy, return to positive energy and nitrogen balance, and a return to or preservation of quality of life.

References

Armstrong PJ, Hardie EM. Percutaneous endoscopic gastrostomy: A retrospective study of 54 clinical cases in dogs and cats. J Vet Intern Med 4:202, 1990.

Buffington T. Feeding the aged dog. In 4th Friskies-Carnation Symposium on Canine Disease and Nutrition, 1991, p 1.

DeBowes LJ, Coyne B, Layton CE. Comparison of French-Pezzar and Malecot catheters for percutaneously placed gastrostomy tubes in cats. J Am Vet Med Assoc 202:1963–1965, 1993.

Diamond P, Brondel L, LeBlanc J. Palatability and postprandial thermogenesis in dogs. Am J Physiol 248:E75, 1985.

Donohue S. Nutritional support of hospitalized patients. Vet Clin North Am 19:475, 1989.

Dudrick SJ, Wilmore DW, Vars HM, et al. Long-term total parenteral nutrition with growth, development, and positive nitrogen balance. Surgery 64:134, 1968.

Goldston RT. Geriatrics and gerontology. Vet Clin North Am 19:1, 1989.

Hand MS, Armstrong PJ, Allen TA. Obesity: Occurrence, treatment, and prevention. Vet Clin North Am 19:447, 1989.

Hoskins JD. Nutritional disorders of the aging dog and cat. In Morgan RV, ed. Handbook of Small Animal Practice. 2nd ed. New York, Churchill Livingstone, 1992, p 1295.

Kronfeld DS. Geriatric diets for dogs. Compend Contin Educ Pract Vet 5:136, 1983.

Laflamme DP. Body condition scoring and weight maintenance. Proc North Am Vet Conf 7:290, 1993.

Laflamme DP, Kuhlman G. Obesity management: It can work. Proc North Am Vet Conf 7:291, 1993.

LeBlanc J, Diamond P. Effect of meal size and frequency on postprandial thermogenesis in dogs. Am J Physiol 250:E144, 1986.

Lippert AC, Faulkner JE, Evans AT, et al. Total parenteral nutrition in clinically normal cats. J Am Vet Med Assoc 194:669, 1989.

Lippert AC, Fulton RB, Parr AM. A retrospective study of the use of total parenteral nutrition in dogs and cats. J Vet Intern Med 7:52, 1993.

Markwell PJ, van Erk W, Parkin GD, et al. Obesity in the dog. J Small Anim Pract 31:533, 1990.

Mashuma Y. Effect of calorie overload on puppy livers during parenteral nutrition. J Parenter Enteral Nutr 3:139, 1979.

Mosier JE. Effect of aging on body systems of the dog. Vet Clin North Am 19:1, 1989.

National Research Council. Nutrition requirements of cats. Washington, DC, National Research Council, 1978, p 1.

Nicholson LJ. Declogging small bore feeding tubes. J Parenter Enteral Nutr 11:594, 1987.

Ogilvie GK. Alterations in metabolism and nutritional support for veterinary cancer patients: Recent advances. Compend Contin Educ Pract Vet 15:925–937, 1993.

Remillard RL, Thatcher CD. Parenteral nutritional support in the small animal patient. Vet Clin North Am 19:1287, 1989.

Roe DA. Drugs and nutrition in the elderly. In Geriatric Nutrition. 2nd ed. Englewood Cliffs, NJ, Prentice-Hall, 1987, p 176.

Sheffy BE, Williams AJ. Nutrition and aging animal. Vet Clin North Am 11:669, 1981.

Sheffy BE, Williams AJ, Zimmer JF, et al. Nutrition and metabolism of the geriatric dog. Cornell Vet 75:324, 1985.

Sibley KW. Diagnosis and management of the overweight dog. Br Vet J 140:124, 1984.

Thompson JS, Hodges RE. Preventing hypophosphatemia during total parenteral nutrition. J Parenter Enteral Nutr 8:137, 1984.

Wheeler SL, McGuire BM. Enteral nutritional support. In Kirk RW, ed. Current Veterinary Therapy X. Philadelphia, WB Saunders, 1989, p 30.

CHAPTER 5

Cancer and Its Therapy

BARBARA E. KITCHELL

Increasing age represents the single leading risk factor for the development of cancer (Lyman, 1992). In human and veterinary medicine, advancing age is associated with an increasing incidence of malignant and benign neoplasms and greater rates of cancer-associated deaths (Dorn and Priester, 1987; Silverberg and Lubera, 1988). The prevalence of cancer in veterinary practice is climbing as a result of greater longevity of pet animals. Better nutrition, widespread use of immunizations, improved preventive medicine measures, and overall better care of animals have resulted in this greater longevity. With longer life span comes the challenge of geriatric medicine, including the treatment of cancer. Figure 5–1 illustrates the age distribution of cancer patients referred to Special Veterinary Services, Berkeley, CA, from 1990 to 1992. Although veterinarians are diagnosing and treating more cases of malignant disease in geriatric patients, the primary veterinary literature has not kept pace in this field. Little information specific to the older dog and cat exists regarding issues such as biologic behavior of cancer, response rates, and morbidity associated with treatment (Kitchell, 1989, 1993; Morrison, 1989).

ONCOGENESIS AND AGING

Multistep Carcinogenesis. The mechanisms by which cancers are initiated and progress to full clinical consequence constitute a field of intense study. The fundamental basis of cancer is change in the genetic material of the cell, with morphologic alterations of chromosomes detectable in some cases and transforming DNA sequences identified in many other cases. Most, but not all, neoplasms originate from a single cell and hence are considered monoclonal. The transformation of cells from normalcy to the malignant state requires sequential steps, referred to as a *multistage process*. An *initiation step* is the first occurrence on this pathway. Initiation fixes the cell at a low level of differentiation and preserves the proliferative potential by genomic mutation. After the initiation step, one or several events occur that are referred to as tumor *promotion*. In promotion, toxins or environmental or other insults induce cell damage and cause cell replication to occur, resulting in progression to full-blown cancer (Anisimov, 1992). Over the lifetime of an animal, many exposures to cancer-causing agents may occur, and damage to DNA then accumulates. Cells that turn over continually during the lifetime of the animal, such as cells of the skin, blood, gastrointestinal tract, and respiratory tract, have a higher propensity to express this DNA damage as uncontrolled proliferation and cancer. Although DNA damage may accrue at the same rate in all cells of the body, those cells that undergo periodic or constant cell divisions during the lifetime of the animal are more likely to have DNA damage that manifests as malignant transformation. Because of this, the absolute number of malignancies of cells of endodermal

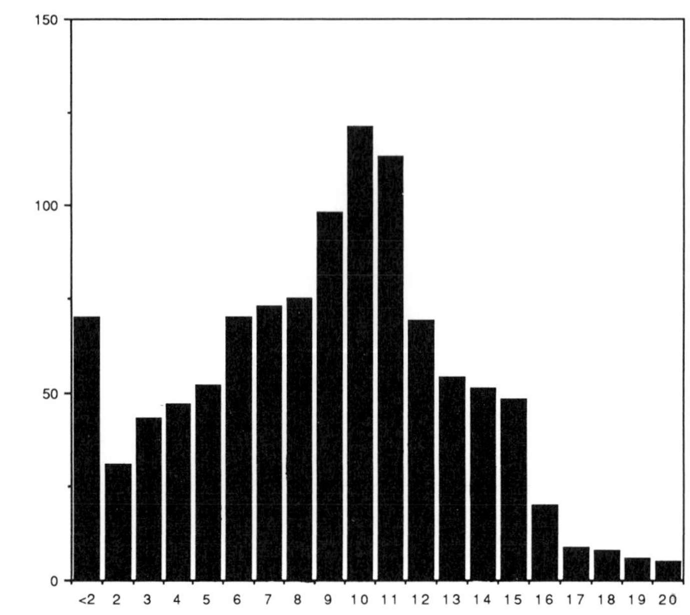

Figure 5–1. Age distribution of cancer-bearing animals seen at Special Veterinary Services, Berkeley, CA, between 1990 and 1992. Note that the peak age of dogs and cats seen is 10 to 11 years.

and ectodermal origin (carcinomas) greatly exceeds the incidence of cancers arising from tissues of mesodermal origin (sarcomas) (Lipshitz et al, 1985).

Molecular Biology of Cancer and Aging. Alterations in cells occur as a result of aging and contribute to susceptibility to cancer. These age-related changes have been extensively studied at the molecular level (Fig. 5–2). Aging cells lose replicative capacity and have impaired ability to repair damage to DNA. Aged cells lose highly repetitious DNA sequences thought to be important for DNA repair. Old cells are deficient in excision repair, in which damaged pieces of DNA are cut out and the DNA is "filled in" (Anisimov, 1992; Oppenheimer, 1985). Aged cells demonstrate decreased methylation of repeated genetic sequences, which may have an impact on which genes in a cell are expressed or "turned on" (Ebbesen, 1984; Jones, 1986). Disposal of free radicals is less efficient in older mammalian cells, which may contribute to cancer via DNA damage, as well to the process of normal aging (Harman, 1971). In contrast, some age-related changes serve to counteract the development of cancer, including loss of proliferative stimulation by hormones and depletion of the pool of immature cells at greatest risk (Ebbesen, 1984). After initiation with a chemical agent or irradiation, it usually takes an average of 10 to 20 per cent of the species' maximum life span before a mass of tumor equivalent to 10^9 cells (1 g of tumor) is detected (Oppenheimer, 1985). This lag time to clinical detection may contribute to recognition

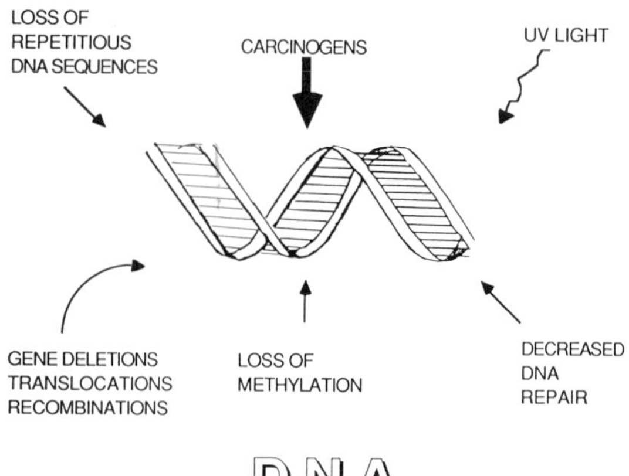

Figure 5–2. Many agents are capable of causing damage to DNA, which results in uncontrolled cell proliferation and cancer.

of cancer in greater numbers in aged individuals (Fig. 5–3) (Ershler, 1992).

Carcinogenesis and Age. Susceptibility to carcinogenic substances may also differ with age. Fetuses (after completion of organogenesis), the very young, and adolescents are more susceptible to cancer induction by some agents than are adult humans and animals. Rapid cell proliferation in these age groups may account for this sensitivity (Anisimov, 1992). On the other hand, aging cells may be more susceptible than young cells to the impact of other specific cancer-causing agents. In humans exposed to atomic bomb fallout, risk of subsequent cancer increased with age. In BALB/c mouse skin exposed to small doses of carcinogens, there is an increase in susceptibility of old skin as compared with young adult skin. Skin grafted from older individuals to young mice demonstrated increased sensitivity to carcinogens, indicating that the age of the tissue, rather than the age of the host, determines susceptibility to carcinogens (Anisimov, 1992). In another experimental animal model, the incidence of neoplasms in mice receiving transplanted splenic or thymic lymphocytes from syngeneic donors was related to the age of the donor, but not to the age of the recipient (Ebbesen, 1971).

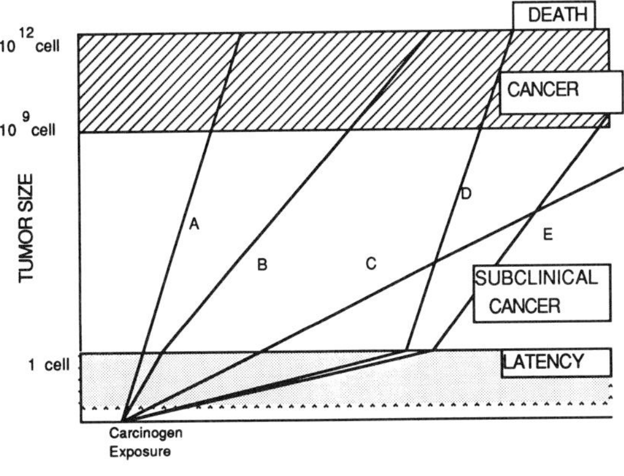

Figure 5–3. A single cell is exposed to a carcinogen early in the life of an animal. Line A represents a very aggressive, fast-growing tumor that is clinically apparent at an early age. An example of this type of neoplasm is lymphosarcoma in young cats, with the feline leukemia virus representing the carcinogenic stimulus. Line B shows a slow-growing tumor that presents in middle age and has a slowly progressive, relatively benign course. An example of this tumor type is the canine hemangiopericytoma. Line C represents a situation in which a carcinogenic stimulus has been applied to the cell, but the replication rate of this tumor cell is so low that cancer is never clinically apparent during the lifetime of the animal. There may be a myriad of such subclinical cancers during the life of an individual. Line D is the situation in which a second strongly carcinogenic event occurs, such as development of abnormal chromosome number in the affected cell, with rapid growth of tumor and patient death. Line E represents a second carcinogic event resulting in a tumor with a long latency period and relatively benign behavior in the elderly animal, such as a low-grade, malignant, mixed mammary tumor in a geriatric dog.

Cellular immune reactivity declines with age, leading to a tendency to fail to eradicate early clones of malignant cells. Although the total number of T lymphocytes does not change with age (possibly because of the long life span of T cells), the distribution of the T-cell subpopulations is altered in humans. The percentage of helper T cells increases and the relative percentage of cytotoxic T cells declines (Makinodan and Kay, 1980). Thymic involution is at least partially responsible for these T-cell changes. Also, subtle metabolic shifts and neurohormonal changes associated with aging may have an impact on development of immune response to malignant cells, as well as on the development of hormonally mediated cancers (Lipshitz et al, 1985).

Biologic Behavior of Tumors in the Elderly. Although the incidence of cancer in elderly individuals may be higher than that seen in young people, the biologic behavior of cancer may be less aggressive for some tumor types (Ershler, 1992). Opinions vary in the human cancer literature, with some investigators holding the opinion that cancers are slower growing in older patients and others holding the contrary view (Ebbesen, 1971). In experimental animal systems, local tumor growth and metastasis are reduced in older animals for certain tumor types (e.g., in mice, B16 melanoma, teratocarcinoma, Lewis's lung carcinoma, murine mammary tumors) (Ershler, 1992). In other tumor types, tumor growth and spread are more aggressive in the elderly than in the young (e.g., ultraviolet light– and methylcholanthrene-induced sarcomas) (Ershler, 1992). Some investigators have proposed that immune senescence may slow the rate of tumor proliferation in the elderly by unknown mechanisms. In certain experimental systems, manipulation of the immune system to mimic changes seen with aging may result in slower tumor growth rate. When young tumor-bearing mice received syngeneic transplants of the immune system of elderly mice, tumors grew less rapidly than in mice bearing their native immune system or transplanted with the immune system of young mice (Ershler et al, 1984; Tsuda et al, 1987). The impression that survival advantage may be conferred by age to human cancer patients has been difficult to confirm statistically, perhaps because of the confounding variables of high rate of concurrent illness and the tendency to treat elderly patients less aggressively than young patients with similar malignancies (Ershler, 1992; Holmes, 1992; Weksler et al, 1988). Studies have not specifically addressed these questions in the veterinary literature.

APPROACH TO THE GERIATRIC CANCER PATIENT

Aging, Cancer, and the Veterinary Patient. Aging is characterized by progressive impairment of vital functions such as glomerular filtration rate, maximal respiratory capacity, and maximal exercise capacity. The net result of the many physiologic changes associated with aging is that the geriatric patient is less resilient and less able to survive physical stress (Balducci et al, 1986). The oncologist brings to this setting of limited life span and decreasing tolerance the tools of the cancer medicine trade, which include many forms of therapy that are noxious to the patient under the best of circumstances. Aggressive surgery, radiation therapy, and cytotoxic chemotherapy are necessary to treat local and metastatic cancer. The goals of such treatment include cure, decrease in overall tumor burden, prolonged disease-free interval, and improved quality of life for the patient by providing relief of symptoms associated with cancer. Although patients of all ages afflicted with locally confined malignant disease have a chance of being cured by appropriate surgery or radiotherapy techniques, it is unlikely that patients with disseminated disease will be cured by chemotherapy as it is currently practiced in veterinary medicine, regardless of age (Rosenthal, 1989). The situation in the elderly patient with disseminated disease is especially difficult. There may be general reluctance to use aggressive chemotherapy in older patients, as there is a paucity of knowledge about drug metabolism in the elderly and much concern for increased toxicity in this population. Most studies in human patients have shown that although there are age-associated changes in pharmacokinetics and drug metabolism, chemotherapy can be a safe and effective modality in the treatment of the aged cancer patient (Joseph, 1988). Happily, the rate of toxicity seen with most chemotherapy protocols appears to be considerably lower in dogs and cats than in humans treated with the same drugs (Couto, 1990).

Strategies for treatment of the aging dog or cat patient must take into account the impact of intercurrent diseases such as cardiac or renal insufficiency on life expectancy and treatment tolerance of the patient. Drug and anesthetic regimens may have to be modified to accommodate intercurrent medical problems, and therapies may have to be tailored to individual patients. The veterinarian must have a good basic knowledge of and familiarity with chemotherapy to adapt drug treatment and anticipate side effects. The *performance status* of the patient, a term referring to the overall quality of the patient's life, must be considered in determining therapy. In human medicine, patients with higher initial performance status generally have better outcomes. A performance status scale modified for veterinary use was described by Misdorp (1987) (Table 5–1).

Screening and Early Detection. Often the single most important prognostic factor for the successful treatment of cancer is early detection. Survival rates for patients diagnosed with extensive disease are much lower than those for patients diagnosed with small tumor burdens and locally confined disease (American Cancer Society, 1987; Misdorp, 1987). The stage of cancer at diagnosis is determined by two sets of variables: the biologic behavior of the cancer and the host, and the factors that influence owner and veterinarian behavior in the process of diagnosis. The early detection of cancer in geriatric patients is complicated by the presence of concurrent chronic illnesses that mask early clinical signs of neoplastic disease (Kitchell, 1993; Morrison, 1989; Robie, 1989). Signs that would draw immediate attention and concern in a young animal are often accepted as a consequence of aging or a result of other known medical problems in the patient (e.g., "His arthritis must be acting up again, Doc"). Pet owners and veterinarians alike may acknowledge the severity of clinical signs in

TABLE 5–1. PERFORMANCE STATUS CRITERIA FOR ANIMALS WITH CANCER

GRADE	CRITERIA
0	Fully active, leading a normal life, with normal body weight
1	Able to exercise but may have fatigue or dyspnea with severe exertion
2	Fatigue or respiratory distress after moderate to severe exertion; may be emaciated
3	Fatigue or dyspnea at rest
4	Recumbent, unable to care for basic needs
5	Moribund

From Misdorp W. The impact of pathology on the study and treatment of cancer. In Theilen GH, Madewell BR, eds. Veterinary Cancer Medicine. 2nd ed. Philadelphia, Lea & Febiger, 1987, pp. 53–70.

an elderly dog or cat but harbor the fatalistic attitude that nothing can be done to definitively treat the patient or to palliate the clinical signs once the patient has reached a certain age ("After all, she is 11 years old") (Goodwin et al, 1986).

Studies of owner attitudes toward diagnostic testing in geriatric dogs and cats are unavailable in the veterinary cancer literature. Several studies are available regarding the stage of disease at cancer diagnosis and the age of human patients (Goodwin et al, 1986; Goodwin and Samet, 1992; Mor et al, 1988). Patients in New Mexico were followed in a retrospective study from 1969 to 1982. Tumors of the urinary bladder, breast, cervix, ovary, thyroid, and uterus and dermal melanomas were found to be more advanced at diagnosis in elderly patients. Conversely, cancers of the lung, pancreas, rectum, and stomach were diagnosed at earlier stages in elderly than in younger patients. No significant trends could be discerned for cancers of the colon, kidney, liver, and prostate gland (Goodwin et al, 1986; Goodwin and Samet, 1992). These findings were attributed to several factors involving patient and physician attitudes and the biologic behavior of cancer in the elderly. First, some tumor types may have presented in a more advanced stage because of increased aggressive behavior of the tumor, failure of patients to seek medical attention when initial signs developed, and less aggressive diagnostic testing applied to this patient population than to their younger counterparts. Tumors diagnosed at a lower stage may have been due to less aggressive behavior of some cancers in the elderly. Also, physicians may have a higher index of suspicion when treating the elderly population, prompting earlier diagnostic work-ups with certain presenting signs (Goodwin et al, 1986; Goodwin and Samet, 1992).

In another study of geriatric patients in Rhode Island, no association between extent of disease and age of the patient at diagnosis was found for lung, breast, and colorectal cancer (Mor et al, 1988). The authors suggest that early detection of these cancers in the elderly could be ascribed to wide application of screening measures, including breast self-examination and mammograms for breast cancer, fecal occult blood tests for colorectal cancer, and chest radiographs for populations at greatest risk for lung cancer, such as smokers and asbestos workers (Mor et al, 1988). Similar studies have not been performed to link stage of disease at diagnosis and patient age in veterinary medicine.

Cancer screening programs are widely used and are considered very successful for many types of common human cancers. Papanicolaou cytologic tests for cervical cancer; mammography and breast self-examinations for breast cancer; and fecal occult blood tests, colonoscopy, or sigmoidoscopy for colorectal cancer are all very useful programs. For screening procedures to be helpful, they must be specific, sensitive to early disease, free of morbidity, cost effective, and available for use in populations at risk of disease. Improvement in quality of life may be even more important than increase in longevity as a criterion for success of such screening programs (Robie, 1989). In veterinary medicine, routine cancer screening measures have not been developed and applied, in part because of the lack of consensus on diseases appropriate for such screening and the difficulty inherent in designing programs that meet all of the previously listed criteria for success. The feline leukemia virus antigen test might be considered a screening test in wide use clinically, as it allows for the detection of viral infection before the onset of clinical signs, alerts the veterinarian and owner to the potential for further disease consequences, and allows early intervention (Kitchell, 1989).

A better approach for the veterinary setting may be the institution of earlier detection of problems through owner education. Pet owners should be made aware of the fact that animals do develop cancer. The most common sites of malignant disease in animals include the skin, mammary glands, lymph nodes, and oral cavity (Dorn and Priester, 1987). Educated owners may seek medical care sooner for their pets. A list of signs analogous to the American Cancer Society's "Seven Warning Signs of Cancer" has been developed by the Veterinary Cancer Society and is applicable to both dogs and cats (Table 5–2) (Kitchell, 1989).

Diagnosis. Malignant disease is diagnosed through histopathologic or cytologic evaluation of tumor tissues. There is no difference in the tech-

TABLE 5–2. COMMON SIGNS OF CANCER IN ANIMALS

1. Abnormal swellings that persist or continue to grow
2. Sores that do not heal
3. Weight loss
4. Loss of appetite
5. Bleeding or discharge from any body opening
6. Offensive odor
7. Difficulty eating or swallowing
8. Hesitation to exercise or loss of stamina
9. Persistent lameness or stiffness
10. Difficulty breathing, urinating, or defecating

Developed by the Veterinary Cancer Society, College of Veterinary Medicine, North Carolina State University, Raleigh, NC 27606.

niques applied to young and old animals. In fact, ". . . even the most clever pathologist cannot determine the age of the patient by microscopic examination of his or her cancer" (Holmes, 1992). Histopathology offers the advantage of allowing a pathologic grade of malignancy to be assigned to the lesion. Histopathologic grading is helpful in predicting the degree of aggressiveness of a tumor and the potential for response to therapy (Misdorp, 1987; Morrison, 1989). Excisional biopsy specimens are examined for complete excision by evaluating the tumor tissue margin.

After the diagnosis of malignant disease is completed, the extent of disease in the patient is defined by a staging work-up. Staging is essential for determining appropriate therapy and can include such tests as thoracic and abdominal radiographs, evaluation of regional and distant lymph nodes, and bone marrow examination. Staging protocols for various tumor types are available elsewhere (Owen, 1980).

The evaluation of the geriatric cancer patient is completed by investigating for concurrent age-related illness through a careful history, thorough physical examination, and clinical laboratory testing. Discovery of underlying chronic diseases, such as renal, hepatic, or cardiac insufficiency, is crucial to treatment planning and accurate prognostication of potential therapeutic outcomes. Debilitating conditions such as arthritis and dental disease may be addressed to improve the patient's quality of life during therapy (Kitchell, 1989, 1993).

CANCER THERAPY FOR THE GERIATRIC PATIENT

Once the diagnosis of cancer has been made and staging completed, definitive therapy can be conducted. Factors to be considered in establishing a treatment protocol include the presence of other life-limiting illnesses, patient performance status, owner attitudes and expectations, and cost of treatment. In addition, aged patients have decreased physiologic reserve and thus increased potential for toxicity during therapy with cancer drugs (Joseph, 1988). Because of these considerations, physicians and veterinarians have opted for conservative treatment regimens for elderly patients, and in some human studies age was found to be inversely related to number of patients treated with chemotherapy or radiotherapy (Joseph, 1988; Mor et al, 1985). The proportion of human patients with locally confined cancer who received treatment with curative intent declined with age, and the proportion of these patients who received no therapy increased with age (Mor et al, 1985). This is even more likely to be the case in veterinary medicine, where euthanasia exists as an option that is not available, at least overtly, to human patients.

Surgery

The basic principles of cancer treatment apply equally to all cancer patients regardless of age at diagnosis. Locally confined tumors achieve the best cure rates when appropriate oncologic surgery principles are applied to their removal. The first surgery represents the best chance to achieve a complete cure, and for this reason careful surgical planning is paramount. Furthermore, geriatric patients are less likely to tolerate repeated subcurative surgeries, so this principle certainly applies to them. En bloc resection techniques should be carried out, followed by careful evaluation of the submitted surgical margins by the pathologist. Descriptions of specific surgical techniques are available elsewhere (Harvey, 1987; Withrow, 1989). Veterinarians should contact surgical specialists for guidance before undertaking a procedure, and patients that would benefit from referral should be availed of that option, regardless of age (Kitchell, 1993).

Human patients older than 70 years have increased surgical mortality rates. It has also been reported that mortality rates correlate with the number of pre-existing medical conditions and not with age as an isolated factor (Becker et al, 1989; Joseph, 1988). Careful pretreatment planning and anesthetic management are essential to successful outcome, as is aggressive supportive care in the pre- and postoperative periods (Joseph, 1988).

Radiotherapy

Radiation therapy is equally effective in killing cancer cells in elderly and young patients. However, radiation therapy can be expected to have 10 to 15 per cent greater adverse effects on normal tissues in the elderly (Gunn, 1980; Joseph, 1988). Some authors feel that the associated side effects of radiation treatment are no worse in the elderly, but the older patient is less able to compensate for the temporary dysfunction caused by radiation damage to tissues and organs (Greenberg and Trotti, 1992). Individuation of treatment programs by changes in fractionation, du-

TABLE 5–3. IMPACT OF PHARMACOKINETIC CHANGES ASSOCIATED WITH AGING

PARAMETER	CHANGE	POSSIBLE DRUGS AFFECTED
Absorption	Possible slight decrease	Oral drugs (cyclophosphamide, methotrexate, melphalan, chlorambucil)
Volume of distribution	Relative decrease in water-soluble drugs and increase in fat-soluble drugs; decreased plasma protein	BCNU, CCNU, doxorubicin, melphalan, cisplatin
Hepatic metabolism	Decreased microsomal activation/inactivation	Cyclophosphamide, dacarbazine (decreased activity); doxorubicin, vinca alkaloids (increased toxicity)
Renal excretion	Declines with age	Cisplatin, methotrexate, bleomycin, melphalan, cyclophosphamide

BCNU, Bis-chlorethyl-nitrosourea; CCNU, chloroethyl-cyclohexyl-nitrosourea.
From Kitchell BE. Cancer therapy for geriatric dogs and cats. J Am Anim Hosp Assoc 29:41–48, 1993.

ration of therapy, total dose delivered, or total tissue volume treated are recommended for human cancer patients (Joseph, 1988). Veterinary patients need brief anesthesia with each fraction of radiotherapy; this may be deleterious in elderly dogs and cats. With appropriate management and precautions, however, potentially curative or palliative radiation therapy may be administered. Also, as most radiotherapy in veterinary medicine is delivered in cancer treatment centers, experienced radiotherapists and anesthesiologists are available to optimize the care of these animals (Kitchell, 1993).

Cancer Chemotherapy

Cancer chemotherapy agents have a low therapeutic index—that is, the dose that produces a desired treatment response is very close to the dose that produces an undesired toxic response. With careful management and clear treatment goals, it is possible to use these drugs safely and effectively. Several excellent discussions of chemotherapy use (Helfand, 1990; Rosenthal, 1989; Theilen and Madewell, 1987) and toxicity (Couto, 1990) in veterinary medicine are available. There is little information specific to geriatric dogs and cats, but general principles of pharmacokinetics and pharmacodynamics should apply (Kitchell, 1993).

Many physiologic alterations occur with advancing age. Alterations in response or toxicity to many classes of drugs have been studied in human medicine, but little information is available specific to veterinary patients (Aucoin, 1989; Balducci et al, 1992). Because of the historical reluctance of physicians to treat elderly patients with aggressive chemotherapy regimens, studies regarding anticancer drug metabolism in this population are only currently being performed (Joseph, 1988). In a study conducted by the Eastern Cooperative Oncology Group, patients over 70 years of age had rates of severe toxicity identical to those of their younger counterparts on 19 different treatment protocols studied. The exception to this was that greater rates of hematologic toxicity were seen when the drugs methotrexate and lomustine were administered to aged patients (Begg and Carbone, 1983).

Age and Pharmacokinetics

Several known pharmacokinetic changes associated with aging may have to be considered in establishing treatment protocols for this patient population. Altered drug absorption, distribution, hepatic metabolism, and renal clearance may be experienced by aged patients (Table 5–3) (Aucoin, 1989; Balducci et al, 1992; Begg and Carbone, 1983; Phister et al, 1989).

Absorption. In general, although maximal absorption of food and drugs may be restricted in the older patient, these changes are of little clinical significance owing to the intestinal absorptive reserve capacity. The possible exception to this is in the use of high-dose L-leucovorin in human patients, which has been documented to vary with age (Balducci et al, 1992).

Distribution. Drug distribution can be altered in the geriatric individual owing to a decrease in lean body mass, an increase in total body fat, and a decrease in plasma proteins (Aucoin, 1989; Phister et al, 1989). Fat-soluble drugs such as nitrosourea (bis-chloroethyl-nitrosourea [BCNU] and chloroethyl-cyclohexyl-nitrosourea [CCNU]) may be retained, resulting in increased myelotoxicity. In humans, there is an age-associated prolongation in the early distribution phase of doxorubicin, with a potential for higher peak plasma concentrations and resulting increased cardiotoxicity (Begg and Carbone, 1986). Because serum albumin concentrations decline with age, drugs that are highly protein bound (melphalan, cisplatin) may have a higher free plasma concentration with altered drug effect. Serum albumin levels may be lowered by concurrent renal, hepatic, and neoplastic diseases (Balducci et al, 1992; Kitchell, 1993; Phister et al, 1989).

Metabolism. The major pathways of elimination of cancer chemotherapeutic agents are listed in Table 5–4 (Balducci et al, 1992). The liver is the main site of metabolism for the majority of cancer drugs. Hepatic drug metabolism changes with age. Liver mass and blood flow through the liver decline, and microsomal oxidative metabolism is impaired. Oxazophosphorines (cyclophosphamide and ifosfamide), nitrosoureas, dacarbazine, and mitomycin C are activated in the liver. These drugs may be less effective in geriatric patients owing to inadequate activation from prodrug (Balducci et al, 1992; Helfand, 1990; Phister et al, 1989). Liver oxidative enzymes are susceptible to inhibition by drugs such as cimetidine or to induction by drugs such as phenobarbital. Polypharmacy is more common in older patients, and use of concurrent drugs must be considered in elderly patients (Balducci et al, 1992).

The conjugative reactions of the liver are responsible for the inactivation of several drugs, including the anthracyclines, mitoxantrone, mitomycin C, and the vinca alkaloids. Decreased elimination of these drugs in patients with abnormal liver function can lead to increased acute toxicity. Dose reduction is suggested when liver function tests are abnormal (Begg and Carbone, 1986; Phister et al, 1989; Susaneck, 1983). Fortunately, the conjugative reactions of the liver are relatively unaffected by age. Concern for abnormal liver metabolism is limited to patients with abnormal liver function due to concurrent disease, regardless of age (Balducci et al, 1992).

TABLE 5–4. ELIMINATION PATHWAYS FOR CANCER CHEMOTHERAPY DRUGS USED IN VETERINARY MEDICINE

PATHWAY	DRUGS
Primarily renal	Methotrexate, bleomycin, carboplatin, cisplatin
Primarily hepatic	Anthracyclines, mitoxantrone, vinca alkaloids
Mixed	Cyclophosphamide, nitrosourea, dacarbazine
Spontaneous degradation	Melphalan, 5-fluorouracil cytarabine, L-asparaginase

From Balducci L, Mowrey K, Parker M. Pharmacology of antineoplastic agents in older patients. In Balducci L, Lyman GH, Ershler WB, eds. Geriatric Oncology. Philadelphia, JB Lippincott, 1992, pp 169–180.

Excretion. A decline in glomerular and tubular function is seen with age and can result in abnormal elimination of renally excreted drugs. A decline in glomerular filtration rate (GFR) is probably the most consistent physiologic change observed with aging (Balducci et al, 1992; Brenner, 1986). Reduced GFR can lead to increased toxicity from drugs such as methotrexate, bleomycin, cisplatin, and possibly cyclophosphamide (Balducci et al, 1992; Couto, 1990). Because there can be great variation in renal function level among elderly patients, renal function should be assessed prior to administration of drugs requiring renal elimination (Kitchell, 1993; Phister et al, 1989). Dose reduction may be indicated because of decreased renal function, but not because of advanced age alone (Hrushesky et al, 1984).

Organ-Specific Toxicity

Myelotoxicity is the most universal adverse effect of chemotherapy owing to the constant and relatively rapid replication of hematopoietic precursor cells. In theory, replacement of chemotherapy-destroyed hematopoietic elements may be delayed in the elderly because of exhaustion of pluripotent hematopoietic stem cells, impaired production of hematopoietic growth factors, and a dysfunctional hematopoietic microenvironment (Balducci et al, 1992). After aggressive treatment of various types of human leukemias, lymphomas, and breast cancer, myelodepression was more prolonged and severe in older patients (Balducci et al, 1992; Gelman and Taylor, 1984; Lazarus et al, 1989). The administration of other myelodepressive drugs such as sulfamethoxazole-trimethoprim may contribute to delayed regeneration (Balducci et al, 1992). Recombinant hematopoietic growth factors may further aid in preventing myelotoxicity in the elderly (Shank, 1992).

Elderly human patients are at risk for mucositis after administration of methotrexate, 5-fluorouracil, bleomycin, and cytarabine. Mucositis is caused by the destruction of rapidly proliferating cells of the gastrointestinal tract. Elderly patients should be treated aggressively if symptoms of vomiting or diarrhea develop after treatment with anticancer drugs. Fluid and electrolyte support, glucocorticoids, and sucralfate may be indicated in these patients (Balducci et al, 1992).

Nausea and vomiting may occur as a result of several mechanisms. Drugs may have direct action on the chemoreceptor trigger zone of the medulla, or mucositis may occur as described previously. Anticipatory nausea and vomiting may be triggered in people by thoughts or sensory input related to the chemotherapy experience. Fortunately, anticipatory nausea has not been reported in veterinary patients. Delayed nausea and vomiting may occur 2 days after treatment and may persist for days. The pathogenesis of this complication is not certain, but older human patients may respond to scopolamine transdermal patches (Balducci et al, 1992). Dexamethasone (0.25 mg/kg IV or SC) and metaclopramide (0.1 to 0.3 mg per kilogram body weight IV, SC, or PO three times daily) have been used successfully as antiemetics in veterinary cancer therapy (Couto, 1990; Rosenthal, 1989). Torbugesic (0.4 mg/kg IM) has been used specifically to block nausea and vomiting associated with the administration of cisplatin in dogs (Moore et al, 1990).

Cardiotoxicity can be a complication of therapy with anthracyclines, mitoxantrone, mitomycin C, or high-dose cyclophosphamide (Balducci et al, 1992). Controversy exists in human medicine as to the potential of doxorubicin for increased cardiotoxicity in the elderly. In two studies, age alone was not found to be a factor, while in two other studies, age was associated with increased risk (Joseph, 1988). Because anthracycline cardiotoxicity may be associated with increased free radical formation in the sarcoplasm, geriatric heart muscle may be at greater risk owing to decreased numbers of free radical scavengers (Balducci et al, 1992). Certainly the presence of pre-existing cardiac disease is a major factor in induction of doxorubicin cardiotoxicity, and careful cardiac evaluation should precede use of this drug (Susaneck, 1983). Mitoxantrone, an anthracenedione derivative of the anthracyclines, is approximately 10 times less cardiotoxic and thus may be useful in geriatric patients (Balducci et al, 1992). Mitoxantrone appears to have a spectrum of anticancer activity similar to that of doxorubicin in dogs and cats (Helfand, 1990; Ogilvie et al, 1991).

Bleomycin may cause increased pulmonary toxicity in the elderly, possibly because of decreased hydrolase activity in aging lungs. Mitomycin C, busulfan, and nitrosoureas may also be associated with pulmonary toxicity in people (Balducci et al, 1992; Joseph, 1988). The decreased vital capacity and forced expiratory volume that occur with age may cause clinical manifestations of pulmonary toxicity to appear sooner in these patients than in the young. Cats are affected by pulmonary edema from systemic administration of cisplatin, and the use of this drug in cats is not appropriate (Knapp et al, 1987).

Similarly, neurotoxicity from vinca alkaloids (vincristine and vinblastine) and epipodophyllotoxins (etoposide and teniposide) may be more significant in elderly individuals because of the effect of unmasking subclinical neuropathies (Joseph, 1988). Manifestations include paresthesias, weakness, and loss of deep tendon reflexes (Balducci et al, 1992). Vincristine neurotoxicity is reversible over time. Cisplatin neurotoxicity is an idiosyncratic effect that is not dose related in people and is often irreversible. Veterinarians should be aware that vincristine and cisplatin may induce acoustic neuropathy with associated hearing loss (Balducci et al, 1992). Geriatric dogs in particular may manifest deafness when treated with these agents, perhaps through unmasking of underlying hearing loss. Central neurotoxicity may be seen in patients receiving high-dose cytarabine, 5-fluorouracil, nitrosoureas, and dacarbazine. The central nervous system of older patients may be more sensitive owing to age-related neuron loss (Balducci et al, 1992). Again, cats are exquisitely sensitive to the neurotoxic effects of 5-fluorouracil, and its use is contraindicated in cats (Theilen and Madewell, 1987).

Nephrotoxicity may be induced by cisplatin, mitomycin C, nitrosoureas, and ifosfamide. Clinical studies with cisplatin in humans have failed to demonstrate increased toxicity in elderly persons, perhaps because of a relatively advantageous decrease in GFR (Gelman and Taylor, 1984). Carboplatin, a non-nephrotoxic analogue of cisplatin, may be substituted in patients with abnormal renal function. Because carboplatin is renally excreted, the dose must be lowered in patients with reduced creatinine clearance to avoid myelosuppression from prolonged exposure (Balducci et al, 1992). Feline patients also have a tendency to develop renal insufficiency on high-dose doxorubicin therapy (Cotter et al, 1985).

Unfortunately, no specific information relative to the rates of toxicity seen in older dogs and cats is available (Kitchell, 1993). However, it is safe to assume that because the majority of chemotherapy patients are older dogs and cats, the veterinary literature is probably an accurate reflection of toxicity in this group of patients. In my practice, no difference in toxicity in the very old has been appreciated, except for an increased tendency toward anorexia in chemotherapy-treated geriatric cats. Further prospective or retrospective analysis of veterinary cancer patients might help elucidate this matter. Similarly, there are no specific data pertinent to differential response rates of geriatric animals to chemotherapy treatment. In a recent New York City Animal Medical Center study of canine lymphosarcoma, age was not found to be a factor in response or survival rates (Greenlee et al, 1990).

Supportive Care

Adequate supportive care is paramount to successful management of all cancer patients, but this principle is particularly applicable to the care of elderly individuals. All aspects of care that optimize quality of life should be used in treatment. Monitoring food intake, water consumption, and elimination is important in managing geriatric patients. Cats especially will benefit from grooming when they are debilitated (Kitchell, 1989).

Pain may be managed with various approaches, including aspirin, corticosteroids, nonsteroidal anti-inflammatory drugs, and even acupuncture in select cases. Corticosteroids may have direct anticancer activity against lymphoma, myeloma, lymphocytic leukemia, and mast cell disease. They are useful for stimulating appetite and promoting a general sense of well-being in human patients, and the same effects appear to be present in dogs and cats. However, corticosteroid administration may compound immune suppression and liver toxicity and has been implicated in the development of pleiotropic drug resistance (Pastan and Gottesman, 1988). The potential benefits of corticosteroid administration should be weighed against these detrimental aspects. Nonsteroidal anti-inflammatory drugs such as piroxicam (Feldene) have been used as palliative agents in the treatment of a variety of canine malignancies (Knapp et al, 1992). Piroxicam has been reported to induce partial remissions in a few dogs treated with this drug as a single agent (Knapp et al, 1992; Morrison, 1989). Most dogs that receive piroxicam at a dose of 0.3 to 0.5 mg per kilogram body weight once daily for 1 week, then on alternate days thereafter, experience enhanced quality of life owing to decreased pain from arthritis and inflammation. This drug should be used very cautiously because it can cause severe gastrointestinal ulceration. Piroxicam should not be used in conjunction with agents such as corticosteroids and aspirin to avoid compounding the ulcerogenic effects (Knapp et al, 1992; Morrison, 1989).

Cancer-induced malnutrition may be a more severe problem for geriatric patients (Balducci et al, 1986). Nausea and vomiting can exacerbate pre-existing nutritional deficits. Food aversions may form as a result of receiving chemotherapy after a meal; in these cases the animal associates the sensation of nausea with the food rather than with the treatment (Kitchell, 1989, 1993). A change in diet, hand feeding, and the use of appetite-stimulating agents such as diazepam (0.05 to 0.4 mg/kg IV or PO) may prove helpful. Metaclopramide (0.1 to 0.3 mg/kg IV, SC, or PO three times daily) may help with appetite support by suppressing subclinical nausea and overt vomiting (Couto, 1990; Kitchell, 1989, 1993). Aggressive nutritional support with enteral or parenteral hyperalimentation in human patients has not proved to have a positive impact on treatment tolerance, immunocompetence, postoperative mortality, or survival (Joseph, 1988). Similar studies have yet to be conducted in geriatric veterinary populations, but it would seem logical that maintenance of adequate nutritional status is important to all cancer patients. The potential negative consequences of aggressive nutritional support (sepsis from feeding tubes or hyperalimentation) should be weighed against the benefits (Ogilvie and Vail, 1990).

Assessing Response to Therapy

The most concrete statistical means of assessing the success of a treatment program in cancer medicine are survival time and remission duration. Analysis of survival becomes especially difficult in the geriatric patient (Holmes, 1992). Competing causes of death and the availability of euthanasia as an end point in veterinary medicine make it especially difficult to determine the efficacy of cancer treatment for geriatric patients. Perhaps owner evaluation of improved quality of life should be weighed as heavily as remission and survival times in assessing the response to cancer therapy in geriatric veterinary patients. In a survey of owners whose pets received chemotherapy treatment at The Ohio State University Veterinary Teaching Hospital, 85 per cent of respondents felt that their pet achieved a quality of life that was equal to or better than that prior to initiation of therapy (Couto, 1990).

CONCLUSION

Veterinary oncology has advanced greatly in recent years. Veterinarians are better able to treat animals with cancer, and clinical outcomes are better than in the past. Therapeutic decisions in the case of elderly cancer patients should be made not on the basis of chronologic age but on the basis of evaluation of the individual's general state of health and quality of life.

References

American Cancer Society. Cancer Facts and Figures—1987. New York, American Cancer Society, 1987.

Anisimov VN. Age as a factor of risk in multistage carcinogenesis. In Balducci L, Lyman GH, Ershler WB, eds. Geriatric Oncology. Philadelphia, JB Lippincott, 1992, pp 53–59.

Aucoin DP. Drug therapy in the geriatric animal: The effect of aging on drug disposition. Vet Clin North Am (Small Anim Pract) 19:41–48, 1989.

Balducci L, Mowrey K, Parker M. Pharmacology of antineoplastic agents in older patients. In Balducci L, Lyman GH, Ershler WB, eds. Geriatric Oncology. Philadelphia, JB Lippincott, 1992, pp 169–180.

Balducci L, Wallace C, Khansur T, et al. Nutrition, cancer and aging: An annoted review. I. Diet, carcinogenesis, and aging. J Am Geriatr Soc 34:127–136, 1986.

Becker TM, Goodwin JS, Hunt WC, et al. Survival after cancer surgery of elderly patients in New Mexico, 1969–1982. J Am Geriatr Soc 37:154–159, 1989.

Begg CB, Carbone PP. Clinical trials on drug toxicity in the elderly. Cancer 52:1986–1992, 1983.

Brenner BM. Effects of aging on the renal glomerulus. Am J Med 80:435–442, 1986.

Cotter SM, Kanki PJ, Simon M. Renal disease in five tumor-bearing cats treated with Adriamycin. J Am Anim Hosp Assoc 21:405–407, 1985.

Couto CG. Management of complications of cancer chemotherapy. Vet Clin North Am (Small Anim Pract) 20:1037–1054, 1990.

Dorn CR, Priester WA. Epidemiology. In Theilen GH, Madewell BR, eds. Veterinary Cancer Medicine. 2nd ed. Philadelphia, JB Lippincott, 1987, pp 27–52.

Ebbesen P. Reticulosarcoma and amyloid development in BALB/c mice inoculated with syngeneic cells from young and old donors. J Natl Cancer Inst 47:1241–1245, 1971.

Ebbesen P. Cancer and normal aging. Mechanisms Aging Dev 25:269–283, 1984.

Ershler WB. Mechanisms of age-associated reduced tumor growth and spread in mice. In Balducci L, Lyman GH, Ershler WB, eds. Geriatric Oncology. Philadelphia, JB Lippincott, 1992, pp 76–85.

Ershler WB, Moore AL, Shore H, et al. Transfer of age advantage in B16 melanoma growth rate by old to young bone marrow transplantation. Cancer Res 44:5677–5680, 1984.

Gelman RS, Taylor SG. Cyclophosphamide, methotrexate and 5-fluorouracil chemotherapy in women more than 65 years old with advanced breast cancer: The elimination of age trends in toxicity by using doses based on creatinine clearance. Clin Oncol 21:1406–1414, 1984.

Goodwin JS, Samet JM. Factors affecting the diagnosis and treatment of older patients with cancer. In Balducci L, Lyman GH, Ershler WB, eds. Geriatric Oncology. Philadelphia, JB Lippincott, 1992, pp 42–50.

Goodwin JS, Samet JM, Kay CR, et al. Stage at diagnosis of cancer varies with the age of the patient. J Am Geriatr Soc 34:20–26, 1986.

Greenberg HM, Trotti AM. Radiotherapy of cancer in the older aged person. In Balducci L, Lyman GH, Ershler WB, eds. Geriatric Oncology. Philadelphia, JB Lippincott, 1992, pp 160–168.

Greenlee, PG, Filippa DA, Quimby FW, et al. Lymphomas in dogs: A morphologic, immunologic and clinical study. Cancer 66:480–490, 1990.

Gunn WG. Radiation therapy for the aging patient. Cancer 30:337–347, 1980.

Harman D. Free radical theory of aging: Effect of the amount and degree of unsaturation of dietary fat on the mortality rate. J Gerontol 26:451–457, 1971.

Harvey HJ. Surgery. In Theilen GH, Madewell BR, eds. Veterinary Cancer Medicine. 2nd ed. Philadelphia, JB Lippincott, 1987, pp 121–128.

Helfand SC. Principles and applications of chemotherapy. Vet Clin North Am (Small Anim Pract) 20:986–1014, 1990.

Holmes FF. Clinical evidence for change in tumor aggressiveness with age. In Balducci L, Lyman GH, Ershler WB, eds. Geriatric Oncology. Philadelphia, JB Lippincott, 1992, pp 86–91.

Hrushesky WJM, Shimp W, Kennedy BJ. Lack of age dependent cisplatin nephrotoxicity. Am J Med 76:579–584, 1984.

Jones PA. DNA-methylation and cancer. Cancer Res 46:461–467, 1986.

Joseph RR. Aggressive management of cancer in the elderly. Clin Geriatric Med 4:29–42, 1988.

Kitchell BE. Feline geriatric oncology. Compend Contin Educ Pract Vet 11:1079–1084, 1989.

Kitchell BE. Cancer therapy for geriatric dogs and cats. J Am Anim Hosp Assoc 29:41–48, 1993.

Knapp DW, Richardson RC, Bottoms GD, et al. Phase I trial of piroxicam in 62 dogs bearing naturally occurring tumors. Cancer Chemother Pharmacol 29:214–218, 1992.

Knapp DW, Richardson RC, DeNicola DB, et al. Cisplatin toxicity in cats. J Vet Intern Med 1:29–35, 1987.

Lazarus HM, Vogler WR, Burns CP, et al. High dose cytosine arabinoside and daunorubicin as primary therapy in elderly patients with acute myelogenous leukemia. Cancer 63:1055–1059, 1989.

Lipshitz DA, Goldstein S, Reis R, et al. Cancer in the elderly: Basic science and clinical aspects. Ann Intern Med 102:218–228, 1985.

Lyman GH. Decision analysis: A way of thinking about health care in the elderly. In Balducci L, Lyman GH, Ershler WB, eds. Geriatric Oncology. Philadelphia, JB Lippincott, 1992, pp 8–19.

Makinodan T, Kay MMB. Age influence on the immune system. Adv Immunol 29:287–330, 1980.

Misdorp W. The impact of pathology on the study and treatment of cancer. In Theilen GH, Madewell BR, eds. Veterinary Cancer Medicine. 2nd ed. Philadelphia, JB Lippincott, 1987, pp 53–70.

Moore AS, Cardona A, Shapiro W, et al. Cisplatin (cis-diaminedichloroplatinum) for treatment of transitional cell carcinoma of the urinary bladder or urethra. J Vet Intern Med 4:148–152, 1990.

Mor V, Guadagnoli E, Masterson-Allen S, et al. Lung, breast and colorectal cancer: The relationship between extent of disease and age at diagnosis. J Am Geriatr Soc 36:873–876, 1988.

Mor V, Masterson-Allen S, Goldberg RJ, et al. Relationship between age at diagnosis and treatments received by cancer patients. J Am Geriatr Soc 33:585–589, 1985.

Morrison WB. Diagnosis and treatment of cancer in aged animals. Vet Clin North Am (Small Anim Pract) 19:137–154, 1989.

Ogilvie GK, Obradovich JE, Elmslie RE, et al. Efficacy of

mitoxantrone against various canine neoplasms. J Am Vet Med Assoc 198:1618–1621, 1991.

Ogilvie GK, Vail DM. Nutrition and cancer: Recent developments. Vet Clin North Am [Small Anim Pract] 20:969–986, 1990.

Oppenheimer SB. Theories of the cause of cancer. In Oppenheimer SB, ed. Cancer: A Biological and Clinical Introduction. 2nd ed. Boston, Jones and Bartlett, 1985, pp 28–36.

Owen LN. TNM Classification of Tumors in Domestic Animals. Geneva, Switzerland, World Health Organization, 1980.

Pastan IH, Gottesman MM. Molecular biology of multidrug resistance in human cells. In DeVita VT, Hellman S, Rosenberg SA, eds. Important Advances in Oncology 1988. Philadelphia, JB Lippincott, 1988, pp 3–16.

Phister JE, Jue SG, Cusack BJ. Problems in the use of anticancer drugs in the elderly. Drugs 37:551–565, 1989.

Robie PW. Cancer screening in the elderly. J Am Geriatr Soc 37:888–893, 1989.

Rosenthal RC. Topics in drug therapy: Clinical application of vinca alkaloids. J Am Vet Med Assoc 179:1084–1086, 1981.

Rosenthal RC. Chemotherapy. In Withrow SJ, MacEwen EG, eds. Clinical Veterinary Oncology. Philadelphia, JB Lippincott, 1989, pp 63–87.

Shank W. Clinical use of hematopoietic growth factors in older patients with cancer. In Balducci L, Lyman GH, Ershler WB, eds. Geriatric Oncology. Philadelphia, JB Lippincott, 1992, pp 208–220.

Silverberg E, Lubera JA. Cancer statistics, 1988. Cancer 38:11–23, 1988.

Susaneck SJ. Topics in drug therapy: Doxorubicin therapy in the dog. J Am Vet Med Assoc 182:70–72, 1983.

Theilen GH, Madewell BR. Clinical application of cancer chemotherapy. In Theilen GH, Madewell BR, eds. Veterinary Cancer Medicine. 2nd ed. Philadelphia, JB Lippincott, 1987, pp 183–196.

Tsuda T, Kim YT, Sisking GW, et al. Role of the thymus and T-cells in slow growth of B16 melanomas in old mice. Cancer Res 47:3097, 1987.

Weksler ME, Tsuda, T, Ershler WB, et al. Immune senescence contributes to the slow growth of tumors in elderly subjects. Ann NY Acad Sci 521:177–181, 1988.

Withrow SJ. Surgical oncology. In Withrow SJ, MacEwen EG, eds. Clinical Veterinary Oncology. Philadelphia, JB Lippincott, 1989, pp 58–62.

Appendix: CHEMOTHERAPY PROTOCOLS

PROTOCOL	DRUGS AND DOSAGES
Canine Lymphosarcoma	
VCP-6MP	Vincristine: 0.030 mg/kg IV, days 1 and 8 Cyclophosphamide: 5.0 mg/kg/day PO, days 15 to 21 Prednisone: 2.0 mg/kg/day PO, days 1 to 8; then 1.0 mg/kg/day PO, days 9 to 21 6-Mercaptopurine: 5.0 mg/kg/day PO, days 15 to 21 (Repeat protocol every 30 days.)
Madewell	*Induction of remission* Vincristine: 0.5 mg/m² IV, single dose Cyclophosphamide: 50.0 mg/m² PO, 4 days/week Prednisone: 10.0 mg/m² PO, bid for 7 days, every other day thereafter Maintenance A Cyclophosphamide: 50.0 mg/m² PO, 4 days/week 6-Mercaptopurine: 50.0 mg/m² PO, sid Methotrexate: 2.5 mg/m² PO, bid once a week Maintenance B Prednisone: 10.0 mg/m², bid every other day Cyclophosphamide: 50.0 mg/m², 4 days/week
COAP-L	Cyclophosphamide: 50.0 mg/m² PO, sid, 4 times/week for 8 weeks Vincristine: 0.5 mg/m² IV, once a week for 8 weeks Cytosine arabinoside (A): 100 mg/m² IV, sid, first 4 days of therapy (approx.) Prednisone: 20 mg/m² PO, bid for 7 days; then 10 mg/m², bid every other day for 7 weeks L-Asparaginase: 20,000 IU/m² SC, once on weeks 9 and 10
COAP-L + autologous vaccine	Same as above plus autologous tumor vaccine on weeks 10, 11, 12, 14, and 16.
AMC	Vincristine: 0.025 mg/kg IV, days 1 and 14 L-Asparaginase: 400 IU/kg SC, days 1, 7, 14, and 21 Cyclophosphamide: 10 mg/kg IV, day 7 Methotrexate: 0.8 mg/kg IV, day 21
COP	Cyclophosphamide: 300 mg/m² PO, day 1 Vincristine: 0.75 mg/m² IV, days 1, 8, and 15 Prednisone: 1 mg/kg PO, sid for 22 days, then every other day
Canine Lymphosarcoma Rescue Protocol	
Day 1	Dexamethasone: 0.5 mg/kg SC Dactinomycin: 0.7 mg/m² IV Cytarabine (ara-C): 200 mg/m² IV drip in 0.9% saline solution over 4 hr
Day 8	Dexamethasone: 0.5 mg/kg SC Melphalan: 20 mg/m² PO (Repeat cycle on day 15 and administer continuous consecutive cycles until relapse.)
Feline Lymphosarcoma	
INDUCTION OF REMISSION	
COAP	Cyclophosphamide: 50 mg/m² PO, 4 days/week (or every other day) Vincristine: 0.5 mg/m² IV, once a week Cytosine arabinoside: 100 mg/m²/day IV drip or SC, for 2 days only Prednisone: 40 mg/m² PO, sid for 1 week; then 20 mg/m² PO, every other day (This protocol is used for 6 weeks; at the end of the induction phase, the cat is started on maintenance therapy.)
INTENSIFICATION	L-Asparaginase: 10,000 to 20,000 IU/m² SC (one dose)
MAINTENANCE	
LMP	Chlorambucil: 2 mg/m² PO, every other day; or 20 mg/m² PO, every other week Methotrexate: 2.5 mg/m² PO, two to three times per week Prednisone 20 mg/m² PO, every other day
COAP	Use as under Canine Lymphosarcoma every other week for six treatments, then every third week for an additional six treatments; try to maintain the cat on one treatment every fourth week.
RESCUE	
First relapse	COAP therapy
Second relapse	Doxorubicin: 30 mg/m² IV, once every 3 weeks

Appendix continued on following page

Appendix: CHEMOTHERAPY PROTOCOLS *Continued*

Nonresectable/Metastatic Feline Squamous Cell Carcinoma
Bleomycin: 10 mg/m^2 IV or SC, every day for 3 to 4 days; then every 7 days to maximum dose of 200 mg/m^2. (Pretreat with diphenhydramine 0.5 mg/lb 15 min before drug injection.)

Chronic Granulocytic Leukemia
Busulfan: 3 to 4mg/m^2 PO, daily

Chronic Lymphocytic Leukemia
Chlorambucil: 2 to 4 mg/m^2 PO, every other day
Prednisone: 20 to 40 mg/m^2 PO, every other day, given on nonchlorambucil days

---

Canine Osteosarcoma, Squamous Cell Carcinoma, Transitional Cell Carcinoma, Pulmonary Carcinoma
Cisplatin: 60 to 70 mg/m^2 IV, every 30 days
Administration procedure:
- Secure IV catheter and administer 0.9% saline solution at 8 ml/lb/hr for 4 hr
- Administer butorphanol at 0.4 mg/kg IM, 30 min before cisplatin injection
- Administer cisplatin (1 mg/ml saline solution) IV over 20 min
- Administer 0.9% saline solution at 8 ml/lb/h for additional 2 hr

(Give two treatments following suture removal in osteosarcoma amputees with no pulmonary metastasis and in cases of pulmonary carcinoma, squamous cell carcinoma, and transitional cell carcinoma with lymphatic or blood vessel invasion. If contaminated surgical margins exist, attempt a second surgical procedure; if this is not possible, treat twice with cisplatin.)

Canine and Feline Fibrosarcoma, Mammary Gland Carcinoma, Intestinal Carcinoma, Pulmonary Carcinoma, Canine Thyroid Carcinoma
Doxorubicin: 30mg/m^2 IV, every 3 weeks
Administration procedure:
- Administer diphenhydramine at 0.5 mg/lb IM, 15 min before drug infusion
- Secure IV catheter
- Administer doxorubicin (0.5 mg/ml saline solution) IV over 7 to 10 min

(Give two treatments beginning at suture removal if there is tumor invasion into lymphatics or blood vessels.)

Multiple Myeloma
Melphalan: 2 to 4 mg/m^2 PO, every other day
Prednisone: 20 to 40 mg/m^2 PO, every other day, given on nonmelphalan days.

Nonresectable Mast Cell Tumors
Prednisone: 20 to 40 mg/m^2 PO, every day for 21 days, then every other day

---

Transmissible Venereal Tumor
Vincristine: 0.025 mg/kg IV, every 7 days until tumor not grossly visible

CHAPTER 6

Behavioral Disorders

BARBARA L. CHAPMAN

Behavior problems in geriatric dogs and cats may be the continuation of problems that developed earlier in life or new problems acquired in old age in animals that were previously well behaved. In a review of behavior problems in old dogs (defined as 10 years of age or older), 77 per cent of dogs developed the behavior problem for which they were presented to an animal behaviorist after they were 10 years old (Chapman and Voith, 1990a). Most of the dogs in this study had been owned for many years before behavioral problems began (mean, 8.3 ± 4.0 years; range, 0 to 14 years). In a similar review of behavior problems in old cats, 60 per cent of cats developed the behavior problem for which they were presented to an animal behaviorist after they were 10 years of age (Chapman and Voith, 1987).

Behavior problems develop in older animals for the same reasons as they do in younger animals (e.g., exposure to a fear-eliciting stimulus such as a loud noise) as well as for reasons peculiar to older animals (e.g., deterioration in sensory and motor capabilities). Although the same types of behavior problems develop in older animals as in younger ones, the frequency of the different types of problems varies. Aggressive behavior is by far the most common reason dogs less than 10 years of age are taken to an animal behaviorist (Borchelt and Voith, 1985a), whereas separation anxiety was the most common behavior problem in dogs over 10 years of age (Chapman and Voith, 1990a).

The behavioral history for old dogs and cats must include details of behaviors earlier in life. An owner may report that a behavior problem has only just developed when in fact it has been developing for some time and has only just become serious enough to prompt a visit to the veterinarian. A good example would be dominance aggression in a dog in which an owner may have ignored early signs of the problem, such as the dog's growling when made to get off the bed, and only become concerned when the aggression escalated to the point where someone was bitten. Separation anxiety may also be a long-standing problem. Two of the 13 dogs with this problem in the previously mentioned study began to show signs as early as 5 or 6 years of age. With cats, elimination behavior problems are frequently long-standing, with 50 per cent of the cats in the study mentioned beginning to eliminate in inappropriate locations in the house before they were 10 years of age (Chapman and Voith, 1987).

All animals presented to veterinarians because of behavior problems should receive a thorough physical examination. Veterinarians are ideally placed to reassure clients that their pets with behavior problems are healthy or to accurately assess how a medical problem may be affecting behavior and to manage concurrent medical problems. However, most behavior problems in old dogs and cats are clearly behavioral and not the result of a disease process. In some instances medical problems do exacerbate behavioral problems and can certainly complicate and compromise case management. This is particularly true for elimination behavior problems in dogs and cats, in which degenerative joint disease, urinary tract infection, gastrointestinal disease, and polydipsia/polyuria may be contributing factors.

Techniques for managing behavioral problems in old dogs and cats are similar to those used for younger animals but with some special considerations and constraints. Physical disabilities in old animals, such as blindness, deafness, and degenerative joint disease, may make it very difficult to institute behavior modification or may preclude surgery. Drugs to modify behavior must be chosen carefully and given in appropriate doses with full knowledge of their potential side effects and age-associated changes in drug distribution, metabolism, and excretion (Aucoin, 1989). In healthy geriatric animals, previous learning may interfere with learning new responses to familiar commands or stimuli. Teaching an old dog new responses may require new commands or signals, powerful reinforcers, and persistence and ingenuity. The owner's physical and intellectual capabilities also should be taken into consideration in planning case management; for example, it may not be possible for someone who works 10 hours a day to avoid leaving a dog that suffers with separation anxiety on its own for long periods of time.

DISORDERS OF GERIATRIC DOGS

The most frequent presenting complaints among 26 dogs 10 years of age and older brought to an animal behavior clinic were destructive behavior, elimination behavior problems (i.e., urination or defecation in the house), excessive vocalization, and aggressive behavior toward people (Chapman and Voith, 1990a). The most common causes of destructive behavior were separation anxiety and fear of thunder and loud noises; the most common cause of excessive vocalization was separation anxiety. Causes of inappropriate elimination included separation anxiety, breakdown of house-training, urine marking, fear of thunder and loud noises, and incontinence secondary to neurologic disease. Although only two dogs were presented for aggressive behavior, the behavioral histories revealed two additional dogs who demonstrated significant aggressive behavior toward people. Such behavior was diagnosed as dominance aggression in three of these cases and playful aggression in the remaining case.

Anorexia and inappetence, sleep disturbances and restlessness, and disobedience and failure to learn have also been reported.

Destructive Behavior

The most common cause of destructive behavior in old dogs is separation anxiety (Chapman and Voith, 1990a). In addition to damaging walls, doors, and furnishings by digging, chewing, and scratching, dogs experiencing separation anxiety frequently urinate and defecate in the house and bark, whine, or howl excessively when left alone (Voith and Borchelt, 1985a). The salient features of separation anxiety and other behaviors in which destruction is the presenting complaint have been reviewed by McCrave (1991). Destructive behavior owing to separation anxiety occurs only in the owner's absence, is often directed at exit points, and usually begins shortly after the owner's departure. Separation anxiety may develop in dogs of any age that have never experienced being left alone. It can also occur in dogs that have previously tolerated being left alone when there is a change in the owner's routine, such as returning to work after a long vacation (Borchelt and Voith, 1982a). It can also be precipitated by the death of a family member or another pet to which the dog was attached (Chapman and Voith, 1990a). It can develop secondary to the occurrence of a frightening experience, such as a thunderstorm, when the dog was alone that subsequently generalizes to the dog's being afraid whenever it is left alone. Most cases of separation anxiety in old dogs are new problems of relatively recent onset (Chapman and Voith, 1990a).

Strategies for managing separation anxiety include desensitization and counterconditioning programs, anxiolytic medications, management changes, or a combination of these approaches (Voith and Borchelt, 1985a). Perhaps the simplest approach is to ensure that the dog is never left alone in a situation in which it is likely to experience separation anxiety. Options include taking the dog to work or leaving it with friends or a dog-sitter. In some situations obtaining another pet, not necessarily a dog, may provide the solution. I know of one family that solved the problem of their dog's destructive behavior caused by separation anxiety by purchasing a guinea pig and keeping it safe in a cage where the dog could see it.

Drug therapy alone is unlikely to resolve other than very mild cases of separation anxiety without other concurrent management changes. Drugs that have been shown to be helpful in reducing the signs of separation anxiety in some dogs include amitriptyline (Voith and Borchelt, 1985a), buspirone (Marder, 1991), and the benzodiazepines (Marder, 1991) (Table 6–1). Phenothiazines (e.g., acetylpromazine) are not recommended unless it is necessary to sedate a dog to prevent extreme destruction or self-trauma. Anxiolytic drugs have different mechanisms of action, and individuals will vary in their response. Therefore, if one drug is ineffective in reducing anxiety it may be appropriate to proceed with a clinical trial with another drug of the same or different class.

Amitriptyline (Elavil) is one of a group of tricyclic antidepressant drugs used in human medicine to treat anxiety and depression. In people its antidepressant effects require several weeks of therapy, but when it is used in dogs for separation anxiety, a reduction in barking and anxiety occurs within hours (Voith and Borchelt, 1985a; Marder, 1990b). Potentially troublesome side effects, especially in old dogs, include tachycardia and arrhythmias, hypotension, and anticholinergic effects such as constipation, urinary retention, and dry mouth. It has a greater tendency to cause sedation than many other tricyclic antidepressants, but in canine patients this is an advantage and possibly explains its efficacy and rapid onset of action. The drug is contraindicated in patients with a history of seizures, urinary retention, cardiac disease, or glaucoma. Medication should be started at the low end of the dosage range and continued for at least 2 weeks. The

TABLE 6–1. DRUG DOSAGES AND REPORTED USES IN BEHAVIORAL DISORDERS

DRUG	DOSE	INDICATIONS	REFERENCE
Acetylpromazine	D: 0.5–1.0 mg/kg SQ	Sedation	
Amitriptyline	D: 2.2–4.4 mg/kg PO, once daily	Separation anxiety, sedation	Voith (1989)
	C: 5–10 mg PO, once daily	Urine marking, separation anxiety	Voith (1989)
Bromocriptine	C: 2–4 mg SQ, every 2–4 wk	Urine marking	Seksel (1992)
Buspirone	D: 2.5–10 mg PO, 2–3 times daily	Separation anxiety, noise phobia	Marder (1991)
	C: 2.5–5 mg PO, 2–3 times daily	Anxiety states	Marder (1991)
Clorazepate	D: 5.6–22.5 mg PO, 1–2 times daily	Separation anxiety, noise phobia	Shull-Selcer and Stagg (1991)
Diazepam	D: 0.55–2.2 mg/kg PO, as needed	Separation anxiety, noise phobia	Voith (1989)
	0.2 mg/kg IV, every 12–24 hr	Appetite stimulant	Macy and Ralston (1989)
	C: 1.0–2.0 mg PO, twice daily	Urine marking	Marder (1991)
	0.2 mg/kg IV, every 12–24 hr	Appetite stimulant	Macy and Ralston (1989)
Flurazepam hydrochloride	C: 0.2–0.4 mg/kg PO, every 4–7 days	Appetite stimulant	Lulich and O'Brien (1988)
Medroxyprogesterone acetate	D: 5.0–10.0 mg/kg SQ or IM	Dominance aggression, urine marking	Voith (1989)
	C: 10.0–20.0 mg/kg SQ or IM	Urine marking	Hart (1980)
Megestrol acetate	D: 2.2–4.4 mg/kg PO, once daily for 2 weeks, halve dose every 2 weeks	Dominance aggression, urine marking	Voith (1989)
	C: 2.5–5.0 mg PO, daily for 7 days, then once weekly	Urine marking	Hart (1980)
Oxazepam	C: 2.5 mg PO, every 24 hr	Appetite stimulant	Macy and Ralston (1989)
Prednisolone	D, C: 0.25–0.5 mg/kg PO per day	Appetite stimulant	Macy and Ralston (1989)

C, Cat; D, dog; IM, intramuscular; IV, intravenous; PO, oral; SQ, subcutaneous.

dose may then be increased gradually to the upper end of the dosage range if the response has been inadequate. Withdrawal of medication after the problem has resolved or because the drug is ineffective should be gradual, over a period of 2 to 4 weeks.

Buspirone (BuSpar) is a relatively new anxiolytic agent that is nonsedative and has a very wide safety margin. It can be combined safely with other medications, including other anxiolytics (Gammans et al, 1986), and appears to be a very safe medication for use in elderly patients. It has been helpful in the management of mild cases of separation anxiety in the dog, with antianxiety effects apparent within 2 weeks of commencing medication (Marder, 1991).

Behavioral modification for the treatment of separation anxiety involves getting the dog used to being alone during very short separations that do not produce anxiety and then gradually increasing the duration of the departures (Voith and Borchelt, 1985a).

Fear of loud noises may also result in destructive behavior. However, in this situation the fearful behavior will occur regardless of whether the owner is present and will be related to the occurrence of the fear-eliciting stimulus and not the departure of the owner (McCrave, 1991). Benzodiazepines (e.g., diazepam, clorazepate) appear to be the most useful of the psychoactive drugs used in dogs for reducing the signs of fear of loud noises and thunderstorms (Voith and Borchelt, 1985b; Marder, 1991; Shull-Selcer and Stagg, 1991). Buspirone may be beneficial in the treatment of low-intensity fear responses, and clinical trials with propranolol suggest that it partially attenuates the fear response during simulated thunderstorms (Shull-Selcer and Stagg, 1991). Ideally, in the treatment of noise phobias, the dog should be medicated every time the fear-eliciting noise is encountered and, if possible, beforehand. This may mean continuous medication throughout the thunderstorm season. The long-acting benzodiazepine clorazepate dipotassium (Tranxene-SD) has been used successfully for this purpose (Voith and Borchelt, 1985b; Shull-Selcer and Stagg, 1991). As with separation anxiety, drugs such as acetylpromazine or phenobarbital are probably of benefit only because they sedate the animal to the extent that it cannot injure itself or property, and so they are not generally recommended, especially for chronic administration in old dogs.

Successful behavioral therapy for noise phobias depends largely on being able to realistically reproduce the fear-eliciting sound and circumstances and being able to present these stimuli in a graded manner for effective desensitization and counterconditioning (Shull-Selcer and Stagg, 1991; Voith and Borchelt 1985b). In some old dogs, advancing age and deterioration in hearing may be advantageous in the resolution of noise phobias.

Other less likely causes of destructive behavior in old dogs include digging to make a sleeping or resting place, play behavior, and accidental damage to property through excitement and overactivity.

Elimination Behavior Problems

Loss of house-training was the most common diagnosis for old dogs urinating or defecating in the house (Chapman and Voith, 1990a). In cases in which house-training has broken down, dogs are not incontinent but fail to inhibit normal urination and defecation in inappropriate locations. Elimination is unrelated to the presence or absence of the owner, and large amounts of urine and/or feces may be found in one or more areas of the house. The occurrence of elimination in the house may be related to the length of time since the dog last had an opportunity to urinate or defecate in an appropriate place (Marder, 1990a). In many cases a specific event may precipitate the loss of house-training (e.g., an episode of diarrhea in which the dog is unable to inhibit defecation in the house). Other possible precipitating factors or events include (1) a physical disability that makes it difficult for the dog to get up and go outside quickly enough to avoid eliminating in the house or makes the dog unwilling to go outside and (2) polydipsia, resulting in the need to urinate more frequently. A thorough medical history and physical examination are particularly important for dogs with elimination behavior problems. Age-related degenerative changes in the central nervous system (senility) may cause behavior changes that include loss of house-training (Fenner, 1988; Luttgen, 1990).

A dog that is urinating or defecating in the house because of a breakdown in house-training will assume typical postures for elimination (Voith and Borchelt, 1985c) and tend to confine elimination to certain locations. Relatively large volumes of urine and/or feces may be found. In contrast, an incontinent dog will tend to pass small volumes of excrement in varied locations and without any effort to squat or lift its leg. Distinguishing loss of house-training from incontinence can be difficult, especially if the owner has not observed the dog in the act of urinating or defecating in the house. However, a careful history may distinguish the two; for example, an owner may complain that the dog has lost control of its urinary bladder, but the history reveals that the dog gets up out of its bed at night to urinate near the door rather than wet its bedding while sleeping. Urine marking can also result in the deposition of small volumes of urine in the house, but this is usually in a few regular locations, especially on vertical objects (Voith and Borchelt, 1985c). An otherwise well-house-trained dog can engage in urine marking.

Separation anxiety and fear of thunder and loud noises can also cause some dogs to eliminate in the house when they are distressed. In separation anxiety, elimination occurs only in the absence of the owner and usually within 30 minutes of the owner's departure (McCrave, 1991).

Re-house-training old dogs follows the same principles used in house-training young puppies (Voith and Borchelt, 1985c), but the older dog's physical limitations and health problems should be taken into consideration. Punishment for eliminating in the house is inappropriate in the case of a dog that cannot help itself. In cases in which the dog should be able to control urination and defecation, punishment should be used only if it can be applied at the time of the misdemeanor. In some cases all that might be required is to let the dog outside more frequently or make it easier for it to go outside (e.g., replacing steps with a ramp or installing a dog door). In other cases medical problems will have to be addressed (e.g., pain relief for a dog with degenerative joint disease or management of polydipsia and polyuria). When an owner cannot be present to let a dog out as frequently as required, training the dog to eliminate on papers might be an acceptable option. In some cases rescheduling feeding times and access to water may facilitate elimination at certain times of the day when the owner can be present to let the dog outside or assist it into and out of the house.

Castration is the usual treatment for suppression of urine marking in intact male dogs but may not be the treatment of choice in an older dog. Castration suppressed or significantly reduced the frequency of urine marking in 5 of 10 male dogs between the ages of 2.5 and 7 years at the time of surgery (Hopkins et al, 1976), but its efficacy in older dogs has not been assessed. When castration is not the preferred option in an old male dog that urine marks in the house, treatment with progestins should be considered (Hart, 1979) (see Table 6–1).

Excessive Vocalization

Separation anxiety is a common cause of excessive barking, howling, and whining in old dogs (Chapman and Voith, 1990a). Old dogs may also bark because they are bored, hungry, seeking attention, or reacting to noises and disturbances around them. Behavioral changes associated with senility may include barking and whining for no apparent reason. Failing eyesight, hearing, and cognitive function contribute to social isolation, reduced mobility, and lack of environmental stimulation. One explanation put forward for this disruptive vocalization is that it provides self-stimulation and compensation for low ambient environmental stimulation.

When excessive vocalization is a distress response, such as in separation anxiety or fear of thunderstorms, the cause of the distress must be addressed rather than simply trying to suppress the vocalization. It is inappropriate and cruel to punish a dog that is fearful and may further contribute to anxiety. Punishment is also inappropriate and probably ineffective when excessive vocalization is the result of senility or central nervous system disease. Fortunately, deterioration in hearing with advancing age may result in a reduction in vocalization associated with fear of loud noises or in barking in response to disturbances. Drug therapy, as discussed in the section on destructive behavior, might be helpful in the management of excessive vocalization associated with separation anxiety or fear of noises.

Before attempts are made to suppress excessive vocalization that is not a distress response, a dog's need for social interaction and activity must be taken into consideration. This is especially true for an old dog that might not see and hear very well. It may be difficult to achieve a balance between providing enough attention to meet a dog's social needs and reinforcing problem behavior. Providing more frequent exercise, attention, and tactile stimulation on a regular basis, or as differential reinforcement at times when the dog is quiet, may help reduce excessive barking for attention and obviate the need for punishment.

When a dog barks excessively to get attention, an owner should take care not to inadvertently reinforce the behavior. Insufficiently aversive punishment may be perceived as rewarding for a dog desperate for any kind of interaction. An effective punisher must be consistently applied immediately and only when the barking begins, be sufficiently startling and intense to stop the barking, and not prone to habituation (Borchelt and Voith, 1985b). Instead of having the owner verbally or physically reprimand a dog, remote punishers such as a short, sharp blast from a foghorn or a bark collar are more likely to meet these criteria. Verbal punishment and startling noises will be ineffective with a deaf dog. Another approach might be to punish barking and reward quiet behavior by confining a barking dog in a small room and letting it out only after it stops barking (Houpt and Beaver, 1981). Initially the dog should be rewarded for brief pauses in barking, but the length of time that it is required to be quiet before release can be gradually extended. In situations in which excessive barking occurs in response to disturbances and noises, it may be possible to identify stimuli that trigger barking and remove or avoid them. For example, a dog that barks when someone walks past the front of the house might not bark if it is kept at the back of the house. Houpt and Beaver (1981) describe a case of excessive barking in a Pomeranian dog that abated when the dog became deaf and could no longer hear the doorbell and other stimuli that triggered barking.

Aggressive Behavior

Aggressive behavior toward people is the most common reason dogs are presented to animal behaviorists (Borchelt and Voith, 1985a), but it is a relatively infrequent presenting complaint among old dogs (Chapman and Voith, 1990a). Possible explanations for aggressive behavior as an infrequent presenting complaint in old dogs are that known aggressive dogs are disposed of before they reach old age and that other types of behavior problems such as separation anxiety occur with much greater frequency in old dogs.

Although only a small number of dogs was involved, dominance aggression was the most common cause of aggressive behavior in one study of behavior problems in old dogs (Chapman and Voith, 1990a). Dominance aggression appears to be the most common diagnosis in cases of aggressive behavior toward people, regardless of the age of the dog (Beaver, 1983). In all three dogs in the previously mentioned study, the behavioral history indicated that aggressive behavior had been observed for a number of years in circumstances compatible with dominance (Line and Voith, 1986). Two dogs began to be aggressive at 7 years of age, and the third dog was displaying aggressive behavior when it was acquired at 9 years of age. These findings are consistent with the fact that dominance aggression usually begins to be manifest around 2 to 3 years of age and tends to increase in intensity and frequency with age.

Painful disease processes in old dogs (e.g., degenerative joint disease) are commonly suggested as a cause of aggressive behavior in old dogs. Pain might be expected to increase irritability, resulting in a lower threshold for aggressive behavior when a dog is disturbed, the painful area is manipulated, or the dog anticipates pain. With failing eyesight and hearing, a dog may be more easily startled and might respond aggressively when disturbed. Central nervous system diseases such as brain tumors and cerebrovascular accidents appear to be an uncommon cause of aggressive behavior in old dogs and would be expected to induce other personality and behavior changes such as seizures, depression, visual deficits, and circling.

When a painful disease condition is identified in an old dog that has become aggressive, this should not automatically be assumed to be the cause of the aggressive behavior. Many dogs do not respond aggressively when in pain or discomfort. In those that do, a careful history may reveal that the dog has responded aggressively in other situations unrelated to handling and pain and that the behavior is, in fact, compatible with dominance aggression.

A major component of the management of dominance aggression is teaching the owner to modify interactions with the dog so as not to elicit aggressive behavior (e.g., teaching the dog to come when called rather than physically trying to get it away from a favored resting place). This prevents the owner from being bitten and avoids the dog's learning to anticipate the occurrence of the eliciting stimuli and escalating its aggressive behavior (Borchelt and Voith, 1986a). Depending on the owner's physical skills, ability to correctly interpret signals from the dog that might predict aggression, and need to interact with the dog in certain ways, stimuli that elicit aggression may be reintroduced in a graded manner so that the dog learns to tolerate them without exhibiting aggression. Through counterconditioning, the dog learns to anticipate a reward associated with the interaction rather than feel threatened or challenged. The goal of these procedures is to gradually and permanently achieve dominance on the part of the owner and submission on the part of the dog in circumstances that previously elicited aggression (Voith and Borchelt, 1982). With an older dog that has engaged in aggressive behavior over a long period of time or that has physical problems that would make it difficult for it to perform the required exercises, changes in the dominance relationship may be harder to achieve. In some cases it may be appropriate for the owner not to attempt to reverse the dominance hierarchy, but to permanently change the way he or she interacts with the dog and learn to live around it. When it is not possible to accommodate the dog safely, euthanasia should be considered. Castration is indicated to reduce dominance aggression in sexually intact male dogs but its efficacy in older dogs is not known. Progestins, as an alternative to or in addition to castration, may reduce dominance aggression (Voith and Borchelt, 1982) (see Table 6–1). If pain-induced aggression has been identified, the dog should receive whatever treatment is needed to make it as comfortable as possible and the owners advised how to interact with the dog in a safe manner. Special care should be exercised in a household with small children; for example, child gates can be used to separate children from a dog that is irritable and/or unable to easily move away when approached.

Anorexia and Inappetence

Obvious causes of anorexia or inappetence include disease problems such as renal failure, cardiac cachexia, and dental problems. Anorexia as a consequence of fever conserves energy normally consumed during foraging for the fight against pathogens (Hart, 1991). Many drugs that are used for medical problems in older dogs can suppress appetite (e.g., digoxin, captopril). Central nervous system disease (Houpt, 1991) and senility can result in anorexia or inappetence. Age-associated reductions in taste and smell contributing to decreased enjoyment of food, reduced activity level and metabolic rate, and reductions in the amount of digestive enzyme production and gastrointestinal motility are some of the factors thought to contribute to inappetence in frail elderly people (Holt, 1991). Another potential cause of anorexia in animals is separation anxiety. In this situation food may remain uneaten in the absence of the owner but consumed soon after the owner returns. Anorexia may follow the death of a family member or another pet to which the dog was attached.

A thorough medical evaluation is required for any anorexic pet, even when the history indicates separation anxiety as the problem. Where there is no obvious physical or behavioral cause for the inappetence, the dog should be fed soft, moist, palatable food with increased caloric density. More frequent smaller meals and flavor enhancers such as spices and gravy may encourage greater intake overall. Regular physical exercise and opportunities to eliminate should be provided.

Appetite stimulants may be appropriate in some cases (e.g., diazepam in the case of separation anxiety). Oral diazepam is considered to be much less effective as an appetite stimulant than intravenously administered diazepam. However, increased appetite was noted as a side effect in a dog given oral diazepam to treat a noise phobia (Voith VL, personal communication). Oxazepam, available for oral administration only, has been used in cats and is considered a more potent appetite stimulant than oral diazepam (Macy and Ralston, 1989). Appetite stimulation and weight gain are frequently reported side effects of antidepressant treatment, especially amitriptyline, in people (Bernstein, 1988). The appetite-stimulating properties of glucocorticoids are well known and could be beneficial when there are no contraindications to their use; relatively low doses of prednisolone are recommended for dogs with poor appetite and weight loss (Macy and Ralston, 1989) (see Table 6–1).

Sleep Disturbances and Restlessness

Sleep occupies up to 80 per cent of the day in normal dogs and cats and occurs in many short cycles throughout the day and night with intervening periods of waking activity (Hendricks, 1988). A dog that remains quiet during the night while the rest of the family is in bed is not necessarily sleeping the entire time. Barking, howling, and restlessness in a dog that was previously quiet through the night may signal that the dog needs to eliminate. Many previously well-housetrained dogs become quite distressed when they cannot get outside to eliminate or have eliminated inside because of incontinence. Barking or howling may also be a manifestation of separation anxiety in the case of a dog isolated from the family at night. The dog may have slept quietly away from the family in the past, but some event has precipitated separation anxiety, or the dog may have been made to sleep elsewhere because of the development of a problem such as incontinence. Pain or physical discomfort (e.g., orthopnea associated with congestive heart failure) and senile dementia should also be considered as possible causes of restlessness and changing sleeping patterns. In demented geriatric people, sleep disturbances often co-occur with other abnormal behaviors such as increased activity and vocalization.

If a thorough medical evaluation fails to disclose a cause for restless behavior or sleep disturbances, drug therapy may be considered. Benzodiazepines are the primary choice in people owing to their safety and efficacy (Gillin and Byerley, 1990) and appear to be a logical first choice in dogs. Diazepam, oxazepam, or the longer acting clorazepate could be used. Antidepressants with sedative properties (e.g., amitriptyline) could also be helpful. (The essential amino acid L-tryptophan, a precursor of serotonin, may act as a weak natural hypnotic [Gillin and Byerley, 1990] and has been used in the treatment of nocturnal restlessness and howling in nonhyperthyroid cats [Marder, 1990b]. However, L-tryptophan has caused problems in people and has been taken off the market.) Drugs such as acetylpromazine should be used with caution because of their prolonged action and tendency to cause hypotension.

Excessive sleepiness appears to be a common occurrence in geriatric dogs; owners often comment that their dogs sleep more than they used to. Factors such as decreased alertness, deafness, reduced nocturnal sleep, and degenerative neurologic disorders could contribute to excessive daytime sleepiness in old dogs. In an otherwise healthy dog, excessive sleepiness is rarely considered a significant problem.

Disobedience and Failure to Learn

Dogs with failing eyesight and hearing may appear to become disobedient through failure to perceive signals and commands and because of physical inability or pain that results in a reluctance to respond. However, dogs without physical limitations may appear to begin ignoring their owners or deliberately disobeying them. In one case in which the presenting complaint was disobedience, the cause was determined to be fear of the owner. The dog had begun running away when called because it feared being punished for eliminating in the house (Chapman and Voith, 1990a).

In attempts to train or retrain an older dog, it may be hard to get the dog's attention with commands that have become meaningless through habituation and/or lack of appropriate reinforcement. New, distinct commands or signals, such as a novel sound or word, should be used. Tasks the dog is required to learn should be simple and within the dog's physical capabilities. Deafness and visual deficits may make it difficult for a dog to perceive the usual spoken commands or hand signals, and pain or weakness may make it difficult for the dog to respond. Powerful reinforcers, such as morsels of highly palatable food, will usually work better than petting and praise.

DISORDERS OF GERIATRIC CATS

Among 25 cats 10 years of age or older examined by an animal behaviorist, the most frequent presenting complaints were urination and/or defecation outside the litterbox and urine spraying. Less common complaints were aggression toward other cats, hyperactivity and excessive vocalization, and scratching furniture (Chapman and Voith, 1987). Inappetence and anorexia have also been reported.

Urination and/or Defecation Outside the Litterbox

Elimination in inappropriate locations appears to be the most common reason owners of cats of all ages consult animal behaviorists. At the Animal Behavior Clinic of the Veterinary Hospital University of Pennsylvania (ABC-VHUP) between 1981 and 1986, 209 of 276 consultations (76 per cent) regarding cats concerned elimination outside the litterbox, urine marking, or both (Voith VL, unpublished data). Of the 25 cats in the study previously mentioned, 20 (80 per cent) were presented for elimination outside the litterbox, urine spraying, or both. Eleven of these 20 cats (55 per cent) were urine spraying. Behavioral descriptions and historical information that enable the establishment of diagnoses such as urine marking and spraying and surface and location preferences/aversions have been reviewed (Borchelt and Voith, 1986b).

Elimination behavior problems in old cats may be long-standing problems or of recent onset. In the study by Chapman and Voith (1987), half the cats eliminating outside the litterbox began to do so after they were 10 years of age, including one cat that had recently begun spraying. Thus, elimination behavior problems can begin in cats of any age that were previously well house-trained.

In any case of urination or defecation outside the litterbox, a thorough medical evaluation is indicated. It is not uncommon for an illness such as cystitis or an episode of diarrhea to precipitate elimination outside the litterbox owing to a sense of urgency or avoidance of the litterbox. If the cat then finds that elimination in this alternative location is not aversive and may in fact be preferable to the litterbox, it may continue to urinate or defecate in this location. A cat with polyuria may also begin to avoid the litterbox if, as a result of excessive urination, the litter is too wet. Only three of the older cats presented with elimination behavior problems in the study by Chapman and Voith (1987) had concurrent or historical medical problems that could have precipitated or exacerbated the behavior problem. Problems identified in these cases were intermittent cystitis, renal insufficiency, and neoplasia.

Once elimination outside the litterbox has been initiated, it may continue as a result of the development of surface or location preferences or the persistence of factors that make the litterbox an unappealing site for elimination. Techniques for manipulating surface and location preferences to correct elimination behavior problems have been reviewed (Borchelt and Voith, 1986b). The goal is to make the litterbox the most attractive place in the house to eliminate while at the same time making the inappropriate locations unsuitable. Changes to enhance the attractiveness of the litterbox include making it bigger or getting more litterboxes, using more or less litter, cleaning more frequently, using different types or textures of litter, removing liners or covers, changing the location of the litterbox, and avoiding strong-smelling deodorants and disinfectants. It is not always possible to predict what features will appeal to a cat, and more than one change may be needed before a successful result is achieved. One study has compared cat preferences for different brands of commercially available cat litter and for litter alternatives such as sand and topsoil (Borchelt, 1991). Cats in this study preferred a finely textured clay litter material over coarse clay litter and litter substitutes. Decreasing the attractiveness of inappropriate locations may be achieved by changing the surface, odor, or significance of the locations (e.g., placing heavy plastic covers on carpeted areas, using repellent odors, and using the area for feeding).

Castration is the first line of treatment for intact male cats that urine mark. However, there is no information on its efficacy specifically in old cats. Presumably, many older cats that urine mark have already been desexed, and other methods, such as environmental manipulations and drug therapy, will be needed to suppress urine marking. Environmental manipulations alone, such as making a sprayed area aversive, are unlikely to stop spraying, as the cat may simply shift to new areas to spray. The progestins megestrol acetate and medroxyprogesterone acetate are the drugs most frequently used to suppress urine marking and spraying (see Table 6–1). These drugs are reported to suppress urine marking and spraying in 30 per cent of cases (Hart, 1980). Short-term administration of progestins in healthy mature cats is unlikely to be associated with significant side effects, but chronic administration of megestrol acetate has been reported to induce diabetes mellitus in a 4-year-old cat (Kwochka and Short, 1984) and a 12-year-old cat (Peterson et al, 1981). Other reported side effects of progestins in cats include mammary hyperplasia and neoplasia, pyometra, depression, lethargy, polyphagia, and weight gain (Romatowski, 1989). Significant adrenocortical suppression can occur in as little as 8 days in cats treated with megestrol acetate and may continue to worsen for as long as a week after discontinuation of the drug. Abrupt cessation of treatment with this drug should be avoided (Chastain et al, 1981; Middleton et al, 1987). Progestins should be used with caution to suppress urine marking behaviors in older cats, as treatment often must be prolonged or repeated. Because diabetes mellitus tends to occur more frequently in older cats (Schaer, 1977), it is recommended that the blood glucose concentration be checked in older cats before commencing treatment with progestins and at intervals thereafter.

Diazepam has been used to suppress urine marking and spraying in desexed male and female cats, including many that were previously unresponsive to progestins (Marder, 1991; Cooper and Hart, 1992). Of 23 cats treated with diazepam over a 2-month period, 17 (74 per cent) experienced at least a 75 per cent reduction in the frequency of urine marking. However, most of the cats that responded favorably to diazepam treatment resumed spraying at some time after cessation of treatment (Marder, 1991). After this study was completed it was observed that with continued use of diazepam, some cats appeared to develop tolerance to the drug and resumed spraying while still on medication. In a different study there was no evidence of the development of tolerance in cats treated with diazepam for 6 months to 4 years (Cooper and Hart, 1992). Diazepam appears to be a safe drug for long-term treatment of behavior problems in cats. In a review of eight cats treated with diazepam for an average duration of 19 months (range, 7 to 28 months) the most frequently reported side effects were calmer behavior, increased affection, and increased appetite. Many owners considered these behavior changes desirable even if the urine marking problem was not completely controlled. Weight gain, drowsiness, incoordination, and lethargy were reported less frequently. At the time of follow-up all cats were in good health, with no apparent ill effects of long-term diazepam treatment (Chapman BL, unpublished observations). Side effects such as weakness and incoordination usually resolved within 3 days of commencing treatment. Because cholestasis, icterus, and hepatocellular damage have been reported in people and dogs receiving high doses of clorazepate, regular serum biochemical profiles should be considered in cats on long-term diazepam treatment.

Clinical trials have shown that injectable bromocriptine, a dopaminergic agonist, can suppress urine marking and spraying in cats (Seksel, 1992).

Aggressive Behavior

Among cats of all ages aggression is the second most frequently reported feline behavioral problem (Borchelt and Voith, 1985a; Beaver, 1989). Although aggressive behavior toward people is more likely to result in the offending cat's being presented to an animal behaviorist, aggressive behavior between cats appears to be a much more common occurrence. Of three cases of aggressive behavior in cats 10 years of age or older, all involved intercat aggression (Chapman and Voith, 1987). In the two cases of recent onset, the older cats retaliated against younger playful cats in the household. In the third case the owner was seeking advice on how to introduce a cat with a history of aggressive behavior into a household with other mature cats.

Aggressive behavior in older cats, as for cats of any age, could occur in a number of other circumstances (e.g., territorial aggression, fearful or defensive aggression, or redirected aggression) (Chapman, 1991). Although older cats are less likely to be playfully aggressive, they may display fearful aggressive behavior in response to overly enthusiastic or persistent playful attacks from a younger cat.

The treatment of intercat aggression varies with the cause. Territorial aggression is particularly difficult to manage and unlikely to respond to drug therapy; progestins and diazepam administered to the aggressor are usually ineffective. Other options include finding another home for one of the cats, keeping the cats separate at all times, and using techniques that gradually expose the cats to each other in nonaggressive circumstances until they learn to tolerate each other (Borchelt and Voith, 1982b). When territorial aggression is triggered by the introduction of a new cat, the cats will sometimes learn to tolerate each other without any special interventions over a periods of weeks to months. However, in some cases tolerance never develops. In cases of fear or defensive aggression, habituation to the fear-eliciting stimulus may occur over time but frequently does not. Desensitization and counterconditioning techniques can be used to overcome fear aggression between cats or when a cat is afraid of a particular person. Aggressive behavior redirected to people can be particularly frightening, and successful management will depend largely on identification and avoidance of arousing stimuli or on the owner's ability to recognize and avoid the cat when it is in an aroused state (Chapman and Voith, 1990b).

Irritability, resistance to restraint, and aggressive behavior can occur in association with hyperthyroidism in cats (Meric, 1989). Sudden blindness secondary to retinal detachment in cats with hyperthyroidism can make them very fearful and difficult and dangerous to handle. Medicating such cats must be done with great care to avoid being scratched or bitten.

Hyperactivity and Increased Vocalization

Hyperthyroidism has been reported in cats as young as 4 years of age, but the average age at the time of diagnosis is approximately 13 years (Meric, 1989). Even in the absence of physical abnormalities such as weight loss and thyroid enlargement, hyperthyroidism should always be considered as a potential cause of hyperactive behavior in older cats. Behavioral changes associated with hyperthyroidism in cats include restlessness, nervousness, increased appetite, irritability, and aggressive behavior (Meric, 1989). Diabetes mellitus should also be considered as a potential cause of restlessness and crying for food. Neurologic disease (e.g., cerebral tumors) can induce restlessness in the form of pacing and circling but usually causes other clinical signs such as depression and seizures as well. Yowling has been reported as a manifestation of separation anxiety in cats (Houpt and Beaver, 1981). Although more likely to occur in young cats, hyperactivity, running around, and knocking things over may be exuberant play behavior. Because there are some distinct medical causes of restlessness and excessive vocalization in cats (e.g., hyperthyroidism), drug therapy to suppress these behaviors should not be used until such medical causes have been ruled out (see Table 6–1).

Anorexia and Inappetence

Healthy adult cats exhibit cyclic changes in appetite and body weight (Houpt, 1991). Anorexia and weight loss of several hundred grams in cycles of several months' duration can be normal. Behavioral causes of anorexia in cats include separation anxiety; other fear or anxiety, such as when cats are hospitalized or in boarding kennels; and preferences for novel foods, with refusal to eat the familiar diet. However, if the novel food is less palatable than the familiar diet, the cat may return to the familiar diet after a few days (Houpt, 1991). The lesser palatability of some prescription diets and home-cooked restricted-protein diets is a significant problem in trying to manage specific diseases such as renal failure. Benzodiazepines, especially intravenous diazepam and oral oxazepam, are effective appetite stimulants in cats (Macy and Ralston, 1989). Flurazepam hydrochloride is also reported to be an effective appetite stimulant in cats and has the advantage of a much longer duration of action (Lulich and O'Brien, 1988). Glucocorticoids and progestins may also be effective, but their side effects should be carefully considered before use.

References

Aucoin DP. Drug therapy in the geriatric animal: The effect of aging on drug disposition. Vet Clin North Am [Small Anim Pract] 19:41, 1989.

Beaver B. Clinical classification of canine aggression. Appl Anim Ethol 10:35, 1983.

Beaver B. Feline behavioral problems other than housesoiling. J Am Anim Hosp Assoc 27:465, 1989.

Bernstein JG. Psychotropic drug induced weight gain: Mechanisms and management. Clin Neuropharmacol 11:S194, 1988.

Borchelt PL. Cat elimination behavior problems. Vet Clin North Am [Small Anim Pract] 21:257, 1991.

Borchelt PL, Voith VL. Diagnosis and treatment of separation-related behavior problems in dogs. Vet Clin North Am [Small Anim Pract] 12:265, 1982a.

Borchelt PL, Voith VL. Diagnosis and treatment of aggression problems in cats. Vet Clin North Am [Small Animal Pract] 12:665, 1982b.

Borchelt PL, Voith VL. Aggressive behavior in dogs and cats. Compend Contin Educ Pract Vet 8:42, 1985a.

Borchelt PL, Voith VL. Punishment. Compend Contin Educ Pract Vet 7:780, 1985b.

Borchelt PL, Voith VL. Dominance aggression in dogs. Compend Contin Educ Pract Vet 8:36, 1986a.

Borchelt PL, Voith VL. Elimination behavior problems in cats. Compend Contin Educ Pract Vet 8:197, 1986b.

Chapman BL. Feline aggression. Classification, diagnosis and treatment. Vet Clin North Am [Small Animal Pract] 21:315, 1991.

Chapman BL, Voith VL. Geriatric behavior problems not always related to age. DVM Mag Vet Med 18:32, 1987.

Chapman BL, Voith VL. Behavioral problems in old dogs: 26 cases (1984–1987). J Am Vet Med Assoc 196:944, 1990a.

Chapman BL, Voith VL. Cat aggression redirected to people: 14 cases (1981–1987). J Am Vet Med Assoc 196:947, 1990b.

Chastain CB, Graham CL, Nichols CE. Adrenocortical suppression in cats given megestrol acetate. Am J Vet Res 42:2029, 1981.

Cooper L, Hart BL. Comparison of diazepam with progestin for effectiveness in suppression of urine spraying behavior in cats. J Am Vet Med Assoc 200:797, 1992.

Fenner WR. Neurology of the geriatric patient. Vet Clin North Am [Small Anim Pract] 18:711, 1988.

Gammans RE, Mayol RF, Labudde JA. Metabolism and disposition of buspirone. Am J Med 80(suppl 3B):41, 1986.

Gillin JC, Byerley WF. The diagnosis and management of insomnia. N Engl J Med 322:234, 1990.

Hart BL. Problems with objectionable sociosexual behavior of dogs and cats: Therapeutic use of castration and progestins. Compend Contin Educ Pract Vet 1:461, 1979.

Hart BL. Objectionable urine spraying and urine marking in cats: Evaluation of progestin treatment in gonadectomized males and females. J Am Vet Med Assoc 177:529, 1980.

Hart BL. The behavior of sick animals. Vet Clin North Am [Small Anim Pract] 21:225, 1991.

Hendricks JC. Sleep and respiratory control. Proc Am Coll Vet Intern Med 6:97, 1988.

Holt PS. Anorexia in the elderly. Geriatr Med Today 10:34, 1991.

Hopkins SG, Schubert TA, Hart BL. Castration of adult male dogs: Effects on roaming, aggression, urine marking and mounting. J Am Vet Med Assoc 168:1108, 1976.

Houpt KA. Feeding and drinking behavior problems. Vet Clin North Am [Small Animal Pract] 21:281, 1991.

Houpt KA, Beaver B. Behavioral problems of geriatric dogs and cats. Vet Clin North Am [Small Animal Pract] 11:643, 1981.

Kwochka KW, Short BG. Cutaneous xanthomatosis and diabetes mellitus following long-term therapy with megestrol acetate in a cat. Compend Contin Educ Pract Vet 6:185, 1984.

Line S, Voith VL. Dominance aggression of dogs towards people: Behavior profile and response to treatment. Appl Anim Behav Sci 16:77, 1986.

Lulich JP, O'Brien TD. Feline idiopathic polycystic kidney disease. Compend Contin Educ Pract Vet 10:1029, 1988.

Luttgen PJ. Disease of the nervous system in older dogs. Part 1. Central nervous system. Compend Contin Educ Pract Vet 12:933, 1990.

Macy DW, Ralston SL. Cause and control of decreased appetite. In Kirk RW, ed. Current Veterinary Therapy X. Philadelphia, WB Saunders, 1989, p 18.

Marder AR. Canine elimination problems. Proc Am Coll Vet Intern Med 8:383, 1990a.

Marder AR. Psychotropic drugs and behavioral therapy. Proc Am Coll Vet Intern Med 8:97, 1990b.

Marder AR. Psychotropic drugs and behavioral therapy. Vet Clin North Am [Small Anim Pract] 21:329, 1991.

McCrave EA. Diagnostic criteria for separation anxiety in the dog. Vet Clin North Am [Small Anim Pract] 21:247, 1991.

Meric S. Diagnosis and management of feline hyperthyroidism. Compend Contin Educ Pract Vet 11:1053, 1989.

Middleton DJ, Watson ADJ, Howe CJ, et al. Suppression of cortisol responses in cats during megestrol acetate and prednisolone therapy. Can J Vet Res 51:60, 1987.

Peterson ME, Javanovic L, Petersen CM. Insulin resistant diabetes mellitus associated with elevated growth hormone concentrations following megestrol acetate treatment in a cat. (Abstract) Proc Am Coll Vet Intern Med, p 63, 1981.

Romatowski J. Use of megestrol acetate in cats. J Am Vet Med Assoc 194:700, 1989.

Schaer M. A clinical survey of thirty cats with diabetes mellitus. J Am Anim Hosp Assoc 13:23, 1977.

Seksel K. Feline urine elimination problems—and spraying. Proc Aust Small Anim Vet Assoc, p 49, 1992.

Shull-Selcer EA, Stagg W. Advances in the understanding and treatment of noise phobias. Vet Clin North Am [Small Anim Pract] 21:353, 1991.

Voith VL. Behavioral disorders. In Ettinger SJ, ed. Textbook of Veterinary Internal Medicine. Philadelphia, WB Saunders, 1989, p 227.

Voith VL, Borchelt PL. Diagnosis and treatment of dominance aggression in dogs. Vet Clin North Am [Small Animal Pract] 12:655, 1982.

Voith VL, Borchelt PL. Separation anxiety in dogs. Compend Contin Educ Pract Vet 7:42, 1985a.

Voith VL, Borchelt PL. Fears and phobias in companion animals. Compend Contin Educ Pract Vet 7:209, 1985b.

Voith VL, Borchelt PL. Elimination behavior and related problems in dogs. Compend Contin Educ Pract Vet 7:537, 1985c.

CHAPTER 7

The Respiratory System

JOSEPH TABOADA

Few diseases of the respiratory system, other than neoplasia, are exclusive to geriatric dogs and cats. This chapter will discuss the effects of senescence on respiratory function and the diseases of the respiratory system that may occur in the geriatric dog and cat.

EFFECTS OF AGING ON THE RESPIRATORY SYSTEM

The determinants of static lung volumes are the elastic properties of the lungs and chest wall and the forces that can be generated by the muscles of respiration. With advancing age there is progressive loss of pulmonary elasticity, which results in changes in lung volumes, expiratory flow rates, and arterial blood gas values (Murray, 1986). Chest wall compliance gradually decreases with age (Mittman et al, 1965). Age-related decreases in chest wall compliance, pulmonary compliance, and pulmonary elastic fiber properties are well tolerated. In one study of lung recoil pressure in elderly individuals, decreased recoil was evident only at lung volumes greater than 40 per cent of total lung capacity (TLC) (Kundson et al, 1977). TLC remains virtually constant as aging occurs, but vital capacity decreases by about 25 per cent and residual volume increases by about 50 per cent.

Dynamic properties of airway resistance and respiratory muscle function are also affected by aging. As an animal reaches middle age, forced vital capacity and maximal expiratory flow rates decline (Rea et al, 1982). Smaller airway caliper plays an important role in increased airway resistance. Lower levels of cyclic adenosine monophosphate (cAMP) may contribute to bronchial constriction, whereas decreased mucociliary transport function results in increased quantities of small airway mucus. The amount of smooth muscle in the walls of dog bronchi also decreases with age.

Distribution of ventilation changes with age. Closing capacity (closing volume [the lung volume at which dependent lung zones cease to ventilate] plus residual volume, expressed as a percentage of TLC) increases until dependent airways are not routinely ventilated. This change is more important in bipedal animals such as humans but probably occurs in large, deep-chested quadrupeds as well. Uniformity of ventilation is improved by increasing the depth of respiration and may account for observations of increased respiratory depth in aging patients. Membrane diffusing capacity has also been shown to decrease with advancing age (Georges et al, 1978). These changes in closing capacity, ventilation, and diffusing capacity are important determinants of age-related changes in arterial P_{O_2}.

Senescence results in a gradual reduction of 15 to 20 per cent in arterial P_{O_2} (Murray, 1986). The most important cause would appear to be ventilation-perfusion inequities associated with the age-related changes discussed previously. Despite changes in arterial P_{O_2}, arterial P_{CO_2} and

TABLE 7–1. EFFECTS OF AGING ON THE NORMAL RESPIRATORY SYSTEM

FUNCTION	AGE-RELATED EFFECT	EXPLANATION
Static lung volumes		
Total lung capacity	Unchanged	Caused by changes in chest wall compliance, pulmonary compliance, pulmonary elasticity, and pulmonary fibrosis
Vital capacity	Decreased	
Compliance		
Chest wall compliance	Decreased	Caused by decreased muscle strength, costal and costochondral ossification, and changes in rib conformation
Pulmonary compliance	Decreased	Caused by remodeling of pulmonary elastic fibers and pulmonary fibrosis
Airway resistance	Increased	Caused by decreased airway caliper resulting from bronchoconstriction and increased small airway mucus
Respiratory muscle function	Decreased	Caused by decreases in muscle mass and strength, as well as increases in body fat content
Forced vital capacity	Decreased	
Maximal expiratory flow rate	Decreased	
Distribution of ventilation		
Closing capacity	Increased	Dependent areas of lung are aerated less efficiently, resulting in ventilation-perfusion mismatch
Membrane diffusing capacity	Decreased	Caused by morphologic changes in the alvelolar-capillary membrane and inhomogeneities in ventilation and/or blood flow
Arterial blood gases		
Pa_{O_2}	Decreased	Caused by ventilation-perfusion inequities
Pa_{CO_2}	Unchanged	
pH	Unchanged	
Ventilatory responses to hypoxia and hypercapnia	Decreased	Diminution of both peripheral and central chemoreception and decreased CNS integration appear to be involved
Pulmonary defense mechanisms		
Alveolar macrophage function	Decreased	
Circulating phagocyte function	Unchanged	
Humoral immunity	Decreased	Decreased concentrations of both immunoglobulin G and immunoglobulin M, but mucosal immunity appears to be unaffected by age
Mucosal immunity	Unchanged	
Cell-mediated immunity	Decreased	Helper T-cell function is decreased, and suppressor T-cell function is enhanced

arterial pH remain constant. Ventilatory response to hypoxia and hypercapnia is diminished with age (Kronenberg and Drage, 1973). Attenuation of response of both peripheral and central chemoreceptors and decreased central nervous system integrative functions are probably involved. This aging change results in diminution of an important protective mechanism in those patients that are most likely to be afflicted with chronic pulmonary diseases.

Respiratory muscle mass decreases with age, as does total muscle mass, resulting in decreased respiratory efforts during exercise or hypoxia from respiratory disease. Pulmonary intravascular pressure also progressively increases during exercise in the aged (Ehrsam et al, 1983). This can increase the potential risks of pulmonary hypertension or pulmonary thromboembolism as seen in hyperadrenocorticism, renal amyloidosis, or immune-mediated hemolytic anemia. The consequences of aging on the normal respiratory system are summarized in Table 7–1.

DISEASES OF THE NASAL CAVITY

History and Clinical Findings

Sneezing and nasal discharge are the most common clinical signs associated with nasal cavity disease. Nasal disease can occur in any aged dog and is of particular concern because of the high incidence of nasal or paranasal sinus neoplasia and chronic rhinitis secondary to dental disease (Ogilvie and LaRue, 1992; Manfra Marretta, 1992). When nasal discharge is reported, the veterinarian should question the owner about the color and consistency of the discharge. Any changes in the discharge after treatment should also be noted. The initial character of the discharge or the character after antimicrobial therapy is important to determine, as it probably more accurately reflects the primary underlying disease process than does the discharge present in chronic diseases with secondary bacterial infection. Secondary bacterial infection results in purulent or mucopurulent discharge regardless of the primary underlying cause.

Diagnostic Evaluation of the Nasal Cavity

A complete physical examination should be part of the evaluation of every patient with nasal disease. Complete evaluation of the nasal cavity requires general anesthesia and should include a complete dental examination, radiographs of the nasal cavity, rhinoscopy, and visual examination of the nasopharynx and internal nares. Radiography is an important diagnostic tool in the evaluation of the nasal cavity; however, radiographs are virtually useless if appropriate views are not taken with the dog or cat under general anesthesia. Lateral, open-mouth ventrodorsal, rostrocaudal projection through the frontal sinuses, and dorsoventral (occlusal) projections should be taken (Fig. 7–1). If dental disease is suspected, lateral oblique projections will help diagnose periapical abscessation or destruction of periodontium. Advanced diagnostic imaging techniques, such as computed tomography (CT) and magnetic resonance imaging (MRI), can also be used to evaluate the nasal cavity and are often available on a referral basis (George and Smallwood, 1992; Moore et al, 1991).

Rhinoscopy can be performed using an otoscope, a rigid arthroscope, or a flexible endoscope (Table 7–2) (Ford, 1990). An otoscope will allow visualization of only the rostral 20 per cent of the nasal cavity, whereas an arthroscope or flexible endoscope will allow more complete visualization of the rostral nasal cavity (50 per cent or more) and occasionally of the caudal nasal cavity and nasopharynx. Rhinoscopy is most useful when it affords both visual recognition of lesions and the ability to obtain sample material directly from sites of disease. It is especially useful in differentiating fungal from neoplastic nasal disease. The caudal portion of the nasopharynx should be examined with a dental mirror placed in the pharynx or with an endoscope equipped with tip deflection of greater than or equal to 180 degrees in at least one direction (Fig. 7–2). Tissue samples from the nasal cavity should be collected for fungal culture, cytology, and histopathologic evaluation. Material for culture should be obtained from within the nasal cavity; swabs of the discharge are rarely useful. Bacterial culture of the nasal cavity is rarely of benefit, as the nasal environment is normally a rich source of bacteria. In

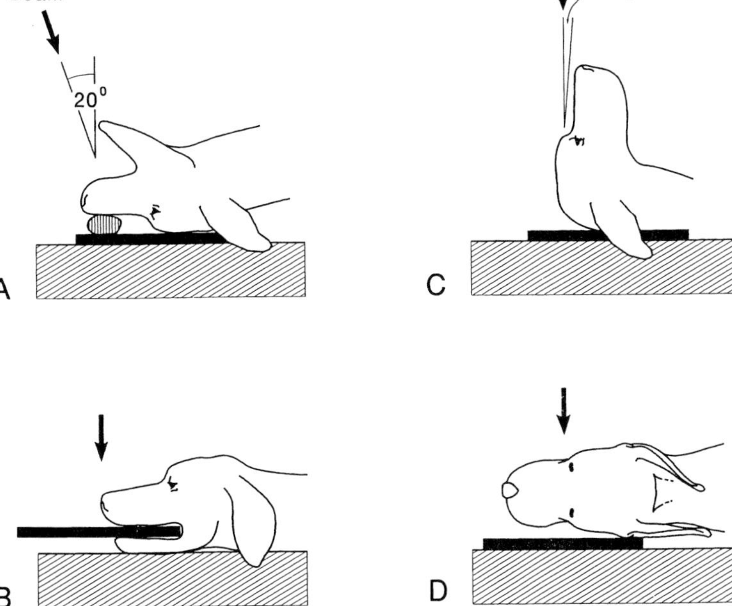

Figure 7–1. Positions for radiographic views of the nasal cavity. *A*, Open-mouth ventrodorsal position. *B*, Occlusal dorsoventral position. *C*, Rostrocaudal skyline position for frontal sinus projection. *D*, Lateral position.

TABLE 7–2. RHINOSCOPIC INSTRUMENTATION ALTERNATIVES

INSTRUMENT	GENERAL ADVANTAGES	LIMITATIONS
Otoscope	Inexpensive tool that can be used for many routine procedures. Multiple tip sizes (2 to 9 mm) allow for flexibility of use in different sizes of dogs and cats. Biopsy and foreign body retrieval are possible through larger sized tips, but are cumbersome.	Visualization is only fair and is limited to the rostral 20 per cent of the nasal cavity, which does not allow visualization of the nasopharynx. The viewing angle is limited by the tip diameter.
Rigid endoscopy (arthroscope)	Good visualization of the rostral 50 per cent or more of the nasal cavity is allowed. The angle of view varies from 5 to 70 degrees with equipment. This may be the easiest system for visualization of the nasal cavity.	Relatively expensive and requires a separate light source and visualization equipment. Through-the-scope biopsy and foreign body retrieval are not possible. Does not allow visualization of the nasopharynx.
Flexible endoscopy (bronchoscope or pediatric gastroscope)	Good visualization of the rostral 50 per cent or more of the nasal cavity and the nasopharynx. The angle of view is generally greater than with other instrumentation alternatives (up to 100 degrees). Through-the-scope biopsy and suction, as well as saline flush, are usually available.	Expensive and requires a separate light source and visualization equipment. Generally, the larger diameter tube limits usefulness in small dogs and cats. Technique is more difficult to learn.

most cases, histopathologic evaluation is critical in the definitive diagnosis of nasal disease (Sullivan, 1987). Methods of obtaining nasal samples for fungal culture, cytology, and histopathology include deep nasal swab, nasal flush, nasal suction biopsy, pinch biopsy, curettage biopsy, and rhinotomy (Figs. 7–3 and 7–4).

Nasal flushing procedures are done with the animal under general anesthesia and with the cuff on the endotracheal tube inflated. The animal should be in lateral recumbency and tilted toward the floor or a sink so that excess fluid or blood flows out of the mouth and nose. Like nasal swabs, nasal flushing procedures are generally noninvasive and tend to be less diagnostic than more aggressive biopsy techniques. Aspiration biopsy (Fig. 7–5) is the best technique for diagnosis of nasal tumors and diseases that result in a large amount of thick exudate (Withrow et al, 1985). The outer casing of a stiff intravenous catheter is connected to a 10- to 12-ml syringe and aggressively inserted into the nasal cavity to the level of the medial canthus of the eye or to the level of radiographically apparent disease. Care must be taken not to extend the casing beyond the medial canthus of the eye. As the plastic casing is inserted, negative pressure is applied to the syringe to aspirate a core of tissue. The tissue is then submitted for culture and histopathologic evaluation. Bleeding is common with this technique but rarely requires more than a few minutes to stop. If bleeding persists, diluted epinephrine (1:100,000) can be flushed over the bleeding area, or roll gauze can be inserted into the nasal cavity. In severe cases a Foley catheter can be inserted into the nasal cavity until the cuff is at the level of the biopsy site; the cuff is then inflated to apply pressure to the bleeding area. I have also had a good success using the pituitary cup forceps technique.

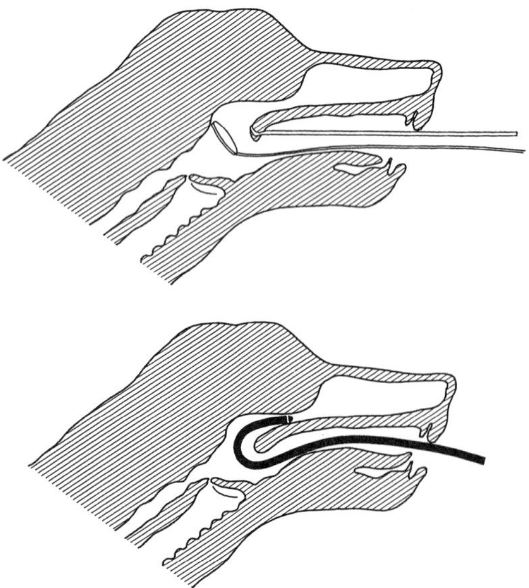

Figure 7–2. A dental mirror *(top)* or a flexible endoscope with a 180-degree tip deflection *(bottom)* can be used to visualize nasal disease in the caudal portion of the nasal cavity.

Nasal cavity exploratory surgery is still occasionally needed for a definitive diagnosis. Indica-

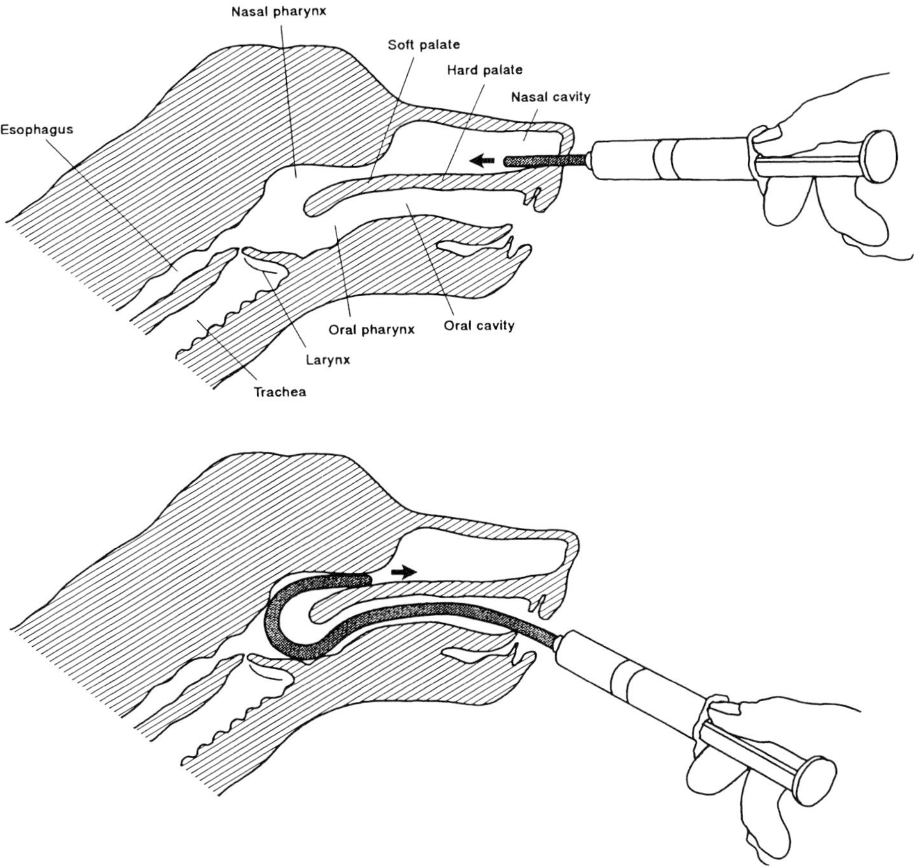

Figure 7–3. Two techniques for nasal flush. Sterile saline is flushed through a catheter into the nasal cavity either from the nares *(top)* or from the nasopharynx *(bottom)*. Diagnostic samples can be collected in gauze at the back of the nasopharynx *(top)*, or the nose can be lowered and samples collected as saline falls from the nares. Samples of mucus, tissue, and other debris can be used for cytologic and histopathologic analysis, and fungal culture. Nasal flushing techniques are generally not as diagnostically effective as biopsy techniques. Note that this procedure should not be performed unless a cuffed endotracheal tube is in place.

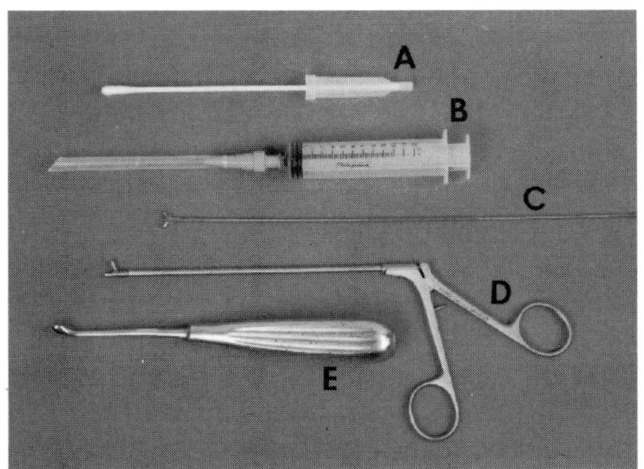

Figure 7–4. Tools for obtaining biopsy and cytology samples from the nasal cavity. *A*, Swab for collecting material for cytologic analysis and culture. *B*, Material for suction biopsy. *C*, Endoscopic biopsy forceps for pinch biopsy. *D*, Pituitary forceps for larger biopsy samples. *E*, Bone curette for largest biopsy samples.

tions include diagnosis of intranasal disease not diagnosed by other means and resection of lesions (Harvey, 1983). Samples should always be obtained from the nasal cavity for both histopathology and fungal culture.

Nasal Diseases

Chronic Rhinitis. Dental disease–induced chronic rhinitis is common in older dogs and cats. It can be caused by periodontal or endodontal disease and by sequelae such as osteomyelitis, bony sequestra, and intranasal tooth migration. Communication between the oral and nasal cavity is referred to as *oronasal fistula*, whereas communication between the oral cavity and the maxillary sinus is referred to as *oroantral fistula*. Oronasal and oroantral fistulas often occur after

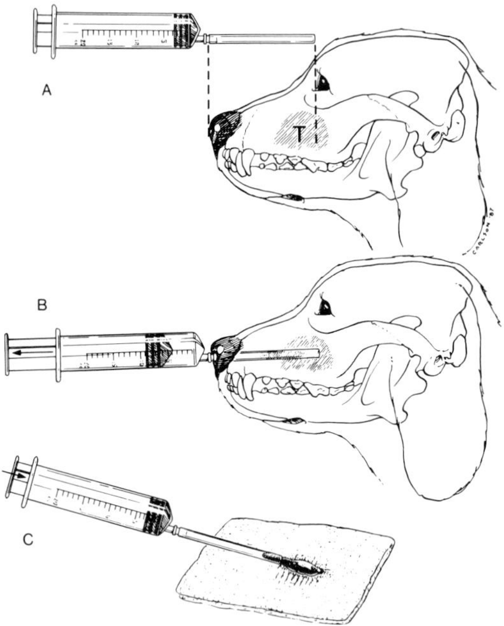

Figure 7–5. Nasal suction biopsy technique. A plastic cannula is connected to a syringe and measured to the medial canthus of the eye *(A)*. The cannula is inserted into the nasal cavity *(B)* through the nares and advanced to the level of the radiographically defined mass while suction is applied to the syringe. The suction is then released, and the cannula is withdrawn. The sample will be in the cannula and can be expressed onto gauze *(C)* or into a formalin container. (From Withrow SJ. Tumors of the respiratory system. In Withrow SJ, MacEwen EG, eds. Clinical Veterinary Oncology. Philadelphia, JB Lippincott, 1989, pp 215–233.)

dental extractions. Extension of periodontal pockets into the nasal cavity or maxillary sinus also may result in oronasal or oroantral fistulas. Therapy for oronasal and oroantral fistulas involves recreating the barrier between the oral and nasal cavities. If periapical tissue is involved or the veterinarian is not skilled in endodontal management, the tooth can be extracted and the oronasal barrier recreated using a mucoperiosteal flap (Ellison et al, 1986; Manfra Marretta, 1988). Tetracycline therapy has been recommended (22 mg/kg PO tid) for 3 weeks after repair to treat infection (Grove, 1990). Alternatively, metronidazole (30 to 60 mg/kg PO sid) or clindamycin (11 mg/kg PO bid) can be used.

Lymphoplasmacytic rhinitis, a steroid-responsive chronic nasal disease, should be considered in the evaluation of a dog with clinical signs of chronic nasal disease. Although not limited to geriatric dogs, the disease should be considered in any middle-aged to older dog that presents with signs of sneezing, upper airway stertor, or nasal discharge. The clinical signs are similar to those of other nasal diseases; sneezing and stertor predominate. Nasal discharge may be serous to mucopurulent. The diagnosis is based on histologic changes characterized by mixed inflammatory cell infiltration of nasal mucosa and submucosa comprising predominantly mature lymphocytes and plasma cells. Because the underlying pathogenesis and cause are unknown, treatment recommendations are usually based on trial-and-error experience. Antimicrobial therapy using ampicillin, chloramphenicol, trimethoprim-sulfamethoxazole combination, or cephalexin are unsuccessful (Burgener et al, 1987). I have had some success using metronidazole (30 to 60 mg/kg PO sid). If the disease does not respond to antibacterials, immunosuppressive therapy should be considered. Immunosuppressive doses of prednisone (2 to 4 mg/kg) should be given initially, followed by a tapering course to the lowest dose that will successfully control the clinical signs. Most dogs will improve, although they may not become completely normal. Other immunosuppressive drugs should be used to treat dogs that cannot tolerate prednisone or in which the disease can be controlled only with high daily doses. Azathioprine (2 mg/kg q 24 hr for 1 week, then 1 to 2 mg/kg q 48 hr), chlorambucil (2 to 4 mg/m^2 q 48 hr), or 6-mercaptopurine (50 mg/m^2 q 24 hr for 1 week, then q 48 hr) can be used.

Fungal Diseases. Fungal diseases of the nasal cavity should also be considered in aged dogs and cats that have signs referable to the nasal cavity (Sharp et al, 1991b). Most pathogenic or opportunistic fungi can infect the nasal cavity, but *Aspergillus* spp., *Penicillium* spp., and *Cryptococcus neoformans* are the most common. Canine aspergillosis and penicilliosis occur most commonly in young to middle-age dogs with dolichocephalic conformation; brachycephalic breeds are rarely affected. Radiographs of the nasal cavity reveal a mixed pattern of osteolysis and increased radiodensity, and rhinoscopic examination may reveal hyperemic nasal mucosa with plaque-like yellow-green to gray-black *Aspergillus* colonies on the mucosal surface (Mortellaro et al, 1989). Positive fungal cultures should be interpreted together with the results of cytology and histopathology, because *Aspergillus* and *Penicillium* are both common contaminants of cultures collected from the nasal cavity. Serologic techniques to detect serum antibodies against *Aspergillus* are widely available. Positive results support active infection, but an incidence of up to 15 per cent false-positive results have been reported (Wolf, 1992). Antibody titers are often negative early in the disease course. Treatment of nasal aspergillosis or penicilliosis may entail systemic or topical therapy. Topical therapy with either enilconazole (10 mg/kg bid for 7 to 10 days) or clotrimazole (1 g in 100 ml polyethylene glycol applied over 1 hour) appears to be most effective (Davidson et al, 1992; Sharp et al, 1993). Systemic therapy using ketoconazole (5 to 10 mg/kg PO bid), itraconazole (5 to 10 mg/kg PO sid), fluconazole (5 to 10 mg/kg PO sid), or thiabendazole (10 mg/kg PO bid) for 6 to 8 weeks appears to be less efficacious (Sharp and Sullivan, 1986; Sharp et al, 1991a; Sharp, 1992).

Cryptococcosis is rhinotropic to the nasal cavity in geriatric cats. Feline leukemia virus (FeLV) antigen and feline immunodeficiency virus (FIV) antibody tests are usually negative in cats with cryptococcosis restricted to the nasal cavity, but cats with disseminated disease may be infected with FIV. Radiographs of the nasal cavity will likely reveal increased soft tissue density early in the course of disease with nasal turbinate and nasal bone destruction occurring later. Definitive diagnosis of cryptococcosis can be made based on cytologic identification of cryptococcal organisms from aspirates or swabs of the nasal cavity. The organisms are 1 to 7 μm in diameter with a non-staining 1- to 30-μm capsule (Wolf, 1992). Detection of cryptococcal capsular polysaccharide antigen in serum and cerebrospinal fluid via a latex cryptococcal antigen test (LCAT) has been shown to be highly sensitive and specific in the diagnosis of cryptococcosis. In addition, antigen titers increase with the severity of the disease, and decline can be used to monitor response to therapy (Medleau et al, 1990b). Treatment with ketoconazole (10 mg/kg sid to bid) and itraconazole (10 mg/kg PO sid) both appear to be effective (Medleau et al, 1990a). Treatment should be continued for 1 month after the remission of clinical signs. Alternatively, the LCAT can be used to monitor response to therapy, and treatment can be discontinued when the test becomes negative.

Neoplasia. Nasal and paranasal neoplasias in the dog are uncommon; however, they are the most common cause of unilateral epistaxis and facial deformity in geriatric dogs (average age of onset, 10 years). Clinical signs of nasal and paranasal tumors are similar to those seen with other chronic nasal diseases (Madewell et al, 1976; Patnaik, 1989). Neurologic signs (seizures, postural reaction deficits, blindness, circling, behavior changes, alterations of consciousness, and contralateral facial hypalgesia) may be the predominant or only sign noted in some dogs (Moore et al, 1991; Smith et al, 1989).

Adenocarcinoma and squamous cell carcinoma are most common, but other carcinomas are occasionally encountered (Ogilvie and LaRue, 1992; Patnaik, 1989). A wide variety of sarcomas are diagnosed; skeletal origin tumors (chondrosarcoma, osteosarcoma) make up about 18 per cent, and soft tissue sarcomas (lymphosarcoma, fibrosarcoma, hemangiosarcoma, fibrous histiocytoma, myosarcoma, nerve sheath tumor, undifferentiated sarcoma) make up about 16 per cent (Patnaik, 1989). Transmissible venereal cell tumor (TVT), neuroendocrine tumors, melanoma, esthesioneuroblastoma, and extramedullary plasmacytoma are seen rarely (Patnaik, 1989). Despite the fact that most nasal tumors are malignant, clinical evidence of metastasis is rare. In one study, 41 per cent of 120 dogs with sinonasal neoplasia diagnosed at necropsy had evidence of distant metastasis (Patnaik, 1989); only 17.6 per cent of soft tissue sinonasal neoplasias (lymphosarcoma, hemangiosarcoma) in a follow-up study had metastasized. Metastasis to local lymph nodes, lung, bone, and brain may occur late in the disease course (Hahn and Matlock, 1990; Patnaik, 1989). Although nasal tumors are slow to metastasize, they are locally very aggressive, making surgical resection largely unrewarding.

Radiographic abnormalities that may be seen in an animal with nasal neoplasia include loss of nasal and fine trabecular turbinate pattern, increased soft tissue density in the nasal cavity and frontal sinus, deviation or destruction of the vomer bone or surrounding nasal and maxillary bones, periosteal new bone formation, and the presence of an external soft tissue mass (Gibbs et al, 1979) (Fig. 7–6). However, it is difficult or impossible to consistently differentiate neoplasia from an inflammatory process solely by radiographic criteria. CT imaging is becoming a widely used tool in the evaluation of nasal cavity disease in many referral institutions. In one study of dogs with malignant tumors and advanced clinical signs of nasal disease, CT imaging was not shown to be more sensitive than conventional radiography for detection of nasal cavity abnormalities. Increased nasal cavity opacity was observed radiographically in all of the dogs in the study (Thrall et al, 1989). However, CT images were more sensitive than radiographs at demonstrating bony lysis and predicting the extent of nasal cavity involvement in early disease (Thrall et al, 1989). MRI is optimal for demonstration of detailed anatomic features of nasal neoplasia and involvement of the nasal cavity and central ner-

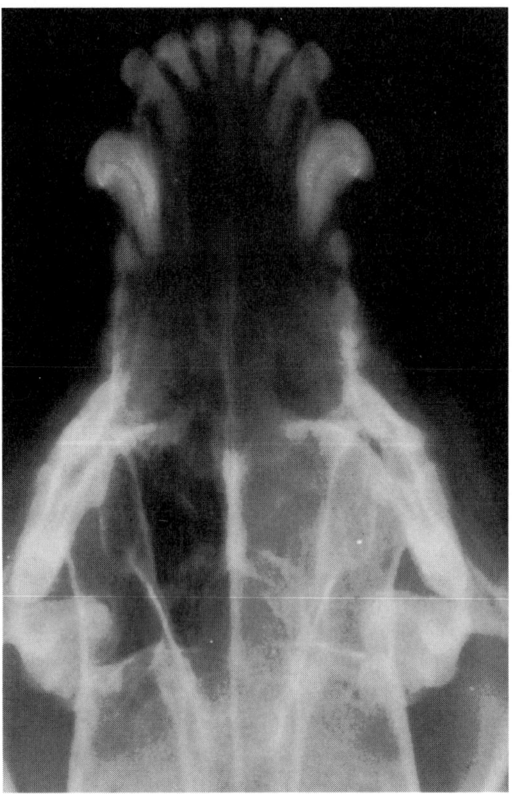

Figure 7–6. Open-mouth ventrodorsal radiograph of the nasal cavity of dog with a nasal adenocarcinoma.

vous system (Moore et al, 1991). Availability of MRI is presently limited to referral practices, and it is generally more expensive than CT.

Reported life expectancies are generally 2 to 5 months without treatment (MacEwen et al, 1977). Chemotherapy, immunotherapy, cryosurgery, and conventional nasal surgery alone do not appear to increase survival times (Ogilvie and LaRue, 1992; MacEwen et al, 1977; Madewell et al, 1976). One study evaluated the response of nasal adenocarcinoma to cisplatin (60 mg/m^2 of body surface, IV, given at 3-week intervals for two to eight doses) in 11 dogs (Hahn et al, 1992). Median survival was only approximately 4 months.

Radiation therapy is the only treatment modality that effectively increases survival times of dogs with nasal tumors (Adams et al, 1987; Evans et al, 1989; McEntee et al, 1991). Orthovoltage x-rays, megavoltage gamma rays produced by a cobalt 60 source, and high-energy x-rays produced by a linear accelerator have all been used to treat nasal tumors. Protocols call for animals to be treated multiple times a week (often on a Monday-Wednesday-Friday schedule) for 3 to 4 weeks.

Orthovoltage radiation is delivered from a therapeutic x-ray machine that delivers low milliampere values (5 to 20 mA) and high kilovolt peak values (150 to 300 kVp). Orthovoltage radiation is absorbed by the bone of the nasal cavity and delivers a high dose of radiation at the level of the overlying skin, resulting in epilation, mucositis, and desquamating dermatitis. Median survival times of 16 to 23 months have been reported when orthovoltage radiation is used in conjunction with aggressive cytoreduction (Evans et al, 1989). The 1- and 2-year survival rates were 54 to 57 per cent and 43 to 48 per cent, respectively. Orthovoltage radiation without surgical cytoreduction resulted in shorter survival times.

Megavoltage radiation is higher energy gamma rays and high-energy x-rays produced by a cobalt 60 source or a linear accelerator. The maximum delivered dose is 5 mm below the skin surface, thereby limiting the mucocutaneous side effects that are prevalent when orthovoltage radiation is used. Ocular complications are the side effects most often reported when megavoltage radiation is used in treatment of nasal tumors. Complications include keratitis, corneal ulceration, keratoconjunctivitis sicca, conjunctivitis, and cataracts (Roberts et al, 1987). Median survival times for dogs treated with megavoltage radiation and no surgical cytoreduction are generally shorter than for orthovoltage radiation after surgical cytoreduction, ranging from 8 to 12.8 months (Adams et al, 1987; McEntee et al, 1991). Longer survival times in McEntee et al's study (1- and 2-year survival rates of 59 and 22 per cent, respectively) were attributed to the use of CT for tumor localization and computer-generated treatment plans.

A third form of radiation therapy that is being used is brachytherapy, which is the local delivery of radiation at the tumor site. It is usually accomplished by implanting radioactive material directly into the tumor bed. The nasal tumor is aggressively removed, and iridium 192 is implanted into the nasal cavity. The iridium implants are left in the nasal cavity for an average time of 4 to 9 days and then removed (Thompson et al, 1992). In the single study reporting the results of iridium 192 nasal implants in dogs with nasal neoplasia, eight dogs were treated. The median survival time was only 3.1 months, but one of the dogs was alive at 587 days (Thompson et al, 1992).

Nasal and paranasal tumors in cats are uncommon compared with such tumors in dogs (Cox et al, 1991; Madewell et al, 1976). Nasal tumors occur more commonly in older male cats (mean age, approximately 9 years) (Cox et al, 1991; Evans and Hendrick, 1989). The clinical signs seen in cats with nasal and paranasal tumors are similar to those seen in dogs; sneezing and nasal discharge are common. Nasal tumors in cats are more likely to cause facial and/or oral deformity and epiphora (Evans and Hendrick, 1989). Systemic evidence of disease (depression, anorexia) is more common in cats than in dogs (Evans and Hendrick, 1989). Diagnosis is based on biopsy results and histopathologic demonstration of tumor type.

Adenocarcinomas (or undifferentiated carcinomas) and lymphosarcoma are the most common feline nasal tumors. Although benign tumors such as chondroma and hemangioma have been reported (Anderson et al, 1989; Cox et al, 1991), most nasal tumors of cats are malignant; distant metastasis is rare. When metastasis occurs, regional lymph nodes are the primary site (Cox et al, 1991). Feline nasal tumors are locally very aggressive and commonly result in facial deformity and bony lysis. Type C retroviral expression has been demonstrated in three olfactory neuroblastomas from cats with FeLV infection (Schrenzel et al, 1990). The diagnostic evaluation of cats suspected of having a nasal tumor is the same as previously mentioned for the dog; however, the smaller nasal cavity makes rhinoscopic evaluation less rewarding. Increased nasal cavity opacity is most commonly seen radiographically, with frontal bone, vomer bone, or palatine lysis occurring less commonly (Cox et al, 1991; Evans and Hendrick, 1989). The veterinarian is more dependent on blind nasal biopsy procedures because of the difficulty encountered with rhinoscopy, although cats have a higher incidence of facial and/or oral lesions, which may make extranasal biopsy sites easy to identify. Care must be taken when interpreting nasal biopsy results, as inflammation is common and biopsies may not include representative areas of neoplasia. Nasal lymphosarcoma may be especially difficult to confirm on nasal biopsy (Evans and Hendrick, 1989).

In general, cats respond well to radiotherapy (Straw et al, 1986). In one study, orthovoltage radiation therapy after rhinotomy resulted in a median survival time of 20.8 months (Evans and Hendrick, 1989). A mean survival time of 19 months was achieved without rhinotomy using high-energy x-ray radiation generated by a linear accelerator (Straw et al, 1986). Localized nasal lymphoma is ideally suited for radiation therapy (Elmslie et al, 1991). With the exception of lymphosarcoma, the use of chemotherapy has not been reported for nasal tumors in cats. An algorithm for approaching the geriatric patient with nasal disease is given in Figure 7–7.

DISEASES OF THE LARYNX

Disease of the larynx is uncommon in the aged patient. When present, it is usually obstructive in nature and most frequently a result of degenerative (idiopathic laryngeal paralysis) or neoplastic causes (Venker-van Haagen, 1992).

History and Clinical Findings

Laryngeal disease is suggested by failure of laryngeal function that results in stridor, inspiratory dyspnea, loss or change of voice, exercise intolerance, or coughing. Stridor is a wheeze or noise that occurs typically during inspiration. In mild disease it may occur only when the animal is exerted or excited and is noticeable only during inspiration. In severe disease it may be heard at rest and during both inspiration and expiration. The wheeze is soft and rasping with mild obstructive disease and becomes loud and high pitched when severe, life-threatening disease is present. Severe, high-pitched stridor is usually accompanied by relentless inspiratory and expiratory dyspnea and cyanosis. In most cases the lungs function normally, and transtracheal or endotracheal intubation results in rapid relief of the dyspnea, stridor, and cyanosis. Hyperthermia may be occasionally noted in animals with significantly increased respiratory efforts or pneumonia. Pneumonia is seen in animals in which poor laryngeal and pharyngeal function has led to tracheal aspiration of foreign material.

Diagnostic Evaluation

The combined signs of inspiratory dyspnea and stridor should lead the veterinarian to suspect laryngeal disease. Diagnostic evaluation includes a thorough physical examination followed by sedation and laryngoscopy. If the patient has severe dyspnea or is rapidly deteriorating, emergency tracheal or transtracheal intubation should precede diagnostic evaluation. If dyspnea is severe but not considered life threatening, sedation may alleviate anxiety and frantic behaviors that tend to traumatize the larynx, contribute to laryngeal swelling, and result in a vicious spiral of dyspnea

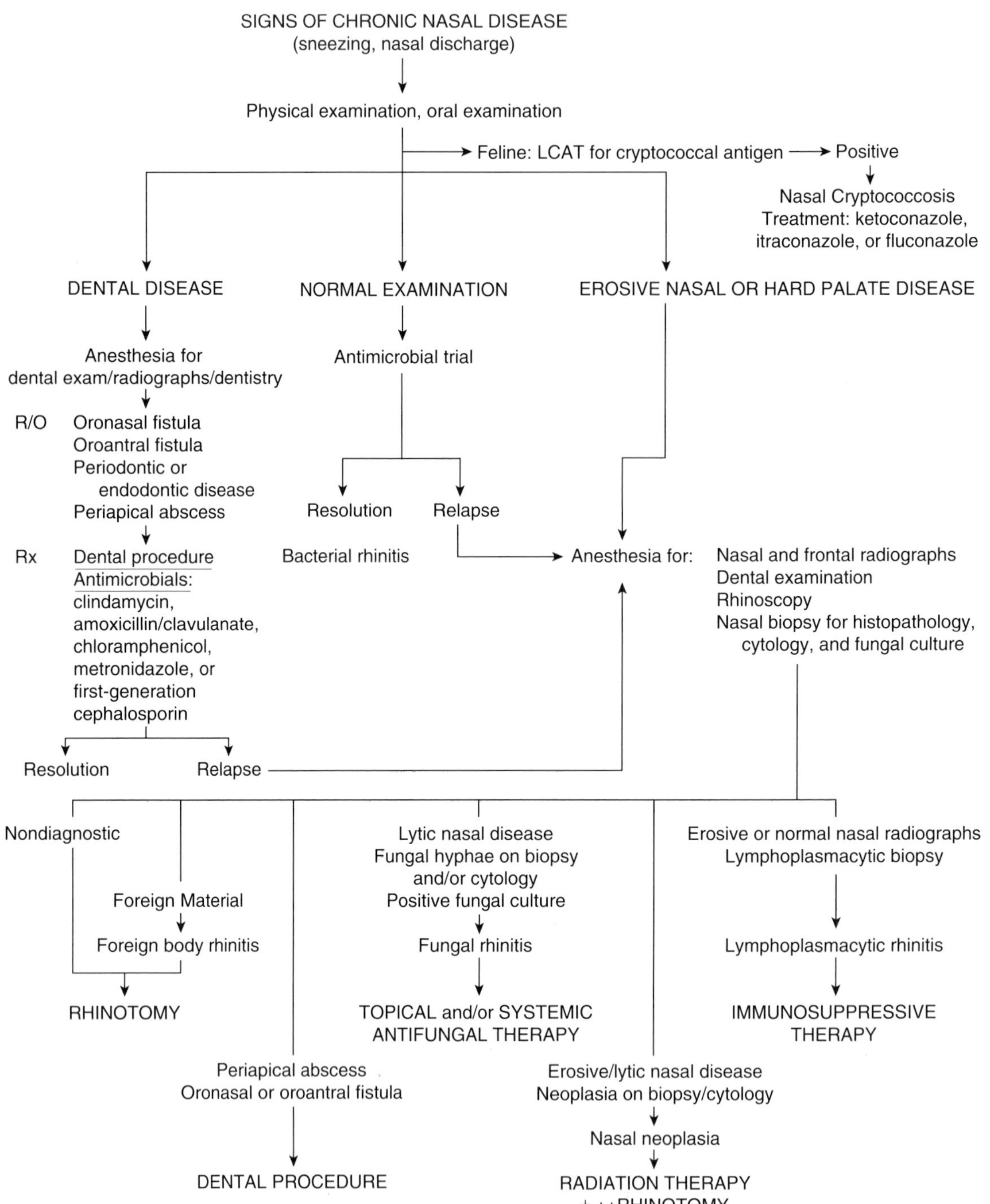

Figure 7–7. Diagnostic algorithm for nasal disease.

and stridor. Neuroleptanalgesic combinations are recommended for this purpose (Aron and Crowe, 1985). Oxygen therapy may be useful early, but once dyspnea and stridor have become life threatening, oxygen therapy alone is rarely of much benefit.

Lateral radiographs of the cervical region may confirm the presence of ossified laryngeal cartilages or laryngeal neoplasia but otherwise are rarely helpful in the diagnosis of laryngeal disease (Wykes, 1983). However, radiography may be useful in ruling out proximal tracheal collapse or intraluminal obstructive disease. Care must be taken when interpreting mild laryngeal distortion or air pockets in and around the laryngeal structures, as even moderate respiratory distress can influence these findings. Thoracic radiographs should be obtained in all animals with laryngeal disease to rule out aspiration pneumonia, metastatic neoplasia, or pulmonary edema secondary to upper airway obstruction. The most important diagnostic test in the evaluation of the larynx is direct inspection via oropharyngeal laryngoscopy. The veterinarian should inspect the glottis for both anatomic and functional abnormalities. The animal must be sedated for satisfactory evaluation, but functional movements are suppressed by cortical or vagal depression. A light plane of anesthesia, therefore, is important for accurate evaluation of glottis function. Dogs may be sedated with oxymorphone or an ultrashort-acting barbiturate without premedication; cats may be sedated with ketamine (Aron and Crowe, 1985). Laryngeal inspection should take place as soon as the animal begins to lose resistance to opening of the mouth. The movement of the arytenoid cartilages and vocal folds should be correlated with respiration. The arytenoid processes and attached vocal folds should symmetrically abduct during inspiration and relax to form a relatively small glottic opening during expiration.

Laryngeal Diseases of the Dog

Laryngeal Paralysis. Laryngeal paralysis occurs most commonly as a slowly progressive disease in middle-age to older dogs (Greenfield, 1987). Laryngeal paralysis may be acquired or congenital (Venker-van Haagen, 1992), but only the acquired form is of concern in the geriatric patient. Acquired laryngeal paralysis may be caused by central or peripheral vagal nerve lesions; recurrent or caudal laryngeal nerve lesions; intrathoracic masses; cervical trauma or masses; laryngeal trauma; previous surgery affecting the recurrent laryngeal nerve; mono- or polyneuropathies affecting the recurrent laryngeal, caudal laryngeal, or vagus nerves; or myopathies affecting the intrinsic laryngeal musculature (Greenfield, 1987).

Idiopathic acquired laryngeal paralysis occurs most commonly in older, large and giant breed, male dogs. The mean age ranged from 7 to 12.2 years (Greenfield, 1987). Labrador and golden retrievers, Afghan hounds, and Irish setters are seen most commonly (Greenfield, 1987).

Respiratory distress and stridor are the most consistent clinical signs of idiopathic laryngeal paralysis. Gagging, coughing, cyanosis, phonation changes, exercise intolerance, and vomiting are also commonly seen. Syncope or collapse may be noted historically. Diagnosis is dependent on visual demonstration of decreased functional integrity of the glottis during inspiration. Most dogs with laryngeal paralysis are affected bilaterally, but unilateral disease is also seen. A complete neurologic examination is important in all animals with laryngeal paralysis, because the paralysis may be the only sign of an underlying polyneuropathy (Braund et al, 1989). Hypothyroidism should be ruled out as a potential cause of laryngeal paralysis (Jaggy, 1990). However, the evidence linking laryngeal paralysis and hypothyroidism is tenuous at best (Duncan, 1991). Thyroid supplementation does not appear to resolve laryngeal paralysis in most cases.

Definitive treatment of laryngeal paralysis is dependent on surgical relief of the glottic obstruction. Initial medical treatment designed to stabilize the dog will depend on the severity of the clinical signs at the time of presentation. The patient in severe respiratory distress will require aggressive emergency therapy, whereas the patient presented with less severe, chronic dyspnea may require minimal initial medical therapy before surgical correction of the airway obstruction. Dogs with severe stridor may require endotracheal intubation or transtracheal intubation via tracheostomy (Taboada et al, 1992).

Surgical widening of the glottic opening is the definitive treatment of canine laryngeal paralysis (Hedlund, 1990; Petersen et al, 1991). Three types of procedures have been advocated: partial laryngectomy (ventriculocordectomy and partial arytenoidectomy) performed either through the mouth or through a ventral laryngotomy incision (Aron and Crowe, 1985; Greenfield, 1987; Petersen et al, 1991; Ross et al, 1991; Wykes, 1983), castellated (step-like) laryngofissure and vocal cord resection (Gourley et al, 1983; Greenfield, 1987), and unilateral or bilateral arytenoid lateralization (Aron and Crowe, 1985; Bedford, 1990; Gilson and Crane, 1990; Greenfield, 1987; White, 1989; Wykes, 1983).

All surgical procedures have been shown to open the glottis and improve airflow. Aspiration pneumonia is the most serious complication during the postoperative period. Partial laryngectomy has been shown to have an exceptionally high incidence of aspiration pneumonia (Ross et al, 1991). Other complications associated with partial laryngectomy include coughing, hemorrhage, hematemesis, failure to effectively alleviate the dyspnea and stridor, and obstructive scar tissue formation (Ross et al, 1991). Because of the high incidence of complications and the greater success reported with arytenoid lateralization, partial laryngectomy is not recommended. Unilateral arytenoid lateralization is a proven technique that consistently provides relief from respiratory distress, improves oxygenation, and has a low complication rate.

During the first 48 hours after laryngeal surgery, the patient should be monitored closely for respiratory dysfunction secondary to laryngeal hemorrhage and/or edema and aspiration pneumonia. If a tracheostomy tube is used, postoperative care should include aseptic aspiration and cleaning of the tube at frequent intervals. To prevent postoperative aspiration pneumonia, food and water should be reintroduced slowly while the patient is closely monitored.

Laryngeal Neoplasia. Laryngeal neoplasia is a rare cause of upper airway dyspnea and stridor in the older dog (Carlisle et al, 1991; Saik et al, 1986). Clinical signs of laryngeal neoplasia are caused by obstruction of the glottic opening. Early clinical signs include voice change, increased respiratory noise, and snoring. Hemoptysis and oral cavity hemorrhage are occasionally seen and are suggestive of a neoplasia. Inspiratory dyspnea, stridor, cyanosis, exercise intolerance, coughing, and gagging also may be noted.

Laryngeal tumors include rhabdomyoma, undifferentiated carcinoma, adenocarcinoma, squamous cell carcinoma, mast cell tumor, osteosarcoma, melanoma, lipoma, chondrosarcoma, leiomyoma, fibrosarcoma, fibropapilloma, myxochondroma, undifferentiated myoblastoma, and oncocytoma (Carlisle et al, 1991; Withrow, 1989). Rhabdomyoma, carcinoma, and squamous cell carcinoma make up almost half of the reported cases (Carlisle et al, 1991). Invasive perilaryngeal or metastatic tumors will occasionally cause upper airway obstruction and dyspnea in older dogs (Withrow, 1989).

Diagnosis of laryngeal neoplasia is dependent on visualization of a laryngeal mass and histologic confirmation of neoplasia. Perilaryngeal tumors such as thyroid carcinoma may cause similar clinical signs but are usually obvious on physical examination (Harari et al, 1986). Partial and total laryngectomy has been reported as a treatment option for small localized tumors (Crowe et al, 1986). Permanent tracheostomy must be maintained after surgery, and hypoparathyroidism is a likely complication (Henderson et al, 1991).

Laryngeal Diseases of the Cat

Laryngeal disease is much less common in older cats than in older dogs. The clinical signs, diagnostic evaluation, and management considerations are very similar, however.

Laryngeal Neoplasia. Laryngeal neoplasia in the cat is rare. Twenty-one laryngeal tumors have been reported (Carlisle et al, 1991; Saik et al, 1986). Carcinomas and lymphosarcoma are most commonly seen. Squamous cell carcinoma, adenocarcinoma, epidermoid carcinoma, and undifferentiated carcinoma have also been reported.

Laryngeal Paralysis. Laryngeal paralysis is rare in the cat, with 13 cases having been reported (Busch et al, 1992; Hardie et al, 1981; White et al, 1986). Of these, six were considered idiopathic, three were congenital, two were thought to be related to a generalized neurologic disorder, and two were secondary to neoplastic involvement of the vagus nerve. Lymphosarcoma was reported to infiltrate the vagal nerve in an 11-year-old cat (Schaer et al, 1979), and a ceruminous gland adenocarcinoma involving the tympanic bulla was reported to cause compression and degeneration of the vagus nerve in a 4-year-old cat (Busch et al, 1992).

Clinical signs of laryngeal paralysis in cats include voice change, change in purr, and inspiratory dyspnea. Cats are usually sensitive to stress and become severely dyspneic during examination or attempted radiography. Diagnosis is dependent on demonstration of laryngeal dysfunction. Failure of arytenoid abduction during inspiration, paradoxical arytenoid movements, and paramedian displacement of the aryepiglottic folds are diagnostic. Care must be taken to differentiate poor laryngeal function from laryngospasm.

Partial laryngectomy (Hardie et al, 1981; White et al, 1986), arytenoid lateralization procedures (White et al, 1986), and castellated laryngofissure with vocal fold resection (Cribb, 1986) have all been reported in the cat. Successful alleviation of dyspnea has been reported with all three surgical procedures. Iatrogenic trauma to the recurrent laryngeal nerves, a potential postoperative complication in the surgical management of hyperthyroidism, may result in laryngeal paralysis (Birchard and Bradley, 1989). Voice change without severe dyspnea is noted most commonly, but complete bilateral paralysis has resulted in severe stridor and death in a few cats (Meric, 1991). The paralysis is usually temporary.

DISEASES OF THE TRACHEA

Tracheal disease is common in the geriatric dog but uncommon in the geriatric cat. Cough, the most common sign noted, is usually nonproductive and resembles a goose honk. Dyspnea may be seen if severe tracheal obstructive disease is present. The dyspnea is most pronounced on inspiration if the disease is affecting primarily the proximal trachea but may be most pronounced on expiration if the distal trachea is more severely involved.

Diagnostic Evaluation

A complete physical examination is warranted to identify abnormalities that may be concurrently or secondarily affecting the trachea. Thoracic and soft tissue cervical radiographs are indicated. Extraluminal compression, tracheal stenosis, intraluminal masses, and tracheal collapse may be apparent radiographically. Expiratory and inspiratory radiographs are useful when evaluating the trachea for dynamic compression, as may occur in tracheal collapse. Other dynamic airway studies include fluoroscopy and tracheoscopy. Tracheoscopy is useful in the evaluation of the trachea when obstructive or mucosal disease is suspected. A flexible pediatric bronchoscope (3.5 to 5 mm diameter) or a rigid arthroscope can be used to visualize the tracheal lumen (Fig. 7–8).

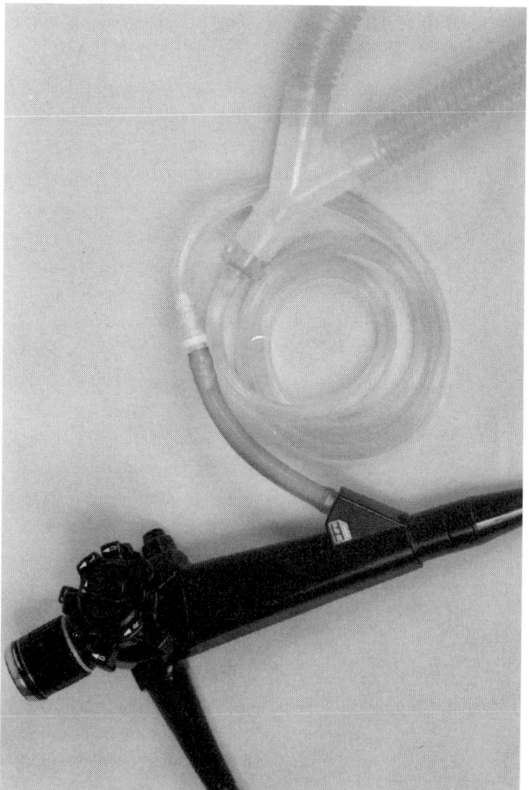

Figure 7–8. Attachment of oxygen line to the biopsy channel of the bronchoscope.

Tracheal Diseases of the Dog

Tracheal Collapse. Tracheal collapse is the most common disease affecting the trachea in the geriatric dog, especially toy and miniature breeds (Hawkins, 1992; Padrid and Amis, 1992); pomeranians, miniature and toy poodles, Yorkshire terriers, and chihuahuas are affected most often (Nelson, 1985). Although the disease is seen in dogs of all ages, the average age at diagnosis is 7.5 years (Hedlund, 1987; Padrid and Amis, 1992). The cause of tracheal collapse is not known. Dorsoventral flattening is typically seen, with the ratio of tracheal width to tracheal height significantly increased when compared with that in normal dogs (Done and Drew, 1976). Lateral collapse is rarely noted.

Diagnosis of tracheal collapse is usually based on the signalment, case history, and exclusion of other causes of dyspnea and cough. Some authors consider fluoroscopy the diagnostic test of choice (Padrid and Amis, 1992), but I believe definitive diagnosis is best made by tracheoscopy. Both medical and surgical treatment have been advocated for the management of tracheal collapse (Hedlund, 1987; Padrid and Amis, 1992). Most dogs can be managed medically, especially during the initial stages. The goals of medical therapy include weight reduction, avoiding stress and pressure on the trachea, minimizing inflammation of the tracheal mucosa, controlling cough, and treating concurrent or secondary conditions. Surgical treatment should be considered for dogs that no longer respond to medical management. Methods of surgical repair include dorsal tracheal membrane plication, the use of internal stents, tracheal ring transection, and external support with spiral or ring-shaped prostheses (Fingland et al, 1987; Hedlund, 1987; Nelson, 1985) (Fig. 7–9). Surgery can be expected to lessen the dog's clinical signs but rarely eliminates them completely.

Tracheal Neoplasia. Tracheal neoplasia is extremely rare in the geriatric dog. Osteochondroma, mast cell tumor, leiomyoma, chondro-

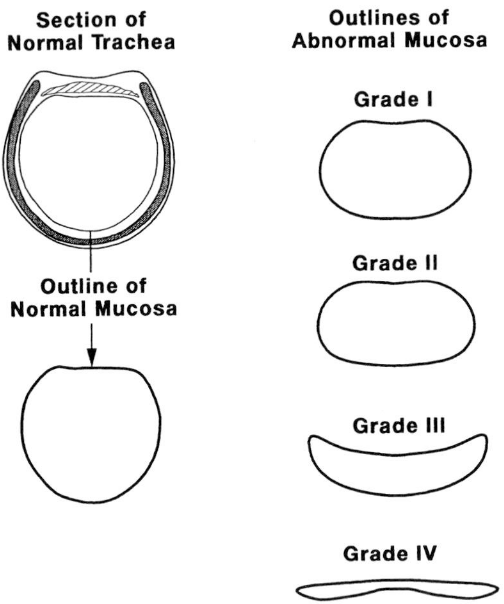

Figure 7–9. Classification of collapsed trachea by grade. Grade I: The tracheal lumen is reduced by approximately 25 per cent. The tracheal membrane (trachealis muscle) protrudes slightly into the lumen, but the tracheal cartilage maintains a normal C shape. Grade II: The tracheal lumen is reduced by approximately 50 per cent. The tracheal membrane is widened and pendulous, and the tracheal cartilages are partially flattened. Grade III: The tracheal lumen is reduced by approximately 75 per cent. The tracheal membrane almost contacts the ventral surface of the trachea, and the tracheal cartilages are nearly flat. Grade IV: The tracheal lumen is nearly obliterated. The tracheal membrane contacts the ventral surface of the trachea, and the tracheal cartilages are flattened and may invert dorsally.

sarcoma, adenocarcinoma, osteosarcoma, chondroma, and undifferentiated carcinoma have all been reported (Carlisle et al, 1991). The median age at diagnosis is 8.6 years (Carlisle et al, 1991). Clinical signs are related to tracheal obstruction and include dyspnea, wheezing, stridor, coughing, and cyanosis. Surgical treatment can be attempted.

Tracheal Diseases of the Cat

Tracheal disease in the geriatric cat is rare. Clinical signs are similar to those seen in the dog, although cough is a less consistent sign, and respiratory distress and stridor are seen more commonly.

Tracheal Neoplasia. Tracheal neoplasia is extremely rare in the cat and includes lymphosarcoma, adenocarcinoma, undifferentiated carcinoma, squamous cell carcinoma, and seromucinous carcinoma. The median age at diagnosis is 8 years. Tracheal tumors are distinct intraluminal masses radiographically, but annular thickening may occur. Surgery should be considered for small locally contained tumors.

Tracheal Collapse. Tracheal collapse is extremely rare (Hendricks and O'Brien, 1985). Cats present for chronic signs of dyspnea and inspiratory stridor. A cranial cervical obstructive lesion may be noted.

DISEASES OF THE SMALL AIRWAYS AND LUNGS

Geriatric dogs and cats with lower airway disease usually present for coughing and/or dyspnea. Various degrees of both cough and dyspnea are typically seen.

History and Clinical Findings

Geriatric animals with disease affecting the small airways and lung parenchyma represent a diagnostic and therapeutic challenge to the veterinarian and pet owner. These animals tolerate stress poorly. Dogs and cats with bronchial disease will typically have cough as a component of the history. Cats are less likely to be presented for cough and more commonly show increased respiratory efforts when afflicted with chronic lower airway disease. Typically, dyspnea caused by lower airway disease will be most pronounced on expiration but may also be noted during inspiration.

Both respiratory and cardiac disease should be considered when evaluating the geriatric animal presented for cough and/or respiratory distress. A cardiac murmur or a rhythm abnormality might be noted with cardiac disease, whereas pulmonary diseases usually cause abnormal lung sounds. Geriatric animals evaluated for lower airway disease may include thoracic radiography; bronchoscopy; cytology and culture (bacterial and fungal) of samples obtained by tracheal wash, bronchoalveolar lavage, or transthoracic aspiration; and histopathology of lung biopsy. Arterial blood gas analysis may be useful for diagnosis as well as to predict severity of disease and monitor response to therapy. A heartworm test, fecal examination, and fungal or protozoal serology tests may be indicated.

Thoracic radiography is integral to the diagnostic evaluation of most older animals with lower airway disease. Radiographs are helpful in localizing and determining extent of disease, prioritizing differential diagnosis lists, and monitoring disease progression. Two views should always be taken (usually a lateral view and a ventrodorsal or dorsoventral view). The radiographic appearance of the lungs should be viewed for alveolar, interstitial, peribronchial, or vascular abnormalities (Table 7–3). Disseminated or diffuse interstitial pulmonary patterns are common in older dogs (Reif and Rhodes, 1966). Calcification of small airways and small fissure lines between lung lobes are frequently seen.

Bronchoscopy is useful for evaluation of major airway diseases, allowing visual assessment of airway inflammation, structural abnormalities, and pulmonary hemorrhage, and is a valuable means of specimen collection for cytology and culture (see Fig. 7–8). The bronchial mucosa of older dogs and cats with chronic airway disease appears erythematous, with excessive mucus secretions that may plug or span the lumen of the airways (Ford, 1990; Padrid, 1992). The mucosa may appear thickened and have an irregular contour, with mucosal vessels appearing hyperemic. Dogs with chronic airway disease often will have collapse of the dorsal tracheal membrane into the tracheal lumen or collapse of intrathoracic airways during passive expiration. Cats with chronic airway disease will have collapse of the airways less commonly.

Bronchoalveolar lavage is useful for obtaining samples from the small airways, terminal bronchioles, and alveoli for cytology and culture (Hawkins et al, 1990; Padrid et al, 1991). It can be performed during bronchoscopy or via endotracheal intubation. Tracheobronchial lavage from the larger airways can be performed in a like manner. Bronchoalveolar lavage samples are collected by instilling sterile 0.9 per cent saline solution (25-ml aliquots in dogs or 10-ml aliquots in cats) through a bronchoscope that has been lodged snugly into a bronchus, then immediately retrieving the solution via gentle suction. In general, total nucleated cell counts from bronchoalveolar lavage solutions are fewer than 500/μl in healthy animals. The predominant cell type is the macrophage, with inflammatory cells occurring less frequently. Lymphocytes, neutrophils, and eosinophils should each make up less than 5 to 10 per cent of the total cell count in dogs (Hawk-

TABLE 7–3. DIFFERENTIAL DIAGNOSIS OF RADIOGRAPHIC ABNORMALITIES IN THE GERIATRIC DOG AND CAT

Abnormal Vascular Pattern
- Enlarged arteries
  - Heartworm disease*
  - Thromboembolic disease*
  - Pulmonary hypertension
- Enlarged veins
  - Left heart failure*
- Small arteries and veins
  - Hyperinflation of the lungs
    - Allergic bronchitis*
    - Feline asthma†
    - Chronic bronchitis*
    - Pulmonary emphysema
  - Hypovolemia
    - Shock*†
    - Dehydration*†
    - Hypoadrenocorticism*†

Nodular Interstitial Pattern
- Neoplasia
  - Metastatic*
- Inflammatory
  - Pulmonary infiltrates with eosinophils
  - Lymphomatoid granulomatosis
  - Idiopathic granulomatous pneumonia
  - Fungal pneumonia
  - Parasitic pneumonia

Peribronchial Pattern
- Allergic bronchitis*
- Chronic bronchitis*
- Feline asthma†
- Bronchiectasis
- Chronic bacterial bronchitis
- Respiratory parasites

Mixed Interstitial/Alveolar Pattern
- Neoplasia
  - Metastatic carcinoma
  - Lymphosarcoma
- Inflammatory disease
  - Infection
    - Bacterial pneumonia*†
    - Protozoal pneumonia
    - Fungal pneumonia
    - Parasitic pneumonia
  - Aspiration pneumonia*†
  - Pulmonary infiltrates with eosinophils
  - Lymphomatoid granulomatosis
- Pulmonary edema
  - Cardiogenic edema*
  - Neurogenic edema
  - Upper airway obstructive edema
  - Lymphatic obstruction
- Pulmonary hemorrhage
  - Thromboembolic disease*
  - Neoplasia
  - Systemic clotting disorders
  - Pulmonary contusions

*Common in the geriatric dog.
†Common in the geriatric cat.

ins et al, 1990). Up to 25 per cent eosinophils may be normal in cats (Padrid et al, 1991).

Tracheobronchial lavage samples can be collected with a through-the-needle jugular catheter via a transtracheal approach or with a No. 3.5 French male urinary catheter passed down the lumen of an endotracheal tube. When a transtracheal approach is used, the needle of the jugular catheter is placed into the tracheal lumen through the cricothyroid ligament (in small or medium dogs) or between tracheal rings (in large dogs). The catheter is then passed to the level of the carina (fourth intercostal space), and 3 to 10 ml of sterile 0.9 per cent saline solution is infused into the tracheal lumen, causing the animal to cough. Gentle suction is used to retrieve a sample of the solution. In small dogs or cats, it is best to intubate the animal, then pass a urinary catheter through the sterile endotracheal tube and instill saline solution, as noted earlier for the transtracheal approach. Tracheal wash fluid from healthy dogs and cats will contain primarily respiratory epithelial cells and a few macrophages; inflammatory cells are noted in diseases.

Cytologic and bacterial/fungal culture samples can be obtained by direct transthoracic aspiration of pulmonary tissue. The procedure is indicated in the evaluation of pulmonary or pleural mass lesions or in cases of diffuse pulmonary disease in which tracheobronchial and bronchoalveolar lavage have failed to yield a diagnosis. Lung aspiration can be performed with a 22-gauge needle and a 10- to 12-ml syringe. The needle should be inserted into the lung in the area of suspected disease. Spinal needles are useful if added length is required to reach the desired location. Multiple needle passes into the area of suspected disease should be attempted to maximize the procedure's diagnostic yield. The animal should be manually restrained for transthoracic aspiration. Sedation is necessary in some animals, but general anesthesia is not recommended, because potential hemorrhage created by the procedure is not cleared as readily from the lungs (Hawkins, 1992).

Lower Airway Diseases of the Dog

Chronic Bronchial Disease. Chronic bronchial disease is a complex, progressive inflammatory disease of uncertain cause that involves the small airways. It is characterized by excessive secretion of mucus in the bronchial tree and frequent coughing, persisting for at least 2 months. Most dogs with chronic bronchial disease are older than 8 years (Padrid and Amis, 1992). Small and toy breeds, such as poodles, Shetland sheepdogs, Pomeranians, Pekingese, chihuahuas, and Yorkshire terriers, are affected most often (Padrid and Amis, 1992). Cough and abnormal lung sounds are the most likely abnormalities noted on physical examination. Inspiratory and expiratory crackles are heard most commonly.

Diagnosis of chronic bronchitis is dependent on a history of chronic cough and on ruling out other causes of a chronic cough (Table 7–4). The most helpful diagnostic tests include thoracic radiographs and tracheal or bronchial lavage for cytology tests and bacterial or fungal culture. Thoracic radiographs of most dogs with chronic bronchitis reveal a prominent bronchointerstitial pattern; on radiographs thickened bronchial structures have an end-on or parallel orientation characterized as a "doughnut" or "tram line" pattern, respectively. Bronchiectasis may be seen (Fig. 7–10) (Brownlie, 1990; Padrid et al, 1990). Excessive mucus with neutrophils and smaller numbers of lymphocytes and eosinophils will characterize tracheal and bronchoalveolar lavage samples. Aerobic bacterial culture should be performed on all lavage samples. Positive cultures should alert the veterinarian to the possibility of bacterial infection, but it must be remembered that neither the lower airway nor the lung parenchyma of healthy dogs is sterile (Lindsey and Pierce, 1978; McKiernan et al, 1984).

Bronchoscopic studies generally reveal a roughened airway surface, with loss of the glis-

TABLE 7–4. DIFFERENTIAL DIAGNOSIS FOR THE GERIATRIC DOG PRESENTED FOR CHRONIC (2 MONTHS' DURATION) COUGH

Common Differential Diagnoses
Heartworm disease
Chronic bronchial disease
Tracheal or mainstem bronchial collapse
Left-sided heart failure (chronic mitral valve insufficiency)
Uncommon Differential Diagnoses
Infectious bronchopneumonia (especially *Bordetella*)
Allergic or eosinophilic bronchitis
Bronchiectasis
Rare Differential Diagnosis
Bronchial foreign body
Parasitic bronchitis
Fungal pneumonia
Bronchopulmonary neoplasia
Eosinophilic or lymphomatoid granulomatosis
Pulmonary thromboembolism
Drug-induced cough (captopril)

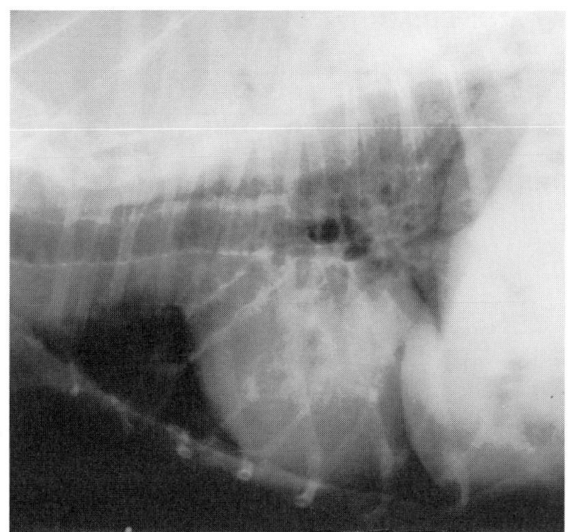

Figure 7–10. Lateral thoracic radiograph of a dog with bronchiectasis secondary to chronic bronchial disease.

tening character of the normal airway mucosa, and excessive mucus secretions. The mucosa is often thickened and granular. Hyperemia of mucosal vessels is noted in most cases. Partial collapse of the mainstem or segmental bronchi may be noted during expiration and is generally considered a poor prognostic finding (Padrid et al, 1990).

EOSINOPHILIC BRONCHITIS. Eosinophilic bronchitis is a pulmonary disease of potential allergic origin (Taboada, 1991); its cause is usually unknown. The clinical signs, radiographic findings, and gross bronchoscopic findings can be identical to those seen in dog with chronic bronchitis, but the age at onset is generally younger. Tracheal or bronchoalveolar lavage reveals excessive mucus and eosinophilic inflammation. Eosinophilia may be noted (Brownlie, 1990).

TREATMENT. Treatment of chronic bronchitis and eosinophilic bronchitis is similar. Symptomatic management for bronchoconstriction and cough and specific management of inflammation are important (Table 7–5). If bacteria are cultured from lavage samples, antimicrobial treatment should be based on appropriate sensitivity tests. Chloramphenicol, tetracycline, enrofloxacin, and amoxicillin-clavulanate are appropriate antimicrobial agents if *Bordetella* infection is suspected. Bronchodilators are used in the long-term management of dogs with chronic bronchial disease. Methylxanthines (salts of theophylline) may improve bronchial relaxation and contractility of fatigued diaphragm muscle (Howell and Roussos, 1984; McKiernan et al, 1981). Theophylline (11 mg/kg orally bid to tid) should be used in dogs with exercise intolerance. Beta$_2$-adrenoceptor agonists such as albuterol and terbutaline will cause excellent bronchial smooth muscle relaxation. They are appropriate for use in dogs, because airway smooth muscle in dogs is primarily innervated only by the beta$_2$ subclass of adrenoceptors. Albuterol is used at a dosage of 0.02 to 0.04 mg/kg orally bid to tid. Tremors and hyperactivity are dose-related side effects of the drug.

Cough suppression is indicated in some dogs with chronic bronchial disease, but judicious use of antitussive medication is recommended. Butorphanol (0.05 to 0.1 mg/kg orally bid to tid) and hydrocodone bitartrate (0.22 mg/kg orally bid to qid) are the most effective cough suppressants to use in the dog. The most effective drugs in ameliorating the signs of chronic bronchial disease are glucocorticoids. Before glucocorticoids are administered, however, airway infection should be ruled out. Prednisone is used at a dose of 1 mg/kg orally bid and tapered to the lowest effective alternate-day dose.

Granulomatosis. Eosinophilic or lymphomatoid granulomatosis is a progressive condition of unknown cause that occurs in middle-age and older dogs. The disease is usually slowly progressive, with cough, dyspnea, anorexia, and weight loss (Berry et al, 1990; Calvert et al, 1988; Fitzgerald et al, 1991). Lymphomatoid granulomatosis is difficult to diagnose. Radiographically the disease is characterized by a diffuse interstitial and/or alveolar pattern with indistinct nodular pulmonary densities, lobar pulmonary consolidation, and hilar lymphadenopathy (Berry et al, 1990). Bronchoalveolar lavage may reveal a suppurative, granulomatous, eosinophilic, or mixed inflammatory pattern. The definitive diagnosis is dependent on lung biopsy findings. Histopathologic findings have included angiitis and angiocentric and angiodestructive granulomatous cellular infiltrates composed of mononuclear "lymphoreticular" cells, lymphocytes, plasma cells, macrophages, mast cells, and eosinophils. Affected dogs are usually poorly responsive to corticosteroids. A few dogs have been treated with cyclophosphamide, vincristine, and prednisone, with some response.

Thromboembolism. Pulmonary thromboembolism is increasingly being recognized in older dogs. Affected dogs typically present with coughing, dyspnea, hemoptysis, tachycardia, lethargy, anorexia, and fever (LaRue and Murtaugh, 1990). Physical examination may reveal a split S_2 sound, and distended jugular pulses caused by pulmonary hypertension may be noted. The most common cause of pulmonary thromboembolism in

TABLE 7–5. DRUGS USED IN THE TREATMENT OF CANINE AND FELINE CHRONIC BRONCHIAL DISEASE

DRUG	DOSE	COMMENTS
Bronchodilators		
Sympathetic amines		
Terbutaline (Brethine)	0.625 mg PO q 12 hr (C) 0.04–0.1 mg/kg IV (C) 0.05–0.1 mg/kg PO q 8 hr (D)	Long-term use is not recommended.
Albuterol	0.02–0.04 mg/kg PO q 8–12 hr (D)	Side effects include muscular tremors.
Isoproterenol (Isuprel)	0.1–0.2 ml SQ (C)	Tachycardia may occur.
Epinephrine (Adrenaline) 1:1000	0.5 ml of 1:10,000 dilution IM or SQ (C)	Use only in emergency situations and if isoproterenol is unavailable.
Methylxanthines		
Aminophylline	4 mg/kg PO, IM, slow IV q 8–12 hr (C) 6–11 mg/kg PO, IM, slow IV q 8 hr (D)	
Sustained-release theophylline (Slo-bid; Theo-Dur)	25 mg/kg PO q 24 hr (C)	
Dyphylline (Dilor)	4 mg/kg IM (C)	Neutral salt of theophylline; less painful.
Corticosteroids		
Prednisolone sodium succinate (Solu-Delta-Cortef)	1–10 mg/kg IV, IM	
Dexamethasone	0.2–1 mg/kg IV, IM	
Prednisone	1 mg/kg PO q 12 hr	Taper to lowest dose that controls signs.
Methylprednisolone acetate (Depo-Medrol)	10–20 mg IM	Rule out infectious causes before administration.
Triamcinolone	0.25–0.5 mg q 24 hr	Taper to lowest dose that will control signs. Once-weekly administration can often be achieved.
Parasympatholytics		
Atropine	0.05 mg/kg SQ, IM (C)	May decrease mucociliary action.
Sedatives		
Ketamine	0.1–1 mg/kg IV (C)	Intubate and administer 100% O_2 if necessary.
Acepromazine	0.05–0.1 mg/kg IV (C,D) to maximum of 1 mg (C) or 3 mg (D)	Heart rate, pulse character, and perfusion should be monitored closely in geriatric dogs.
Antitussives (Canine)		
Hydrocodone bitartrate	0.22 mg/kg PO q 6–12 hr (D)	Use as needed; antitussives are most important in dogs with nonproductive cough or collapsing airway.
Butorphanol	0.05–0.1 mg/kg PO, SQ q 8–12 hr (D)	Use as needed.
Antimicrobials		With efficacy against *Bordetella* and *Mycoplasma*.
Amoxicillin-clavulanate	10–20 mg/kg PO q 12 hr (C,D)	
Tetracycline	10–20 mg/kg PO q 8 hr (C,D)	
Chloramphenicol	50 mg/kg PO, IV q 6–8 hr (D) 25 mg/kg PO, IV q 12 hr (C)	

C, cat; D, dog; PO, oral administration; IV, intravenous administration; SQ, subcutaneous administration.

dogs of all ages is dirofilariasis. Other causes include nephrotic syndrome, hyperadrenocorticism, immune-mediated hemolytic anemia, neoplasia, bacterial endocarditis, septicemia, surgery, trauma, hyperviscosity syndrome, polycythemia, vasculitis, disseminated intravascular coagulopathy, pancreatitis, hypothyroidism, and primary hypercoagulable states (Dennis, 1991; Green and Kabel, 1982; Klein et al, 1989; LaRue and Murtaugh, 1990). Thromboemboli may occur in the dog with hyperadrenocorticism owing to a hypercoagulable state produced by increased plasma concentrations of coagulation factors V, VIII, IX, X, ATIII, fibrinogen, and plasminogen.

The diagnosis of pulmonary thromboembolism is based on consistent radiographic changes in an animal with arterial blood gases that suggest ventilation-perfusion mismatch. Blood gas findings include severe hypoxemia while breathing room air, with little improvement while breathing 100 per cent oxygen. Radiographic changes include increased alveolar densities that are usually fluffy and indistinct but may be lobar or triangular. Mild pleural effusion may occur in some cases (Fluckiger and Gomez, 1984). Heartworm-induced thromboemboli are seen in animals with moderate to severe radiographic evidence of dirofilariasis and primarily affect the caudal lung lobes. Selective angiography is the gold standard for the diagnosis of pulmonary thromboembolism but is invasive and requires general anesthesia. Ventilation-perfusion scintigraphy is technically easier to perform than angiography in the conscious animal and has been shown to have a high sensitivity when compared with angiography (Koblik et al, 1989).

Treatment of severe pulmonary thromboembolism is difficult and often unrewarding. Oxygen and bronchodilators are initially given but may have limited efficacy in animals with severe ventilation-perfusion mismatch. Glucocorticoids are important in the treatment of heartworm-induced disease but may be contraindicated in treatment of thromboembolism from other causes. If ongoing thrombosis owing to a hypercoagulable state is suspected, heparin is indicated to prevent further thrombus formation. Heparin at a dose of 200 U/kg IV followed by a continuous infusion of 15 to 20 U/kg/hr has been recommended (Wall, 1992). Dissolution of existing thrombi can be accomplished using recombinant tissue plasminogen activator (r-TPA) at a dose of 1 mg/kg IV over 15 minutes (Schiffman et al, 1988). Platelet inhibitors such as aspirin or dipyridamole are probably less effective than heparin. Cage rest is always recommended. If the underlying cause of thromboembolism can be determined, it should be treated specifically. The prognosis for heartworm-induced thromboembolism is good to excellent with strict cage confinement and corticosteroid, oxygen, and bronchodilator therapy. The prognosis for other causes is always guarded, especially if the underlying cause cannot be identified or resolved.

Pneumonia. Age-related changes in pulmonary defense mechanisms predispose the geriatric dog to bacterial pneumonia. Pneumonia is especially prominent in dogs with bronchial disease in which the chronic degenerative process has resulted in bronchiectasis and decreased mucociliary clearance. *Klebsiella, Escherichia coli, Pasteurella, Enterobacter, Pseudomonas, Streptococcus,* and *Bordetella bronchiseptica* organisms are common bacterial isolates (Stone and Pook, 1992). Aspiration of food, gastric contents, or foreign material in dogs with diseases that cause chronic vomiting, megaesophagus, laryngeal paralysis, or pharyngeal dysfunction also predisposes to bacterial pneumonia. Bacterial pneumonia should be suspected in any dog presented with fever and cough. Other clinical signs include lethargy, anorexia, dyspnea, exercise intolerance, and mucopurulent nasal discharge. Thoracic radiographs are generally characterized by alveolar and interstitial disease, most prominent in the cranial, middle, and ventral lung fields. If radiographic evidence is supportive of bacterial pneumonia, a tracheal or bronchoalveolar lavage should be performed and samples submitted for cytology tests, Gram staining, and aerobic bacterial culture, and in vitro sensitivity testing.

Antimicrobials, airway hydration, and physiotherapy are the keys to successful management of dogs with bacterial pneumonia. Because the causative organisms and the antimicrobial sensitivities of those organisms vary significantly, antimicrobial choice should be based on in vitro sensitivity tests, whenever possible. In uncomplicated cases of bacterial pneumonia, trimethoprim-sulfamethoxazole, amoxicillin-clavulanate, and first-generation cephalosporins are recommended for initial treatment while waiting for culture results (Stone and Pook, 1992). Enrofloxacin, a cephalosporin-aminoglycoside combination, and chloramphenicol are recommended for life-threatening or nosocomial infections. Clinical improvement should be noted in 48 to 72 hours if an appropriate antimicrobial has been chosen. Radiographic improvement may lag behind clinical improvement. Antimicrobials should be continued for at least 1 week beyond clinical and radiographic resolution.

After rehydration, physiotherapy for pneumonia is the process whereby mechanical attempts are made to promote coughing and facilitate clearance of exudate from the airways. Mild forced exercise and coupage are useful forms of physiotherapy. Coupage, in which a cupped hand is used to forcefully strike the chest over the affected lung fields, is generally safer in the severely compromised patient. The mechanical force induces coughing and helps to loosen secretions in consolidated areas.

If aspiration pneumonia is suspected, a thorough diagnostic evaluation looking for underlying diseases (usually related to esophageal or pharyngeal dysfunction) should be performed. Radiographic findings seen in aspiration pneumonia 12 to 24 hours after aspiration include consolidation and alveolar and interstitial infiltration of dependent lung lobes. Aspiration pneumonia should be treated similarly to other types of pneumonia. If

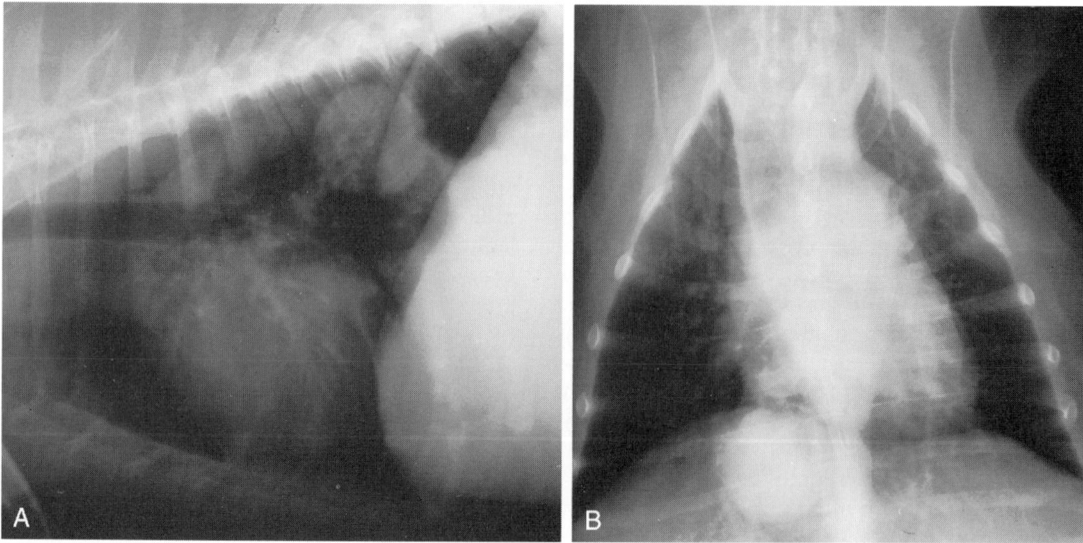

Figure 7–11. Lateral *(A)* and ventrodorsal *(B)* radiographs of a dog with a primary lung tumor in the right caudal lung lobe.

the animal is seen shortly after aspiration has occurred, mechanical suction of the airways should be attempted. Bronchodilator therapy and a single dose of corticosteroids may reduce bronchoconstriction. Antimicrobials with efficacy against gram-negative and anaerobic bacteria should be used if secondary infection is suspected.

Neoplasia. Primary pulmonary neoplasia is rare in the dog; mean age at diagnosis is approximately 9 to 11 years (Madewell and Theilen, 1987; Mehlhaff and Mooney, 1985; Ogilvie et al, 1989). Cough (52 per cent), dyspnea (24 per cent), lethargy (18 per cent), and weight loss (12 per cent) are the most common clinical findings associated with primary lung tumors (Ogilvie et al, 1989). Reported paraneoplastic syndromes included hypertrophic osteopathy (3 per cent), hypercalcemia (1 per cent), and ectopic adrenocorticotropic hormone (ACTH) secretion (1 per cent). Adenocarcinoma is the most commonly diagnosed primary lung tumor (75 per cent of cases), followed by differentiated and anaplastic alveolar carcinomas (20 per cent of cases), and squamous cell carcinomas and bronchial carcinomas (5 per cent of cases).

Presumptive diagnosis of primary lung neoplasia is usually made radiographically (Mehlhaff and Mooney, 1985; Miles, 1988). The characteristic radiographic finding is a solitary nodular lesion involving a single lung lobe (Miles, 1988); infrequently multiple nodules or diffuse involvement of one or more lung lobes are seen. The right caudal lung lobe is most commonly affected (Fig. 7–11). A single nodular lesion is suggestive of primary pulmonary neoplasia, whereas multiple nodules more likely represent metastatic disease (Fig. 7–12). Definitive diagnosis is dependent on cytologic or histologic confirmation of neoplasia. Surgical biopsy and/or fine-needle aspiration is often necessary to confirm the specific neoplastic type. Wide surgical resection of the pulmonary mass is the treatment of choice for primary pulmonary neoplasia. The average survival is about 19 months postoperatively for dogs with adenocarcinoma and 8 months for those with squamous cell carcinoma (Mehlhaff et al, 1984). Little information on the chemoresponsiveness of canine primary lung tumors is available. Improved survival has been reported in four dogs in which a combination of cisplatin and vindesine was used (Mehlhaff et al, 1984). Cisplatin alone may be of benefit in some dogs (Moore, 1992).

Lower Airway Diseases of the Cat

Neoplasia. Primary pulmonary neoplasia is rare in the cat. The clinical signs are usually nonspecific and include weight loss, lethargy, anorexia, and weakness (Barr et al, 1987; Koblik, 1986; Mehlhaff and Mooney, 1985). The mean age of affected cats is 11 to 12 years. Adenocarcinoma is the most common tumor type (two thirds of primary lung tumors), followed by bronchoalveolar and anaplastic carcinomas) (15 per cent) and squamous cell carcinomas (14 per

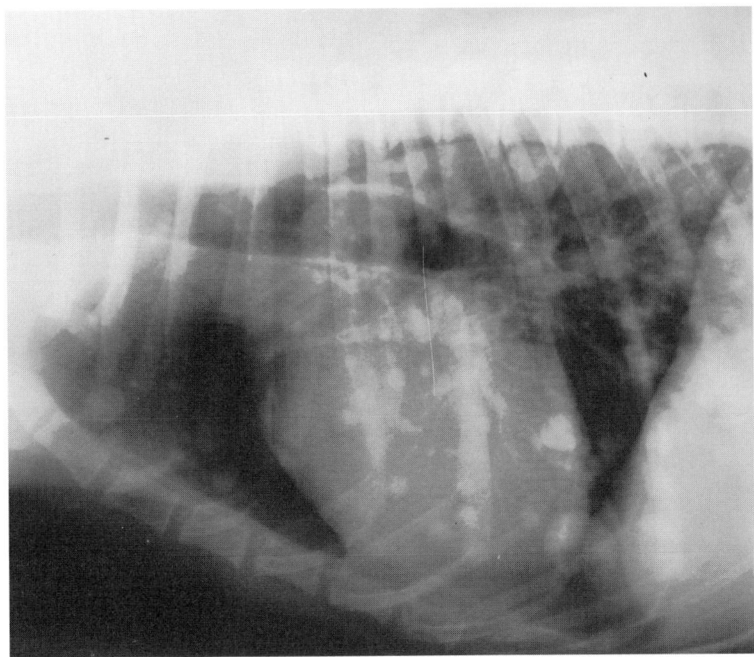

Figure 7–12. Lateral radiograph from a dog with metastatic neoplasia.

cent). The most common radiographic pattern consists of focal, well-circumscribed solitary mass lesions or multiple poorly circumscribed masses. Adenocarcinoma affects all lung lobes equally, whereas squamous cell carcinoma tends to affect the middle and peripheral portions. Little is known about treatment of primary lung tumors in cats. Solitary mass lesions should probably be surgically removed, but metastasis is common, making the prognosis poor in most cases. Chemotherapeutic protocols for use in cats with pulmonary neoplasia have not been reported. It should be noted that cisplatin, a recommended agent in dogs, should not be used in cats, because it produces severe, usually fatal pulmonary edema (Knapp et al, 1987).

Bronchitis and Asthma. Feline chronic bronchitis or feline asthma occurs in young to middle-age female cats; Siamese cats are predisposed to asthma (Moise et al, 1989). Clinical signs include wheezing, gagging, dyspnea, tachypnea, coughing, and vomiting. A chronic history of coughing or respiratory difficulty may be present, but severe signs often occur acutely without a previous history that would support respiratory disease. Wheezes and increased breath sounds are heard on thoracic auscultation of most cats with chronic bronchial disease. Diagnosis is based on clinical signs and radiographic evidence of peribronchial interstitial infiltrates (Fig. 7–13). Care should be taken not to stress affected cats. Severely affected cats should be initially treated based on clinical suspicion rather than risk the stress of thoracic radiographs. Increased bronchial markings are the most common radiographic abnormality noted (Moise et al, 1989). A tracheal wash should be performed on all stable cats with radiographic evidence of peribronchial disease. Bacterial bronchitis and aelurostrongylosis should be ruled out. Most cats will have cytologic evidence of a nonseptic exudate. Eosinophilic, neutrophilic, granulomatous, and mixed infiltrates are all seen with about equal frequency.

Treatment of feline chronic bronchitis relies on anti-inflammatory drugs, bronchodilators, and, occasionally, antimicrobials (see Table 7–5). Chronic outpatient therapy is usually sufficient, but overt cyanosis or status asthmaticus is occasionally seen and should be considered a medical emergency requiring immediate therapeutic action. Dramatic response can usually be expected within 15 to 30 minutes of initiating therapy. Dexamethasone sodium phosphate or prednisolone sodium succinate should be used initially, with bronchodilators such as the methylxanthine derivatives or the beta$_2$-adrenoceptor agonist terbutaline used to augment the response. Less severely affected cats will usually respond to oral glucocorticoids with or without augmentation from oral bronchodilator use. Dosage of glucocorticoids should be tapered to the lowest possible dose that controls the clinical signs. Alterna-

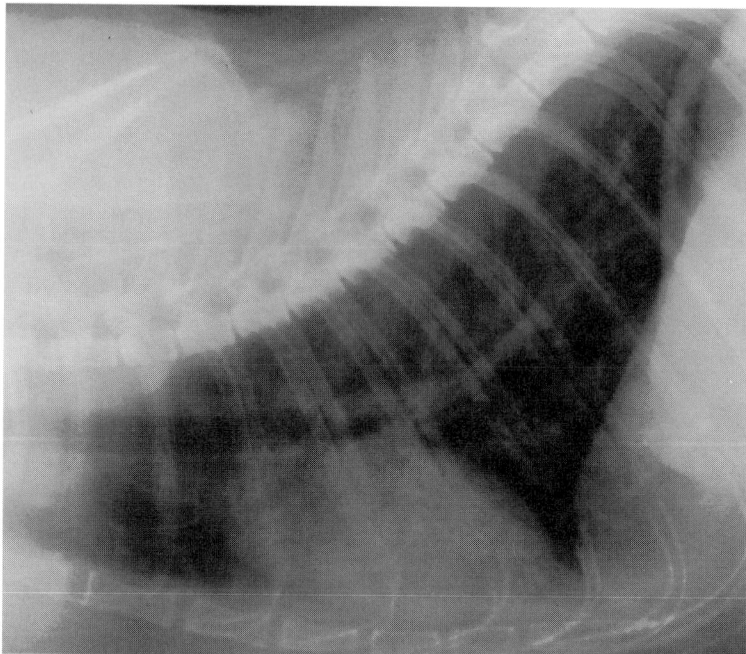

Figure 7–13. Lateral radiograph demonstrating diffuse peribronchial infiltrates in a cat with feline asthma.

tively, long-acting or reposital steroids such as prednisolone acetate may provide better long-term management.

DISEASES OF THE PLEURA

Neoplastic pleural effusions are a primary concern in the geriatric patient (Table 7–6). Neoplastic pleural effusions can be of any type. Neoplastic involvement of the pleura may disrupt capillary integrity, allowing fluid and protein leakage into the pleural space, resulting in modified transudate. Protein and fluid accumulation can also be secondary to lymphatic obstruction. If the thoracic duct or other primary lymphatic structures are involved, a chylous effusion may be seen. Hemorrhagic effusion can occur if vascular integrity is severely disrupted. Neoplasia should be high on the differential diagnosis list for any bloody effusion that is not due simply to hemorrhage. Lymphosarcoma often results in pleural fluid that contains many neoplastic cells. The diagnosis of lymphosarcoma can usually be confirmed via thoracocentesis and cytologic evaluation of the fluid.

Neoplastic diseases that may result in pleural effusion include metastatic disease, mesothelioma, lymphosarcoma (especially of mediastinal origin), thymoma, and tumors involving the right heart. Thymoma is derived from thymic epithelial tissue that frequently contains numerous lymphocytes; it may be either benign and noninvasive or malignant and invasive (Bellah et al, 1983). Diagnosis is based on radiographic evidence of a cranial mediastinal mass and cytologic or histologic confirmation of thymoma. Thoracotomy may be necessary for definitive diagnosis (Moore, 1992). Canine thymomas are locally aggressive, whereas feline thymomas tend to be less invasive (Bellah et al, 1983; Carpenter and Holzworth, 1982). Paraneoplastic syndromes are commonly associated with thymomas. Treatment of thymoma is dependent on the invasiveness of the tumor. Surgical resection is the treatment of choice in cats, in which the tumor is usually benign and well encapsulated. However, the invasive nature of most thymomas in dogs makes surgical resection difficult to impossible.

Mesotheliomas are rare neoplasms that arise as papillomatosis growths on the pleural, pericardial, and peritoneal surfaces (Madewell and Theilen, 1987). Clinical signs are usually related to massive fluid accumulation in affected body cavities. Dyspnea, tachypnea, and weight loss are the primary clinical signs. Diagnosis is dependent on demonstration of the malignant cells in the pleural fluid or on biopsy findings. The effusion is usually characterized as a nonseptic, hemorrhagic exudate with numerous reactive or neoplastic mesothelial cells. Cytologic analysis of pleural fluid alone is unreliable as a method of confirming a diagnosis of malignancy because of

TABLE 7–6. DISEASES CAUSING PLEURAL EFFUSION IN THE DOG AND CAT

DISEASE	FLUID EVALUATION
Neoplastic disease Mesothelioma Lymphosarcoma (mediastinal or diffuse pulmonary) Primary pulmonary neoplasia Metastic neoplasia	Modified transudate, nonseptic exudate, chylous effusion, hemorrhagic effusion, and neoplastic effusion are all possible. Reactive mesothelial cells in the effusion make definitive diagnosis of neoplasia difficult from cytology.
Right heart failure	Transudate initially, then modified transudate when chronic
Hypoalbuminemia	Transudate.
Diaphragmatic hernia	Modified transudate or nonseptic exudate.
Lung lobe torsion	Modified transudate, nonseptic exudate, chylous or hemorrhagic effusion.
Chylothorax Idiopathic Neoplasia Trauma Dirofilariasis Heart disease	Chylous effusion; triglyceride content is higher than in serum, while cholesterol content is usually lower.
Hemothorax Vitamin K antagonist rodenticide toxicity Systemic coagulopathy Trauma	Hemorrhagic effusion.
Pyothorax	Septic exudate.
Pancreatitis	Modified transudate or nonseptic exudate.
Pulmonary thromboembolism	Modified transudate or nonseptic exudate.

the difficulty in distinguishing reactive mesothelial cells from those that are neoplastic. Therapy includes frequent thoracocentesis. Intracavitary chemotherapy with cisplatin (50 mg/m^2) infused into the pleural space has resulted in reduction or resolution of pleural effusion (Moore, 1992). The combination of intracavitary cisplatin and systemic doxorubicin may prove to be the most effective treatment for mesothelioma in dogs.

References

Effects of Aging on the Respiratory System

Ehrsam RE, Perruchoud A, Oberholzer M, et al. Influence of age on pulmonary haemodynamics at rest and during supine exercise. Clin Sci 65:653, 1983.

Georges R, Sauman G, Loiseau A. The relationship of age to pulmonary membrane conductance and capillary blood volume. Am Rev Respir Dis 117:1069, 1978.

Kundson RJ, Clark DF, Kennedy TC, et al. Effect of aging alone on mechanical properties of the normal adult human lung. J Appl Physiol 43:1054, 1977.

Kronenberg RS, Drage CW. Attenuation of the ventilatory and heart rate responses to hypoxia and hypercapnia with aging in normal men. J Clin Invest 52:1812, 1973.

Mittman C, Edelman NH, Norris AH, et al. Relationship between chest wall and pulmonary compliance and age. J Appl Physiol 20:1211, 1965.

Murray JF. Aging. In The Normal Lung: The Basis for Diagnosis and Treatment of Pulmonary Disease. 2nd ed. Philadelphia, WB Saunders, 1986, p 339.

Rea H, Becklake MR, Ghezzo H. Lung function changes as a reflection of tissue aging in young adults. Bull Eur Physiopathol Respir 18:5, 1982.

Diseases of the Nasal Cavity

Adams WM, Withrow SJ, Walshaw R, et al. Radiotherapy of malignant nasal tumors in 67 dogs. J Am Vet Med Assoc 191:311, 1987.

Anderson WI, Parchman MB, Cline JM, et al. Nasal cavernous haemangioma in an American short haired cat. Vet Rec 124:41, 1989.

Burgener DC, Slocombe RF, Zerbe CA. Lymphoplasmacytic rhinitis in five dogs. J Am Anim Hosp Assoc 23:565, 1987.

Cox NR, Brawner WR, Powers RD, et al. Tumors of the nose and paranasal sinuses in cats: 32 cases with comparison to a national database (1977 through 1987). J Am Anim Hosp Assoc 27:339, 1991.

Davidson A, Komtebedde J, Pappagianis D, et al. Treatment of nasal aspergillosis with topical clotrimazole. Proc Am Coll Vet Intern Med 10:807, 1992.

Ellison GW, Mulligan TW, Fagan DA, et al. A double reposition flap technique for repair of recurrent oronasal fistulas in dogs. J Am Anim Hosp Assoc 22:803, 1986.

Elmslie RE, Ogilvie GK, Gillette EL, et al. Radiotherapy with and without chemotherapy for localized lymphoma in 10 cats. Vet Radiol 32:277, 1991.

Evans SM, Goldschmidt M, McKee LJ, et al. Prognostic factors and survival after radiotherapy for intranasal neoplasms in dogs: 70 cases (1974–1985). J Am Vet Med Assoc 194:1460, 1989.

Evans SM, Hendrick M. Radiotherapy of feline nasal tumors: A retrospective study of nine cases. Vet Radiol 30:128, 1989.

Ford RB. Endoscopy of the upper respiratory tract of the dog and cat. In Tams TR, ed. Small Animal Endoscopy. St. Louis, CV Mosby, 1990, p 297.

George TF, Smallwood JE. Anatomic atlas for computed tomography in the mesaticephalic dog: Head and neck. Vet Radiol 33:217, 1992.

Gibbs C, Lane JG, Denny HR. Radiographical features of intranasal tumor lesions in the dog: A review of 100 cases. J Small Anim Pract 20:515, 1979.

Grove TK. Problems associated with the management of periodontal disease in clinical practice. Prob Vet Med 2:110, 1990.

Hahn KA, Knapp DW, Richardson RC, et al. Clinical response of nasal adenocarcinoma to cisplatin chemotherapy in 11 dogs. J Am Vet Med Assoc 200:355, 1992.

Hahn KA, Matlock CL. Nasal adenocarcinoma metastatic to bone in two dogs. J Am Vet Med Assoc 197:491, 1990.

Harvey CE. Surgery of the nasal cavity and sinuses. In Bojrab MJ, ed. Current Techniques in Small Animal Surgery. 2nd ed. Philadelphia, Lea & Febiger, 1983, p 253.

MacEwen EG, Withrow SJ, Patnaik AK. Nasal tumors in the dog: Retrospective evaluation of diagnosis, prognosis, and treatment. J Am Vet Med Assoc 170:45, 1977.

Madewell BR, Priester WA, Gillette EL, et al. Neoplasms of the nasal passages and paranasal sinuses in domesticated animals as reported by 13 veterinary colleges. Am J Vet Res 37:852, 1976.

Manfra Marretta S. The diagnosis and treatment of oronasal fistulas in three cats. J Vet Dent 5:4, 1988.

Manfra Marretta S. Chronic rhinitis and dental disease. Vet Clin North Am [Small Anim Pract] 22:1101, 1992.

McEntee MC, Page RL, Geidner GL, et al. A retrospective study of 27 dogs with intranasal neoplasms treated with cobalt radiation. Vet Radiol 32:135, 1991.

Medleau L, Green CE, Rakich PM. Evaluation of ketoconazole and itraconazole for treatment of disseminated cryptococcosis in cats. Am J Vet Res 51:1454, 1990a.

Medleau L, Marks MA, Brown J, et al. Clinical evaluation of a cryptococcal antigen latex agglutination test for diagnosis of cryptococcosis in cats. J Am Vet Med Assoc 196:1470, 1990b.

Moore MP, Gavin PR, Kraft SL, et al. MR, CT, and clinical features from four dogs with nasal tumors involving the rostral cerebrum. Vet Radiol 32:19, 1991.

Mortellaro CM, Della Franca P, Caretta G. *Aspergillus fumigatus*, the causative agent of infection of the frontal sinuses and nasal chambers of the dog. Mycoses 32:327, 1989.

Ogilvie GK, LaRue SM. Canine and feline nasal and paranasal sinus tumors. Vet Clin North Am [Small Anim Pract] 22:1133, 1992.

Patnaik AK. Canine sinonasal neoplasms: Clinicopathological study of 285 cases. J Am Anim Hosp Assoc 25:103, 1989.

Roberts SM, Lavach JD, Severin GA, et al. Ophthalmic complications following megavoltage irradiation of the nasal and paranasal cavities in dogs. J Am Vet Med Assoc 190:43, 1987.

Schrenzel MD, Higgins RJ, Hinrichs SH, et al. Type C retroviral expression in spontaneous feline olfactory neuroblastomas. Acta Neuropathol 80:547, 1990.

Sharp NJH. Nasal aspergillosis: Treatment with enilconazole. Proc Am Coll Vet Intern Med 10:253, 1992.

Sharp NJH, Harvey CE, O'Brien JA. Treatment of canine nasal aspergillosis/penicilliosis with fluconazole (UK-49,858). J Small Anim Pract 32:513, 1991a.

Sharp NJH, Harvey CE, Sullivan M. Canine nasal aspergillosis and penicilliosis. Compend Contin Educ Pract Vet 13:41, 1991b.

Sharp NJH, Sullivan M. Treatment of canine nasal aspergillosis with systemic ketoconazole and enilconazole. Vet Rec 118:560, 1986.

Sharp NJH, Sullivan M, Harvey CE, et al. Treatment of canine nasal aspergillosis with enilconazole. J Vet Intern Med 7:40, 1993.

Smith MO, Turrel JM, Bailey CS, et al. Neurologic abnormalities as the predominant signs of neoplasia of the nasal cavity in dogs and cats: Seven cases (1973–1986). J Am Vet Med Assoc 195:242, 1989.

Straw RC, Withrow SJ, Gillette EL, et al. Use of radiotherapy for the treatment of intranasal tumors in cats: Six cases (1980–1985). J Am Vet Med Assoc 189:927, 1986.

Sullivan M. Differential diagnosis of chronic nasal disease in the dog. In Pract Nov:217, 1987.

Thompson JP, Ackerman N, Bellah J, et al. ^{192}Ir brachytherapy, using an intracavitary afterload device, for the treatment of intranasal neoplasms in dogs. Am J Vet Res 53:617, 1992.

Thrall DE, Roberton ID, McLeod DA, et al. A comparison of radiographic and computed tomographic findings in 31 dogs with malignant nasal cavity tumors. Vet Radiol 30:59, 1989.

Withrow SJ, Susaneck SJ, Macy DW, et al. Aspiration and punch biopsy techniques for nasal tumors. J Am Anim Hosp Assoc 21:551, 1985.

Wolf AM. Fungal diseases of the nasal cavity of the dog and cat. Vet Clin North Am [Small Anim Pract] 22:1119, 1992.

Diseases of the Larynx

Aron DN, Crowe DT. Upper airway obstruction general principles and selected conditions in the dog and cat. Vet Clin North Am [Small Anim Pract] 15:891, 1985.

Bedford PG. Unilateral arytenoid lateralization in the dog. In Bojrab MJ, ed. Current Techniques in Small Animal Surgery. 3rd ed. Philadelphia, Lea & Febiger, 1990, p 335.

Birchard SJ, Bradley RL. Surgery of the respiratory tract. In Sherding RG, ed. The Cat: Diseases and Clinical Management. New York, Churchill Livingstone, 1989, p 851.

Braund KG, Steinberg HS, Shores A, et al. Laryngeal paralysis in immature and mature dogs as one sign of a more diffuse polyneuropathy. J Am Vet Med Assoc 194:1735, 1989.

Busch DS, Noxon JO, Miller LD. Laryngeal paralysis and peripheral vestibular disease in a cat. J Am Anim Hosp Assoc 28:82, 1992.

Carlisle CH, Biery DN, Thrall DE. Tracheal and laryngeal tumors in the dog and cat: Literature review and 13 additional patients. Vet Radiol 32:229, 1991.

Cribb AE. Laryngeal paralysis in a mature cat. Can Vet J 27:27, 1986.

Crowe DT, Goodwin MA, Greene CE. Total laryngectomy for laryngeal mast cell tumor in a dog. J Am Anim Hosp Assoc 22:809, 1986.

Duncan ID. Peripheral neuropathy in the dog and cat. Prog Vet Neurol 2:111, 1991.

Gilson SD, Crane SW. Bilateral arytenoid lateralization by ventral midline approach in the dog and cat. In Bojrab MJ, ed. Current Techniques in Small Animal Surgery. 3rd ed. Philadelphia, Lea & Febiger, 1990, p 336.

Gourley IM, Paul H, Gregory C. Castellated laryngofissure and vocal fold resection for the treatment of laryngeal paralysis in the dog. J Am Vet Med Assoc 182:1084, 1983.

Greenfield CL. Canine laryngeal paralysis. Compend Contin Educ Pract Vet 9:1011, 1987.

Harari J, Patterson JS, Rosenthal RC. Clinical and pathologic features of thyroid tumors in 26 dogs. J Am Vet Med Assoc 188:1160, 1986.

Hardie EM, Kolata RJ, Stone EA, et al. Laryngeal paralysis in three cats. J Am Vet Med Assoc 179:879, 1981.

Hedlund CS. Treatment of laryngeal paralysis. In Bojrab MJ,

ed. Current Techniques in Small Animal Surgery. 3rd ed. Philadelphia, Lea & Febiger, 1990, p 329.

Henderson RA, Powers RD, Perry L. Development of hypoparathyroidism after excision of laryngeal rhabdomyosarcoma in a dog. J Am Vet Med Assoc 198:639, 1991.

Jaggy A. Neurologic manifestations of hypothyroidism in dogs. Proc Am Coll Vet Intern Med 8:1037, 1990.

Meric SM. Therapeutic options for hyperthyroidism. In August JR, ed. Consultations in Feline Medicine. Philadelphia, WB Saunders, 1991, p 243.

Petersen SW, Rosin E, Bjorling DE. Surgical options for laryngeal paralysis in dogs: A consideration of partial laryngectomy. Compend Contin Educ Pract Vet 13:1531, 1991.

Ross JT, Matthiesen DT, Noone KE, et al. Complications and long-term results after partial laryngectomy for the treatment of idiopathic laryngeal paralysis in 45 dogs. Vet Surg 20:169, 1991.

Saik JE, Toll SL, Diters RW, et al. Canine and feline laryngeal neoplasia: A 10-year survey. J Am Anim Hosp Assoc 22:359, 1986.

Schaer M, Zaki FA, Harvey HJ, et al. Laryngeal hemiplegia due to neoplasia of the vagus nerve in a cat. J Am Vet Med Assoc 174:513, 1979.

Taboada J, Hoskins JD, Morgan RV. Respiratory emergencies. In Emergency Medicine and Critical Care in Practice. Trenton, NJ, Veterinary Learning Systems, 1992, p 50.

Venker-van Haagen AJ. Diseases of the larynx. Vet Clin North Am [Small Anim Pract] 22:1155, 1992.

White RA. Unilateral arytenoid lateralisation: An assessment of technique and long term results in 62 dogs with laryngeal paralysis. J Small Anim Pract 30:543, 1989.

White RA, Littlewood JD, Herrtage ME, et al. Outcome of surgery for laryngeal paralysis in four cats. Vet Rec 118:103, 1986.

Withrow SJ. Tumors of the respiratory system. In Withrow SJ, MacEwen EG, eds. Clinical Veterinary Oncology. Philadelphia, JB Lippincott, 1989, p 215.

Wykes PM. Canine laryngeal diseases. II. Diagnosis and treatment. Compend Contin Educ Pract Vet 5:105, 1983.

Diseases of the Trachea

Carlisle CH, Biery DN, Thrall DE. Tracheal and laryngeal tumors in the dog and cat: Literature review and 13 additional patients. Vet Radiol 32:229, 1991.

Done SA, Drew RA. Observations on the pathology of tracheal collapse in dogs. J Small Anim Pract 17:783, 1976.

Fingland RB, DeHoff WD, Birchard SJ. Surgical management of cervical and thoracic tracheal collapse in dogs using extraluminal spiral prostheses. J Am Anim Hosp Assoc 23:163, 1987.

Hawkins EC. Respiratory disorders. In Nelson RW, Couto CG, eds. Essentials of Small Animal Internal Medicine. St. Louis, Mosby–Year Book, 1992, p 153.

Hedlund CS. Surgical disease of the trachea. Vet Clin North Am [Small Anim Pract] 17:301, 1987.

Hendricks JC, O'Brien JA. Tracheal collapse in two cats. J Am Vet Med Assoc 187:418, 1985.

Nelson AW. Lower respiratory system. In Slatter DH, ed. Textbook of Small Animal Surgery. Philadelphia, WB Saunders, 1985, p 990.

Padrid P, Amis TC. Chronic tracheobronchial disease in the dog. Vet Clin North Am [Small Anim Pract] 22:1203, 1992.

Diseases of the Small Airways and Lung

Barr F, Gruffydd-Jones TJ, Brown PJ, et al. Primary lung tumors in the cat. J Small Anim Pract 28:1115, 1987.

Berry CR, Moore PF, Thomas WP, et al. Pulmonary granulomatosis in seven dogs (1976–1987). J Vet Intern Med 4:157, 1990.

Brownlie SE. A retrospective study of diagnosis in 109 cases of canine lower respiratory disease. J Small Anim Pract 31:371, 1990.

Calvert CA, Mahaffey MB, Lappin MR, et al. Pulmonary and disseminated eosinophilic granulomatosis in dogs. J Am Anim Hosp Assoc 24:311, 1988.

Dennis JS. The pathophysiologic sequelae of pulmonary thromboembolism. Compend Contin Educ Pract Vet 13:1811, 1991.

Fitzgerald SD, Wolf DC, Carlton WW. Eight cases of canine lymphomatoid granulomatosis. Vet Pathol 28:241, 1991.

Fluckiger MA, Gomez JA. Radiographic findings in dogs with spontaneous pulmonary thrombosis or embolism. Vet Radiol 25:124, 1984.

Ford RB. Endoscopy of the lower respiratory tract of the dog and cat. In Tams TR, ed. Small Animal Endoscopy. St. Louis, CV Mosby, 1990, p 309.

Green RA, Kabel AL. Hypercoagulable state in three dogs with nephrotic syndrome: Role of acquired antithrombin III deficiency. J Am Vet Med Assoc 181:914, 1982.

Hawkins EC. Respiratory disorders. In Nelson RW, Couto CG, eds. Essentials of Small Animal Internal Medicine. St. Louis, Mosby–Year Book, 1992, p 153.

Hawkins EC, DeNicola DB, Kuehn NF. Bronchoalveolar lavage in the evaluation of pulmonary disease in the dog and cat. J Vet Intern Med 4:267, 1990.

Howell S, Roussos C. Isoproterenol and aminophylline improve contractility of fatigued canine diaphragm. Am Rev Respir Dis 129:118, 1984.

Klein MK, Dow SW, Rosychuk RAW. Pulmonary thromboembolism associated with immune-mediated hemolytic anemia in dogs: Ten cases (1982–1987). J Am Vet Med Assoc 195:246, 1989.

Knapp DW, Richardson RC, DeNicola DB, et al. Cisplatin toxicity in cats. J Vet Intern Med 1:29, 1987.

Koblik PD. Radiographic appearance of primary lung tumors in cats: A review of 41 cases. Vet Radiol 27:66, 1986.

Koblik PD, Hornof W, Harnagel SH, et al. A comparison of pulmonary angiography, digital subtraction angiography, and ^{99m}Tc-DTPA/MAA ventilation-perfusion scintigraphy for detection of experimental pulmonary emboli in the dog. Vet Radiol 30:159, 1989.

LaRue MJ, Murtaugh RJ. Pulmonary thromboembolism in dogs: 47 cases (1986–1987). J Am Vet Med Assoc 197:1368, 1990.

Lindsey JO, Pierce AK. An examination of the microbiologic flora of normal lung of the dog. Am Rev Respir Dis 117:501, 1978.

Madewell BR, Theilen GH. Tumors of the respiratory tract and thorax. In Theilen GH, Madewell BR, eds. Veterinary Cancer Medicine. 2nd ed. Philadelphia, Lea & Febiger, 1987, p 535.

McKiernan BC, Neff-Davis CA, Koritz GD, et al. Pharmacokinetic studies of theophylline in dogs. J Vet Pharmacol Ther 4:103, 1981.

McKiernan BC, Smith AR, Kissil M. Bacteria isolated from the lower trachea of clinically healthy dogs. J Am Anim Hosp Assoc 20:139, 1984.

Mehlhaff CJ, Leifer CE, Patnaik AK, et al. Surgical treatment of primary pulmonary neoplasia in 15 dogs. J Am Anim Hosp Assoc 20:799, 1984.

Mehlhaff CJ, Mooney S. Primary pulmonary neoplasia in the dog and cat. Vet Clin North Am [Small Anim Pract] 15:1061, 1985.

Miles KG. A review of primary lung tumors in the dog and cat. Vet Radiol 29:122, 1988.

Moise NS, Wiedenkeller D, Yeager AE, et al. Clinical, radiographic, and bronchial cytologic features of cats with bronchial disease: 65 cases (1980–1986). J Am Vet Med Assoc 194:1467, 1989.

Moore AS. Chemotherapy for intrathoracic cancer in dogs and cats. Prob Vet Med 4:351, 1992.

Ogilvie GK, Haschek WM, Withrow SJ, et al. Classification of primary lung tumors in dogs: 210 cases (1975–1985). J Am Vet Med Assoc 195:106, 1989.

Padrid P. Chronic lower airway disease in the dog and cat. Prob Vet Med 4:320, 1992.

Padrid P, Amis TC. Chronic tracheobronchial disease in the dog. Vet Clin North Am [Small Anim Pract] 22:1203, 1992.

Padrid PA, Feldman BF, Funk K, et al. Cytologic, microbiologic, and biochemical analysis of bronchoalveolar lavage fluid obtained from 24 healthy cats. Am J Vet Res 52:1300, 1991.

Padrid PA, Hornof WJ, Kurpershoek CJ, et al. Canine chronic bronchitis: A pathophysiologic evaluation of 18 cases. J Vet Intern Med 4:172, 1990.

Reif JS, Rhodes WH. The lungs of aged dogs: A radiographic-morphologic correlation. J Am Vet Radiol Soc 7:5, 1966.

Schiffman F, Ducas J, Hollett P, et al. Treatment of canine embolic pulmonary hypertension with recombinant tissue plasminogen activator. Circulation 78:214, 1988.

Stone MS, Pook H. Lung infections and infestations: Therapeutic considerations. Prob Vet Med 4:279, 1992.

Taboada J. Pulmonary diseases of potential allergic origin. Semin Vet Med Surg 6:278, 1991.

Wall RE. Respiratory complications in the critically ill animal. Prob Vet Med 4:365, 1992.

Diseases of the Pleura

Bellah JR, Stiff ME, Russell RG. Thymoma in the dog: Two case reports and a review of 20 additional cases. J Am Vet Med Assoc 183:306, 1983.

Carpenter JL, Holzworth J. Thymoma in 11 cats. J Am Vet Med Assoc 181:248, 1982.

Madewell BR, Theilen GH. Tumors of the respiratory tract and thorax. In Theilen GH, Madewell BR, eds. Veterinary Cancer Medicine. 2nd ed. Philadelphia, Lea & Febiger, 1987, p 535.

Moore AS. Chemotherapy for intrathoracic cancer in dogs and cats. Prob Vet Med 4:351, 1992.

CHAPTER 8

The Cardiovascular System

JOHN E. RUSH and LISA M. FREEMAN

Management of cardiovascular disease in geriatric dogs and cats can be challenging. Aging changes affecting the heart and blood vessels result in diminished cardiovascular reserves. Lacking these normal reserves, geriatric dogs and cats are more likely to experience adverse reactions to cardiac medications. In addition, older dogs and cats commonly have concurrent diseases that may complicate therapy. Successful control of the cardiovascular diseases affecting geriatric dogs and cats requires a knowledge of these aging phenomena, an understanding of drug effects and toxicities, and a good owner and veterinarian relationship allowing for therapeutic adjustments as needed.

AGING CHANGES IN THE CARDIOVASCULAR SYSTEM

Several alterations in the structure and function of the cardiovascular system are known to attend advancing age. In dogs and cats, accumulation of intracytoplasmic lipofuscin within myocytes occurs with increasing age (Baskin et al, 1981), although this is not known to impair function. Amyloid deposition within the myocardium is recognized microscopically in aged dogs (Jonsson, 1974), but infiltrative cardiomyopathy resulting from amyloidosis is rare in dogs and cats. More important are the age-related changes in responsiveness of the cardiovascular system to neural stimulation. Diminished responsiveness to adrenergic stimulation may significantly change cardiac performance. Adrenergic stimulation usually causes an increase in heart rate and inotropy (strength of myocardial contraction) and a shortened duration of contraction. Studies have demonstrated an age-associated diminution in the maximal response of the heart to beta-adrenergic stimulation (Wei, 1992; Yin et al, 1979). The limited ability of the aging cardiovascular system to increase heart rate, inotropic state, and cardiac output in crisis situations is important in the management of cardiac disease. In addition, the lack of response to beta-adrenergic stimulation may limit the utility of certain cardiovascular medications or alter the dose required to achieve a therapeutic response.

Concurrent decreases in the responsiveness of vascular smooth muscle to sympathetic stimulation have also been demonstrated (Yin et al, 1981). The vasodilatory response to $beta_2$ stimulation is blunted with advancing age. These changes lead to diminished exercise capacity and increases in the resistance (or afterload) faced by the left ventricle. Additional changes that are recognized in older humans and animals include increased basal catecholamine concentrations, diminished affinity of the beta-adrenergic receptor for catecholamines, and blunted baroreceptor reflexes (Wei, 1992). These factors also contribute to a reduction in cardiovascular reserves. Young, healthy patients may have an increased cardiac output of up to 25 per cent in response to stress, but such cardiac reserves are often lacking in the geriatric population (Wei et al, 1984). Arteriosclerosis of intramural cardiac arteries has been reported to be a frequent necropsy finding in aged dogs (Jonsson, 1972). These lesions result from vascular hyalinosis and amyloidosis, are limited to the vessels of the heart, and may lead to multifocal intramural myocardial infarction (MIMI). The associated electrocardiographic (ECG) finding is notching in the downstroke of the QRS complex, a common finding in dogs with chronic valvular disease (Fig. 8–1).

GENERAL MANAGEMENT

Older dogs and cats often have diminished cardiovascular and respiratory reserves and are prone to deterioration with excessive stress or exertion. Exercise limitation is often required, as many dogs fail to realize their cardiovascular limitations and will continue to exercise.

Cardiovascular Drug Therapy. Most drugs used to treat cardiovascular disease have narrow therapeutic windows, significant side effects, and the potential for serious toxicities (Table 8–1). Toxicities may be prevalent in geriatric dogs and cats as a result of diminished muscle mass, renal blood flow or renal function, and hepatic function. Some respiratory medications (e.g., aminophylline, theophylline, terbutaline) also affect the heart and contribute to arrhythmias. Thyroid hormone replacement therapy should be initiated in a stepwise fashion in cardiovascular patients to avoid arrhythmias or excessive cardiac stimulation. Some chemotherapeutic agents (e.g., doxorubicin, prednisone) may adversely affect dogs and cats with cardiac disease. Some cardiovascular drugs should be administered at reduced doses to older dogs and cats. Digoxin is an example. Digoxin pharmacokinetics are also altered by concurrent therapy with quinidine or verapamil. Other drug combinations (furosemide and enalapril) must be used cautiously with pre-existing renal dysfunction. Doses of drugs such as beta blockers and calcium channel blockers should be increased in a stepwise fashion, when possible, to avoid decompensation of congestive heart failure and/or bradyarrhythmias.

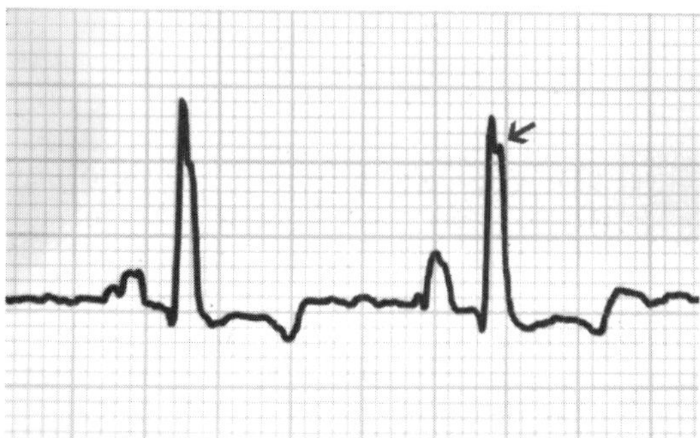

Figure 8–1. Electrocardiogram (ECG) obtained from an aged dog with chronic valvular disease. P mitrale (left atrial enlargement) is noted, as the P wave is notched and has a duration of 0.06 second. Notching in the downstroke of the QRS complex *(arrow)* was seen in all ECG leads and resulted from multifocal intramural myocardial infarction (MIMI). Recorded at 50 mm/sec and 1 cm/mV.

Nutritional Support. Dietary sodium restriction has long been recommended for patients with congestive heart failure and hypertension (Hamlin and Buffington, 1989; LaKatta, 1992). The stage of heart disease at which to institute a sodium-restricted diet is debated. Early institution of sodium restriction may delay the onset of congestive heart failure. Many dogs and cats will eat commercial sodium-restricted diets, especially when such diets are introduced gradually (Lewis et al, 1987). Although sodium-restricted diets are probably the optimal diet to feed dogs and cats with congestive heart failure, another important consideration is that the animal consumes adequate calories to meet energy requirements. Decreased nutrient intake can be caused by anorexia associated with congestive heart failure or resulting from cardiac medications (e.g., digoxin, captopril). Current areas of research involving nutrition and heart disease include the use of omega-3 fatty acids and antioxidants. Omega-3 fatty acids may decrease the susceptibility to cardiac arrhythmias (Leaf and Hallaq, 1992; McLennan, 1993). The use of antioxidant vitamins (e.g., beta-carotene, vitamin C, vitamin E) holds promise for prevention of oxidative damage to cells.

DISORDERS OF THE DOG

Chronic Valvular Disease (Endocardiosis)

The most common cardiovascular abnormality in older dogs is chronic valvular disease (Hamlin, 1990; Maher and Rush, 1990). Chronic valvular disease results in nodular thickening of the mitral

TABLE 8–1. COMMON CARDIOVASCULAR DRUGS, DOSES, AND SIDE EFFECTS

DRUG	INDICATIONS	DOSE	SIDE EFFECTS
Furosemide	CHF/edema formation	Dog: 1–4 mg/kg sid–tid Cat: 0.5–2 mg/kg qod–bid	Dehydration, azotemia, hypokalemia
Enalapril	CHF	0.5 mg/kg sid to bid	Hypotension, renal insufficiency
Captopril	CHF	0.5–2 mg/kg tid	Anorexia, vomiting, hypotension
Nitroglycerine	Pulmonary edema	⅛–1 inch transcutaneously	Hypotension, irritability, headache?
Hydralazine	Refractory CHF	1–3 mg/kg bid	Hypotension, vomiting
Digoxin	Myocardial failure, refractory CHF, supraventricular arrhythmias	Dog: 0.011 mg/kg bid Cat: ¼ of a 0.125 mg tab q o d	Vomiting, diarrhea, anorexia, depression, arrhythmias
Propranolol	Supraventricular or ventricular arrhythmias	Dog: 0.2–2 mg/kg q 8–12 hr Cat: 0.25–10 mg q 8–12 hr	Worsening CHF, lethargy, bradycardia, bronchospasm
Atenolol	Supraventricular or ventricular arrhythmias	Dog: 2.5–1 mg/kg bid Cat: ¼ of a 25-mg tab q d	Hypotension, bradycardia, worsening CHF
Metoprolol	Supraventricular or ventricular arrhythmias	Dog: 0.25–1 mg/kg bid	Hypotension, worsening CHF, bradycardia
Diltiazem	Supraventricular arrhythmias or hypertrophic cardiomyopathy	0.5–1.5 mg/kg tid	Hypotension, bradycardia
Verapamil	Supraventricular arrhythmias without CHF	1–2 mg/kg q 8–12 hr	Hypotension, bradycardia, CHF, constipation
Lidocaine	Ventricular arrhythmias	1–4 mg/kg bolus; 40–80 μg/kg/min CRI	Vomiting, seizures, hypotension
Procainamide SR	Ventricular arrhythmias	Dog: 6–20 mg/kg tid Cat: 62.5 mg/cat tid	Hypotension, vomiting, agranulocytosis
Quinidine	Ventricular arrhythmias, atrial fibrillation without underlying heart disease	Dog: 6–20 mg/kg tid Cat: 4–8 mg/kg tid	Hypotension, vomiting, diarrhea, weakness
Tocainide	Ventricular arrhythmias	Dog: 10–20 mg/kg tid	Hypotension, GI distress
Aspirin	Antithrombotic	Dog: 5 mg/kg sid Cat: ¼ of a 325 mg tab PO q 2–3 d	Vomiting, GI ulceration

CHF, Congestive heart failure; CRI, continuous rate infusion; GI, gastrointestinal; PO, oral administration.

and/or tricuspid valves. The mitral valve is most commonly affected, followed by a combination of mitral and tricuspid valve involvement and isolated tricuspid valve insufficiency.

Clinical Features. Chronic valvular disease is often slowly progressive. Cough, dyspnea, exercise intolerance, anorexia, syncope, or abdominal distention are common complaints. Of these, cough is the most common finding. As the disease progresses, signs of exercise intolerance, nocturnal dyspnea or tachypnea, anorexia, or abdominal distention may develop. Syncope is more common in dogs with concurrent respiratory disease and in some cases may precede the development of congestive heart failure. Dogs that have syncopal episodes during or just after coughing may have "cough drop" syndrome. Paroxysmal coughing increases the intrathoracic pressure and impedes venous return, which leads to a decrease in cardiac output. Paroxysmal coughing may increase intracranial pressure and diminish cerebral blood flow. Coughing may also increase vagal tone and cause bradycardia. Antitussive therapy with hydrocodone or butorphanol should be considered in these patients. Drug therapy should also be considered as a contributing cause of hypotension (vasodilators) or bradycardia (calcium channel blockers and beta blockers).

ECG and Radiographic Findings. ECG findings include enlargement or widening of the P wave (P pulmonale and P mitrale, respectively), tall QRS complexes in lead II (greater than 2.5 mV) indicating left ventricular enlargement, or widened QRS complexes with deep Q waves indicating biventricular enlargement. A right ventricular enlargement pattern may be seen in cases of isolated tricuspid valve endocardiosis. Sinus rhythm or sinus tachycardia may be interrupted by supraventricular or atrial premature depolarizations. When left atrial enlargement is marked, atrial fibrillation may be present. The combination of sinus arrhythmia, a wandering pacemaker, and P pulmonale are uncommon in dogs with heart failure, and such findings should lead to a reconsideration of respiratory diseases (Fig. 8–2). Thoracic radiographic findings usually include generalized cardiac enlargement, left ventricular

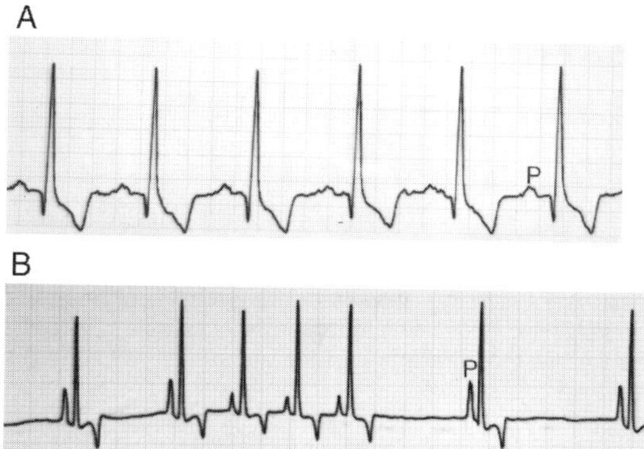

Figure 8–2. Comparison of ECG findings commonly seen in dogs with chronic valvular disease and in dogs with chronic respiratory disease. *A,* ECG, recorded at 50 mm/sec and 1 cm/mV, obtained from a dog with chronic valvular disease or endocardiosis. The ECG abnormalities include P mitrale (P wave duration = 0.06 seconds), and ventricular enlargement, as evidenced by tall R waves (R = 2.6 mV) and a wide QRS complex (0.07 seconds). ST segment slurring and/or depression is also noted. *B,* ECG, recorded at 25 mm/sec and 1 cm/mV, obtained from a dog with respiratory disease. The ECG diagnoses include sinus arrhythmia, a wandering pacemaker, and some tall P waves (0.6 mV) compatible with P pulmonale. These findings are common in animals with chronic respiratory disease.

enlargement, and left atrial enlargement. Compression of the left mainstem bronchus by left atrial enlargement, which is best appreciated on the lateral view, may contribute to coughing (Fig. 8–3). On ventrodorsal view, marked left atrial enlargement commonly causes separation of the bronchi caudal to the carina ("bowlegged cowboy sign"). Pulmonary venous distention, interstitial pulmonary edema, and, as the disease progresses, alveolar pulmonary edema may also be present. Pleural effusion is frequently present in dogs with tricuspid valve endocardiosis and concurrent ascites.

Echocardiographic Findings. Common echocardiographic findings include a volume overload to the left ventricle, thickening of the mitral valve and/or tricuspid valve, and atrial enlargement (Fig. 8–4). The left ventricular shortening fraction (per cent delta D) is typically normal or greater than normal as a result of the volume overload (Fig. 8–5). With chronic or severe valvular disease, the shortening fraction may be diminished, indicating myocardial systolic dysfunction and a poor prognosis. Dogs with rupture of a chorda tendinea may have prolapse of the mitral valve leaflet, often the anterior mitral valve leaflet, into the left atrium (Fig. 8–6). Echocardiography may also document pericardial effusion, resulting from left atrial tear or right-sided heart failure in dogs with pleural effusion and ascites.

Management. Treatment for chronic valvular disease varies (Tables 8–2 and 8–3). Dogs with a cardiac murmur but no clinical signs do not require any therapy. Dogs with early clinical find-

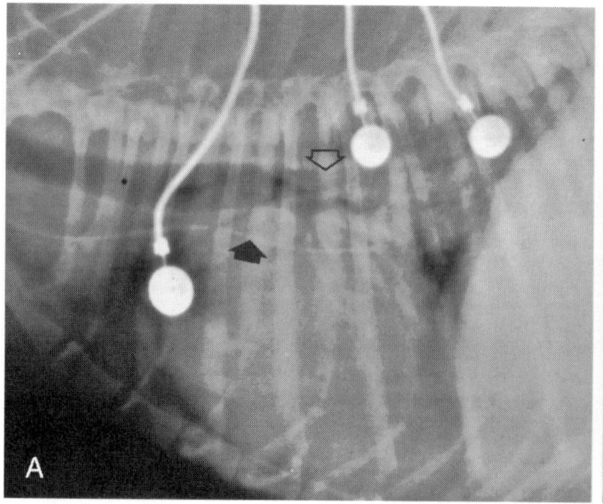

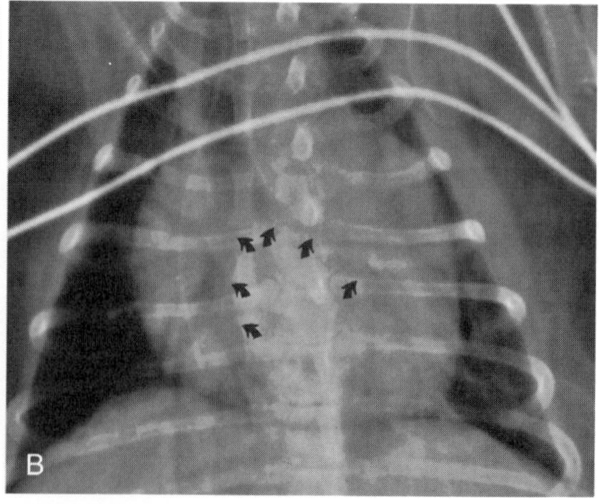

Figure 8–3. Lateral *(A)* and ventrodorsal *(B)* thoracic radiographs obtained from a cocker spaniel with chronic valvular disease and doxorubicin-induced cardiotoxicity. The cardiac silhouette is markedly enlarged, and there is an increased interstitial and alveolar pattern to the lung fields resulting from pulmonary edema, which is especially prominent in the hilar regions. The bright white lines and circles are from ECG leads used for continuous ECG monitoring. Marked elevation of the left mainstem bronchus *(open arrow),* resulting from severe left atrial enlargement, is noted on the lateral view. The jugular catheter *(solid arrow)* is positioned to allow for serial central venous pressure measurements during dobutamine infusion. On the ventrodorsal view, left atrial enlargement results in separation of the bronchi just past the tracheal bifurcation *(arrows),* which has been referred to as the "bowlegged cowboy sign."

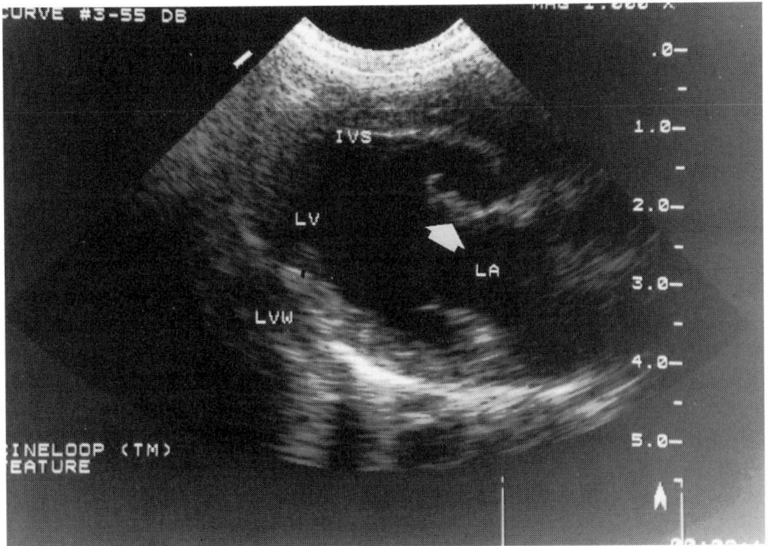

Figure 8–4. Two-dimensional echocardiogram, long-axis view, obtained from a dachshund with chronic valvular disease affecting the mitral valve. The mitral valve is severely thickened *(arrow)*, the left atrium (LA) is enlarged, and the left ventricle (LV) is dilated. IVS, Interventricular septum; LVW, left ventricular free wall.

ings of cough or dyspnea, especially nocturnal cough, may be initially treated with a low-sodium diet, diuretics, or an angiotensin converting enzyme (ACE) inhibitor. In dogs with moderate cardiac enlargement, radiographic evidence of congestive heart failure, or worsening clinical signs, additional therapies may be indicated. In addition to low-sodium diets and furosemide, exercise restriction, and vasodilator therapy should be used. The initial drug therapy choice should be an ACE inhibitor, either enalapril (0.5 mg/kg PO sid) or captopril (0.5 to 2.0 mg/kg PO tid). In dogs concurrently receiving furosemide, conservative doses of furosemide should be used to prevent hypotension. When congestive heart failure improves in response to ACE inhibitor therapy, dogs may develop hypotension, weakness, fainting, and azotemia as a result of excessive diuretic administration—i.e., the congestive heart failure has improved, but the previous dose of furosemide is no longer required. Simply reducing the dose of furosemide will resolve azotemia and improve clinical signs.

Many cardiologists also employ digoxin in dogs with chronic valvular disease and moderate cardiac failure. Some believe that digoxin should be

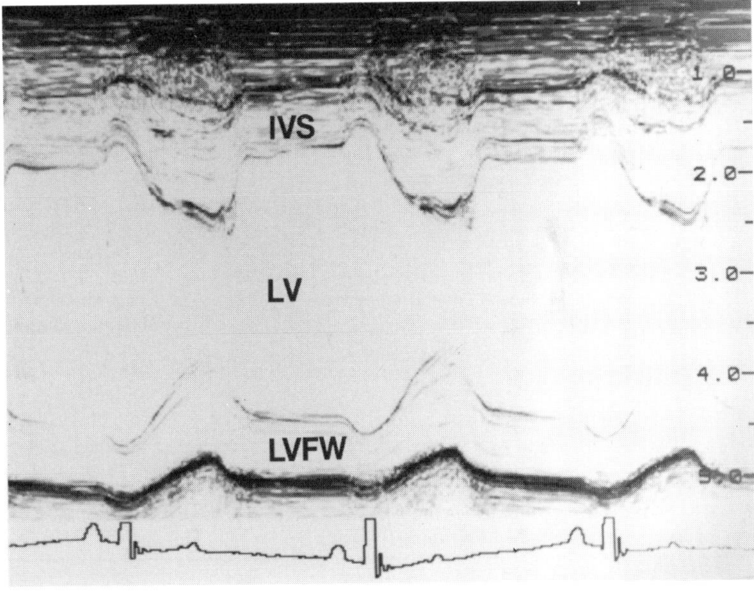

Figure 8–5. M-mode echocardiogram from a dog with chronic valvular disease documents volume overload and preserved myocardial function. The shortening fraction was 52 per cent (per cent delta D = 52 per cent). IVS, Interventricular septum; LV, left ventricular cavity; LVFW, left ventricular free wall.

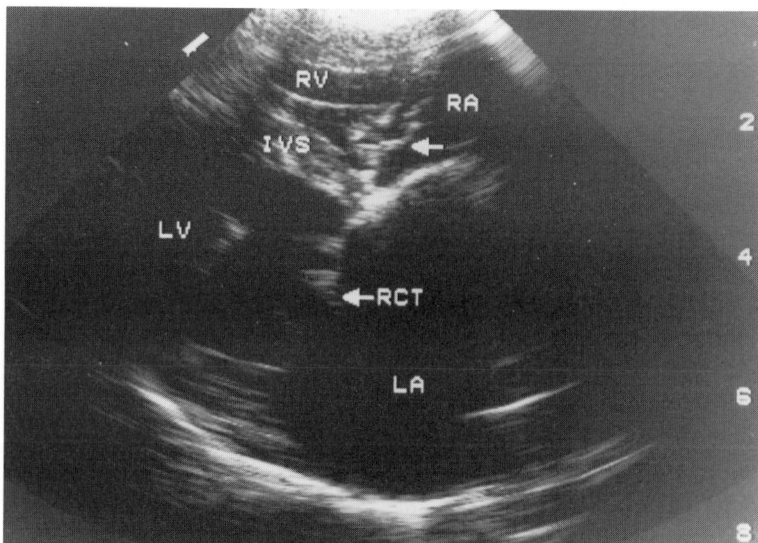

Figure 8–6. Two-dimensional echocardiogram, long-axis view, from a dog with chronic valvular disease and ruptured chordae tendineae (RCT) in both the mitral and tricuspid valves *(arrows)*. The affected leaflets prolapse back into the respective atria. The left atrium (LA) is massively enlarged. IVS, Interventricular septum; LV, left ventricular cavity; RA, right atrium; RV, right ventricle.

limited to the later stages of the disease when heart failure is refractory to therapy or when echocardiographic findings suggest diminished systolic function (Keene and Rush, 1989; Kittleson, 1988). Some evidence suggests that digoxin therapy may be useful for modulation of neural stimulation to the heart and that digitalis's positive inotropic effect is not the only benefit of the drug (Gheorghiade and Ferguson, 1991). In dogs with severe chronic valvular disease, additional therapies include oxygen therapy, digitalis, and, where intensive care monitoring is available, aggressive therapy such as dobutamine, dopamine, or sodium nitroprusside.

Arrhythmias in Chronic Valvular Disease. Arrhythmias may be identified at any stage of chronic valvular disease. Most frequently these arrhythmias are isolated supraventricular prema-

TABLE 8–2. MANAGEMENT OF CANINE CHRONIC VALVULAR DISEASE

CLINICAL SIGNS	THERAPY
Cardiac murmur; no clinical signs	No therapy or moderate sodium-restricted diet
Nocturnal cough, mild exercise intolerance	Furosemide, 1–2 mg/kg sid Enalapril, 0.5 mg/kg sid Moderate sodium-restricted diet Moderate exercise restriction
Dyspnea, frequent cough, moderate exercise intolerance	Furosemide, 2–4 mg/kg sid or bid Enalapril, 0.5 mg/kg sid Strict sodium-restricted diet Moderate exercise restriction ± Hydralazine, 1–2 mg/kg bid ± Digoxin
Severe dyspnea, marked exercise intolerance, severe pulmonary edema, anorexia	Furosemide, 4 mg/kg q 2 hr IV until improved Enalapril, 0.5 mg/kg q 12 hr Marked sodium restriction Cage rest Hydralazine, 1–2 mg/kg bid Nitroglycerine, ¼–½ inch transcutaneously q 6 hr Digoxin Dobutamine infusion, 2.5–10 μg/kg/min IV
If pleural effusion is present, thoracocentesis is performed to remove as much fluid as possible.	
If ascites is compressing the diaphragm, abdominocentesis is performed to remove enough fluid to improve ventilatory effort.	

IV, intravenous administration.

TABLE 8–3. ARRHYTHMIAS AND MANAGEMENT FOR DOGS WITH DILATED CARDIOMYOPATHY AND CHRONIC VALVULAR DISEASE

ARRHYTHMIA	COMMENTS	MANAGEMENT
Supraventricular premature beats	May not require therapy if clinical signs are infrequent or absent	Digoxin or beta blocker or diltiazem
Supraventricular tachycardia	Usually requires therapy	Digoxin or beta blocker or diltiazem or verapamil
Atrial fibrillation	Reduce heart rate/ventricular response to <160 beats/min	Digoxin first; if heart rate >160 beats/min after 5–7 days, add beta blocker or diltiazem
Ventricular premature complexes	May not require therapy if clinical signs are infrequent or absent	Procainamide or quinidine or tocainide or beta blocker
Ventricular tachycardia	Aggressive treatment is indicated; predisposition to sudden death	Procainamide or quinidine or tocainide; add beta blocker if control is inadequate

ture depolarizations. In these instances specific antiarrhythmic drug therapy is usually not required. When supraventricular arrhythmias are sustained, frequent, or contributing to clinical signs, therapy should consist of digoxin, beta blockers, or calcium channel blockers (Table 8–4). For supraventricular arrhythmias and concurrent congestive heart failure, digitalis is usually the preferred drug. When congestive heart failure does not accompany the arrhythmias, calcium channel blockers (diltiazem at 0.5 to 1.5 mg/kg PO tid) or beta blockers (propranolol at 0.2 mg/kg orally, with the dose adjusted upward until the arrhythmia resolves and/or rate reduction occurs) are useful. Although more expensive, $beta_1$-specific blockers such as atenolol or metoprolol (initial dose, 0.5 to 1 mg/kg PO bid for each blocker) may be used. When atrial fibrillation complicates chronic valvular disease, digitalis should be the initial drug of choice. In most instances, routine oral digitalization is adequate. The desired end point of antiarrhythmic therapy is to slow atrioventricular (AV) nodal conduction to a rate of 160 beats/minute or less. When the rate is in excess of 160 beats/min after 5 to 7 days of digoxin administration, a beta blocker or calcium channel blocker (see Table 8–4) is indicated. Because atrial fibrillation is usually accompanied by congestive heart failure, caution is advised when administering beta blockers or calcium channel blockers, as both groups of drugs have significant negative inotropic effects and may worsen the congestive heart failure.

Complications of Endocardiosis. Potential complications of endocardiosis include rupture of a chorda tendinea and left atrial tear. A ruptured chorda tendinea appears to be much more common than previously believed, and immediate death may not occur. However, such rupture is still a common cause for acute deterioration. There is no specific therapy to treat ruptured chorda tendinea other than the therapies indicated earlier. Left atrial tear as another potential complication of endocardiosis results in cardiac tamponade. Clinical findings suggestive of left atrial tear include diminished intensity of the cardiac murmur, tachycardia, recent onset of atrial arrhythmias, jugular vein distention, weak femoral pulses, and evidence of forward heart failure. Radiographic findings include diminished pul-

TABLE 8–4. COMPARISON OF DRUGS USED TO TREAT SUPRAVENTRICULAR ARRHYTHMIAS

DRUG	MECHANISM OF ACTION	INOTROPIC EFFECT	VASODILATOR EFFECT	COMMENTS
Digoxin	Blocks Na^+-K^+-ATPase; vagomimetic effect	+ +	±	First choice if CHF present
Propranolol	$Beta_1$ and $beta_2$ blockade	–	–	Less expensive beta blocker Bronchoconstriction
Atenolol	$Beta_1$, blocker	–	±	Renal elimination
Metoprolol	$Beta_1$ blocker	–	±	Hepatic elimination
Diltiazem	Calcium channel blocker	–	+	Second choice if CHF present
Verapamil	Calcium channel blocker	– – –	+	Avoid in CHF

ATPase, Adenosine triphosphatase; CHF, congestive heart failure.

monary vascular markings in combination with dramatic enlargement of the cardiac silhouette and relative loss of chamber definition, although left atrial enlargement is still commonly seen. Diagnosis may be confirmed by echocardiography. Pericardiocentesis is the therapy of choice when left atrial tear results in life-threatening cardiac tamponade.

Bacterial Endocarditis

Bacterial endocarditis is an uncommon disease in dogs (Woodfield and Sisson, 1989). Bacteremia, a prerequisite for the development of bacterial endocarditis, may result from a variety of infections, including prostate or urinary tract infections, pyoderma, pneumonia, and dental infections. The actual site of original infection, however, is rarely determined. Bacterial colonization of the valve requires bacteremia and occurs more readily in dogs with a pre-existing cardiac lesion, valvular damage, or abnormal blood flow. Dogs with subaortic stenosis, for example, are predisposed. Additional predisposing factors include immunosuppressive therapy, infectious diseases causing immunosuppression, intravenous catheter use, surgical procedures, and concurrent systemic disease. The mitral and aortic valves are most commonly affected in older dogs. Common organisms include *Staphylococcus aureus, Streptococcus, Corynebacterium, Pseudomonas,* and *Escherichia coli.*

Clinical Features. Bacterial endocarditis is difficult to confirm and should be considered in any older dog with cardiac involvement and polysystemic signs, fever, and immunologic disorders. Affected dogs may have fever, a new cardiac murmur, tachypnea, myalgia or shifting leg lameness, poorly localized pain, urinary tract infection, or evidence of embolization. The presence of a diastolic decrescendo murmur of aortic insufficiency is strongly suggestive of bacterial endocarditis.

Diagnostic Testing. Radiographic findings are nonspecific and may include cardiomegaly, congestive heart failure, or pneumonia. ECG findings may include ventricular or supraventricular arrhythmias, atrial or ventricular enlargement patterns, and AV block or bundle branch block. Multiple bright echoes on affected cardiac valves may be noted. Laboratory abnormalities may include hypoproteinemia, elevated levels of serum alkaline phosphatase and liver enzymes, azotemia, pyuria, bacteriuria, and hematuria. The complete blood cell (CBC) count is usually abnormal, with leukocytosis with a left shift, anemia, and/or monocytosis. Blood cultures are needed to confirm the diagnosis and determine appropriate antimicrobial therapy. At least three blood culture specimens should be obtained, with at least 1 hour separation time between specimens. Both aerobic and anaerobic cultures should be obtained. Positive blood cultures are seen in 60 to 85 per cent of confirmed cases.

Treatment. Intravenous broad-spectrum antimicrobials should be initiated while blood culture results are pending. Appropriate empirical choices include combinations of ampicillin and amikacin or cephalothin and gentamicin. When anaerobic infections are suspected, metronidazole may be added to the regimen. Imipenem may be used if the initial therapeutic response is considered inadequate. Treatment should be continued for 6 to 8 weeks based on the results of bacterial culture and sensitivity testing from blood cultures. Congestive heart failure should be treated as previously described for chronic valvular disease. Antimicrobial prophylaxis is recommended for dogs with congenital heart disease or other cardiovascular abnormalities that undergo procedures likely to result in bacteremia (e.g., dentistry and tooth extraction, endoscopy, urogenital manipulations, gastrointestinal surgery).

Dilated Cardiomyopathy

Dilated cardiomyopathy is the second most frequently encountered cardiac disease in geriatric dogs (Van Vleet and Ferrans, 1986). Giant breed dilated cardiomyopathy is recognized in Great Danes, Irish wolfhounds, St. Bernards, German shepherds, Newfoundlands, and other giant breed dogs. Doberman pinschers also commonly develop cardiomyopathy, and some information indicates that subclinical disease may be present in many Dobermans long before signs of congestive heart failure exist (O'Grady and Horne, 1991). Boxers (Keene et al, 1991) and English and American cocker spaniels also develop cardiomyopathy, more often in geriatric individuals (Kittleson et al, 1991).

Clinical Features. Signs of dilated cardiomyopathy may include anorexia, exercise intolerance, episodic rear limb weakness, episodes of collapse or syncope, and difficulty breathing. The most common presenting complaint is coughing or gagging. Tachypnea or dyspnea is common in dogs with congestive heart failure. Mucous membrane color may be normal or slightly gray or

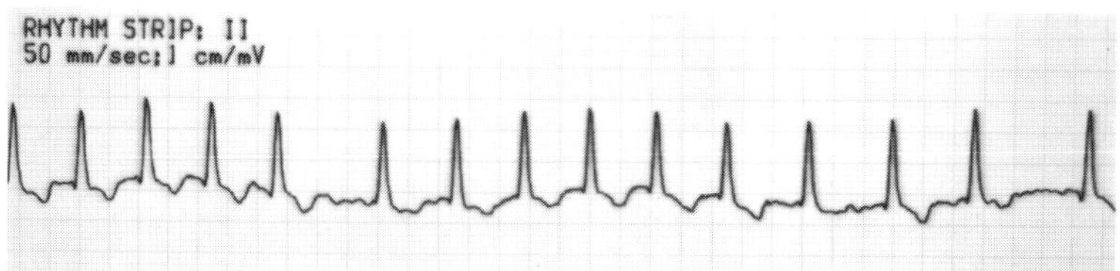

Figure 8–7. ECG obtained from a dog with atrial fibrillation and dilated cardiomyopathy. The heart rate is 250 beats/min. At rapid ventricular rates, the rhythm is more regular; however, the use of calibers helps confirm the irregularity of the rhythm and the lack of P waves in the baseline.

ashen with a slow capillary refill time. Arterial pulses are usually weaker than normal, and in many instances, variable pulse quality is present, signaling the presence of cardiac arrhythmia. Jugular vein distention or a positive hepatojugular reflex may be present. Dogs with right-sided congestive heart failure have hepatomegaly, splenomegaly, and/or ascites. Common abnormalities on auscultation include the presence of a systolic regurgitant murmur, usually over the mitral and/or tricuspid valve locations. Other common findings include the presence of an S_3 gallop, irregular cardiac rhythm, and pulse deficits. Pulmonary crackles may be ausculted in dogs with pulmonary edema, and lung sounds may be absent ventrally in dogs with pleural effusion.

ECG and Radiographic Findings. Typical ECG findings in dogs with dilated cardiomyopathy include P mitrale (prolonged P wave duration), tall and/or widened QRS complexes, nonspecific ST segment changes, and a left axis shift in the frontal plane. Supraventricular premature depolarizations, atrial fibrillation, ventricular premature depolarizations, and ventricular tachycardia are common arrhythmias. Giant breed dogs with dilated cardiomyopathy are more likely to have atrial fibrillation (Fig. 8–7) and/or tall R waves in lead II. Atrial premature complexes are particularly common in cocker spaniels with dilated cardiomyopathy. Doberman pinschers commonly have ventricular arrhythmias, P mitrale, and wide QRS complexes, although atrial fibrillation and tall R waves may also be observed. The ventricular arrhythmias in affected Doberman pinschers often have a negative QRS deflection in lead II, indicating a left ventricular origin (Fig. 8–8). Affected boxers frequently have normal or low-voltage QRS complexes and may present with ventricular arrhythmias as the predominant ECG disturbance. Ventricular premature complexes in boxers are commonly upright, or positive, in lead II, with a left bundle branch block appearance, which indicates origination from the right ventricle.

Thoracic radiographic changes include generalized cardiac enlargement, left atrial enlargement, and signs of either left-sided or right-sided congestive heart failure. Left-sided heart failure may be manifested as pulmonary venous distention, pulmonary interstitial markings resulting from early edema, peribronchial cuffing (especially in Doberman pinschers), or alveolar edema in dogs with severe congestive heart failure (Fig. 8–9). Signs of right-sided heart failure may include a dilated caudal vena cava, hepatomegaly, ascites, and, in some cases, pleural effusion. Cardiac enlargement may not be obvious in affected Doberman pinschers.

Echocardiographic Findings. Echocardiographic findings include two-dimensional evidence of dilation and enlargement of all four chambers (Fig. 8–10). M-mode measurements confirm dilation of the left ventricle and left atrium. Poor myocardial systolic function is most

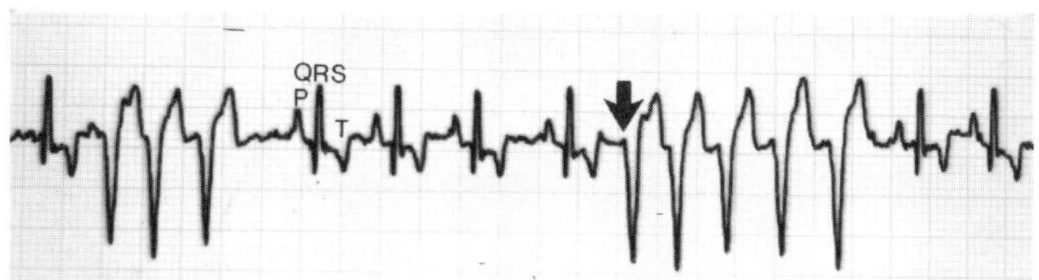

Figure 8–8. Paroxysmal ventricular tachycardia in a Doberman pinscher with dilated cardiomyopathy. Sinus rhythm at a rate of 150 beats/min is interrupted by ventricular tachycardia at a rate of 240 beats/min *(arrow)*. Recorded at 25 mm/sec and 1 cm/mV.

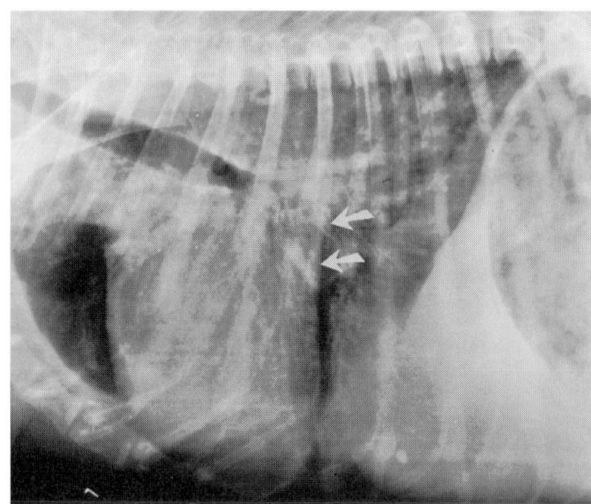

Figure 8–9. Lateral thoracic radiograph from a Doberman pinscher with dilated cardiomyopathy. Moderate generalized cardiomegaly is evident with left atrial enlargement at the caudal aspect of the cardiac silhouette *(arrows).* Hilar pulmonary edema is noted as an increased interstitial, early alveolar, and increased peribronchial pattern.

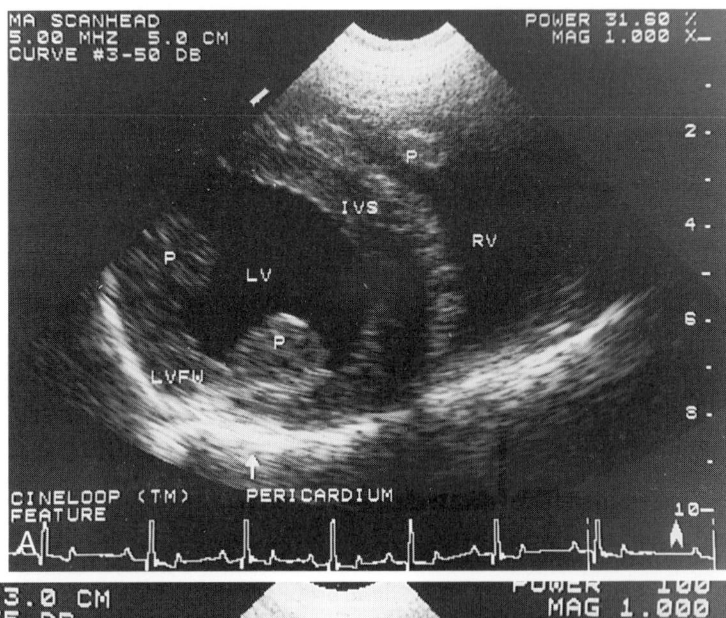

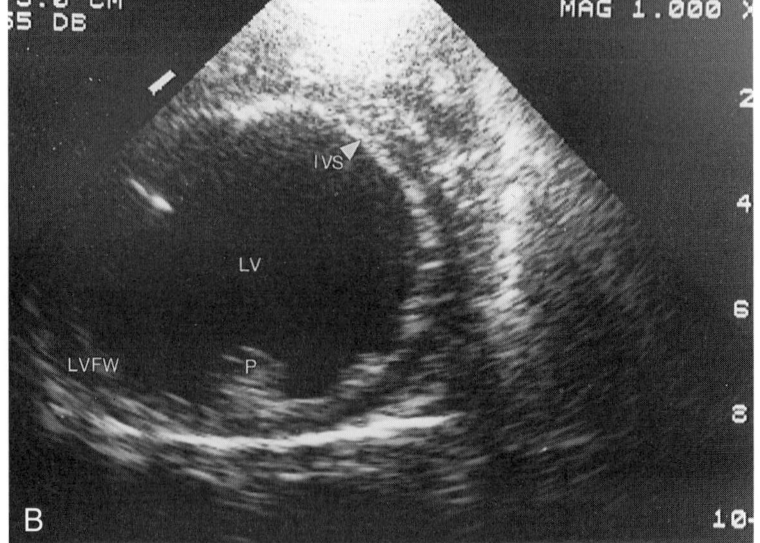

Figure 8–10. Comparison of the echocardiographic findings from the short-axis view through the left ventricle in a healthy dog *(A)* and in a dog with dilated cardiomyopathy *(B).* In comparison with the healthy dog, the dog with dilated cardiomyopathy has thinned ventricular walls (IVS, interventricular septum; LVFW, left ventricular free wall), a dilated left ventricular cavity (LV, left ventricle), and small papillary muscles (P). RV, Right ventricle.

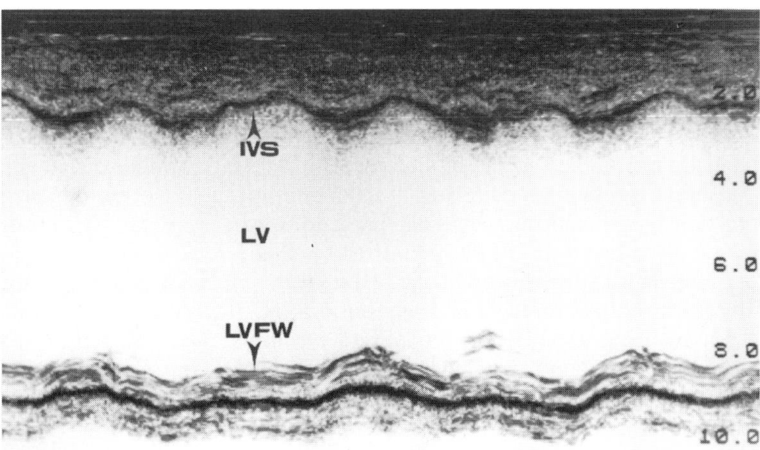

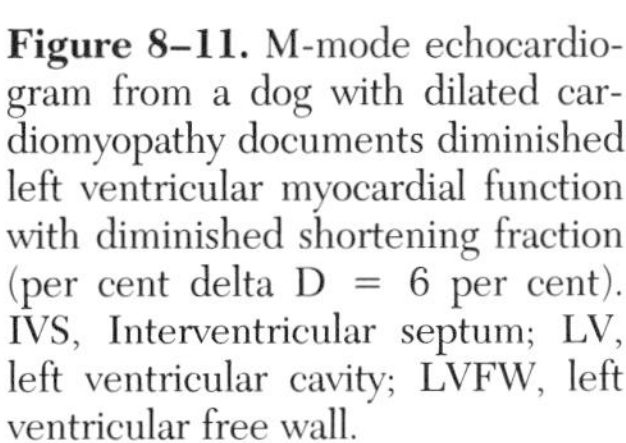
Figure 8–11. M-mode echocardiogram from a dog with dilated cardiomyopathy documents diminished left ventricular myocardial function with diminished shortening fraction (per cent delta D = 6 per cent). IVS, Interventricular septum; LV, left ventricular cavity; LVFW, left ventricular free wall.

evident when evaluating the left ventricle, where the shortening fraction is diminished (per cent delta D = less than 28 per cent) (Fig. 8–11). The normal shortening fraction in Doberman pinschers may be significantly less than other breeds (O'Grady and Horne, 1991), and Doberman pinschers with isolated dilated cardiomyopathy (without concurrent endocardiosis) and congestive heart failure typically have a shortening fraction less than 20 per cent. Additional findings include diminished motion of the aortic root, increased E-point to septal separation, and a dilated end-diastolic left ventricular size.

Management. Treatment of dilated cardiomyopathy depends on the clinical findings and the presence or absence of congestive heart failure and arrhythmias (Table 8–5). Congestive heart failure is typically treated with a low-sodium diet, moderate exercise restriction, furosemide, and an ACE inhibitor or other vasodilator. Most cardiologists would also initiate treatment with digoxin unless ventricular arrhythmias worsen after initiation of the drug (Gheorghiade and Ferguson, 1991). Digoxin is definitely indicated for treatment of atrial fibrillation and frequent or symptomatic supraventricular arrhythmias. Dogs with severe congestive heart failure should be treated with high doses of furosemide in combination with vasodilators and potent inotropic agents. The preferred inotropic agent is dobutamine (administered by continuous-rate infusion at 2.5 to 10 μg/kg/min), which is initiated at 2.5 μg/kg/min in a small volume of intravenous fluids and accompanied by ECG monitoring and, where available, blood pressure monitoring. If the response is inadequate after 1 to 2 hours, the dose is titrated upward, usually at increments of 2.5 μg/kg/min. Effective response

TABLE 8–5. MANAGEMENT OF CANINE DILATED CARDIOMYOPATHY

SIGNS	DRUGS	ANCILLARY
No CHF	Digoxin ± ACE inhibitor	Moderate sodium-restricted diet Moderate exercise restriction
Mild pulmonary edema	Furosemide, 1–2 mg/kg bid ACE inhibitor Digoxin	Moderate sodium-restricted diet
Moderate pulmonary edema	Furosemide, 2–4 mg/kg bid Digoxin ACE inhibitor ± Nitroglycerine	Low-sodium diet Marked exercise restriction ± Oxygen
Severe pulmonary edema with signs of low cardiac output (pallor, hypothermia, weakness)	Furosemide, 4 mg/kg IV q 2 hr until stable ACE inhibitor Digoxin Dobutamine Nitroglycerine	Low-sodium diet Cage rest Oxygen

ACE, Angiotensin converting enzyme; CHF, congestive heart failure; IV, intravenous administration.

includes improved peripheral perfusion, increased body temperature, reduced dyspnea, onset of diuresis, and maintenance of a mean blood pressure above 70 mm Hg and a systolic pressure in excess of 95 mm Hg. Dobutamine infusion is typically maintained for 3 days along with ECG and blood pressure monitoring. As dobutamine infusion is reduced on the third day, additional medications begun on day 1 or 2 of the infusion (e.g., enalapril, digoxin, or other vasodilators or diuretics) should be reaching therapeutic levels.

Carnitine and Taurine. Decreased carnitine levels inhibit adenosine triphosphate (ATP) production and diminish normal myocardial function. Carnitine deficiency in the myocardium may play an important role in contributing to canine dilated cardiomyopathy, at least in some forms (Keene et al, 1991). Although dietary requirements for carnitine are unknown, dogs seem to have a greater need than other species because of the relatively poor reabsorption of carnitine by the renal tubular cells. Although the association between carnitine and canine dilated cardiomyopathy is incomplete, carnitine supplementation (2 g of carnitine PO tid) may be beneficial, especially for large breed dogs. The L isomer of carnitine, the only form that is well utilized by dogs, can be purchased at health food stores. An alternative is to add lean ground beef to the diet several times per week. Although the association of taurine deficiency with cardiomyopathy has been an historical phenomenon in cats, one study found low plasma taurine concentrations in American cocker spaniels with dilated cardiomyopathy (Kittleson et al, 1991). Although this preliminary report had a small number of dogs, it should alert veterinarians to the potential role of taurine and/or carnitine deficiency in cardiomyopathy.

Arrhythmias in Dilated Cardiomyopathy. Atrial fibrillation should be treated as described in the section on chronic valvular disease. Digoxin should be initiated and a beta blocker or calcium channel blocker added, with the dose of the calcium channel blocker or the beta blocker progressively increased until the ventricular rate is reduced to approximately 160 beats/min or less. In general, the lower the heart rate, the better the prognosis, although many dogs with severe heart failure do not tolerate heart rates of 100 beats/min or less. Ventricular arrhythmias may be treated with class I antiarrhythmics (e.g., lidocaine, procainamide, quinidine, mexiletine, tocainide), with or without the addition of beta blockers (e.g., propranolol, metoprolol, atenolol). Our preferred approach is to initially treat with slow-release procainamide (6 to 20 mg/kg tid PO) and determine the response after several days of therapy with procainamide and other medications for congestive heart failure. If the arrhythmia is not controlled, a beta blocker is then added (usually metoprolol for Doberman pinschers and giant breeds with cardiomyopathy and atenolol for boxers with cardiomyopathy and ventricular arrhythmias). The defined end point for adequate treatment of ventricular arrhythmias is unclear; we usually aim to have fewer than 20 ventricular premature complexes per minute and to eliminate repetitive forms of ventricular tachycardia. For dogs with symptomatic arrhythmias or who are predisposed to sudden death (especially Doberman pinschers and boxers), we currently recommend continuing antiarrhythmic therapy for life.

Cardiac Neoplasia

Dogs with cardiac neoplasms may be presented for clinical signs resulting from cardiac arrhythmias, pericardial effusion, or obstruction to blood flow by an intracardiac mass. Common primary cardiac neoplasms include hemangiosarcoma, mesothelioma, fibrosarcoma, myxoma, thyroid carcinoma, rhabdomyosarcoma, and heart base tumors (e.g., chemodectoma). Neoplasms that metastasize to the heart include hemangiosarcoma, lymphosarcoma, mammary and thyroid gland adenocarcinoma, and melanoma.

Clinical Features. Presenting complaints may include weight loss, lethargy, anorexia, tachypnea, or dyspnea; in the case of metastatic disease, the dog may be presented for signs referable to the primary neoplasm. More specific signs resulting from the cardiac neoplasm include weakness, syncope or collapse, and abdominal distention. Potential physical examination findings include arrhythmias, dyspnea or tachypnea, weak arterial pulses, systolic or diastolic cardiac murmur, or signs referable to pericardial effusion, such as ascites or hepatomegaly, jugular distention, muffled heart sounds, or pulsus paradoxus.

ECG and Radiographic Findings. Supraventricular or ventricular arrhythmias may result from irritation of local myocardial tissue. Large cardiac neoplasms can cause conduction blocks through the AV node or bundle branches. Intracardiac masses that cause obstruction to blood flow can lead to atrial or ventricular enlargement patterns as a result of compensatory cardiac enlargement or hypertrophy. Pericardial effusion can cause low-voltage QRS complexes, ST segment elevation, and electrical alternans. The most striking radiographic findings are seen in cases of pericardial effusion, in which a globoid cardiac silhouette, enlarged caudal vena cava, pleural effusion, hepatomegaly, or ascites may be noted. Heart base tumors may cause elevation of the trachea and displacement of the heart or other structures near the heart base. Pulmonary edema is an infrequent occurrence with cardiac neoplasia. When echocardiography is not available, nonselective angiography can be very useful to outline intracardiac filling defects, pericardial effusion, or the vascular "blush" of a cardiac mass.

Echocardiographic Findings. The best diagnostic test for cardiac neoplasia is the echocardiogram. Chamber enlargement resulting from obstruction to blood flow, pericardial effusion, and intracardiac masses are readily identified in most instances (Fig. 8–12). The echocardiogram is less frequently able to document small cardiac metastases originating from extracardiac neoplasms.

Management. Specific management of dogs with cardiac neoplasms is dependent on the presenting complaints, tumor type, and clinical signs that are manifested. Arrhythmias should be treated with appropriate antiarrhythmic drugs. Pericardial effusion should be removed by pericardiocentesis; specific management of cardiac neoplasms causing pericardial effusion is discussed later. Intracardiac masses causing obstruction to blood flow usually require surgical intervention (Bright et al, 1990). These surgeries are usually complex and are often only palliative, as the entire mass can rarely be resected, and regrowth is likely.

Pericardial Effusion

Pericardial disease is an increasingly recognized cause of syncope/collapse and heart failure in the geriatric dog population (Thomas, 1989). The most common cause of pericardial effusion in dogs is cardiac neoplasia. Other causes include idiopathic pericardial effusion, left atrial tear secondary to chronic valvular disease, coagulopathies, uremia, and congestive heart failure. Of the cardiac neoplasms causing pericardial effusion, the most common is hemangiosarcoma located in either the right atrium or at the junction of the right ventricle and the right atrium (Aronsohn, 1985).

Clinical Features. Golden retrievers and German shepherd dogs are predisposed to both idiopathic pericardial effusion and right atrial hemangiosarcoma (Rush and Atkins, 1991). Diseases resulting in hemorrhage into the pericardial space often cause acute collapse and weakness. Effusions of a more chronic nature can also lead to these signs; however, owners more frequently report anorexia, lethargy, exercise intolerance, abdominal distention, or tachypnea. Muffled heart sounds is a common finding. Cardiac murmurs may be present in dogs with chronic valvular disease and left atrial tear, although the murmur may be softer than previously noted. Tachypnea, dyspnea, hepatomegaly, ascites, and

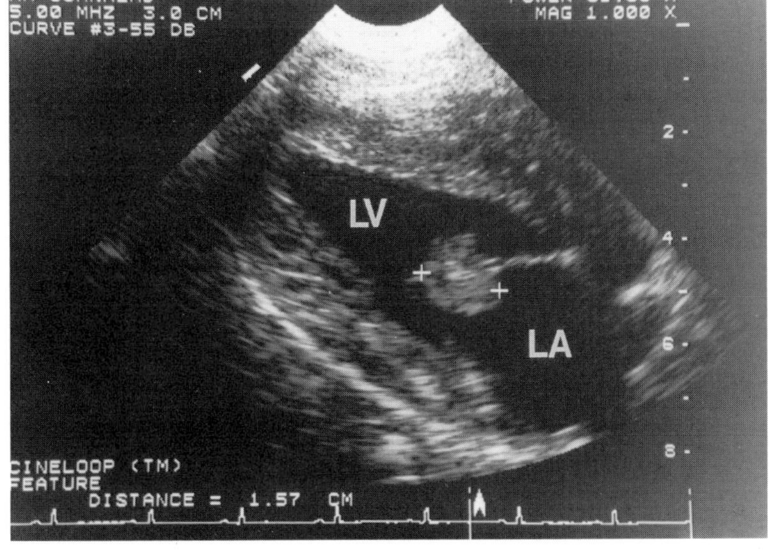

Figure 8–12. Mass lesion on the mitral valve leaflet viewed from a two-dimensional, long-axis echocardiogram. The mass resulted in mitral valve insufficiency. At autopsy the mass was identified as a hemangiosarcoma. LA, left atrium; LV, left ventricle.

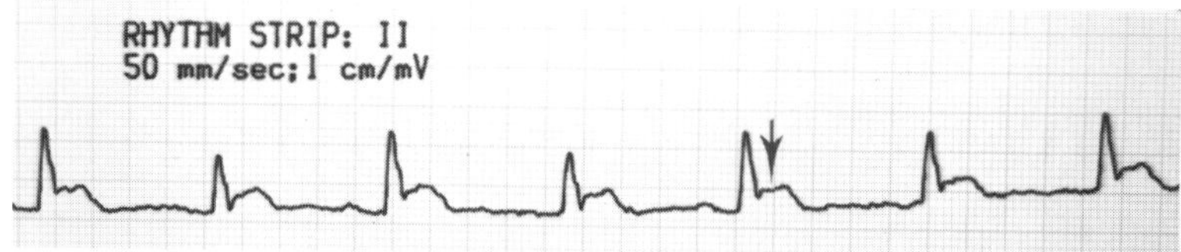

Figure 8–13. ECG obtained from a dog with pericardial effusion. QRS voltage in all leads was less than 1 mV, ST segment elevation is noted *(arrow)* in comparison with the TP baseline, and electrical alternans is also present, noted as an alteration in QRS height on every other beat.

jugular venous distention are more common in cases of chronic pericardial effusion. Changes in ventricular filling that attend respiration may cause pulsus paradoxus, with weaker femoral arterial pulses noted during inspiration.

ECG and Radiographic Findings. ECG findings in pericardial disease include low-voltage QRS complexes, electrical alternans, and ST segment changes (often ST segment elevation) (Fig. 8–13). Although some dogs with pericardial effusion may have all of the aforementioned ECG changes, any combination or none of the findings may be present. Radiographic findings include a globoid cardiac silhouette with lack of cardiac chamber definition (Fig. 8–14). Dogs with acute effusion may have mild to moderate cardiomegaly.

Echocardiographic Findings. Echocardiographic findings characteristic of pericardial effusion include an echo-free space between the pericardium and epicardium (Fig. 8–15). The right ventricle and right atrium are more easily seen than in an unaffected dog. Two-dimensional echocardiography is also useful in determining the cause of the pericardial effusion.

Management. With the exception of dogs with left atrial tear or severe coagulopathy who are tolerating their effusions well, pericardiocentesis is the treatment of choice in dogs with cardiac tamponade. Pericardiocentesis can be performed with relative safety if ECG monitoring can be performed. Pericardiocentesis is performed from the right thorax, usually with the dog in sternal recumbency. The area from above the costochondral junction down to the sternum is clipped and aseptically prepared. A long (2 to 5 cm), large-gauge (14- to 18-gauge) needle or catheter is inserted through the skin at the fifth or sixth intercostal space and is slowly advanced into the pericardial sac. Simultaneous ECG mon-

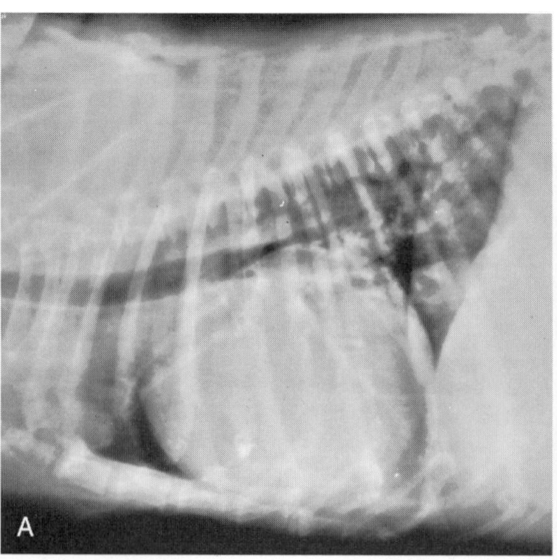

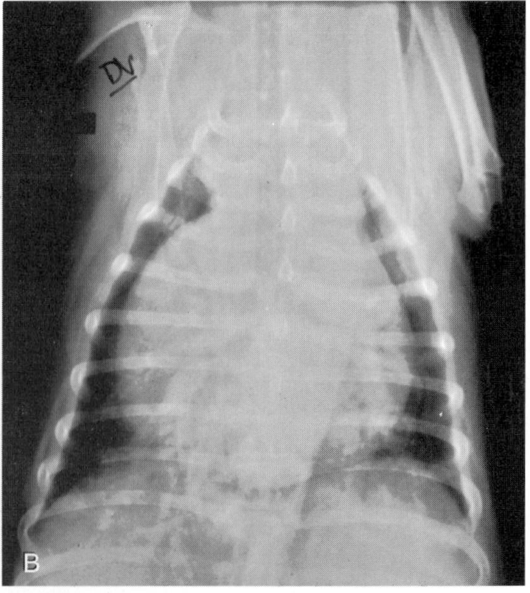

Figure 8–14. Lateral *(A)* and dorsoventral *(B)* thoracic radiographs obtained from a dog with a large volume of pericardial effusion. The markedly enlarged, globe-shaped cardiac silhouette fails to show chamber definition. The caudal vena cava is dilated, and the dog had ascites.

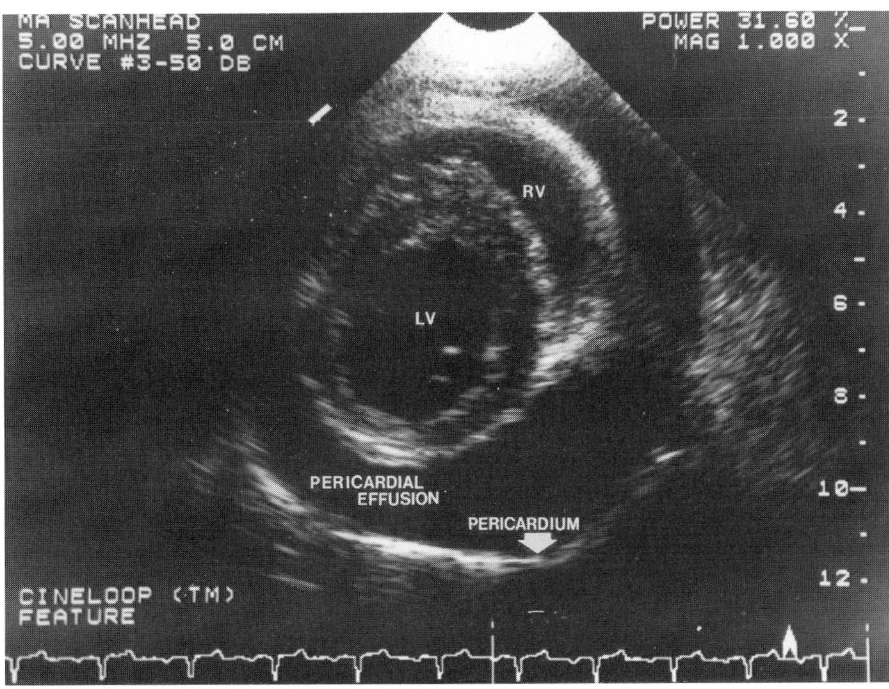

Figure 8–15. Two-dimensional echocardiogram from a dog with pericardial effusion. Note the echo-free space between the pericardium and the ventricular myocardium. LV, Left ventricle; RV, right ventricle.

itoring is performed to monitor for the development of ventricular arrhythmias. Ventricular arrhythmias usually indicate that the needle or catheter is against the ventricular wall and should be retracted a short distance. Pericardiocentesis should be performed as both a therapeutic maneuver to remove effusion and as a diagnostic procedure. Fluid analysis including cytologic analysis should be performed, although cytology is rarely able to discriminate between neoplastic and idiopathic pericardial effusion (Sisson et al, 1984). Bacterial culture and sensitivity testing should be performed if indicated by cytologic analysis or clinical presentation. Blood gas analysis has been proposed as a method to discriminate between neoplastic and inflammatory effusions, with the latter having a pH less than 7.1 (Edwards, 1991).

Specific therapy for pericardial effusion depends on the underlying cause. Those dogs with an identifiable underlying disease (i.e., uremia, coagulopathy, vitamin K antagonist intoxication) should have the underlying disease aggressively treated. Dogs with idiopathic pericardial effusion may respond to a single pericardiocentesis. These dogs may be treated with pericardiocentesis alone or pericardiocentesis in combination with intrapericardial or systemic administration of corticosteroids. Clinical trials demonstrating efficacy of corticosteroids are not currently available. Subtotal pericardiectomy is considered to be the best therapeutic option in cases when pericardial effusion returns after more than one pericardiocentesis (Mattahiesen and Lammerding, 1985). Surgery is often curative, although some dogs have recurrent pleural effusion after pericardiectomy. Dogs with cardiac neoplasms may be managed by sequential pericardiocentesis or surgery. Dogs with heart base tumors often do well for a prolonged time after pericardiectomy, as these masses are usually slow growing and slow to metastasize. Once the pericardium is removed, the pleural cavity can often accommodate the fluid produced by the tumor. Cardiac hemangiosarcomas with pericardial effusion are usually managed with repeated pericardiocentesis performed when needed, as indicated by recurrence of clinical signs. Surgery can be performed in cases whose owners wish to "do everything." The primary hemangiosarcoma may be resectable by amputation of the right atrial appendage. Most are not resectable, however, and simple pericardiectomy may allow for hemorrhagic diathesis into the thoracic cavity. Palliative surgery can be attempted by enclosing the mass within a pericardial "flap" by suturing the pericardium to the epicardial surface of the heart around the mass. This technique prevents cardiac tamponade, and hemorrhage from the mass is held within the "pocket," preventing blood loss into the thoracic cavity.

Cardiac Arrhythmias

Older dogs may be presented for signs related to cardiac arrhythmias. Common arrhythmias in aged dogs include ventricular tachycardia, atrial fibrillation, and bradyarrhythmias (e.g., sick sinus syndrome, AV block).

Ventricular Arrhythmias

ECG Findings. Ventricular arrhythmias, or premature depolarization originating from the ventricles, are identified by their wide and bizarre morphologic appearance (see Fig. 8–8). The QRS complex may be upright, negative, or nearly isoelectric, but the T wave is typically large and in the opposite direction of the largest portion of the QRS complex. The normal ST segment seen in the sinus beats is typically absent in ventricular premature depolarizations. Ventricular arrhythmias in runs or paroxysms of three or more are identified as ventricular tachycardia.

Management. Treatment of ventricular arrhythmias in aged dogs is determined by the presence or absence of clinical signs and accompanying myocardial, valvular, or pericardial disease. The initial goal should be to identify underlying cardiac enlargement, congestive heart failure, or myocardial disease. Dogs with underlying cardiac enlargement or congestive heart failure should be aggressively treated for ventricular arrhythmias. Noncardiac conditions that are commonly associated with ventricular arrhythmias include hypovolemia, splenic mass, gastric dilatation/volvulus, trauma, neurologic disease, hypertension, and adrenal gland disease. When ventricular arrhythmias are found in the absence of underlying cardiac disease, treatment of the arrhythmia may not be required. Isolated ventricular premature depolarizations or ventricular arrhythmias occurring at slow heart rates (less than 140 beats/min) may not require treatment, especially if an underlying cause can be identified and eliminated. Ventricular arrhythmias that result in clinical signs of fainting, weakness, collapse, or diminished forward blood flow should be aggressively treated. Similarly, ventricular tachycardia at rates exceeding 200 beats/min should almost always be treated.

For short-term management of ventricular arrhythmias, an intravenous bolus of lidocaine should be administered (2 to 4 mg/kg IV) and followed by a continuous rate infusion of lidocaine at 40 to 80 μg/kg/min. Many dogs fail to respond to lidocaine or have only an initial transient response. Additional drugs to control ventricular arrhythmias include procainamide, propranolol, and analgesic medications (e.g., butorphanol, buprenorphine). In most instances, ventricular arrhythmias resolve when the precipitating systemic or metabolic disease has been corrected. In rare instances the arrhythmias persist, and long-term management, similar to that described in "Dilated Cardiomyopathy," is required.

Atrial Fibrillation

ECG Findings. The ECG diagnosis of atrial fibrillation is confirmed by the rapid and irregularly irregular ventricular response, the lack of P waves, and the presence of "f" waves in the ECG baseline (see Fig. 8–7).

Management. In dogs, atrial fibrillation is commonly seen in association with underlying cardiac disease and severe atrial enlargement (Manohar and Smetzer, 1992). Management of atrial fibrillation is the same as for chronic valvular disease and dilated cardiomyopathy. Atrial fibrillation is occasionally seen in dogs without cardiac enlargement, usually large or giant breed dogs that have accompanying diseases (e.g., gastrointestinal disease or hypothyroidism) or who have undergone trauma or recent surgery. In these cases conversion of atrial fibrillation to normal sinus rhythm should be attempted to prevent progressive cardiac enlargement and eventual heart failure (Fig. 8–16). Conversion of atrial fibrillation is usually performed immediately after any identifiable underlying disease process has been corrected. This is achieved with intramuscular quinidine at 7 mg/kg every 6 hours. If ventricular response is rapid (>220 beats/min), then digitalization before quinidine is recommended. If quinidine is unsuccessful after six to eight doses, then diltiazem may be used to facilitate conversion to sinus rhythm. If these techniques are unsuccessful, then cardioversion with an ECG-synchronized defibrillator is the final option.Conversion of atrial fibrillation to sinus rhythm with cardioversion is rarely successful if the rhythm is long-standing and previous therapies have been unsuccessful. When conversion to sinus rhythm is unsuccessful and long-term management is required, treatment is similar to that outlined in previous sections.

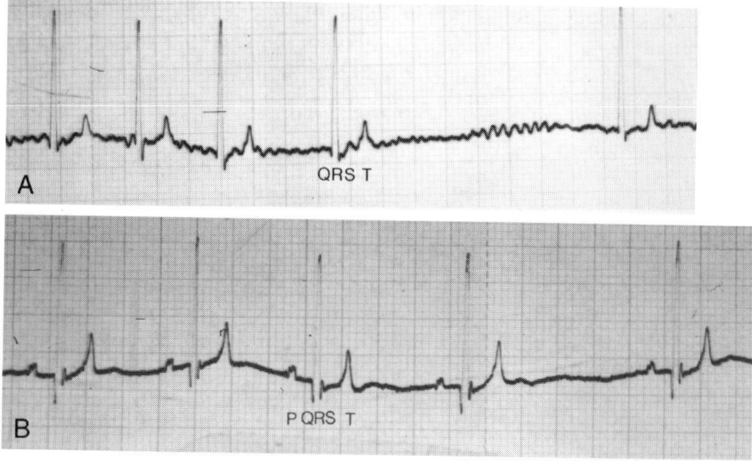

Figure 8–16. ECG obtained from a Great Dane the day after surgery for gastric dilation and volvulus. *A*, Atrial fibrillation is diagnosed by the presence of an irregular rhythm, the lack of P waves, and the irregular motion of the baseline (f waves). An echocardiogram revealed normal cardiac size and function. *B*, Quinidine was initiated, and this ECG was obtained the following morning. Sinus rhythm is now present, as P, QRS, and T complexes are noted. Both ECGs were recorded at 25 mm/sec and 1 cm/mV.

Sick Sinus Syndrome

ECG Findings. Sick sinus syndrome is manifested by bradycardia from sinus arrest, supraventricular tachycardia, or, in many instances, the presence of both bradycardia and runs of supraventricular tachycardia (Fig. 8–17). Sick sinus syndrome is the result of abnormal responsiveness of the sinus node. In many cases, the AV junctional tissue fails to generate an escape beat, which is likely indicative of more widespread disease of the conduction system. Clinical signs may result from bradycardia or tachycardia, although most affected dogs collapse during prolonged periods of sinus arrest.

Management. Sick sinus syndrome can be effectively treated pharmacologically in some cases, but many dogs eventually require pacemaker implantation. Supraventricular tachycardia can be treated pharmacologically, but these dogs must be closely monitored, as the drugs used to treat the supraventricular arrhythmia (e.g., digoxin, beta blockers, calcium channel blockers) may worsen the periods of bradycardia. For dogs with bradycardia, the effectiveness of drug therapy can often be predicted by response to atropine administration. For testing purposes, atropine should be administered both intramuscularly (0.02 mg/kg) and intravenously (0.02 mg/kg). An ECG recorded 20 minutes after drug administration is then compared with the baseline recording. Sinus rhythm and resolution of sinus pauses after the atropine response test are predictive of an acceptable clinical response to long-acting oral anticholinergic therapy with either propantheline (0.25 to 0.5 mg/kg bid to tid) or isopropamide. The prognosis for affected dogs is usually fair to good if pacemaker implantation is possible. Pharmacologic therapies may help some dogs for a few months to a year, but many of these dogs eventually require pacemaker implantation (Fig. 8–18). The typical survival after pacemaker implantation is 1 to 3 years (Rush and Ross, 1992).

Atrioventricular (AV) Blocks

ECG Findings. First-degree AV block is a prolongation of conduction through the AV node, yet all sinus impulses are conducted to the ventricle. First-degree AV block does not cause any clinical signs or require therapy. With second-degree AV block, some of the sinus impulses are blocked at the AV node and not conducted to the ventricles—i.e., some P waves without accompanying QRST complexes are present. Third-degree AV block, or complete heart block, results in total dissociation of the atria from the ventricles. P waves occur without relation to QRST complexes, and the ventricular rhythm results

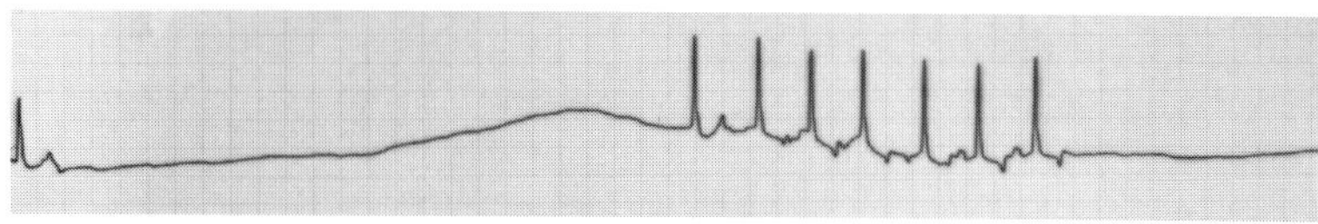

Figure 8–17. ECG obtained from a dog with sick sinus syndrome. A long period of sinus arrest is terminated by a junctional tachycardia. Negative P waves can be seen in the T waves of the previous QRS complexes. The run of junctional tachycardia is followed by another period of sinus arrest.

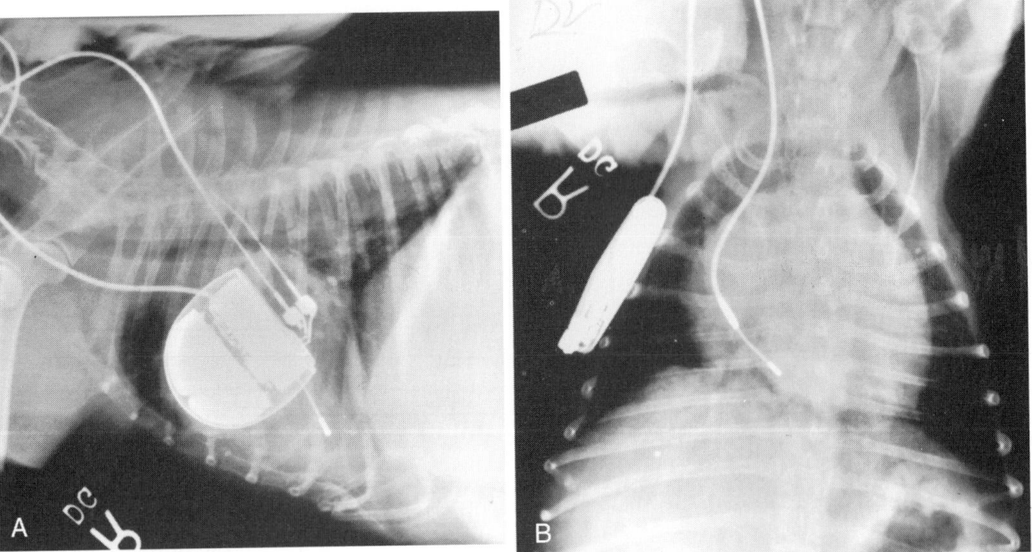

Figure 8–18. Lateral *(A)* and dorsoventral *(B)* thoracic radiographs from a schnauzer with sick sinus syndrome after pacemaker implantation. The dog also had mitral insufficiency as a result of chronic valvular disease (endocardiosis). The transvenous pacemaker lead is located in the right ventricle with the lead wire coursing through the right atrium and cranial vena cava and exiting from the jugular vein. The pulse generator is located in a subcutaneous pocket over the lateral aspect of the thorax.

from either a junctional or ventricular escape focus at a rate of 35 to 60 beats/min.

Management. Dogs with second- and third-degree AV block require treatment. Drug therapy may control the arrhythmia in some cases but is rarely effective in dogs with third-degree AV block. An atropine response test can also be used to identify dogs that may respond well to anticholinergic therapy (i.e., propantheline or isopropamide). Because third-degree AV block may occur secondary to myocarditis, a trial with anti-inflammatory doses of corticosteroids may be useful if pacemaker implantation is not an option. The treatment of choice in dogs with second- or third-degree AV block is pacemaker implantation (see Fig. 8–19).

DISORDERS OF THE CAT

Cardiovascular disease is a significant problem in the geriatric cat population. Many of the disorders seen in older dogs also occur in older cats. Several cardiovascular disorders affect cats almost exclusively (e.g., hyperthyroidism, hypertension, aortic thromboembolism).

Hypertrophic Cardiomyopathy

Hypertrophic cardiomyopathy is the most common myocardial disease in older cats (Medinger and Bruyette, 1992). The primary pathophysiologic process occurring in hypertrophic cardiomyopathy is diminished ventricular compliance (i.e., increased "stiffness"), which leads to elevated diastolic filling pressures. In older cats the clinician should also consider other systemic diseases that could result in a similar clinical appearance.

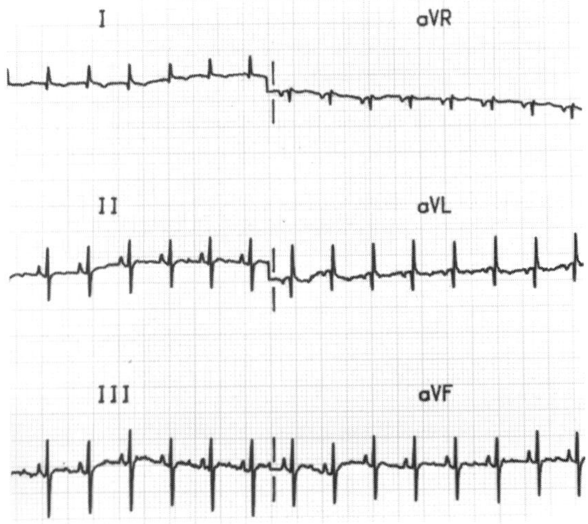

Figure 8–19. ECG recorded from a cat with hypertrophic cardiomyopathy. A left axis shift is present with deep S waves in leads II, III, and aVF, and a qR pattern in leads I and aVL. Recorded at 25 mm/sec and 1 cm/mV.

Clinical Features. Common findings in cats with hypertrophic cardiomyopathy include dyspnea, open-mouth breathing, recent onset of anorexia, and signs resulting from thromboembolism. Cats often present with a strong left apex beat and hyperdynamic precordial impulse. Arterial pulses may be normal or weak, and in cats with long-standing disease and concurrent right-sided heart failure, jugular vein distention may be present. When congestive heart failure is present, dyspnea, tachypnea, open-mouth breathing, pulmonary crackles, or muffled heart and/or ventral lung sounds may be noted. A murmur, usually at the left sternal border, is often heard. A cardiac gallop (S_4, S_3, or summation gallop), which may be intermittent and of varying intensity, may also be present. Cardiac arrhythmias, with or without pulse deficits, are also common.

ECG and Radiographic Findings. ECG abnormalities may include P pulmonale (P wave > 0.2 mV) or P mitrale (P wave > 0.04 sec), tall R waves, or a left axis shift (Fig. 8–19). The left axis shift, which is often identified as a left anterior fascicular block, results from concentric hypertrophy of the left ventricle with or without pathologic abnormality of the left anterior fascicle of the left bundle branches. Supraventricular or ventricular arrhythmias may be noted; however, they are rarely severe enough to require specific antiarrhythmic therapy. Thoracic radiographic findings include generalized cardiomegaly and biatrial enlargement (or valentine-shaped heart). Pulmonary venous distention is common with long-standing disease, and overt interstitial and alveolar pulmonary edema may be present (Fig. 8–20).

Echocardiographic Findings. Concentric hypertrophy of the left ventricle and intraventricular septum are the classic echocardiographic findings in hypertrophic cardiomyopathy. In some cats hypertrophy of the interventricular septum results in a discrete subaortic narrowing (Fig. 8–21). M-mode echocardiography can confirm the small left ventricular endsystolic dimensions and thickened ventricular walls (Fig. 8–22). In some cases hypertrophy and/or dilation of the right ventricular wall may also be present. Pericardial effusion can accurately be diagnosed echocardiographically; however, this is usually seen only in cats with congestive heart failure.

Management. Treatment of hypertrophic cardiomyopathy should be approached with three goals: to improve diastolic compliance and prevent tachycardia, to treat congestive heart failure when present, and to prevent systemic arterial thromboembolization. Improved diastolic compliance is achieved through the use of a beta-adrenergic blocker (e.g., propranolol, used initially at 2.5 mg per cat PO tid and then slowly increased until the heart rate is maintained at less than 160 beats/min, or atenolol, used at ¼ of a 25-mg tablet per cat once daily) or a calcium channel blocker (e.g., diltiazem used at ¼ of a 30-mg tablet PO tid). If a beta blocker is initiated and the response is inadequate, then a calcium channel blocker should be employed. We prefer beta blockers in very young cats and cats with sinus tachycardia and less severe hypertrophy.

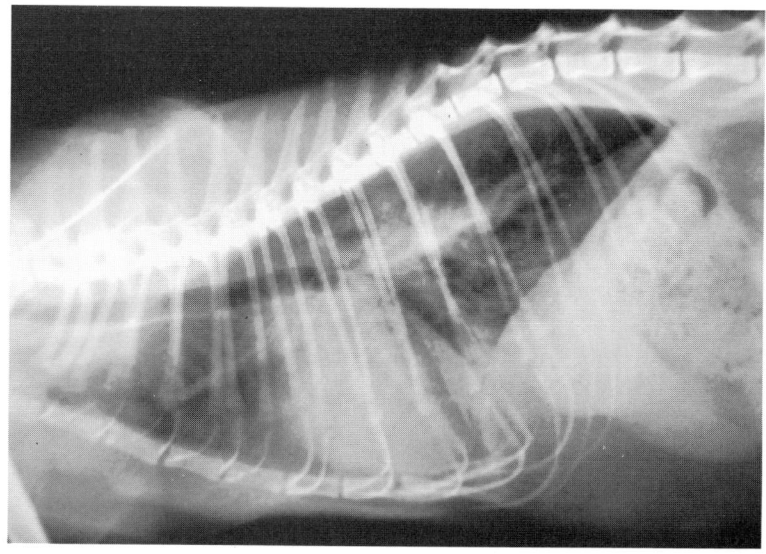

Figure 8–20. Lateral thoracic radiograph from a cat with hypertrophic cardiomyopathy. The pulmonary veins are dilated, and there is an increased interstitial and early alveolar pattern resulting from pulmonary edema. The cat also has hepatomegaly and a very small volume of pleural effusion.

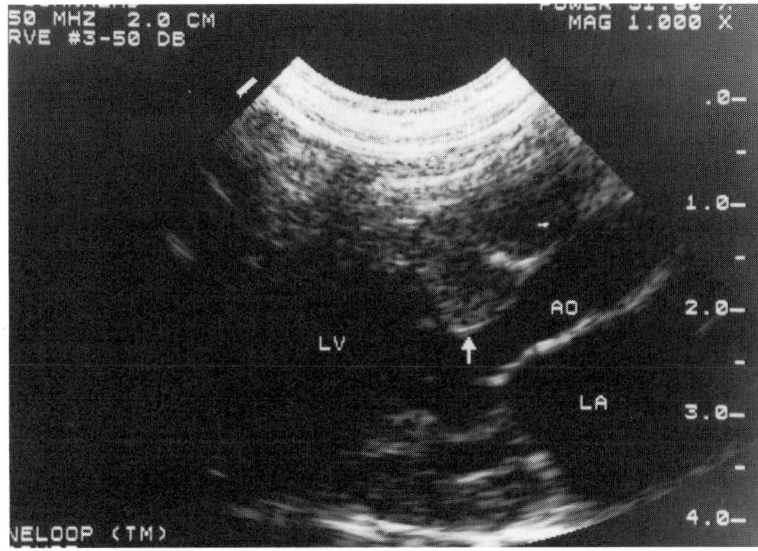

Figure 8–21. Two-dimensional echocardiogram, long-axis view, from a cat with hypertrophic cardiomyopathy. Left atrial enlargement is noted. The subaortic narrowing resulting from hypertrophy of the intraventricular septum *(arrow)* is also remarkable. AO, Aorta; LA, left atrium; LV, left ventricle.

Diltiazem is usually preferred for cats with severe disease and marked left atrial enlargement. In cases of life-theatening pulmonary edema, furosemide can be administered at 4 mg/kg IV every hour until adequate diuresis occurs and dyspnea is improved. Additional therapies for severe pulmonary edema include oxygen and nitroglycerine. Nitroglycerine paste should be applied to any hairless region (⅛ to ¼ inch every 4 to 6 hours), although in hypothermic cats or those with cold ears or extremities, the response is usually superior when the drug is applied in the inner thigh region. Nitroglycerine is discontinued after 2 or 3 days, when diltiazem or beta blockers have been initiated.

When congestion persists despite the use of furosemide in combination with diltiazem or a beta blocker, additional drugs should be added to the treatment regimen. Enalapril (2.5 mg per cat PO sid) or captopril are indicated, especially in cats with pleural effusion or ascites. Cats with any form of cardiomyopathy are predisposed to

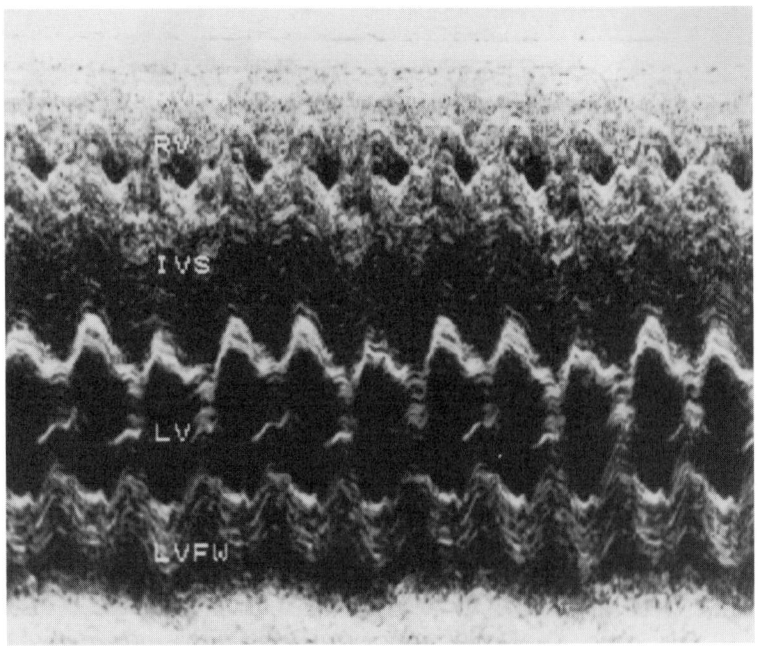

Figure 8–22. M-mode echocardiogram from a cat with hypertrophic cardiomyopathy. Note the remarkable hypertrophy of the interventricular septum (IVS) and the small left ventricular (LV) internal dimensions. LVFW, Left ventricular free wall; RV, right ventricle.

the development of left atrial or left ventricular thrombi, and antithrombotic therapy is indicated. The initial preventive measure is to use aspirin (¼ of a 325-mg tablet per cat PO) every other day or every third day. Although the efficacy of aspirin is unproven, it is the subjective opinion of many cardiologists that aspirin does reduce the incidence of thromboembolism and is indicated. In cats that have had a previous episode of thromboembolism, aspirin therapy alone is probably inadequate to prevent repeat embolization, and coumadin (in a dosage ranging from ¼ of a 2-mg tablet every other day to ¼ tablet once daily) should be initiated. A prothrombin time (increased by 1.25 to 1.5 times above the baseline level) should be obtained on days 0, 3, 6, and 9, then weekly for 2 weeks, and then monthly until a therapeutic dose has been identified.

Dilated Cardiomyopathy

Dilated cardiomyopathy currently is very uncommon. Affected cats may present for weakness, lethargy, difficulty breathing, or clinical signs referable to arterial thromboembolism. A systolic cardiac murmur or cardiac gallop is often present. ECG changes may include tall R waves resulting from left ventricular enlargement, P mitrale, ventricular premature complexes, or supraventricular complexes. The cardiac silhouette is enlarged on thoracic radiographs, and pulmonary edema with pleural effusion is common in untreated individuals. The echocardiographic findings include a diminished left ventricular shortening fraction with dilation of the left ventricle (left ventricle end-diastolic size > 16 mm) and left atrium (Fig. 8–23). The right atrium and

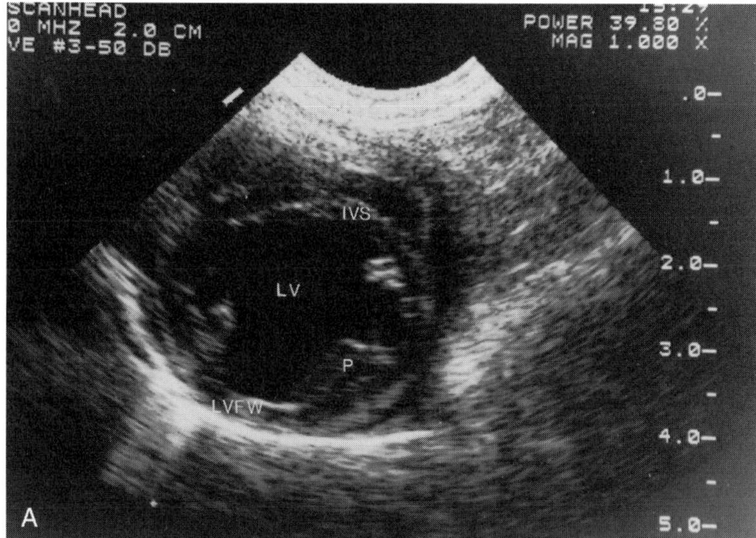

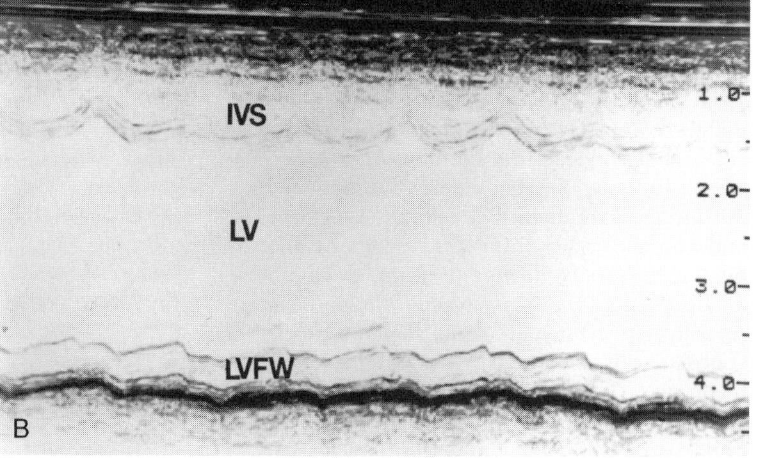

Figure 8–23. Echocardiograms from a cat with dilated cardiomyopathy. The two-dimensional echocardiogram *(A)* documents dilation of the left ventricle (LV), atrophy of the papillary muscles (P), and thinning of the ventricular walls (IVS, interventricular septum; LVFW, left ventricular free wall). The M-mode echocardiogram *(B)* confirms diminished myocardial function and a dilated left ventricle (per cent delta D = 6 per cent).

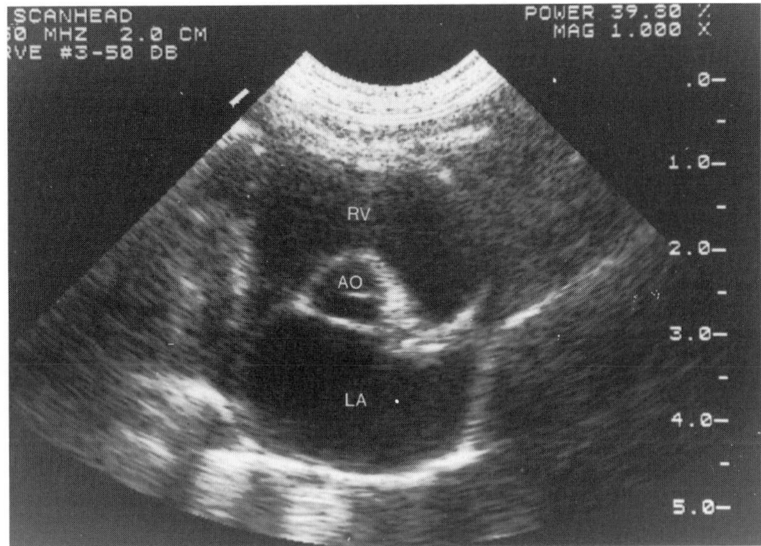

Figure 8–24. Two-dimensional, short-axis echocardiogram from a cat with dilated cardiomyopathy. The left atrium (LA), which normally approximates the size of the aorta (AO) in this view, is moderately dilated. The right ventricle (RV) is also dilated.

ventricle may also be dilated, with diminished motion of the aortic root (Fig. 8–24). Digoxin (¼ of a 0.125-mg tablet PO per cat every other day) and enalapril (2.5 mg PO per cat sid) are often useful adjunctive therapies (Atkins et al, 1990). Plasma taurine levels should be determined, and taurine should be initiated at 250 mg PO sid or bid.

Restrictive Cardiomyopathy

Restrictive cardiomyopathy is an uncommon form of myocardial disease in cats (Harpster, 1986). Affected individuals have marked thickening and fibrosis of the left ventricular endomyocardial surface from previous inflammatory endomyocarditis. Cats may present for dyspnea, weakness, weight loss, or arterial thromboembolism. A cardiac gallop, weak arterial pulses, pulmonary edema, and occasionally a cardiac murmur are present. ECG findings are variable, but atrial premature complexes and ventricular premature complexes are common. Intraventricular conduction defects from the fibrosis are also possible. The angiocardiographic findings include left atrial enlargement with filling defects in the endocardial surface of the left ventricle. Echocardiography also confirms left atrial enlargement and left ventricular hypertrophy. The endocardial surface may be hyperechoic. Left atrial or left ventricular thrombi may be observed using either technique. Because these cats are highly predisposed to arterial thromboembolism, antithrombotic therapy is indicated. Additional treatment for congestive heart failure and/or arrhythmias may be needed.

Intermediate Forms of Cardiomyopathy

Many cats have myocardial disease with clinical and echocardiographic findings that are not typical of hypertrophic, dilated, or restrictive cardiomyopathy (Fox, 1989). Variations may include left ventricular dilation with thickened left ventricular walls and good myocardial function, normal echocardiographic appearance of the left ventricle and mitral valve with significant left atrial enlargement, and excessive left ventricular moderator bands as seen in cats with congenital heart disease and other forms of cardiomyopathy. Clinical signs may include syncope, dyspnea, and other signs resulting from congestive heart failure or thromboembolism. Cardiac murmurs and cardiac gallops are common. ECG and radiographic findings are nonspecific but may include atrial or ventricular enlargement and cardiac arrhythmias. There is no specific therapy for this form of myocardial disease, and treatment should be directed at the predominant clinical findings.

Hyperthyroid Heart Disease

Hyperthyroid heart disease may appear similar to hypertrophic cardiomyopathy and intermediate forms of cardiomyopathy (Moise and Dietze, 1986). Hyperthyroidism should always be considered in older cats with a cardiac murmur or gallop. In addition, hyperthyroid cats typically have a thyroid nodule and tachycardia and frequently have ECG evidence of a left axis shift or left ventricular enlargement. Thoracic radiographs usually demonstrate cardiomegaly occasionally with evidence of congestive heart failure. Echocardiographic findings are variable but usually confirm cardiac enlargement (Moise and Dietze, 1986). In addition to the specific treatment of hyperthyroidism, management of the cardiac changes may be indicated. Sinus tachycardia, especially when it persists after initiation of treatment of hyperthyroidism, and cardiac arrhythmias should be specifically treated and are best managed with a beta blocker (either propranolol or atenolol). Congestive heart failure should be treated in a standard fashion. Most cats have total resolution of the cardiac changes after successful treatment of hyperthyroidism; however, those with heart failure and previous valvular or myocardial disease often have persistent heart failure after therapy. These cats require long-term management of congestive heart failure.

Systemic Hypertension

Systemic hypertension, or arterial hypertension, is another common cause of hypertrophic heart disease in older cats (Kobayashi et al, 1990; Ross, 1989). Arteriosclerosis of vessels throughout the body is a common histopathologic finding in cats with chronic hypertension. The cause of hypertension is unclear. Renal failure is thought to be the cause of hypertension in many cases. It may well be that essential hypertension is the most common cause of increased blood pressure, and the cardiac, renal, ocular, and neurologic manifestations are merely sequelae. We have also identified several cats with aldosterone-producing adrenal carcinomas and secondary hypertension.

Clinical Features. Common findings in hypertensive cats include mild azotemia (creatinine 2 to 3 mg/dl), the presence of a systolic murmur or cardiac gallop, and ophthalmologic abnormalities (e.g., retinal hemorrhages, retinal detachment, or tortuous arterial vessels). Hypertensive cats seem to develop severe congestive heart failure less often than do cats with other causes of hypertrophic heart disease. Seizures or other evidence of neurologic dysfunction are seen in some cats and may result from intracranial hemorrhage or hypertensive encephalopathy. The most common ECG finding is a left axis shift, although many cats with hypertension have a normal ECG. Thoracic radiographs may be normal or document cardiac enlargement (Fig. 8–25). Echocardiographic findings are similar to those seen with hypertrophic cardiomyopathy; however, the left atrium is infrequently enlarged in hypertensive cats.

Hypertension can be documented only by the measurement of blood pressure. Blood pressure measurements in the cat can vary widely depending on the presence or absence of sedation, the environment in which measurements are made, and whether blood pressure is measured directly or indirectly. Indirect blood pressure measurement, using either the Doppler or oscillometric technique, can be performed with relative accuracy in most cats and is preferred over direct blood pressure measurement (Grandy et al, 1992; Hunter et al, 1990). The upper limit of normal systolic blood pressure in cats ranges from 135 to 170 mm Hg (Cowgill and Fallet, 1986; Kobayashi et al, 1990; Ross, 1989). The upper limit of normal diastolic blood pressure ranges from 95 to 135 mm Hg. Most cats with clinical signs resulting from hypertension will have either a systolic blood pressure greater than 165 mm Hg or a diastolic blood pressure greater than 125 mm Hg. Repeated measurements are needed to confirm hypertension.

Management. Treatment of hypertension requires sequential blood pressure measurement. With blood pressures greater than 200 mm Hg and retinal lesions, single-drug therapy is fre-

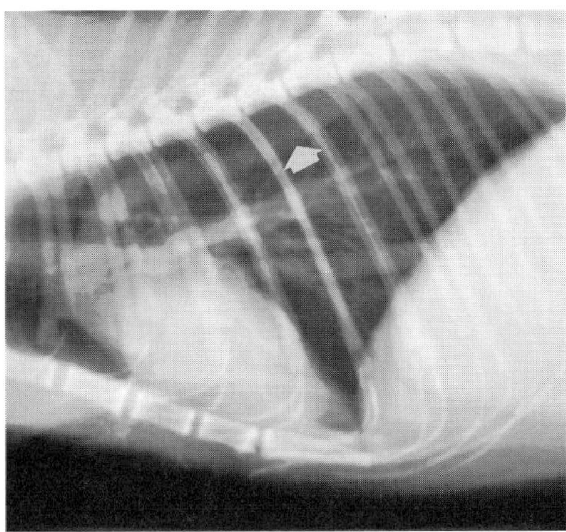

Figure 8–25. Lateral thoracic radiograph from an aged cat with hypertension. Note the tortuous path of the aorta *(arrow)*, the dilated aortic root, and mild ventricular enlargement.

quently unsuccessful. Drug therapy includes calcium channel blockers, beta blockers, ACE inhibitors, alpha blockers, and other vasodilators. Drugs that we have had success with include enalapril, diltiazem, prazosin, and amylodipine. The exact order in which to initiate drug therapy and the desired end points of therapy have not been clearly established. We often start with either diltiazem (¼ of a 30-mg tablet per cat PO tid) or enalapril (2.5 mg per cat PO sid) and measure the blood pressure in 2 to 3 days. A reduction in systolic blood pressure to ≤ 170 mm Hg is considered a satisfactory response. Additional drugs are added if hypertension persists; typically prazosin (0.5 mg per cat PO bid) or amylodipine (0.625 mg PO sid) are the next drugs to be selected. Blood pressure is measured in a serial fashion until an acceptable response is achieved.

Pericardial Effusion

Pericardial effusion occurs infrequently in older cats (Rush et al, 1990). Pericardial effusion is usually diagnosed in association with other systemic disease that causes fluid accumulation, coagulopathy, or increased vascular permeability. Common causes include feline infectious peritonitis, severe systemic infections that extend into the pericardial space, advanced renal failure, and congestive heart failure. Primary and metastatic neoplasia can also cause pericardial effusion. Lymphosarcoma in the heart or extending into the pericardial sac from the mediastinum is another common cause of effusion. Metastatic neoplasms causing pericardial effusion include lymphosarcoma, mammary and pulmonary adenocarcinomas, melanomas, and hemangiosarcoma.

Clinical Features. In most instances cats with pericardial effusion are presented for clinical signs resulting from the underlying disease. Many cats with pericardial effusion have muffled heart sounds and/or murmurs or gallops. ECG findings are usually not diagnostic, although electrical alternans is occasionally present. Radiographic evidence of marked cardiac enlargement with a globoid cardiac silhouette and an enlarged vena cava may be noted (Fig. 8–26). Echocardiography confirms the echo-free space between the epicardium and pericardium. Echocardiographic evidence of diastolic collapse of the right atrium and/or right ventricle may be noted and indicates the presence of cardiac tamponade.

Management. The management of pericardial effusion in the cat depends on the precipitating cause and the presence or absence of cardiac

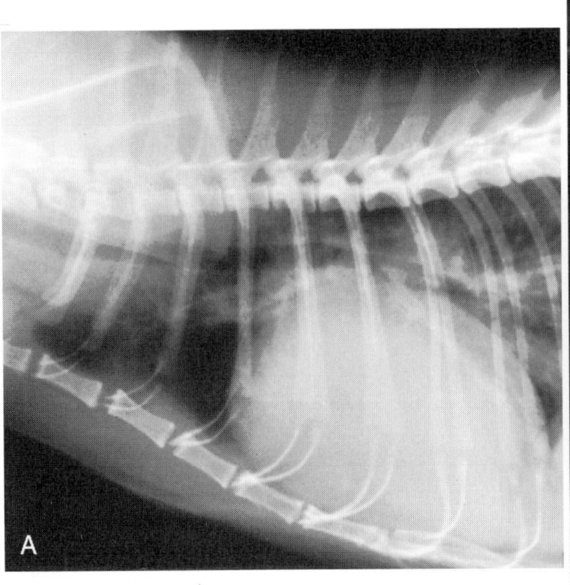

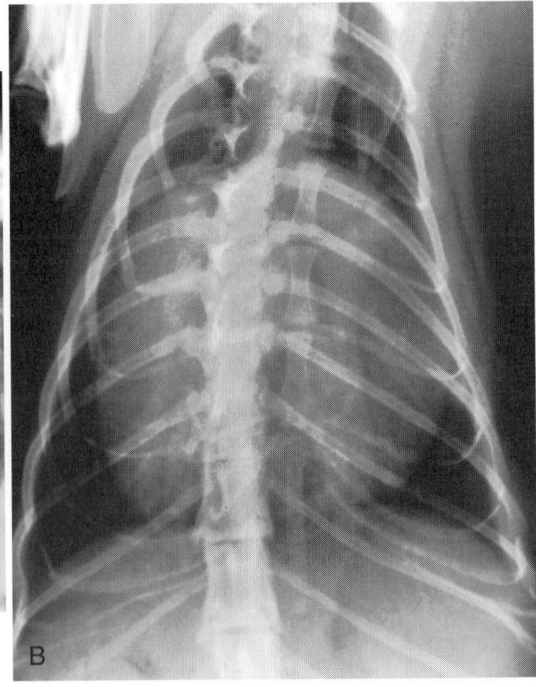

Figure 8–26. Lateral *(A)* and ventrodorsal *(B)* thoracic radiographs from a cat with hypertrophic cardiomyopathy. The cat also had a large volume of pericardial effusion causing severe radiographic cardiomegaly. Mild hilar pulmonary edema is also noted.

tamponade. Therapeutic pericardiocentesis is indicated in cases of cardiac tamponade. If the underlying cause (i.e., congestive heart failure, renal failure, coagulopathy) can be determined without pericardiocentesis and tamponade is not present, treatment of the underlying disorder alone often resolves the effusion. When the cause of effusion is not clear, diagnostic pericardiocentesis is indicated and should be performed in a manner similar to that described for the dog. Pericardial fluid analysis may be more valuable with respect to identification of the underlying cause in the cat, especially in cases of feline infectious peritonitis or bacterial infection.

Valvular Insufficiency

Geriatric cats may also develop heart failure or thromboembolism in association with valvular insufficiency (Bonagura, 1989). The most common cause of mitral and tricuspid valve insufficiency results from myocardial disease. Aging changes in the mitral or tricuspid valve may also occur in older cats but are an infrequent cause of severe heart failure. Bacterial endocarditis is a rare cause of valvular insufficiency in cats. Organisms most frequently identified in cats with bacterial endocarditis are *Staphylococcus* and *Streptococcus* species. The clinical findings and management of bacterial endocarditis in cats are similar to those in dogs. Mitral insufficiency results in a systolic cardiac murmur at the left sternal border, left atrial enlargement, and a volume overload to the left ventricle. The mitral valve is typically thickened in chronic valvular disease, and Doppler studies will confirm mitral insufficiency. The treatment of valvular insufficiency in cats should be directed toward treatment of congestive heart failure, when present.

Arterial Thromboembolism

Systemic thromboembolism in the cat, most frequently aortic thromboembolism, can be a common and devastating complicating factor in cats with any form of cardiac disease that results in significant atrial enlargement. Clinical findings include posterior paresis or paralysis, diminished femoral arterial pulses, cold limbs, cyanotic nail beds that do not bleed when clipped, and firm, painful gastrocnemius muscles (Bonagura, 1989; Harpster, 1986). Management of arterial thromboembolism involves the standard treatment of congestive heart failure, prevention of further thromboembolic occurrences, and treatment of the active thromboembolism (Table 8–6).

TABLE 8–6. MANAGEMENT OF ARTERIAL THROMBOEMBOLISM

Conservative management
Treat CHF if present
Diltiazem or hydralazine
Butorphanol or oxymorphone or acepromazine
Heparin, 200 IU/kg IV followed by 100 IU/kg SC q 6 hr
Physical therapy
Aggressive management
Treat CHF if present
Diltiazem or hydralazine
Butorphanol or oxymorphone or acepromazine
Heparin, 200 IU/kg IV followed by 100 IU/kg SC q 6 hr
Physical therapy
Warfarin, 0.5 mg PO q 24–48 hr
Tissue plasminogen activator, 1–10 mg/kg IV at 0.25–1 mg/kg/hr or streptokinase, 90,000 IU over 20 min then 45,000 IU/hr for 3 hr

CHF, Congestive heart failure; IV, intravenous administration; SC, subcutaneous administration.

Cardiac Arrhythmias

Most cardiac arrhythmias in older cats are not a discrete clinical entity but are seen in conjunction with myocardial, valvular, or pericardial diseases (Harpster, 1992). Therefore, a search for an underlying disease should be conducted. In most instances treatment of the underlying disorder and management of heart failure are adequate to correct or control cardiac arrhythmias. Exceptions to this general rule include atrial fibrillation, AV block, or persistent ventricular arrhythmias.

Atrial fibrillation is seen with hypertrophic or restrictive cardiomyopathy. Digoxin (¼ of a 0.125-mg tablet per cat every other day) should be initiated at the time that other medications are initiated for the underlying myocardial disease. The desired heart rate is 160 beats/min or less. If this goal cannot be achieved with digitalization alone, the addition of propranolol or atenolol may help. AV block, although uncommon in cats, may be seen with intermediate forms of cardiomyopathy, hypertrophic cardiomyopathy, or hyperthyroidism. Pacemaker implantation is indicated for cats with syncope resulting from bradycardia. Cats with AV block with a ventricular rate less than 90 beats/min and heart failure that is resistant to medical management may benefit from pacemaker implantation.

Ventricular arrhythmias may occur with hyperthyroidism, valvular heart disease, or any form of cardiomyopathy. Management of ventricular arrhythmias is rarely required. If treatment of heart failure does not control the arrhythmia, antiarrhythmic therapy should be instituted. Specific antiarrhythmic drug therapy is also indicated for cats with rapid ventricular tachycardia (i.e., rates greater than 200 beats/min). Intravenous lidocaine may cause neurotoxicity in cats and should be used only at low doses (0.5 to 1 mg/kg IV bolus slowly; 10 μg/kg/min IV infusion) and when continuous ECG monitoring can be performed. Oral procainamide (62.5 mg PO tid) or propranolol (2.5 to 7.5 mg PO tid) are the preferred ventricular antiarrhythmics. In general, aggressive management of ventricular arrhythmias should be undertaken with caution; these arrhythmias are unlikely to result in sudden death. Treatment of heart failure or myocardial disease often results in adequate arrhythmia control.

References and Supplemental Reading

Aronsohn M. Cardiac hemangiosarcoma in the dog: A review of 38 cases. J Am Vet Med Assoc 187:922, 1985.

Atkins CE, Snyder PS, Keene BW, et al. Efficacy of digoxin for treatment of cats with dilated cardiomyopathy. J Am Vet Med Assoc 196:1463, 1990.

Baskin SI, Kendrick V, Roberts J, et al. The cardiovascular system. In Johnson JE, ed. Aging and Cell Structure. Vol 1. New York, Plenum Press, 1981, p 305.

Bonagura JD. Cardiovascular diseases. In Sherding RG, ed. The Cat: Diseases and Clinical Management. New York, Churchill Livingstone, 1989, p 649.

Bright JM, Toal RL, Blackford M. Right ventricular outflow obstruction caused by primary cardiac neoplasia. J Vet Intern Med 4:12, 1990.

Cowgill LD, Fallet AJ. Systemic hypertension. In Kirk RW (ed). Current Veterinary Therapy IX. Philadelphia, WB Saunders, 1986, p 360.

Edwards NJ. Pericardial diseases. Proc Acad Vet Cardiol 1991, p 39.

Fox PR. Myocardial diseases. In Ettinger SJ, ed. Textbook of Veterinary Internal Medicine. 3rd ed. Philadelphia, WB Saunders, 1989, p 1097.

Gheorghiade M, Ferguson D. Digoxin: A neurohormonal modulator in heart failure? Circulation 84:2181, 1991.

Grandy JL, Dunlop CI, Hodgson DS, et al. Evaluation of the doppler ultrasonic method of measuring systolic arterial blood pressure in cats. Am J Vet Res 53:1166, 1992.

Hamlin RL. Identifying the cardiovascular and pulmonary diseases that affect old dogs. Vet Med p 483, 1990.

Hamlin RL, Buffington CAT. Nutrition and the heart. Vet Clin North Am 19:527, 1989.

Harpster NK. Feline myocardial diseases. In Kirk RW, ed. Current Veterinary Therapy IX. Philadelphia, WB Saunders, 1986, p 380.

Harpster NK. Feline arrhythmias: Diagnosis and management. In Kirk RW, Bonagura JD, eds. Current Veterinary Therapy XI. Philadelphia, WB Saunders, 1992, p 732.

Hunter JS, McGrath CJ, Thatcher CD, et al. Adaptation of human oscillometric blood pressure monitors for use in dogs. Am J Vet Res 51:1439, 1990.

Jonsson L. Coronary arterial lesions and myocardial infarcts in the dog. ACTA Vet Scand Suppl 38:7, 1972.

Jonsson L. Senile cardiac amyloidosis in the dog. Acta Vet Scand 15:206, 1974.

Keene BW, Panciera DP, Atkins CE, et al. Myocardial L-carnitine deficiency in a family of dogs with dilated cardiomyopathy. J Am Vet Med Assoc 198:647, 1991.

Keene BW, Rush JE. Therapy of heart failure. In Ettinger SJ, ed. Textbook of Veterinary Internal Medicine. 3rd ed. Philadelphia, WB Saunders, 1989, p 939.

Kittleson MD. Management of heart failure: Concepts, therapeutic strategies, and drug pharmacology. In Fox PR, ed. Canine and Feline Cardiology. New York, Churchill Livingstone, 1988, p 171.

Kittleson MD, Pion PD, DeLellis LA, et al. Dilated cardiomyopathy in American cocker spaniels: Taurine deficiency and preliminary results of response to supplementation. Proc Am Coll Vet Intern Med, 1991, p 879.

Kobayashi DL, Peterson ME, Graves TK, et al. Hypertension in cats with chronic renal failure or hyperthyroidism. J Vet Intern Med 4:58, 1990.

LaKatta EG. Interaction between nutrition and aging: A summary of effects on the cardiovascular system. Nutr Rev 50:419, 1992.

Leaf A, Hallaq HA. The role of nutrition in the functioning cardiovascular system. Nutr Rev 50:402, 1992.

Lewis LD, Morris ML, Hand MS. Small Animal Clinical Nutrition III. Topeka, KS, Mark Morris Associates, 1987, p A3-2.

Maher ER Jr, Rush JE. Cardiovascular changes in the geriatric dog. Compend Contin Educ Pract Vet 12:921, 1990.

Manohar M, Smetzer DL. Atrial fibrillation. Compend Contin Educ Pract Vet 14:1327, 1992.

Mattahiesen DT, Lammerding J. Partial pericardiectomy for idiopathic hemorrhagic pericardial effusion in the dog. J Am Anim Hosp Assoc 21:41, 1985.

McLennan PL. Relative effects of dietary saturated, monounsaturated, and polyunsaturated fatty acids on cardiac arrhythmias in rats. Am J Clin Nutr 57:207, 1993.

Medinger TL, Bruyette DS. Feline hypertrophic cardiomyopathy. Compend Contin Educ Pract Vet 14:479, 1992.

Moise NS, Dietze AE. Echocardiographic, electrocardiographic, and radiographic detection of cardiomegaly in hyperthyroid cats. Am J Vet Res 47:1487, 1986.

O'Grady MR, Horne R. Occult dilated cardiomyopathy: An echocardiographic and electrocardiographic study of 193 asymptomatic doberman pinschers. Proc Am Coll Vet Intern Med (9th Annual Meeting), 1991, p 112.

Ross L. Hypertensive disease. In Ettinger SJ, ed. Textbook of Veterinary Internal Medicine. 3rd ed. Philadelphia, WB Saunders, 1989, p 2047.

Rush JE, Atkins CE. Pericardial disease. In Allen DG, ed. Small Animal Medicine. Philadelphia, JB Lippincott, 1991, p 303.

Rush JE, Keene BW, Fox PR. Pericardial disease in the cat: A retrospective evaluation of 66 cases. J Am Anim Hosp Assoc 26:39, 1990.

Rush JE, Ross JN. Cardiac pacing. In Murtaugh RJ, Kaplan PM, eds. Veterinary Emergency and Critical Care Medicine. St. Louis, Mosby-Year Book, 1992, p 657.

Sisson DD, Thomas WP, Ruehl WW, et al. Diagnostic value of pericardial fluid analysis in the dog. J Am Vet Med Assoc 184:51, 1984.

Thomas WP. Pericardial disorders. In Ettinger SJ, ed. Textbook of Veterinary Internal Medicine. 3rd ed. Philadelphia, WB Saunders, 1989, p 1132.

Van Vleet JF, Ferrans VJ. Myocardial diseases of animals. Am J Pathol 124:671, 1986.
Wei JY. Age and the cardiovascular system. N Engl J Med 327:1735, 1992.
Wei JY, Spurgeon HA, Lakatta EG. Excitation-contraction in rat myocardium: Alterations with adult aging. Am J Physiol 246:H784, 1984.
Woodfield JA, Sisson D. Infective endocarditis. In Ettinger SJ, ed. Textbook of Veterinary Internal Medicine. 3rd ed. Philadelphia, WB Saunders, 1989, p 1151.
Yin FC, Spurgeon HA, Greene HL, et al. Age associated decrease in heart rate response to isoproterenol in dogs. Mech Aging Dev 10:17, 1979.
Yin FC, Weisfeldt ML, Milnor WR. Role of aortic input impedance in the decreased cardiovascular response to exercise with aging in dogs. J Clin Invest 68:28, 1981.

CHAPTER 9

The Oral Cavity and Dental Disease

LINDA J. DeBOWES and COLIN E. HARVEY

Significant oral pain, general malaise, and lack of activity are common signs in geriatric animals with advanced periodontal disease. The impact of severe dental disease on a particular animal may not be evident until improvement is observed after treatment. Many owners are unaware that severe dental disease may cause systemic signs and may attribute changes in their pet to "old age" rather than to the dental disease.

Periodontally diseased, fractured, and worn teeth are commonly found and oral neoplasia occurs more frequently in aged patients. Odontoclastic resorptive lesions are a common problem in older cats. A preliminary oral examination may be performed with physical restraint alone. Patients with advanced oral disease may be in too much pain for examination without sedation, and therefore, a complete evaluation of the oral structures requires sedation or general anesthesia.

When clinical signs suggest disease of the oral cavity, a complete examination of the oral cavity should be performed. Such signs include halitosis, changes in eating patterns, behavioral changes (e.g., reclusiveness or aggression), ptyalism, blood-tinged saliva, rubbing the face, nasal discharge, sneezing, facial swelling, and draining tracts (Manfra Marretta, 1989).

Physical examination of the oral cavity should include evaluation of the lips, vestibule of the mouth, dentition, attached gingiva, hard and soft palate, tonsils, sublingual tissue, and tongue. External palpation of the mandible, maxilla, and local lymph nodes should also be included. The lips are retracted while holding the mouth closed to allow inspection of the labial and buccal tooth surfaces and to identify the occlusal pattern (Fig. 9–1). A gloved finger can be used to examine the

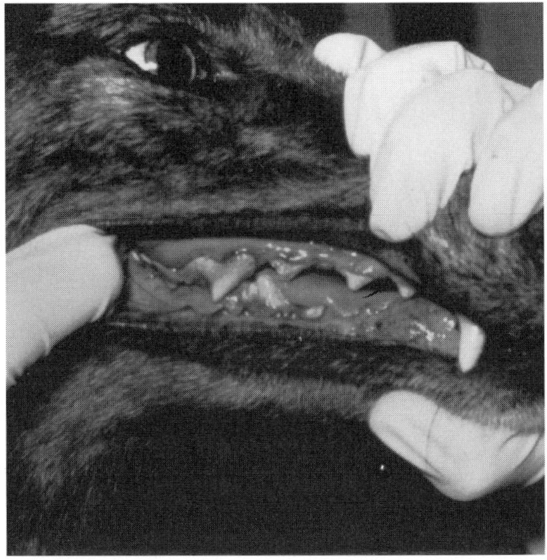

Figure 9–1. Retraction of the lips to allow for examination of the labial and buccal tooth surfaces.

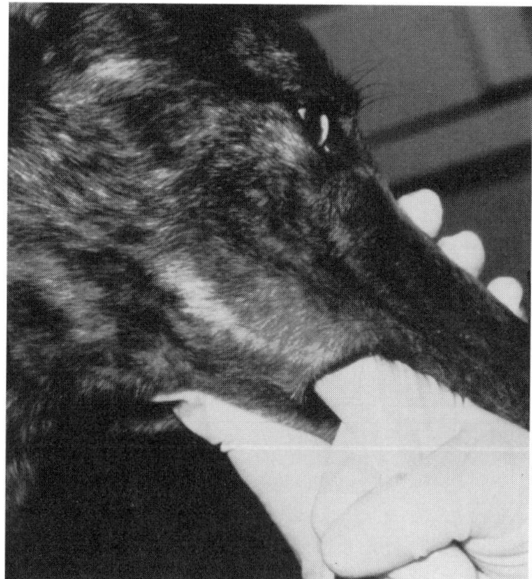

Figure 9–2. Examination of the vestibule of the mouth.

vestibule of the mouth (Fig. 9–2). The mouth is then opened, and the palatal and lingual aspects of the teeth are examined, followed by examination of the hard and soft palate, tongue, sublingual tissues, and tonsils. To examine cats, raise the head vertically with one hand holding the zygomatic arches, and open the mouth by pressing the mandible ventrally with a finger from the other hand (Fig. 9–3). To examine under a cat's tongue, place a finger between the rami of the mandible and push dorsally (Fig. 9–4).

Equipment, instruments, and materials used in small animal dentistry are listed in Table 9–1.

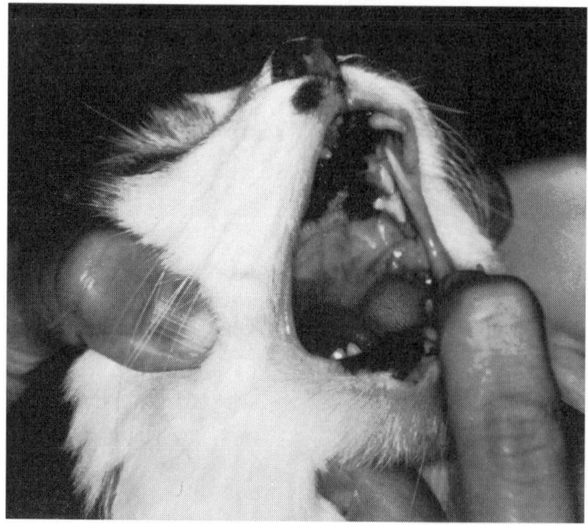

Figure 9–3. Examination of oral cavity in a cat.

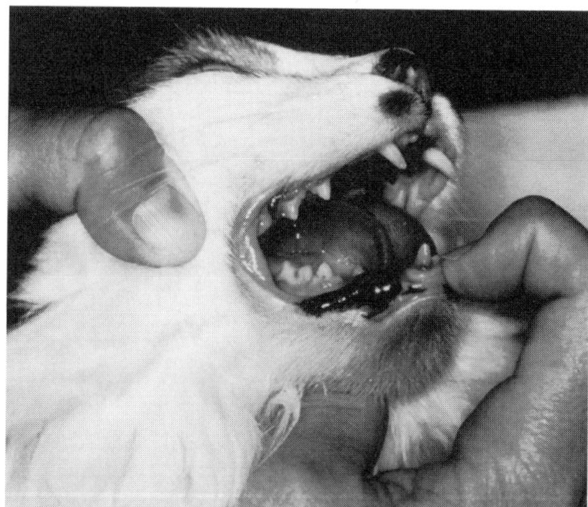

Figure 9–4. Examination of the sublingual area in a cat.

DISORDERS OF DOGS

Periodontal Disease

Cause. Plaque, bacterial by-products, and the resulting inflammatory response lead to periodontal disease. Plaque is composed primarily of bacteria in a matrix of salivary glycoproteins and extracellular polysaccharides. The initial bacterial population in gingivitis is predominantly gram positive with gram-negative bacteria and spirochetes increasing as disease progresses to periodontitis (Hennet and Harvey, 1991). Plaque tends to accumulate more readily on teeth that are crowded, have roughened surfaces (i.e., enamel hypoplasia or fractures) or calculus buildup. Diet may play a role, with soft, nonabrasive diets resulting in plaque buildup more rapidly than more abrasive diets.

Marginal gingivitis, the earliest stage of periodontal disease, occurs when dental plaque accumulates on the tooth crown adjacent to the gingival margin. If supragingival plaque is not removed, it will progress subgingivally, and gingival inflammation will progress beyond marginal gingivitis. Subgingival plaque and the associated inflammatory response may eventually lead to a breakdown of the epithelial attachment to the tooth. As the epithelial attachment moves apically, pocket formation and periodontitis (loss of connective tissue and bone attachment) begins (Holmstrom et al, 1992). Continued loss of attachment results in advanced periodontitis, increased tooth mobility, and eventual tooth loss.

Incidence. Periodontal disease is the most common problem of the oral cavity in dogs (Holmstrom, 1989). The incidence of periodon-

TABLE 9–1. SMALL ANIMAL DENTISTRY: INSTRUMENTS, EQUIPMENT, AND MATERIALS*

DENTAL PROPHYLAXIS
Power equipment: electrically driven or air-driven units
Dental handpieces: high-speed and low-speed handpieces
Ultrasonic and subsonic dental scalers
Roto-Pro scaler bur (295-8151)†
Basic veterinary dental kit (100-5798)
  Explorer/probe ST 4 (100-4807)
  Jacquette 2/3 scaler (100-9848)
  McCalls Starlight curette 13/14 (800-9066)
  #299 Conical sharpening stone (600-6804)
  16A Instrument tray (100-8068)
Sharpening stone oil
Prophylaxis polishing paste or pumice
Endodontic Procedures*
Restorative Procedures*
Extractions
Dental extraction forceps (100-8266, 100-6525)
Dental elevators (100-9235, 100-3332, 100-9415)
Dental luxators (888-3220)
Root tip pick (100-6967)
Home Care Instruments*
Gauze pads
Cotton-tipped applicators
Sponge-tipped applicators
Finger toothbrush
Animal toothbrushes
Oral Hygiene Products*
Pastes (e.g., CET dentrifice)
Rinses (e.g., Nolvadent, Fort Dodge Laboratories)
Gels (e.g., CHX Gel, VRx Products; Maxiguard oral cleansing gel, Addison Biological Laboratory, Inc.)

*See Harvey and Emily (1993) and Aller (1993) for more details.
†Item numbers in parentheses refer to the Henry Schein veterinary and dental supplies catalog (Telephone number: 1-800-V-SCHEIN).

titis increases in aged patients (Harvey and Emily, 1993). Gingival inflammation and calculus formation occur most commonly on the upper teeth, with the upper fourth premolar and first molar having the most extensive calculus deposits (Harvey, 1992).

Clinical Features. Normal gingival tissue is light pink in color, with a sharp edge to the gingival margin. The gingival margin is closely opposed to the tooth crown. Gingival sulcus depth in dogs is normally 3 mm or less. Signs of periodontal disease vary and depend on the extent of disease. Marginal gingivitis is the initial stage, evidenced by erythema of the marginal gingiva only. Established gingivitis is identified clinically by a rounding of the marginal gingival tissue as a result of edema, erythema of the attached gingiva, and an increased tendency to hemorrhage with gentle pressure on probing. In the absence of periodontitis, the epithelial attachment level is unchanged with gingivitis, and the depth of the gingival sulcus is normal unless gingival hyperplasia or edema results in pseudopocket formation. Clinical features of periodontitis include gingival recession, periodontal pocket formation, and increased tooth mobility, as well as signs of gingivitis. Nasal discharge, sneezing, and oronasal fistulas may be present with advanced periodontitis, especially when the maxillary canine tooth is involved. Uncommon signs of periodontal disease include severe hemorrhage of the gingival sulcus, pathologic jaw fracture, contact ulcers, intranasal tooth migration, and osteomyelitis (Manfra Marretta, 1987).

Diagnosis. A complete dental examination is performed with the patient anesthetized and intubated. Each tooth should be evaluated for clinical features of gingivitis or periodontitis. The depth of the gingival sulcus should be evaluated to determine whether periodontal pockets are present. Severe periodontitis may result in deep periodontal pocket formation on the palatal aspect of the maxillary canine tooth. The presence of periodontal pocket formation indicates loss of periodontal ligament and alveolar bone. When the epithelial attachment is in the normal position and gingival edema or hyperplasia results in increased gingival sulcus depth, a pseudopocket results. An explorer is used to identify subgingival calculus and furcation exposure (indicative of alveolar bone loss). Periodontitis may occur without periodontal pocket formation if gingival recession occurs at about the same rate as alveolar bone loss.

Dental radiographs are taken to verify the extent of periodontal disease and assist in treatment planning (Smith et al, 1985; Zontine, 1974). Normal radiographic signs of aging include a narrowed pulp cavity, an increased density and coarseness of the trabeculae of the mandible and maxilla, indistinct lamina dura as a result of changes in alveolar bone, and slight resorption of the alveolar crest (Zontine, 1974). Common radiographic signs of periodontal disease include a rounding of the alveolar crest bone at the cementoenamel junction, increased width of the periodontal space, loss of integrity of the lamina dura, alveolar bone changes (e.g., an increase or decrease in bone density), and loss of alveolar crestal bone (Zontine, 1974). Horizontal bone loss is the most common type of alveolar bone loss (Fig. 9–5). Vertical bone loss may also occur, resulting in infrabony pockets.

Management. The treatment goal is to relieve oral pain, restore the mouth to a healthy condition, and maintain a healthy mouth after treatment. A complete history is obtained and a physical examination is performed on the aged pet to

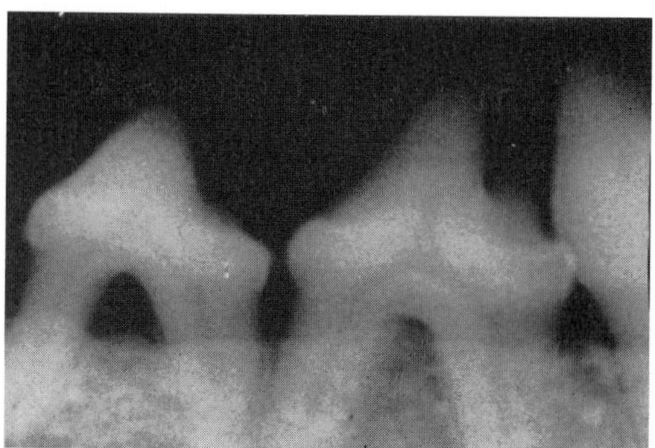

Figure 9–5. Horizontal bone loss in a dog with periodontal disease.

determine the appropriate diagnostic tests that should be done before anesthesia. When determining the most appropriate treatment plan for a geriatric patient, the following factors must be considered:

- the anesthetic risk versus the benefit of the dental procedure,
- the expected life span of the patient,
- the owner's commitment to regular professional dental treatments in severe cases,
- the risk of repeated anesthetic procedures,
- the owner's commitment and ability to perform home care, and
- the patient's temperament (Harvey, 1991b).

In most geriatric patients with moderate to severe periodontitis it is best to extract teeth rather than subject the patient to repeated dental procedures requiring anesthesia.

A complete dental examination and the required treatment are performed with the patient intubated and under general anesthesia. A dental record (Fig. 9–6) should be completed for each patient to assist in owner communication and evaluation of disease progression and for legal purposes.

Antimicrobial administration is recommended before a dental procedure in an aged dog with any stage of periodontal disease if the dog is predisposed to endocarditis or has a compromised immune system and is more susceptible to infections (Sarkiala and Harvey, 1993). Adequate antimicrobial blood concentrations can be achieved by administration of a subcutaneous or intramuscular injection at the time of administration of preoperative medications or by oral administration 24 hours preceding mechanical treatment (Manfra Marretta, 1992b; Sarkiala and Harvey, 1993). Amoxicillin–clavulanate potassium and clindamycin are effective against the anaerobes associated with periodontal disease; amoxicillin-clavulanate is also broadly effective against aerobes (Sarkiala and Harvey, 1993). Depending on the severity of periodontal or oral disease antimicrobials are continued for 0 to 7 days after the procedure. (Manfra Marretta, 1992b; Sarkiala and Harvey, 1993). The combination of amoxicillin and metronidazole is an alternative treatment for dogs with severe periodontitis. Dogs with chronic recurrent periodontitis may also benefit from long-term tetracycline administration (Manfra Marretta, 1992b).

Complete dental prophylaxis is performed when gingivitis is present and calculus has formed. If the disease has not progressed beyond gingivitis, such treatment will result in resolution. Complete dental prophylaxis includes supragingival and subgingival scaling to remove all plaque and calculus, polishing of the teeth, and rinsing the gingival sulcus (Harvey and Emily, 1993; Holmstrom et al, 1992). Scaling may be done with mechanical and hand instruments. Hand instruments may be used for the entire scaling procedure, but such use usually prolongs the length of the procedure. Mechanical instruments used for scaling include ultrasonic, air sonic, and rotary scalers (Holmstrom et al, 1992). Mechanical instruments are used primarily on the crown to remove the majority of plaque and calculus deposits; with care, they can also be used effectively subgingivally. Hand instruments are necessary to remove remaining plaque and calculus deposits on the crown and to scale subgingivally. Scalers are used supragingivally, and curettes are used supragingivally and subgingivally. Maintaining the sharpness of the hand instruments is important. Polishing the teeth is an essential step after scaling to decrease the rate of subsequent plaque accumulation by smoothing the irregular tooth surface left by scaling. A soft rubber prophy cup and fine prophy paste or flour pumice are used to polish the teeth. The gingival sulcus is irrigated after polishing to remove polishing paste and debris that may have accumulated during the procedure; 0.1 to 0.2 per cent chlorhexidine solution is recommended, which may be followed with a fluoride treatment of the teeth.

Established periodontitis requires additional treatment planning beyond routine dental prophylaxis. When periodontitis is present and periodontal pocket depths are less than 4 to 5 mm, "closed" subgingival plaque and calculus removal and root planing can be performed (Harvey and Emily, 1993; Holmstrom et al, 1992). Periodontal pockets greater than 5 mm in depth are difficult to treat conservatively (Harvey, 1991b). When advanced periodontitis is present and periodontal pockets exceed 9 mm in depth, with alveolar bone loss of 70 per cent or greater, the tooth is best treated by extraction.

In geriatric patients moderate to severely periodontically diseased teeth are best treated with extraction. Simple extractions are those involving single-rooted teeth, excluding the canine tooth. Multirooted teeth, especially the maxillary fourth premolar, maxillary first molar, and mandibular first molar, are more difficult to extract. Extraction techniques have been described in detail elsewhere (Holmstrom et al, 1992; Manfra Marretta and Tholen, 1990) and will be presented only briefly here. When performing an extraction, the gingival attachment is first severed with a scalpel blade or a sharp dental elevator. Single-rooted teeth other than the canine tooth are extracted by forcing a dental elevator between the tooth and alveolar bone to stretch and tear the periodontal ligament. Dental extraction forceps may be used to apply gentle force, levering the tooth toward the buccal and then the lingual surfaces, or to gently rotate the tooth on its long axis. Patience is important in performing a successful extraction; when applying pressure on the tooth, the veterinarian should hold the tooth in each position for several seconds to permit the tearing effect to occur.

Sectioning multirooted teeth into single-rooted segments facilitates the extraction procedure (Manfra Marretta and Tholen, 1990). A crosscut fissure bur on a high-speed handpiece with water irrigation may be used to section teeth. Once the crown has been sectioned into single-rooted segments, each segment is removed as for a single-rooted tooth.

Difficult extractions usually include the canines, maxillary fourth premolar, first maxillary molar, and first mandibular molars. Extracting these teeth may require gingival flap surgery and buccal bone removal to facilitate extraction (Manfra Marretta and Tholen, 1990). The removal of a canine tooth is less difficult when severe periodontitis is present. When extracting the maxillary canine tooth, it is important to avoid levering the crown in the labial direction, as this causes the root apex to move medially into the nasal cavity and may create an oronasal fistula. If an oronasal fistula is present or is created during extraction, a single- or double-flap procedure should be performed (see "Oronasal Fistula").

Complications that may occur during or after tooth extraction include broken root tips, hemorrhage, jaw fracture, osteomyelitis, and oronasal fistula formation (Manfra Marretta and Tholen, 1990). After tooth extraction the alveolar bone should be carefully evaluated for sharp edges or fractures that may inhibit healing, predispose to development of osteomyelitis, or form sequestra (Manfra Marretta and Tholen, 1990). An alveoloplasty should be performed before suture placement to smooth any bony irregularities. The alveolus should be flushed to remove all bony fragments and debris before suturing. Suturing the gingiva is not required after extraction of the incisors or other teeth if severe periodontal disease was present. When extraction sites are sutured, the gingival tissue should be apposed and sutured without creating tension on the gingival tissue.

Home Care. Home care is necessary after dental prophylaxis for optimal plaque control. The success of home care depends on the owner's schedule and commitment and the patient's cooperation. Daily plaque removal is ideal, but removal every 2 days is adequate (Aller, 1989). Older animals may be trained to allow home care. This training process should be gradual, eventually resulting in the patient allowing the home care to be performed (Aller, 1989). Instruments used by owners should be designed to remove plaque without causing harm to the tooth surface. Suitable products for home care include children's or infant's soft toothbrushes, veterinary toothbrushes, finger toothbrushes, gauze pads, and other products designed for plaque removal (Aller, 1993). Oral hygiene products are available as pastes, liquids, gels, and sprays (Aller, 1989). Hard dog food and soft rubber chew toys may help to mechanically remove plaque. However, these are less likely to be successful in aged dogs that are missing some teeth and are more settled in their dietary and chewing habits. Dogs should not be allowed to chew on hard objects, as this may result in tooth fracture.

Fractured Teeth

Cause. Teeth may be fractured by external trauma (e.g., if the animal is hit by a car) or excessive occlusal forces produced by chewing on hard objects (e.g., stones, sticks, and bones). Dogs with severe malocclusions and dogs that are chronic fence chewers may wear down their canine teeth and weaken them to the point where they eventually fracture.

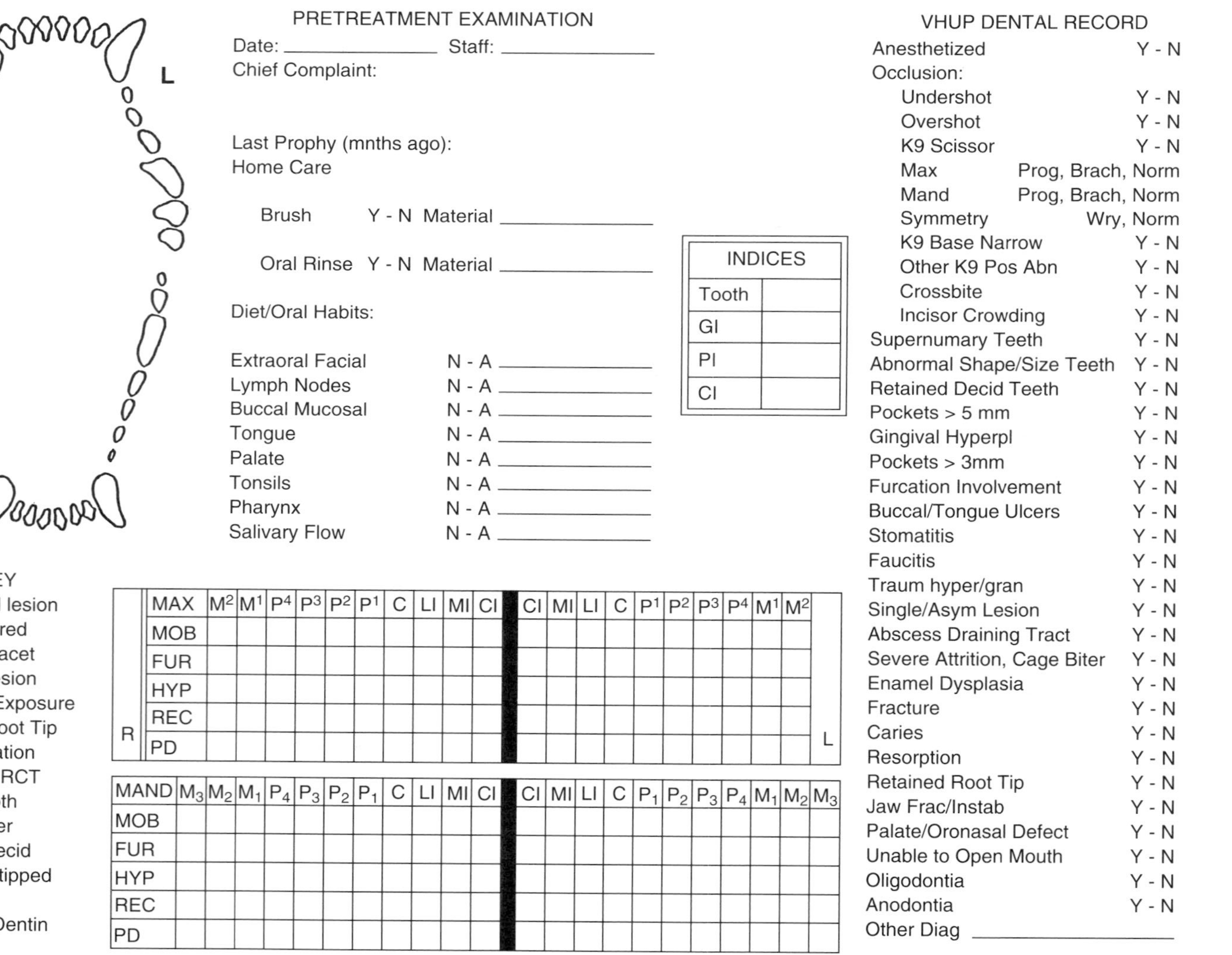

PRETREATMENT EXAMINATION

Date: ______________ Staff: ______________

Chief Complaint:

Last Prophy (mnths ago):

Home Care

Brush Y - N Material ______________

Oral Rinse Y - N Material ______________

Diet/Oral Habits:

Extraoral Facial N - A ______________

Lymph Nodes N - A ______________

Buccal Mucosal N - A ______________

Tongue N - A ______________

Palate N - A ______________

Tonsils N - A ______________

Pharynx N - A ______________

Salivary Flow N - A ______________

INDICES	
Tooth	
GI	
PI	
CI	

VHUP DENTAL RECORD

Anesthetized	Y - N
Occlusion:	
Undershot	Y - N
Overshot	Y - N
K9 Scissor	Y - N
Max	Prog, Brach, Norm
Mand	Prog, Brach, Norm
Symmetry	Wry, Norm
K9 Base Narrow	Y - N
Other K9 Pos Abn	Y - N
Crossbite	Y - N
Incisor Crowding	Y - N
Supernumary Teeth	Y - N
Abnormal Shape/Size Teeth	Y - N
Retained Decid Teeth	Y - N
Pockets > 5 mm	Y - N
Gingival Hyperpl	Y - N
Pockets > 3mm	Y - N
Furcation Involvement	Y - N
Buccal/Tongue Ulcers	Y - N
Stomatitis	Y - N
Faucitis	Y - N
Traum hyper/gran	Y - N
Single/Asym Lesion	Y - N
Abscess Draining Tract	Y - N
Severe Attrition, Cage Biter	Y - N
Enamel Dysplasia	Y - N
Fracture	Y - N
Caries	Y - N
Resorption	Y - N
Retained Root Tip	Y - N
Jaw Frac/Instab	Y - N
Palate/Oronasal Defect	Y - N
Unable to Open Mouth	Y - N
Oligodontia	Y - N
Anodontia	Y - N
Other Diag ______________	

CODE KEY

E-Enamel lesion
Fx-Fractured
W-Wear facet
N-Neck lesion
PE-Pulp Exposure
RT-Ret Root Tip
R-Restoration
RC-Prev. RCT
L-Lost tooth
CH-Chatter
RD-Ret decid
↻Rotated/tipped
C-Caries
SD-Sec. Dentin

	MAX	M^2	M^1	P^4	P^3	P^2	P^1	C	LI	MI	CI	CI	MI	LI	C	P^1	P^2	P^3	P^4	M^1	M^2	
	MOB																					
	FUR																					
	HYP																					
	REC																					
R	PD																					L

MAND	M_3	M_2	M_1	P_4	P_3	P_2	P_1	C	LI	MI	CI	CI	MI	LI	C	P_1	P_2	P_3	P_4	M_1	M_2	M_3
MOB																						
FUR																						
HYP																						
REC																						
PD																						

Figure 9–6. Example of canine *(above)* and feline *(next page)* dental charts used to record oral examination findings.

R L

CODE KEY
E-Enamel lesion
Fx-Fractured
W-Wear facet
N-Neck lesion
PE-Pulp Exposure
RT-Ret Root Tip
R-Restoration
RC-Prev. RCT
L-Lost tooth
RD-Ret decid
ʕ-Rotated/tipped
H-Ging Hyperplas
M-Mobility
#-Perio Pocket
F-Furcation
GR-Ging Recess

PRETREATMENT EXAMINATION

Date: ______________ Staff: ______________

Chief Complaint:

Last Prophy (mnths ago):

Home Care

Brush Y - N Material ______________

Oral Rinse Y - N Material ______________

Diet/Oral Habits:

Extraoral Facial N - A ______________

Lymph Nodes N - A ______________

Buccal Mucosal N - A ______________

Tongue N - A ______________

Palate N - A ______________

Tonsils N - A ______________

Pharynx N - A ______________

Salivary Flow N - A ______________

INDICES	
Tooth	
GI	
PI	
CI	

VHUP DENTAL RECORD

Anesthetized	Y - N
Occlusion:	
Undershot	Y - N
Overshot	Y - N
K9 Scissor	Y - N
Max	Prog, Brach, Norm
Mand	Prog, Brach, Norm
Symmetry	Wry, Norm
K9 Base Narrow	Y - N
Other K9 Pos Abn	Y - N
Crossbite	Y - N
Incisor Crowding	Y - N
Supernumary Teeth	Y - N
Abnormal Shape/Size Teeth	Y - N
Retained Decid Teeth	Y - N
Pockets > 5mm	Y - N
Gingival Hyperpl	Y - N
Pockets > 3mm	Y - N
Furcation Involvement	Y - N
Buccal/Tongue Ulcers	Y - N
Stomatitis	Y - N
Faucitis	Y - N
Traum hyper/gran	Y - N
Single/Asym Lesion	Y - N
Abscess Draining Tract	Y - N
Severe Attrition, eg. Cage Biter	Y - N
Enamel Dysplasia	Y - N
Fracture	Y - N
Caries	Y - N
Resorption	Y - N
Retained Root Tip	Y - N
Jaw Frac/Instab	Y - N
Palate/Oronasal Defect	Y - N
Unable to Open Mouth	Y - N
Other Diag ______________	

Figure 9–6 *Continued*

Incidence. Fractured teeth are common in the dog and occur less frequently in aged dogs than in young dogs. The crowns are affected more often than the roots. The incisors, maxillary fourth premolar, and maxillary canines are most frequently fractured (Harvey, 1989; Rossman et al, 1985).

Clinical Features. A tooth fracture extending into the dentin may be painful. Exposed dentinal tubules are sensitive to stimulation by heat, cold, or pressure (Rossman et al, 1985). A dog with an acute fracture involving the pulp may exhibit signs of pain or may show little evidence of discomfort (Williams, 1986). The exposed pulp may be a source of pain until it dies and becomes necrotic (Manfra Marretta, 1992a). Clinical signs may include refusal to chew or bite down on hard objects or food, refusal to carry objects in the mouth, chewing on one side of the mouth only, and constant licking (Williams, 1986).

Diagnosis. A fractured tooth crown is identified by visual examination. A dental explorer is used to determine whether the pulp has been exposed by the fracture. In a fresh fracture the pulp tissue will bleed when probed. In an old fracture the pulp tissue is dead and appears as a dark spot in the center of the tooth. Dental radiographs are necessary to identify root fractures.

Management. Specific treatment for a crown fracture is not required if pulp tissue is not exposed (Harvey, 1989). Rough tooth edges that might lacerate the buccal mucosa should be smoothed out (Rossman et al, 1985). Significant loss of the crown structure may require a crown buildup procedure with a restorative material to prevent gingival damage. A tooth with pulp exposure may develop a periapical abscess, and therefore treatment of such a tooth is recommended (Harvey, 1989; Rossman et al, 1985). Options for ideal treatment of a fractured tooth with pulp exposure include a root canal procedure or extraction (Harvey, 1989; Rossman et al, 1985). However, root canal treatment in aged patients is more difficult because of their narrow root canal diameters (Harvey and Emily, 1993). The narrow root canal lumens are more difficult to locate and debride, and total debridement to the apex may not be possible. Conventional endodontic therapy may be successful even though radiographic evaluation demonstrates that the obturation is 2 to 3 mm short of the apex (Harvey and Emily, 1993). A surgical root canal procedure can be done to salvage the tooth if a conventional root canal fails.

In most geriatric patients the typical choices for management of a recently fractured tooth are extraction or benign neglect. Teeth with fractures that extend into the root should be extracted. Horizontal root fractures occurring at the level of the alveolar bone crest require extraction (Rossman et al, 1985). The root may be saved after crown extraction by treating it endodontically. A crown may be placed on the remaining root if a crown-lengthening procedure is done. A post-and-core crown restoration is the preferred crown used for restoration (Rossman et al, 1985). Horizontal root fractures that are below the alveolar crest may be sufficiently stabilized by surrounding bone and not require treatment. If the crown is discolored, indicating pulpal trauma or death, the treatment options include extraction of the entire tooth, root canal therapy, or leaving the tooth alone and periodically evaluating it for development of disease (Rossman et al, 1985).

Root fractures occurring along the long axis of the root cannot be treated, and the tooth should be extracted (Emily and Penman, 1990). Root fractures in the coronal third of the root may be endodontically treated, followed by placement of a post in the endodontic system; however, prognosis is poor with this type of fracture (Holmstrom et al, 1992). Teeth should be extracted when root fractures occur in the middle third of the root. The best prognosis for root fractures occurs with fractures in the apical third of the root. Treatment of root fractures in the apical third of the root may not be required (Emily and Penman, 1990). The apical segment may maintain its normal blood supply, and the coronal segment will often receive adequate collateral circulation. A cementodentinal callus develops at the fracture site and prevents pulpal pathology (Emily and Penman, 1990). Pulpal disease, if it develops, is usually in the coronal segment, and conventional endodontic therapy is required only on the coronal segment. The apical segment rarely becomes diseased; if it does, it should be removed and the coronal segment treated with conventional or surgical endodontic therapy. (Emily and Penman, 1990).

Periapical Abscessation

Cause and Incidence. The tooth most commonly affected with a periapical abscess is the maxillary fourth premolar. The problem is most commonly seen in older dogs (Harvey, 1989). Periapical abscesses form secondary to bacterial infection of the pulp tissue. The pulp tissue can be infected after exposure by a crown fracture or hematogenously after trauma.

Clinical Features. Clinical signs may include avoiding chewing on hard food, excessive salivation, jaw chattering, constant licking, reluctance to carry anything in the mouth, and a general feeling of malaise (Emily and Penman, 1990). Working dogs may be reluctant to bite down hard on objects used in training exercises. An apical abscess of the maxillary fourth premolar may lead to a soft tissue swelling or draining fistula ventral to the medial canthus of the eye (Fig. 9–7). These are usually painful until they rupture and drain. A fracture of the affected tooth with exposure of the pulp tissue may be noted on oral examination.

If the palatal root of the maxillary fourth premolar is affected, epistaxis or unilateral nasal discharge may be present. If the maxillary first molar has a periapical abscess, the dog may exhibit pain on opening the mouth. Exophthalmus and maxillary sinusitis may also be present. Periapical abscesses involving the maxillary canine teeth usually cause a facial swelling above the second premolar. A swelling below the mandible at the level of the second or third premolar is present with periapical disease of the mandibular canine teeth. Periapical abscesses in mandibular canine teeth may drain externally through the skin or into the oral cavity.

Diagnosis. The presence of a periapical abscess should be considered when a facial swelling develops over the apex of a tooth root. A dental radiograph is taken to confirm the diagnosis. A radiolucent area surrounding the apex of the tooth affected with a periapical abscess will be present.

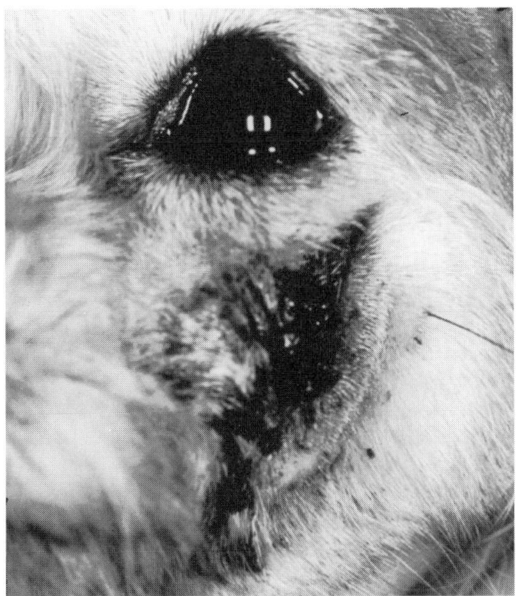

Figure 9–7. Draining tract from periapical abscess involving the maxillary fourth premolar tooth.

Management. If adequate alveolar bone remains, the tooth may be successfully treated endodontically (Harvey, 1989). An alternative to root canal therapy is extraction.

Oronasal Fistula

Cause. Oronasal fistulas occur secondary to severe periodontitis, periapical root abscess formation, or trauma. The distal and palatal aspects of the maxillary canine teeth are frequently sites of severe periodontitis resulting in deep periodontal pocket formation. There is a relatively thin section of bone between the maxillary canine tooth root and the nasal cavity that can be destroyed by a periapical abscess or severe periodontal disease. This thin portion of bone can also be destroyed iatrogenically if the tooth root is levered medially during extraction of a maxillary canine tooth.

Incidence. The tooth most frequently associated with oronasal fistula formation is the maxillary canine.

Clinical Features. Clinical signs associated with an oronasal fistula include nasal discharge and sneezing. The character of the nasal discharge may be serous, serosanguineous, or purulent.

Diagnosis. The diagnosis is made by examining the oral cavity and demonstrating a deep periodontal pocket that communicates with the nasal cavity or by observing the fistula if the tooth is absent (Fig. 9–8). The presence of an oronasal fistula is confirmed if hemorrhage from the nose occurs on the affected side when a periodontal probe is inserted into the pocket or when the tooth is extracted. Dental radiographs are usually not contributory in determining the presence or absence of an oronasal fistula.

Management. Oronasal fistulas may be closed with a single-layer or double-layer mucoperiosteal flap (Harvey and Emily, 1993). A single-layer mucoperiosteal flap is successful in the majority of cases. The first step in the procedure is to debride the epithelial margin of the fistula. Divergent releasing incisions are made down through the periosteum on either side of the fistula, extending above the mucogingival line. The flap is gently raised with a periosteal elevator. The flap is reflected once it is raised, and the attachment tissues of the lip are incised at the

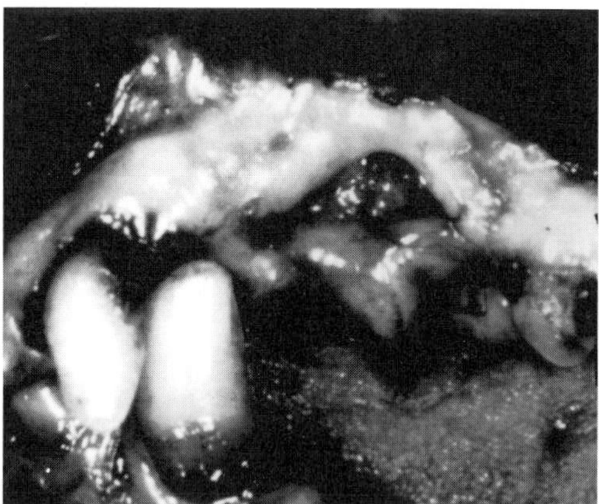

Figure 9–8. Dog with an oronasal fistula secondary to severe periodontal disease involving the maxillary canine, which has been lost.

base of the flap. When excising this tissue, care is taken to leave the mucosa intact. Once the periosteum has been incised, the flap should cover the oronasal fistula without creating any tension on the tissues. If the flap is sutured under tension, it is more likely to dehisce. If buccal bone interferes with tissue apposition, it should be removed with rongeurs or a dental bur. The oronasal fistula should be thoroughly irrigated before closure. The flap is sutured in a single interrupted pattern with absorbable suture material.

A double-layer mucoperiosteal flap may also be used to close an oronasal fistula. This technique provides double-layer coverage of the fistula. A palatal flap and a buccal mucoperiosteal flap are used to cover the fistula.

Gingival Hyperplasia

Cause. Gingival hyperplasia may be a response to chronic irritation or inflammation from plaque and calculus accumulation (Beard and Beard, 1989; Tholen and Hoyt, 1990). However, it is often present in dogs with minimal plaque or calculus that do not have acute gingivitis (Harvey, 1989). Boxers, Great Danes, collies, Doberman pinschers, dalmatians, and Afghan hounds are commonly affected. A heritable predisposition is likely in the commonly affected breeds (Beard and Beard, 1989; Harvey, 1989; Tholen and Hoyt, 1990). Phenytoin has been reported to cause gingival hyperplasia in a dog (Waner and Nyska, 1991). Dogs have also developed gingival hyperplasia under experimental conditions when administered calcium channel blocking drugs (i.e., oxodipine, nitrendipine, and verapamil) and cyclosporine (Waner and Nyska, 1991).

Incidence. Gingival hyperplasia is common in aged dogs (Beard and Beard, 1989).

Clinical Features. Hyperplastic gingival tissue is a firm, nonpainful, proliferative lesion of the free gingival margin (Beard and Beard, 1989; Harvey, 1989). It may be so extensive that the teeth are covered by the excessive gingival tissue. When gingival hyperplasia is present, it leads to the formation of deep periodontal pockets (pseudopockets). When pocket depth is significantly increased, increased subgingival plaque accumulation results (Harvey, 1989).

Diagnosis. Large hyperplastic gingival lesions may resemble an epulis. A definitive diagnosis is made by collecting a biopsy specimen for histopathologic examination (Harvey, 1989).

Management. Gingival hyperplasia is managed with a gingivectomy to remove excessive gingival tissue and return the gingival sulcus to a normal depth. It may be performed with a gingivectomy knife, scalpel blade, or electrocautery (Beard and Beard, 1989). When removing excessive gingival tissue, caution must be taken to avoid damaging the underlying tooth or alveolar bone. To perform a gingivectomy, the pocket depth is first measured with a periodontal probe. The pocket depth is marked on the external surface of the gingiva by creating bleeding points with the periodontal probe that correspond to the bottom of the periodontal pocket. The gingivectomy is performed apical to the bleeding points, creating a normal angle to the gingival margin. A minimum of 2 mm of attached gingiva should remain after the procedure. After gingivectomy the tooth surface is scaled and polished. Postsurgical care includes feeding soft food for a few days if necessary and maintaining a clean oral cavity while the gingiva heals.

Dental Caries

Cause. Dental caries are areas of demineralized tooth enamel caused by toxins released from microorganisms after carbohydrate fermentation.

Incidence. Caries are uncommon in dogs, but they do occur occasionally, especially in older dogs. The occlusal surface of the maxillary and mandibular molars are most commonly affected (Tholen and Hoyt, 1990).

Clinical Features. Caries initially appear as chalky white areas on the enamel. As a caries progresses the site becomes brown to black in color (Tholen and Hoyt, 1990). A dog with a caries may be reluctant to eat and may exhibit chattering of the jaw (Rossman et al, 1985).

Diagnosis. The diagnosis is made on clinical examination, usually while the animal is anesthetized. The caries will be visible as a chalky white or brown-black area. The enamel is soft, and a dental explorer will penetrate and stick in the lesion. By contrast, exposed dentin is hard and is not penetrated by an explorer (Fig. 9–9). Dental radiographs may be required to evaluate the extent of the lesion and determine pulp involvement.

Management. Treatment of dental caries involves removal of all affected tooth structure and placement of a restorative material in the cavity (Tholen and Hoyt, 1990). Amalgam is the preferred restorative material on occlusal surfaces because of its strength. If the pulp is involved, a root canal must be completed before placing such material. Extraction of the affected tooth is recommended if the caries is not treated with restorative therapy.

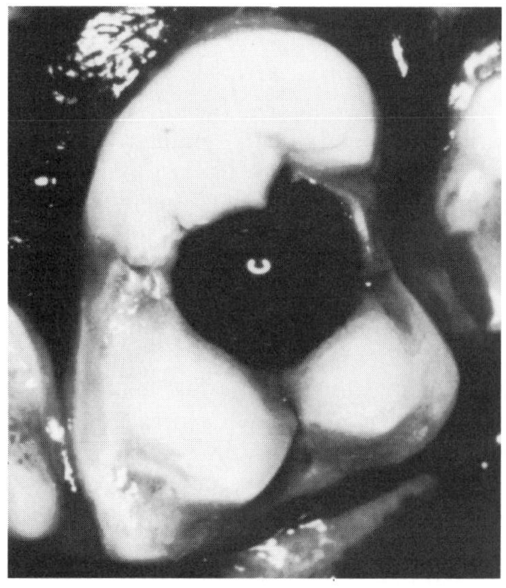

Figure 9–9. Caries on the occlusal surface of the first maxillary molar.

Worn Teeth (Attrition)

Cause and Incidence. A slight amount of tooth wear is normal in aged dogs, with the incisors being the most commonly affected (Harvey, 1989; Rossman et al, 1985). Abnormally rapid loss of crown height or attrition is common (Rossman et al, 1985). Attrition may be associated with a chewing vice or malocclusions (Williams, 1986). Dogs with pruritic dermatologic problems will often chew on themselves excessively and may demonstrate severe attrition of the incisors (Rossman et al, 1985) (Fig. 9–10).

Clinical Features. If the enamel is worn down gradually, reparative dentin is laid down, protecting the pulp from exposure. Reparative dentin is identified as a dark brown spot in the center of the tooth (Harvey, 1989; Williams, 1986). If attrition occurs very rapidly, the pulp tissue may be exposed.

Diagnosis. A dental explorer is used to evaluate the worn tooth for evidence of pulp involvement. If a defect in the central brown area is detected with a dental explorer, then the pulp has been exposed. Reparative dentin is smooth and covers the center of the tooth, so a dental explorer cannot enter the pulp.

Management. Treatment is not necessary when the pulp has not been exposed. If the pulp has been exposed or becomes necrotic, endodontic treatment or extraction should be performed.

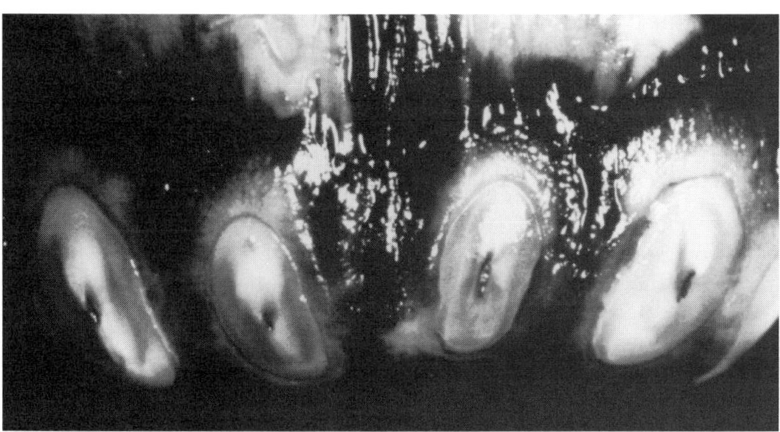

Figure 9–10. Severe attrition of the incisors in a dog.

Mandibular Fractures

Cause. Small breed dogs are especially prone to pathologic mandibular fractures secondary to severe periodontal disease. Minimal stress to the bone (e.g., chewing on a bone) may cause bilateral mandibular fractures if severe periodontal disease is present. Iatrogenic fractures may occur in dogs with severe periodontal disease during attempted extraction of the mandibular first molar or canine tooth (Manfra Marretta, 1987).

Clinical Features. Fractures occur most frequently in the region of the first mandibular molar. Bilateral mandibular fractures in the region of the first molar are usually open fractures, and affected dogs are often presented with the rostral portion of their mandible ventrally displaced (Manfra Marretta, 1987).

Diagnosis. The diagnosis is made by direct examination and radiographic evaluation.

Management. Teeth in the fracture line are generally not extracted until the fracture has healed, unless the teeth are unstable (Harvey and Emily, 1993). Certain mandibular fractures may be managed by placing a tape muzzle around the nose and mandible. However, this technique should be limited to animals with intact canine teeth and unilateral fractures. Additional methods of fixation include dental wiring and splinting, osseous wiring, plates and screws, and pins (Harvey and Emily, 1993).

Oral Tumors

Incidence. The oral cavity is the fourth most common site of tumors in the dog (Oakes et al, 1993) (Table 9–2). Malignant melanoma is the most common malignant oral tumor in dogs, followed by squamous cell carcinoma and fibrosarcoma. Other malignant tumors may also be found in the oral cavity (Oakes et al, 1993). Epulides are the most common benign oral tumors. Odontogenic tumors, also benign, occur infrequently in dogs; ameloblastomas are the most common such tumors (Oakes et al, 1993).

Clinical Features. Hemorrhage from the oral cavity, reluctance to eat or chew, drooling, loose teeth, and a foul oral odor may be associated with oral tumors. Frequently the tumors are large at the time of diagnosis and cause a facial deformity or are visible. Neoplasia should be suspected if a loose tooth is found in a focal area of inflammation or ulceration. The prognosis for long-term survival is poor for malignant melanomas because of local invasiveness and early metastasis (Oakes et al, 1993).

Diagnosis. The diagnostic evaluation should allow for clinical staging according to the World Health Organization (Oakes et al, 1993). A minimum data base (complete blood cell [CBC] count, chemistry profile, and urinalysis) should be obtained for each dog, and specific diagnostic tests should be performed to evaluate the tumor. The tumor may be identified by fine-needle aspiration cytology or biopsy collection with histopathologic evaluation. The local extent of tumor involvement may be determined with skull radiographs, computed axial tomography, or magnetic resonance imaging. Regional lymph node involvement and evidence of distant metastasis should also be determined (Oakes et al, 1993).

Treatment. Surgical excision is generally the recommended treatment for the majority of oral tumors. The reader is referred to the reference list for sources describing the surgical procedures and other treatment modalities (Oakes et al, 1993).

DISORDERS OF CATS

Periodontal Disease

Cause. Gingivitis is inflammation of the marginal gingiva. The inflammation occurs in response to bacteria (plaque) accumulating adjacent to the free gingival margin. If left untreated, gingivitis may progress to periodontitis, or inflammation of the periodontium (gingiva, periodontal ligament, cementum, and alveolar bone). Periodontitis occurs when plaque bacteria accumulate subgingivally, leading to inflammation of the periodontium.

Incidence. Periodontal disease is the most common problem of the oral cavity in cats (Holmstrom, 1989). Aged cats have an increased incidence of severe periodontal disease (i.e., periodontitis). The upper premolar and molar teeth are the most severely affected by gingival inflammation and calculus deposits (Harvey, 1992).

Clinical Features. Clinical signs associated with gingivitis include halitosis, redness of the gingival margins, and gingival edema, which causes rounding of the gingival margin and loss of its sharp edge. Inflamed gingiva tends to bleed either spontaneously or with minimal pressure. Clinical signs associated with periodontitis, in addition to signs of gingivitis, may include gingival recession, increased tooth mobility, gingival sul-

TABLE 9–2. COMMON ORAL TUMORS IN DOGS AND CATS

	CANINE				FELINE	
	SCC	FS	MM	Dental	SCC	FS
Frequency (%)	17–30	7.5–25	30–42	5	70	20
Age (yr)	8–10	7–8.3	10–12	9	10	10
Patient size	Larger	Larger	Smaller	No prevalence	—	—
Site predilection	Gingiva, rostral mandible	Palate, gingiva, maxilla	Gingiva, buccal mucosa	Rostral mandible	Mandible, maxillary bone	Gingiva
Regional lymph node metastasis	Rare (except tonsil and tongue)	Rare	Common	Never	Occasional	Rare
Distant metastasis	Rare (except tonsil and tongue)	Occasional	Common	Never	Rare	Occasional
Prognosis	Rostral, good; caudal, poor	Poor–fair	Poor–fair	Excellent	Poor	Fair–good

FS, fibrosarcoma; MM, melanoma; SCC, squamous cell carcinoma; —, not applicable.

Compiled from Oakes MG, Hedlund CS, Lewis DD, et al. Canine oral neoplasia. Compend Contin Educ Pract Vet 15:1, 15, 1993; and Withrow SJ. Tumors of the gastrointestinal system. In Withrow SJ, Mac Ewen EG, eds. Clinical Veterinary Oncology. Philadelphia, JB Lippincott, 1989, p 177.

cus depth greater than the normal 0 to 1 mm, pain with eating or biting on hard objects, and ptyalism. Owners may report a change in food preference or eating behavior in cats with severe periodontitis.

Diagnosis. Periodontal disease is identified on oral examination. The extent of periodontal involvement is diagnosed by careful oral examination performed with the cat under general anesthesia. A dental probe is used to evaluate for increased periodontal pocket depth indicative of periodontitis. An explorer is used to identify odontoclastic resorptive lesions. Dental radiographs are important to determine the extent of disease and the integrity of tooth roots, pulp tissue, and alveolar bone. They are also essential for identification of root tip fragments that contribute to chronic gingivitis, stomatitis, and faucitis (Fig. 9–11).

Management. Complete dental prophylaxis should be performed to remove all supragingival and subgingival plaque and calculus. Mechanical methods (e.g., ultrasonic, air sonic, and rotary burs on high-speed handpieces) may be used to remove the majority of supragingival plaque and calculus. Hand instruments are used to remove the remaining plaque and calculus and to scale subgingivally. The teeth should be polished after scaling. After completion of dental prophylaxis, the gingival sulcus should be flushed to remove debris and polishing material that may have accumulated during the procedure; 0.1 per cent to 0.2 per cent chlorhexidine solution is recommended, which may be followed with a fluoride treatment of the teeth. Home care is advised to retard plaque accumulation (see discussion of home care for dogs with periodontal disease). Unfortunately, even with a compliant owner, some cats may not be cooperative enough for successful home care.

Odontoclastic Resorptive Lesions

Cause. Odontoclastic resorptive lesions are erosions in the tooth that begin at or near the cementoenamel junction. The underlying cause

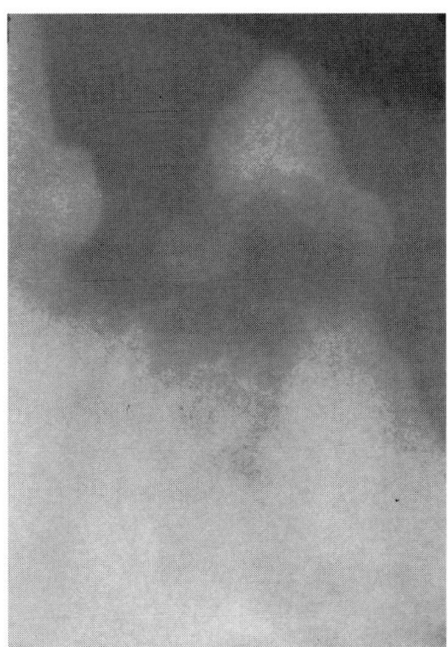

Figure 9–11. Dental radiograph of a tooth with an odontoclastic resorptive lesion showing severe loss of crown and remaining root fragments.

of these lesions has not been identified. Originally the lesions were thought to be caries, but this is not the case.

Incidence. Odontoclastic resorptive lesions are a common problem in domestic cats. The prevalence rate has been as high as 67 per cent in some reports (van Wessum et al, 1992). Siamese, Abyssinian, and Persian cats have been reported to have an increased incidence compared with other breeds. The incidence of resorptive lesions and the number of lesions per cat are increased in older cats (van Wessum et al, 1992). The buccal and labial surfaces of the premolar and molar teeth are most frequently affected.

Clinical Features. Clinical signs may be absent in cats with minor lesions. Cats with advanced lesions have significant oral pain and associated signs such as anorexia, changes in eating behavior, or changes in food preference (i.e., soft versus dry food). Oral examination may suggest the presence of odontoclastic resorptive lesions. Proliferative gingival tissue will frequently cover a lesion (Fig. 9–12), and the tissue usually bleeds very readily. Extensive tooth destruction may result in partial loss of a tooth crown or complete loss with retained root fragments. Gingivitis may be present in areas where root fragments remain.

Diagnosis. Odontoclastic resorptive lesions are classified into four stages based on the extent of the tooth resorption (Table 9–3). Stage 1 lesions are identified by using a dental explorer to locate the defect. Stage 2 lesions are painful, and the cat may respond even under anesthesia when these are explored. In a light plane of anesthesia, the cat will typically exhibit a chattering motion with the jaw when the lesions are probed. Dental radiographs should be taken to determine whether the pulp is involved. Tooth structure is compromised to a variable degree in Stage 3 lesions; dental radiographs are taken to evaluate pulp involvement if there is any doubt. In Stage 4 lesions the roots may be completely transformed by the resorptive process. The crown may be missing, and gingival tissue may have closed over the root remnants. Radiographs may be required to identify retained root fragments. The tooth roots may be ankylosed to the alveolar bone as a result of periodontal ligament loss and cementum remodeling.

TABLE 9–3. CLASSIFICATION OF ODONTOCLASTIC RESORPTIVE LESIONS

Stage 1:	Early lesions with resorption involving enamel and cementum only
Stage 2:	Lesions that extend into the dentin but do not involve the pulp
Stage 3:	Advanced lesions that extend into the pulp
Stage 4:	Chronic lesions with extensive tooth involvement

Canine teeth typically have minimal evidence of disease on the tooth crown, even when the root is totally destroyed (Fig. 9–13). Dental radiographs should be taken of these teeth to diagnose the root resorption (Fig. 9–14).

Management. Treatment of odontoclastic resorptive lesions should be directed at resolving oral pain and returning the cat's oral cavity to a healthy, nonpainful condition. Stage 1 lesions are too small to require restoration. Treatment should include complete dental prophylaxis followed by polishing with a nonfluoridated flour-grade pumice. A fluoride cavity varnish is applied to the clean dry tooth and allowed to air dry. A

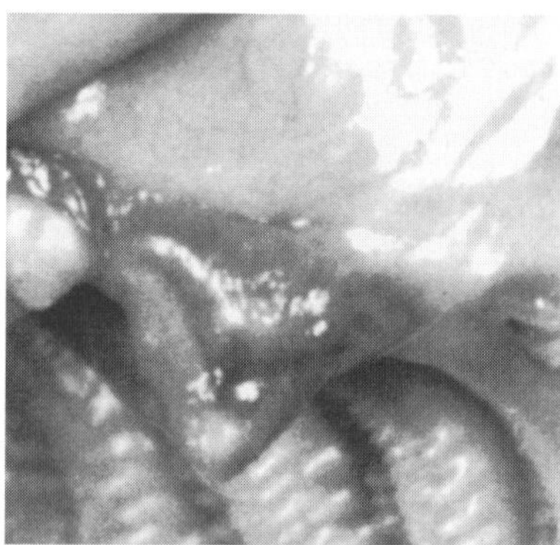

Figure 9–12. Proliferative gingival tissue covering an odontoclastic resorptive lesion.

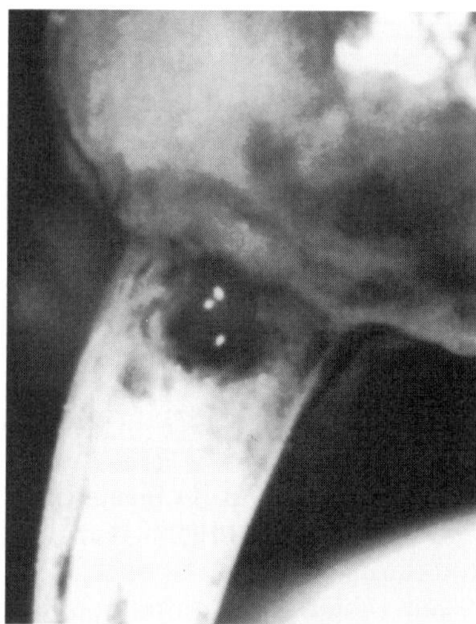

Figure 9–13. Feline canine tooth with evidence of an odontoclastic resorptive lesion at the gingival margin.

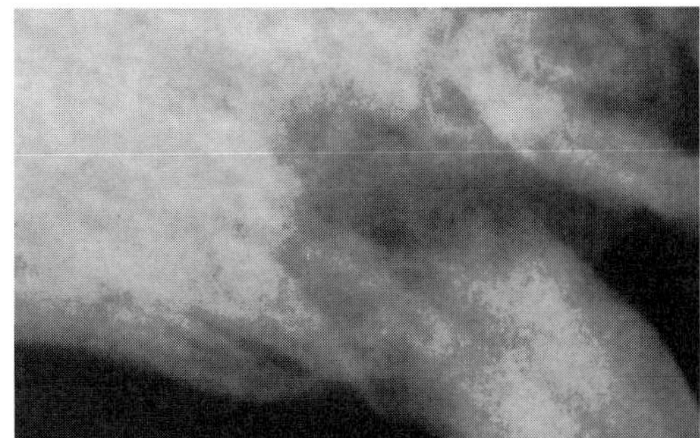

Figure 9–14. Dental radiograph of the cat shown in Figure 9–13 demonstrating complete destruction of the maxillary canine tooth root.

fluoride gel should be applied to the tooth on a regular basis to slow plaque accumulation on the tooth (Lyon, 1992). The treatment of choice for Stage 2, 3, or 4 resorptive lesions in geriatric cats is extraction. Treatment of Stage 2 lesions by placement of restorative material has been described (Lyon, 1992) but is not practical in the aged cat.

Oral Inflammatory Disease

Cause. Gingivitis and periodontitis are the result of plaque and calculus accumulating supragingivally and subgingivally (see preceding discussion of feline periodontal disease). Systemic diseases, immune-mediated diseases, trauma, and oral neoplasms can cause inflammation in the oral cavity. In some cats inflammation involving the oral mucosa (stomatitis), pharynx, palate, tongue, and glossopalatine arches (faucitis) has an undetermined cause. Plasmacytic-lymphocytic gingivitis-stomatitis-pharyngitis has been described as a specific syndrome characterized histologically by an infiltrate of primarily plasma cells and lymphocytes. The cause of this syndrome is unknown, but chronic antigenic stimulation is suggested. A group of cats diagnosed with plasmacytic-lymphocytic gingivitis have been evaluated for serum antibodies directed against known human periodontal pathogens (Sims et al, 1990). An increased serum immunoglobulin G (IgG) titer against these pathogens suggests a bacterial component for the cause of plasmacytic-lymphocytic gingivitis-stomatitis-pharyngitis. An inappropriate or hypersensitivity response to oral bacteria has been suggested as a cause for chronic stomatitis. Inflammation, proliferation, and ulceration of tissue in the glossopalatine arch (faucitis) is a prominent feature in some cats. Viruses have been suggested as potential pathogens causing or contributing to oral inflammation. Feline calicivirus causes acute gingivitis and faucitis and may play a role in chronic faucitis (Reubel et al, 1992). Calicivirus has been isolated from oropharyngeal swabs of the fauces in cats with chronic oral inflammation. Feline leukemia virus (FeLV) probably does not play a significant role as a primary pathogen of oral inflammatory disease (Pederson, 1992). FeLV-infected cats that are immunocompromised and neutropenic may be more likely to have oral disease. Chronic gingivitis, periodontitis, and stomatitis are the most common clinical signs associated with feline immunodeficiency virus (FIV) infection (August, 1989). Cats with concurrent FIV and calicivirus infection are more likely to develop chronic faucitis (Tenorio et al, 1991). The underlying cause of many cases of chronic oral inflammatory disease currently is not known. The reason some cats are more predisposed to the development of chronic oral inflammatory disease is also unknown.

Incidence. The incidence of gingivitis and periodontitis is high and increases as cats get older. Chronic oral inflammatory disease is a relatively common problem in cats.

Clinical Features. Gingivitis is inflammation of the gingiva and is clinically recognized as gingival margin hyperemia, edema (with resulting rounded edges), and a tendency to bleed easily. Periodontitis is inflammation of the gingiva as well as involvement of the periodontal ligament, alveolar bone, and cementum. Clinical signs of periodontitis may include gingival recession, increased periodontal pocket depth, furcation exposure, and tooth mobility. Chronic oral inflammatory disease with gingival and mucosal tissue proliferation and ulceration may cause clinical signs of halitosis, ptyalism, blood-tinged saliva, inappetence, anorexia, and oral pain.

Diagnosis. Gingivitis and periodontitis resulting from dental disease can be diagnosed with a complete oral examination and response to dental prophylaxis. Oral examination, laboratory assessment, and a patient history will help to rule out systemic disease, trauma, and neoplasia as underlying causes for oral inflammation. Oropharyngeal swabs may be used for calicivirus isolation. Serologic tests to determine the presence of antibodies to FIV may also be indicated. A biopsy specimen of the involved oral tissue should be collected for histopathologic analysis. Chronic inflammatory diseases usually show a predominance of neutrophils or plasma cells and lymphocytes (Harvey, 1991a).

Management. A complete dental prophylaxis should be performed in all cases to eliminate any inflammation secondary to plaque and calculus accumulation. Several medical treatments have been suggested for management of chronic oral inflammatory diseases, but the response to such treatments is generally poor (Harvey and Emily, 1993). Antimicrobial agents may provide temporary relief, but generally the inflammation returns after antimicrobials are discontinued. Anti-inflammatory doses of corticosteroids may also be beneficial in decreasing the inflammation. However, the frequency of administration required to alleviate clinical signs and the varied response to therapy make this a less desirable choice. Controversy exists over the use of corticosteroids and its potential harm in immunosuppressed cats with FeLV or FIV. Progestins, gold salt therapy, immunoregulin, cryotherapy, and laser therapy have been recommended, with varying reports of success. Unresponsive or severe cases may benefit from extraction of all the teeth caudal to the canines. Some veterinary dentists have reported excellent success with this therapy.

Oronasal Fistula

Cause. Oronasal fistulas may be associated with dental disease in cats (Manfra Marretta, 1988). They may result from severe periodontal disease or may occur as a complication of extraction (Kapatkin et al, 1990). Periapical lysis secondary to tooth fracture has been reported as a cause of an oronasal fistula in a cat (Manfra Marretta, 1988). Odontoclastic resorptive lesions with pulp exposure can also lead to an oronasal fistula (Manfra Marretta, 1988).

Incidence. Oronasal fistulas secondary to dental problems are less frequent in cats than in dogs (Manfra Marretta, 1988). Oronasal fistulas in the cat are generally associated with the maxillary canine (Wiggs and Lobprise, 1993). Oronasal fistulas of the cat maxillary canine have been considered rare but may be more common than the veterinary literature has suggested (Manfra Marretta, 1988).

Clinical Features. Clinical signs associated with an oronasal fistula may include nasal discharge (purulent or hemorrhagic), mucoid ipsilateral ocular discharge, and signs of upper respiratory tract disease (e.g., sneezing, nasal and ocular discharge) (Manfra Marretta, 1988).

Diagnosis. An oronasal fistula may be identified after tooth extraction or at a site of tooth loss by visualizing the exposed nasal cavity. When the tooth remains, the fistula may be identified by probing a deep pocket or defect and observing bleeding from the ipsilateral nostril. Dental radiographs may reveal bone loss surrounding the root apex, supporting a diagnosis of oronasal fistula.

Management. Uncomplicated cases may be repaired with a mucoperiosteal flap (Manfra Marretta, 1988; Wiggs and Lobprise, 1993). The prognosis for successful corrective procedures may be more guarded in cats with chronic oronasal fistula, which may be associated with severe underlying infections, possibly even osteomyelitis (Wiggs and Lobprise, 1993). Recurrent or large oronasal fistulas may require a double-layer flap technique (Kapatkin et al, 1990).

Fractured Teeth

Cause. Fractured teeth are frequently identified on physical examination, and the cause is usually unknown (Manfra Marretta, 1992a). Trauma (e.g., being struck by a car or falling) is one potential cause of fracture in a normal, healthy tooth (Frost and Williams, 1986; Holmstrom 1992). Teeth that have been weakened by disease (e.g., odontoclastic resorptive lesions) may be fractured by normal occlusal forces (Wiggs and Lobprise, 1993).

Incidence. Fractured teeth are commonly identified in cats (Frost and Williams, 1986; Mills, 1992). Horizontal fractures through the tip or middle of the crown of the canine tooth are the most frequently seen fractures (Frost and Williams, 1986). Vertical fractures are seen occasionally.

Clinical Features. Fractures may involve the crown tip without pulp exposure, the crown with pulp exposure, or the tooth root. A fracture that does not expose or damage the pulp will not cause clinical signs (Wiggs and Lobprise, 1993). An acute fracture with pulp exposure will have a pink or red dot indicating such exposure and will bleed (Wiggs and Lobprise, 1993). Acute pulp exposure may cause discomfort, which usually lasts for 1 to 7 days (Wiggs and Lobprise, 1993). Clinical signs associated with an acute fracture with pulp exposure may include hypersalivation, reluctance to eat, abnormal behavior, and pawing at the mouth (Manfra Marretta, 1992a; Wiggs and Lobprise, 1993). After a fracture that exposes the pulp, a series of events may progressively occur over the ensuing months to years. These events, which can result in a number of clinical signs, include pulpitis, pulpal necrosis, apical granuloma, periapical abscess, acute alveolar periodontitis, osteomyelitis, and sepsis (Manfra Marretta, 1992a). Cats that develop periapical disease may show signs of pain and may develop facial swellings or draining tracts. Cats with fractured teeth and pulp exposure of chronic duration may present with nasal discharge and signs of chronic rhinitis (Manfra Marretta, 1992a).

Diagnosis. A dental explorer is used to probe any fractured tooth with suspected pulp exposure. If the explorer penetrates the suspected site and enters inside the tooth, the pulp has been exposed (Manfra Marretta, 1992a). Dental radiographs are used to identify periapical disease resulting from tooth fracture and pulp exposure.

Management. A fractured tooth with no pulp exposure may not require treatment. Smoothing the fracture to prevent self-trauma and to reduce plaque and calculus accumulation has been recommended (Wiggs and Lobprise, 1993). A fractured tooth with acute pulp exposure may be managed by one of four treatments: extraction, pulpotomy, root canal, or root canal followed by crown placement (Wiggs and Lobprise, 1993). A pulpotomy is performed to maintain the vitality of the tooth. A pulpotomy may be performed in an acute fracture of less than 4 to 6 hours' duration. A complete root canal procedure may be performed to retain the tooth; in cats this is usually performed on canine teeth (Wiggs and Lobprise, 1993). Endodontic procedures in cats have been described (Holmstrom, 1992; Wiggs and Lobprise, 1993).

Oral Neoplasms

Incidence. Oral tumors occur relatively frequently in cats and the majority of the tumors are malignant (Cotter, 1981; Vos and van der Gaag, 1987) (see Table 9–2). Squamous cell carcinoma (SCC) is by far the most frequent oral tumor in cats, followed by fibrosarcomas (Cotter, 1981; Vos and van der Gaag, 1987). Melanomas and other malignant tumors are much less frequently reported (Cotter, 1981; Patnaik and Mooney, 1988; Vos and van der Gaag, 1987). Tumors of dental origin occur rarely in cats (Abbott et al, 1986; Dubielzig, 1982). Benign oral tumors are less common than malignant tumors and have been infrequently reported (Rothwell et al, 1988; Salisbury et al, 1986; Vos and van der Gaag, 1987).

Clinical Features. Anorexia, weight loss, dysphagia, bleeding from the mouth, excessive salivation, halitosis, facial swelling, and loss of teeth may all be associated with the presence of oral neoplasia (Bradley et al, 1984; Madewell et al, 1976; Vos and van der Gaag, 1987). Oral tumors frequently ulcerate and become secondarily infected. Aspiration pneumonia may develop as a consequence of dysphagia with oral tumors (Cotter, 1981). Regional lymph nodes may be enlarged, but cervical lymph node metastases is a late occurring feature in oral tumors (Bradley et al, 1984; Cotter, 1981). Distant metastasis is rare, and local disease is usually the cause of death (Bradley et al, 1984; Brown et al, 1980; Cotter, 1981). Bone involvement is common with SCC, and bone destruction occurs frequently; however, bone proliferation mimicking a primary bone tumor has been reported (Bradley et al, 1984; Cotter, 1981; Madewell et al, 1976). Oral tumors frequently occur under the tongue; this is the most common site for SCC (Vos and van der Gaag, 1987). The gingiva is the second most frequent site for SCC and the most common site for fibrosarcoma (Cotter, 1981; Vos and van der Gaag, 1987). During dental procedures the oral cavity should be evaluated for evidence of neoplastic lesions. Neoplasia should be considered when loose teeth occur in the absence of significant dental disease.

Diagnosis. Oral lesions that may be neoplastic should undergo biopsy, and histopathologic analysis should be performed. The sample collected should be large enough to ensure an accurate diagnosis.

Management. Surgical excision is the treatment of choice. However, at the time of initial diagnosis most tumors are nonresectable (Bradley et al, 1984; Cotter, 1981; Salisbury et al, 1986; Wiggs and Loprise, 1993). Local recurrence after surgical excision is common (Bradley et al, 1984; Cotter, 1981). Combined therapy, including surgery, chemotherapy, and immunotherapy, has been described (Brown et al, 1980). Cryotherapy of oral tumors has been suggested as an adjunct to surgery (Glannone, 1984).

References

Abbott DP, Walsh K, Diters RW. Calcifying epithelial odontogenic tumours in three cats and a dog. J Comp Pathol 96:131, 1986.

Aller S. Basic prophylaxis and home care. Compend Contin Educ Pract Vet 11(12):1447, 1989.

Aller S. Dental home care and preventative strategies. Semin Vet Med Surg 8(3):204, 1993.

August JR. Feline immunodeficiency virus. Vet Med Rep 1:150, 1989.

Beard GB, Beard DM. Geriatric dentistry. Vet Clin North Am [Small Anim Pract] 19:1, 49, 1989.

Bradley RL, MacEwen EG, Loar AS. Mandibular resection for removal of oral tumors in 30 dogs and 6 cats. J Am Vet Med Assoc 184:460, 1984.

Brown NO, Hayes AA, Mooney S, et al. Combined modality therapy in the treatment of solid tumors in cats. J Am Anim Hosp Assoc 16:719, 1980.

Cotter SM. Oral pharyngeal neoplasms in the cat. J Am Anim Hosp Assoc 17:917, 1981.

Dubielzig RR. Proliferative dental and gingival diseases of dogs and cats. 18:577, 1982.

Emily P, Penman S. Periodontal disease, dental prophylaxis and minor periodontal surgery. In Handbook of Small Animal Dentistry. New York, Pergamon Press, 1990, p 35.

Frost P, Williams CA. Feline dental disease. Vet Clin North Am [Small Anim Pract] 16:851, 1986.

Glannone JA. Cryotherapy for oral lesions of dogs and cats. Mod Vet Pract 65(11):833, 1984.

Harvey CE. Oral, dental, pharyngeal, and salivary gland disorders. In Ettinger SF, ed. Textbook of Veterinary Internal Medicine. Vol 2. Philadelphia, WB Saunders, 1989, p 1203.

Harvey CE. Oral inflammatory diseases in cats. J Am Anim Hosp Assoc 27:585, 1991a.

Harvey CE. Treatment planning for periodontal disease in dogs. J Am Anim Hosp Assoc 27:592, 1991b.

Harvey CE. Epidemiology of periodontal conditions in dogs and cats. Annu Vet Dental Forum 6:45, 1992.

Harvey CE, Emily PP. Periodontal disease, oral inflammatory and immune-mediated oral surgery. In Harvey CE, Emily PP, eds. Small Animal Dentistry. St. Louis, Mosby-Year Book, 1993, pp 89, 145, 312.

Hennet PR, Harvey CE. Anaerobes in periodontal disease in the dog: A review. J Vet Dent 8(2):18, 1991.

Holmstrom SE. Periodontal disease. Compend Contin Educ Pract Vet 11(12):1485, 1989.

Holmstrom SE. Feline endodontics. Vet Clin North Am [Small Anim Pract] 22:1433, 1992.

Holmstrom SE, Frost P, Gammon RL. Dental prophylaxis; Periodontal therapy; Exodontics; Endodontics. In Veterinary Dental Techniques. Philadelphia, WB Saunders, pp 105, 137, 174, 207, 1992.

Kapatkin AS, Manfra Marretta S, Schloss AJ. Problems associated with basic oral surgical techniques. Prob Vet Med 2(1):85, 1990.

Lyon KF. Subgingival odontoclastic resorptive lesions: Classification, treatment, and results in 58 cats. Vet Clin North Am [Small Anim Pract] 22:1417, 1992.

Madewell BR, Ackerman N, Sesline DH. Invasive carcinoma radiographically mimicking primary bone cancer in the mandibles of two cats. J Am Vet Radiol Soc 27:213, 1976.

Manfra Marretta S. The common and uncommon clinical presentations and treatment of periodontal disease in the dog and the cat. Semin Vet Med Surg [Small Anim Pract] 2(4):230, 1987.

Manfra Marretta S. The diagnosis and treatment of oronasal fistulas in three cats. J Vet Dent 5:4, 1988.

Manfra Marretta S. History, clinical signs, radiographic changes of dental problems. ACVS Forum 17:254, 1989.

Manfra Marretta S. Chronic rhinitis and dental disease. Vet Clin North Am [Small Anim Pract] 22:1101, 1992a.

Manfra Marretta S. Current perspectives on periodontal disease in dogs and cats. Supplement to Compendium, Veterinary Exchange, Veterinary Learning System, p 5, 1992b.

Manfra Marretta S, Tholen M. Extraction techniques and management of associated complications. In Bojrab MJ, Tholen M, eds. Small Animal Oral Medicine and Surgery. Philadelphia, Lea & Febiger, 1990, p 75.

Mills AW. Oral-dental disease in cats. Vet Clin North Am [Small Anim Pract] 22:1297, 1992.

Oakes MG, Hedlund CS, Lewis DD, et al. Canine oral neoplasia. Compend Contin Educ Pract Vet 15:1, 15, 1993.

Patnaik AK, Mooney S. Feline melanoma: A comparative study of ocular, oral, and dermal neoplasms. Vet Pathol 25:105, 1988.

Pederson NC. Inflammatory oral cavity diseases of the cat. Vet Clin North Am [Small Anim Pract] 22:1323, 1992.

Reubel GH, Hoffman DE, Pederson NC. Acute and chronic faucitis of domestic cats; a feline calicivirus-induced disease. Vet Clin North Am [Small Anim Pract] 22:1347, 1992.

Rossman LE, Garber DA, Harvey CE. Disorders of teeth. In Harvey CE, ed. Veterinary Dentistry. Philadelphia, WB Saunders, 1985, p 79.

Rothwell JT, Valentine BA, Eng VM. Peripheral giant cell granuloma in a cat. J Am Vet Med Assoc 192:1105, 1988.

Salisbury SK, Richardson DC, Lantz GC. Partial maxillectomy and premaxillectomy in the treatment of oral neoplasia in the dog and cat. Vet Surg 15:16, 1986.

Sarkiala E, Harvey C. Systemic antimicrobials in the treatment of periodontitis in dogs. Semin Vet Med Surg 8(3):197, 1993.

Sims TJ, Moncla BJ, Page RC. Serum antibody response to antigens of oral gram-negative bacteria by cats with plasma cell gingivitis-pharyngitis. J Dent Res 69:877, 1990.

Smith MM, Zontine WJ, Willits NH. A correlative study of the clinical and radiographic signs of periodontal disease in dogs. J Am Vet Med Assoc 186(12):1286, 1985.

Tenorio AP, Franti CE, Madewell BR, et al. Chronic oral infections of cats and their relationship to persistent oral carriage of feline calici-, immunodeficiency, or leukemia viruses. Vet Immunol Immunopathol 29:1, 1991.

Tholen M, Hoyt R. Oral pathology. In Bojrab MJ, Tholen M, eds. Small Animal Oral Medicine and Surgery. Philadelphia, Lea & Febiger, 1990, p 25.

van Wessum R, Harvey CE, Hennet P. Feline dental resorptive lesion: Prevalence patterns. Vet Clin North Am [Small Anim Pract] 22:1405, 1992.

Vos JH, van der Gaag I. Canine and feline oral-pharyngeal tumors. J Vet Med 34:420, 1987.

Waner T, Nyska A. Gingival hyperplasia in dogs. Compend Contin Educ Pract Vet 13:81, 207, 1991.

Wiggs RB, Lobprise HB. Dental diseases, Oral disease. In Norsworthy GD, ed. Feline Practice. Philadelphia, JB Lippincott, 1993, pp 290, 438.

Williams CA. Endodontics. Vet Clin North Am [Small Anim Pract] 16:875, 1986.

Withrow SJ. Tumors of the gastrointestinal system. In Withrow SJ, Mac Ewen EG, eds. Clinical Veterinary Oncology. Philadelphia, JB Lippincott, 1989, p 177.

Zontine WJ. Dental radiographic technique and interpretation. Vet Clin North Am 4(4):741, 1974.

CHAPTER 10

The Digestive System

COLIN F. BURROWS

Unlike many other organs, the gastrointestinal tracts of the dog and the cat are not afflicted by any classic age-related disease. In contrast to other organs, the gastrointestinal tract, like some well-oiled machine, continues to churn away. Reasons for this apparent immunity to the ravages of time are unclear. Cell turnover in the gastrointestinal tract is much faster than in any other body organ except the skin. What we do know is that virtually all other organs exhibit signs of aging before the gastrointestinal tract does, and for this the veterinary gastroenterologist can at least be grateful. This is not to say that there are no age-associated changes. Gastric secretion decreases with age in the dog, just as it does in humans, and significant changes in the gastrointestinal flora occur, with an increase in *Clostridia* and a decrease in *Lactobacillus* and *Bacteroides* (Benno and Mitsuoka, 1989). The clinical importance of these changes however, is unclear. There is no information on any age-related changes in feline gastrointestinal function. This is not to say that the veterinarian can remain oblivious to the ravages of time on the gastrointestinal tract of his or her canine and feline patients; a number of conditions give cause for concern (Table 10–1). Most important of these are tumors (both dog and cat). However, idiopathic megaesophagus (dog), gastric motility disorders (including dilatation-volvulus, and gastroparesis in the dog), lymphocytic plasmacytic enteritis (dog and cat), and idiopathic megacolon of the cat are also important. Age-related diseases appear most frequently in the stomach and small intestine, to a lesser extent in the colon, and rarely in the esophagus.

HISTORY

Patients with gastrointestinal disease present with one or more of the signs listed in Table

TABLE 10–1. MAJOR AGE-RELATED DISEASES OF THE GASTROINTESTINAL TRACT

ORGAN	DOG	CAT
Esophagus	Megaesophagus Foreign Body Tumors Esophagitis/stricture	Tumors
Stomach	Tumors Ulcer Gastritis Outlet obstruction Motility disorders Dilatation-volvulus	Tumors Gastritis Hairballs
Small intestine	Lymphocytic-plasmacytic enteritis Eosinophilic enteritis Villous atrophy Tumors	Inflammatory bowel disease Lymphocytic-plasmacytic enteritis Eosinophilic enteritis Tumors
Colon, rectum, and anus	Impaction Tumors Fecal incontinence	Impaction Megacolon Tumors

TABLE 10–2. SIGNS OF GASTROINTESTINAL DISEASE IN THE DOG AND CAT

Vomiting	Constipation
Regurgitation	Flatus
Diarrhea	Salivation
Abdominal pain	Shock
Tenesmus	Weight loss
Dyschezia	Change in appetite
Hematochezia	

10–2. It is important to realize however, that with the exception of dyschezia, none of these are specific for gastrointestinal disease. It is the clinician's interpretation of the various manifestations and combinations of these signs that leads first to a differential diagnosis and diagnostic plan, and then to a specific diagnosis and appropriate therapy.

Vomiting

Vomiting is a complex reflex act controlled by the emetic center in the medulla. The emetic center is in turn influenced by the chemoreceptor trigger zone (CRTZ) in the floor of the fourth ventricle. Vomiting results from stimulation of these areas in one of four ways: (1) gastric disease, (2) abdominal disease, (3) systemic and metabolic disease, or (4) neurologic disease (Table 10–3).

Diagnosis of the cause of vomiting is facilitated by considering the frequency and nature of the vomiting. Specific facts to be elicited in the history include (1) the presence of food in the vomitus and its state of digestion; (2) the temporal relationship of vomiting to eating; (3) the presence of mucus, bile, or blood; and (4) the color and consistency of the vomitus.

Normal gastric emptying time in the dog and cat is about 7 to 8 hours. Vomiting of food more than about 10 hours after a meal therefore suggests delayed gastric emptying. This is usually associated with either gastric outlet obstruction or impaired secretion and motility associated with inflammatory or neoplastic disease of the stomach, pancreas, or proximal duodenum. Bile in the vomitus indicates reflux of duodenal contents and the possibility of reflux gastritis. Fresh or digested blood in the vomitus usually indicates disruption of the gastric mucosal barrier and, if chronic, suggests severe gastric disease. Eating grass and vomiting in a patient that does not ordinarily do this is a reliable sign of abdominal disease.

It is important to differentiate vomiting from regurgitation (Table 10–4) and to appreciate that the pet owner's complaint of vomiting may be erroneous. For example, few owners whose dog has megaesophagus present the dog with the complaint of regurgitation; to them, expulsion of digested food from the mouth means that the animal is vomiting. Also, many dogs with tonsillitis and an accumulation of mucus in the pharynx are presented with the spurious complaint of "vomiting" when in fact what they are doing is gagging or coughing up mucous and saliva that is too painful for them to swallow. Examination of the oropharynx in such patients reveals accumulations of white frothy mucus and enlarged, hyperemic tonsils.

Regurgitation

Regurgitation, defined in clinical veterinary medicine as the expulsion of undigested food from the esophagus or caudal pharynx, is a rela-

TABLE 10–3. MAJOR NONGASTRIC CAUSES OF VOMITING IN THE GERIATRIC DOG AND CAT

Abdominal disorders
- Enteritis
- Pancreatitis
- Peritonitis
- Colitis
- Pyometra
- Paralytic ileus
- Intestinal obstruction/foreign body
- Prostatitis
- Constipation
- Hepatic disorders
- Acute urinary obstruction
- Pancreatic and intestinal tumors

Systemic or metabolic disorders
- Ketoacidosis
- Uremia
- Hepatic encephalopathy
- Adrenal insufficiency
- Drugs (erythromycin, tetracycline, acetaminophen, chloramphenicol, digoxin, adriamycin) or toxins
- Hyperthyroidism (cats)

Neurologic disorders
- Central nervous system tumors
- Encephalitis
- Central nervous system trauma
- Motion sickness
- Autonomic or visceral epilepsy
- Vestibular disease

TABLE 10–4. VOMITING OR REGURGITATION? A CHECKLIST FOR HISTORY TAKING

QUESTION	REGURGITATION	VOMITING
Describe act	Effortless (passive) expulsion	An active process; abdominal contractions pronounced; retching or heaving
Preceding activity	Few premonitory signs	Premonitory signs pronounced
Ptyalism	Ptyalism excessive in esophageal inflammatory or obstructive disase	Ptyalism, pacing, swallowing, tachycardia, (nausea)
Appearance	Semiformed material; food material obvious, may smell "fermented"; often contains mucus (saliva); blood is rare; never bile stained	No characteristic consistency; varies from freshly ingested food to liquid ± bile, blood, and mucus; may also contain grass

tively common complaint that is often confused with vomiting. Regurgitation is a relatively passive event and is seldom associated with marked abdominal contractions. Regurgitated material also appears undigested and does not smell like vomit. The major cause of regurgitation is megaesophagus. The time from ingestion to regurgitation varies widely; animals with swallowing disorders regurgitate almost immediately, while those with megaesophagus can retain food for many hours and occasionally for 1 or 2 days.

Diarrhea

Diarrhea is the most common gastrointestinal complaint and can be either primary or secondary. Primary diarrhea is due to either specific intestinal or colonic disease (e.g., plasmacytic lymphocytic colitis, hookworm infection, or exocrine pancreatic insufficiency) or functional disorders of the gastrointestinal tract (e.g., stress or dietary change). Secondary diarrhea results from systemic disease with gastrointestinal manifestations (e.g., hypoadrenocorticism).

Because diarrhea is a very common sign, it is not the fact that the animal has diarrhea that is important; rather, the nature and frequency of the diarrhea together with its relationship to other signs must be used to formulate a differential diagnosis.

Facts that should be elicited in the history are listed in Table 10–5.

Information gleaned from the history regarding the diarrhea should allow differentiation into acute or chronic and small or large bowel diarrhea. This is important because the diagnostic and therapeutic approaches differ with each category (Table 10–6).

Abdominal Pain

Abdominal pain is a nonspecific sign that can be (1) related to primary gastrointestinal disease, (2) referred from the thoracic cavity or spine, or (3) related to other viscera.

Useful differentiating factors are the localization of pain by palpation and percussion and the attitude of the patient. Abdominal pain is more often associated with acute disease. Pain can sometimes be elicited and localized by deep and

TABLE 10–5. DIARRHEA: KEY FACTS IN THE HISTORY

Duration: The time that diarrhea has been present allows categorization into acute or chronic diarrhea. Persistence during fasting suggests secretory diarrhea, whereas cessation suggests osmotic diarrhea.

Urgency: If defecation is associated with a sense of urgency or "accidents," signs are most likely attributable to large intestinal disease.

Tenesmus or dyschezia: The presence of tenesmus or pain on defecation is usually associated with distal colonic, rectal, or anal disease.

Appearance of the feces: Excessive mucus in the feces usually suggests large intestinal disease, whereas bulky or fatty feces indicate nutrient maldigestion or malabsorption. Fresh blood indicates hemorrhage into the large bowel, whereas melena suggests small intestinal hemorrhage. Small-volume feces suggest colonic disease.

Frequency of defecation: A low frequency of defecation (one to three bowel movements per day) suggests small intestinal disease, whereas a high frequency (more than five bowel movements per day) suggests large intestinal disease.

Past history of diarrhea: Historical association with extraneous factors (e.g., dietary change, stressful situations, parasite-infected environments) can help categorize diarrhea. A history of previous diarrhea and response to treatment also helps avoid therapeutic blunders.

TABLE 10–6. CLASSIFICATION OF DIARRHEA

	ACUTE	CHRONIC
Small intestine	Usually less than 48 hr in duration. Feces are variable in volume; they seldom contain mucus. Fresh or partly digested blood is not uncommon. Patients are usually inappetent or anorexic, so there is no steatorrhea. Feces are brown or red in color. Defecation is accompanied by a sense of urgency and is increased in frequency. Tenesmus may be present. Dyschezia is absent. *Symptomatic therapy is usually effective.*	Usually 7 to 10 days or longer in duration. Feces are large in volume; they contain little or no mucus. Blood, if present, is melena. Steatorrhea is present with maldigestion or malabsorption. Feces are brown in color. There is little urgency; no tenesmus is present. Frequency is two to three times normal. Dyschezia is absent; weight loss may be present. It can often be controlled by dietary manipulation. *Biopsy and specific diagnosis and therapy are essential.*
Large intestine	Uncommon; usually less than 48 hr in duration. Feces are small in volume, mucus may be abundant, and fresh blood is frequent; there is no steatorrhea. Fecal leukocytes are abundant. There is much urgency; accidents in the house are common. Tenesmus is frequent and severe. There is marked increase in frequency of defecation. Dyschezia is variable and may be severe. *Symptomatic therapy is usually effective, although the condition may become chronic.*	Usually 7 to 10 days or longer in duration (may be months). Feces are small in volume, usually with abundant mucus; blood is usually but not invariably present. Defecation is associated with a sense of urgency; accidents in the house are common. Tenesmus is common. Frequency of defecation is markedly increased. Dyschezia is present if the distal colon or the rectum is involved. *Biopsy and specific therapy are essential.*

careful abdominal palpation and is most often associated with pancreatitis, peritonitis, or tumors. Most painful conditions are inflammatory. Dogs (and to a much lesser extent, cats) with cranial abdominal disease may adopt the position of relief (Fig. 10–1). Abdominal pain should be differentiated from the splinting of abdominal muscles that occurs in intervertebral disk disease.

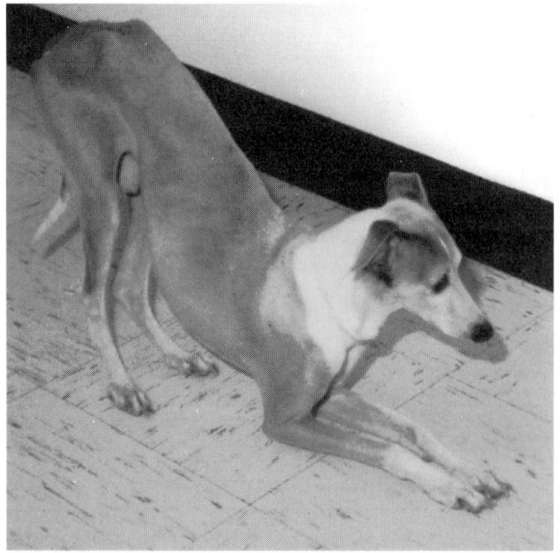

Figure 10–1. Position of relief. This 9-year-old Italian greyhound with eosinophilic gastroenteritis repeatedly adopted this position throughout the day and several times in the examination room. Signs responded to treatment with prednisone, diet change, mucosal protection, and oral antimicrobial agents for secondary small intestinal bacterial overgrowth.

Tenesmus

Tenesmus is common in diseases of the lower gastrointestinal, urinary, or reproductive tracts. The relevant organ system can usually be identified from the history and results of physical examination. The timing of tenesmus in relationship to defecation can be helpful. Dogs with colitis may have tenesmus after defecation, while tenesmus before defecation is usually associated with constipation or an obstructive lesion such as rectal carcinoma.

Dyschezia

Painful or difficult defecation, the only sign specific to the gastrointestinal tract, is usually associated with rectal, anal, or perianal lesions. The animal may cry out as it attempts to defecate and may stop, walk around restlessly, and then repeat the process. Fecal retention and constipation may ensue if pain is severe. Diseases associated with dyschezia include pseudocoprostasis, perianal fistula, rectal tumors, and perineal hernia.

Hematochezia

Fresh blood in the feces is usually a sign of colonic or rectoanal disease. Bloody diarrhea (dysentery) is associated with severe small or large intestinal disease, while streaks of blood in normal feces suggest an isolated bleeding lesion such as a tumor. Digested blood (melena) suggests either gastric or small intestinal hemorrhage or hemoptysis (in which the coughed-up blood is swallowed). Animals with bleeding disorders may also exhibit melena or hematochezia, but bleeding in such patients is seldom confined to the gastrointestinal tract.

Constipation

Constipation, defined as infrequent defecation, passage of excessively hard or dry feces with tenesmus, or an unusually small fecal volume, is perhaps more a disorder with a variety of causes than a sign of gastrointestinal disease. It is included here, however, because many clients equate tenesmus with constipation. Intractable constipation (or obstipation) has a guarded prognosis, as degenerative changes in the colon wall may be irreversible and result in megacolon. Megacolon is defined as a dilated colon that is incapable of contractile activity because of irreversible neuromuscular degeneration. General causes of constipation are listed in Table 10–7.

Flatus

Excessive flatus often occurs in dogs with nutrient maldigestion. Gas is produced by bacterial degradation of unabsorbed dietary carbohydrate in the colon. Diets containing soy are associated with flatus more than other diets, a fact that is attributed to complex carbohydrates in these diets that can be digested only by colonic bacteria. Flatus is normal in brachycephalic dog breeds and probably results from swallowed air.

TABLE 10–7. GENERAL CAUSES OF CONSTIPATION IN THE DOG AND THE CAT

Dietary and environmental causes: Ingestion of bones or foreign material; hospitalization; litterbox dirty or absent.
Painful defecation Anorectal disease; orthopedic disease.
Obstructive lesions: Perineal hernia; healed pelvic fractures; tumors.
Neuromuscular diseases: Spinal cord disease; pelvic nerve dysfunction; smooth muscle contractile defect.
Endocrine and metabolic dysfunctions: Hypothyroidism; hypercalcemia.
Drugs: Barium; anticholinergics; narcotics.

Salivation

Excess salivation (ptyalism) is uncommon. When present it suggests one of the following:

- Chemical poisoning (e.g., organophosphates).
- Pharyngeal or esophageal disease (foreign bodies, inflammation, reflux esophagitis, tumors).
- Oral disease (stomatitis and/or periodontal disease).
- Insect stings in the oral cavity elicit salivation; cats that chew certain insects may also salivate.
- Nausea, especially in the cat.
- Hepatic encephalopathy in cats and, less often, in dogs.

Differentiation of the cause of ptyalism from the history and results of the physical examination is not difficult. Nausea is a subjective sign but should be suspected in animals presented with a history of repeated swallowing and salivation. Nausea may also be observed as a side effect of treatment with drugs such as Adriamycin, cisplatin, ketoconazole, and digoxin.

Shock

Shock in gastrointestinal disease can result from severe fluid or blood loss or from sepsis. Signs of shock are obviously not pathognomic for acute gastrointestinal disturbances, but their presence indicates the severity of the disease. Treatment, at least on a symptomatic basis, is essential while a diagnosis is being pursued.

Weight Loss

Loss of body weight and condition is not specific for gastrointestinal disease. Nevertheless, it occurs with sufficient frequency in chronic conditions to be considered an important prognostic sign.

Loss of weight can be due to (1) decreased nutrient intake (reduced appetite or defective absorption), (2) increased nutrient loss (protein-losing enteropathy, protein-losing nephropathy), and (3) increased utilization (hyperthyroidism, some cancers).

Intestinal parasite infection is a common cause of weight loss (or of a failure to gain weight), especially in young dogs, but should never be forgotten as a possible cause of weight loss in animals of any age.

Anemia

Anemia is uncommon in gastrointestinal disease, but when present it reflects either gastrointestinal hemorrhage (tumor, ulcer, bleeding disorder, parasites) or defective red cell production (malabsorption or bone marrow depression—the anemia of chronic disease).

Anorexia, Polyphagia, or Pica

The appetite of a dog or cat is a good indication of its state of health. A change in appetite is common in gastrointestinal disease. Anorexia is to be expected in acute conditions, while polyphagia occurs in some chronic conditions, particularly those associated with malabsorption. Pica (including coprophagia) occurs in exocrine pancreatic insufficiency. Coprophagia is rarely associated with parasite infections and is usually a vice. Increased appetite, weight loss, and voluminous feces are common in hyperthyroid cats.

PHYSICAL EXAMINATION

Oral Cavity

Examination of the gastrointestinal tract begins in the oral cavity. The mouth should be open and a thorough examination performed. Cell turnover in the mouth is faster than anywhere else in the body, and in animals with protein-calorie malnutrition, particularly in those with hypoproteinemia due to nutrient malabsorption and protein-losing enteropathy, it is not uncommon to find lingual and buccal ulceration. This is presumably due to the body's inability to supply sufficient protein for cell regeneration and to recycle the amino acids in intestinal epithelial sloughed cells. Another possible reason is the decrease in secretory immunoglobulin A (IgA) in the saliva of debilitated and stressed patients, which results in increased numbers of oral bacteria and fungi with a concomitant exacerbation of ulceration. Oral ulcers also occur in uremia, particularly on the buccal mucosa over the upper canine teeth as well as on the dorsal surface and tip of the tongue.

The mouth should also be examined for foreign bodies, particularly in animals presented with a history of anorexia, gagging, and ptyalism. Linear foreign bodies may be found under the tongues of dogs and cats of any age.

If possible the tongue should always be pulled forward to allow examination of the caudal oropharynx. This is very important in patients, usually dogs, presented with a history of gagging, retching, or vomiting. Accumulation of frothy white mucus in the caudal oropharynx suggests tonsillitis. Secondary tonsillitis due to chronic respiratory disease or to chronic vomiting or regurgitation is more common than primary tonsillitis in older dogs. Both conditions are uncommon in cats.

Particles of food in the frothy mucus suggest regurgitation associated with esophageal disease, or less likely, a swallowing disorder. The latter disorder is usually suspected from a history of dysphagia and violent expulsion of food and is seen primarily in young animals. However, clients often present these animals with a history of "vomiting" since few people have the knowledge or vocabulary to distinguish between retching, regurgitation, and vomiting in their dogs or cat.

Esophagus

Physical examination of the esophagus is difficult and gives limited results. Evaluation is best accomplished using radiology or endoscopy. However, careful palpation of the laryngeal area in dogs that are presented with ptyalism, regurgitation, anorexia, or dysphagia may reveal a mass. This could be a foreign body, cervical abscess, or thyroid carcinoma or some other type of tumor. The thoracic inlet should also be carefully palpated for masses or irregularities in older dogs with a history of regurgitation.

In dogs with a history of regurgitation and in which megaesophagus is suspected, the index of suspicion can be increased by what I call the "external Valsalva maneuver." For this, a hand is placed over the mouth and nose to occlude the airway, and an assistant sharply compresses the thoracic cavity. This increases intrathoracic pressure and forces esophageal contents out of the thoracic and into the cervical esophagus. This is evidenced by a ballooning of the neck in the jugular groove on the left side. Obviously, this test works best in short-coated dog breeds.

Stomach

Examination of the stomach is ordinarily impossible in the dog and very difficult in the cat unless there is a large gastric tumor or foreign body such as a hairball larger than 3 cm in diameter. Ordinarily these can be palpated only in thin cats. A tympanitic abdomen suggests gastric dilatation or dilatation-volvulus, particularly in a large or giant breed dog presented with signs of shock.

Small Intestine and Colon

Examination of the small intestine and colon is usually included in a thorough abdominal palpation. In cats and small dogs, the abdomen can best be palpated using one hand. The intestines can usually be slipped between the finger and thumb as the hand is drawn downward. Using this technique, an experienced clinician can detect the sometimes subtle intestinal thickening that is not uncommon in both inflammatory bowel disease and diffuse intestinal lymphoma. The colon can usually be easily differentiated from the small intestine because it contains feces or, if empty, because of its thicker wall. In larger dogs the same technique is applied, but using the tips of the fingers of both hands gently pressing in toward the center and moved slowly toward the ventral abdomen. Palpation should be repeated if the animal is tranquilized or anesthetized, as the relaxed abdomen is much easier to palpate.

Masses in the small intestine suggest the presence of a foreign body, tumor, or granuloma. With care, normal small intestine can usually be palpated on either side of the mass. The mass can sometimes also be fixed and brought to the body wall to allow aspiration cytology. A thickened "sausage loop" suggests intussusception, a disorder not unheard of in older dogs, particularly in the distal ileum or at the ileocolonic junction.

Aggregated loops of bowel suggest a linear foreign body or adhesions, while intraluminal gas or fluid distention suggests obstruction. It is unusual to palpate ingesta in the small intestine, since in the fed state the small intestine usually contains only a thin, watery liquid. Palpable ingesta suggest nutrient malabsorption and mural disease but may also be present in cats with hyperthyroidism.

Palpation may also identify enlarged mesenteric lymph nodes, which suggest inflammation of the small or large intestine, local bacterial or fungal infection, or neoplasia. In the older cat, for example, a generalized thickened intestine with mesenteric lymphadenopathy suggests lymphoma or inflammatory bowel disease, with the former being more likely.

Abdominal effusion can be detected by visual observation if severe or by ballotment if more subtle. In some dogs, particularly in the miniature and toy breeds, and if distention is severe, ascites may be confused with an enlarged gas-filled stomach, since both can be tympanitic. Ascites in small breed dogs may be due to protein-losing enteropathy and lowered plasma oncotic pressure resulting from hypoproteinemia, but there are many other causes. However, for reasons that are unclear, hypoproteinemia, while causing ascites in small dogs, most often results in peripheral edema or anasarca in the larger breeds. Ascites is rare in the cat and is rarely, if ever, associated with gastrointestinal disease.

Rectal Examination

A thorough rectal examination is an essential part of the evaluation of older dogs with signs of gastrointestinal disease, particularly those exhibiting signs of dyschezia, tenesmus, or hematochezia. Rectal examination should be postponed for humane reasons in cats and in very small dogs until the animal is heavily tranquilized or anesthetized.

Rectal examination should begin with a thorough evaluation of the perineum and external anus. Any irregularities, asymmetry, or change in color should be noted. Anal disease is relatively common in older dogs but is rare in cats. The perianal area should then be carefully palpated, again with a view to detecting asymmetries. The anal sacs should be located but should not be evacuated at this time. Next, a lubricated gloved finger is inserted into the anus and a careful palpation begun. The walls of the pelvic diaphragm should be examined for uniformity on both sides. Rectal sacculation and dilation are not uncommon in older male dogs and can be readily palpated when they are not visible as an overt perianal hernia. The walls of the rectum should be smooth and devoid of irregularities. In all but the largest dogs, it should also be possible to move the rectum to the left and right and to feel the walls of the pelvis. Rectal fixation and possible narrowing of the rectum may suggest scar tissue or, more likely, a rectal tumor. Rectal carcinoma is common in German shepherd dogs. The iliac nodes can be palpated in most breeds, as can the prostate gland in male dogs, especially if it is fixed and elevated at the pelvic brim with the clinician's other hand. Careful ventral palpation should also detect the pelvic urethra. It is important to be able to appreciate the texture of a normal urethra so that urethral inflammation can be appreciated. Finally, the anal sacs should be evacuated as the hand is withdrawn and the contents examined for signs of infection. Blood or pus suggests anal sac infection and inflammation.

DIFFERENTIAL DIAGNOSIS

It is not the preceding historical signs themselves that are necessarily important in formulating a differential diagnosis, but rather their various combinations and manifestations. These, together with the results of the physical examination, lead the veterinarian to formulate a list of potential diagnoses—the *differential diagnoses*.

In formulating a differential diagnosis, all available pertinent facts, even subjective impressions, must be considered. The not-always-easy question of whether the presentation is caused by a primary gastrointestinal disease or a gastrointestinal-mimicking disease must also be answered. Any irregularities in the expected presentation must be identified and an attempt made to explain them in the light of the probable diagnosis. If some signs are unexplained, then the diagnosis should be re-examined; *most combinations of signs can usually be explained by a single disease process.*

Above all, it is important for the veterinarian to keep an open mind and to be prepared for the unexpected. An attempt should always be made to be consistent in the approach to the problem and to prescribe treatment from a knowledge of pathophysiology. "Snap" diagnoses or diagnoses based on a "feeling" for the case are often wrong, to the detriment of both the patient and the veterinarian's professional reputation.

Diagnosis

After a list of differential diagnoses has been formulated, a specific diagnosis is made by means of a variety of confirmatory diagnostic procedures that should be selected to eliminate possible diagnoses. In gastrointestinal disease, as well as in diseases of most other organ systems, these procedures fall into three main groups: clinical laboratory studies, radiographic and other imaging procedures, and specific diagnostic procedures (e.g., endoscopy, biopsy).

CLINICAL LABORATORY STUDIES

Some laboratory studies should be carried out in most older patients, whereas others are indicated only to confirm a provisional diagnosis. For convenience such studies can be divided into two classes: essential and confirmatory.

Essential Studies

"Essential" studies usually include the hemogram, blood chemistry panel, fecal examination, and routine urinalysis. The results of the hemogram and blood chemistry panel are rarely diagnostic under these circumstances but can provide an indication of the nature and severity of the disease process. Urinalysis is a useful screening test for a variety of disorders and should be routine in all patients with signs of gastrointestinal disease that require any sort of detailed evaluation.

The most important essential study is the fecal examination. This should be routine in any patient with signs of gastrointestinal disease. The five basic components are as follows:

1. *Appearance:* Fecal volume can help to localize the disease process. Although volume is influenced by the nature of the diet, voluminous feces are most often associated with nutrient malabsorption. Small-volume feces (especially if associated with increased frequency of defecation) suggest colitis.
2. *Microscopic examination:* a direct smear and flotation test help detect parasites, red cells, white cells, mucus, and fat (split and unsplit).
3. *Occult blood:* This is seldom useful unless strongly positive because of the effect of diet and intestinal parasites.
4. *Culture:* This is rarely useful, but feces should be cultured if infection with *Salmonella, Campylobacter* or *Yersinia* is suspected.
5. *Specific enzymatic tests:* A fecal enzyme-linked immunosorbent assay (ELISA) for parvovirus provides a ready means of diagnosis.

Confirmatory Studies

Serum Amylase and Lipase. These tests should be used to help make the clinical diagnosis of acute pancreatitis. Lipase is believed to be more specific than amylase but sometimes reaches peak levels more slowly. It should be appreciated, however, that both lipase and amylase are released from extrapancreatic sources. Normal serum amylase comes from the liver and small intestine. Lipase is stored in large quantities in gastric mucosal epithelial cells and is released into the blood in gastritis (Raphel et al, 1992). Serum amylase may be elevated in the presence of intestinal disease, peritonitis, and renal failure, as well as pancreatitis. Amylase levels should therefore be evaluated in the light of all clinical signs. Both amylase and lipase are excreted by the kidneys, and their concentration is increased in azotemia. Results of these studies therefore should always be interpreted with caution, especially since severe pancreatitis may be present in patients with normal or near-normal values. It should be remembered that serum amylase and lipase concentrations are normal in exocrine pancreatic insufficiency.

Serum proteins. A low serum albumin level reflects either decreased hepatic synthesis or excessive protein loss, while a low total protein level usually indicates gastrointestinal protein loss. Albumin and globulin are both lost into the intestinal lumen in protein-losing enteropathies, because mucosal damage is sufficiently severe to let the larger globulin module escape into the lumen. In protein-losing nephropathy, on the other hand, the membrane damage is such that only the smaller albumin molecule can escape, resulting in hypoalbuminemia with normal or increased globulin. Serum calcium is also low in hypoalbuminemia because some calcium is albumin bound.

Serum Alanine Aminotransferase and Aspartate Aminotransferase. Increased liver enzyme activities indicate hepatocellular damage or biliary obstruction. It is important to realize that a variety of extrahepatic diseases can cause increased enzyme activity. Mild to moderate increases in alanine aminotransferase (ALT) and aspartate aminotransferase (AST) activity occur, for example, after shock, trauma, or sepsis. Increased activity is common in pancreatitis and in acute and chronic enteritis. This is because the liver is a filter, with its reticuloendothelial system removing translocated bacteria, endotoxins, and macromolecules and the subsequent chemical reaction causing hepatocellular damage. Chronic pancreatitis may also be associated with an increase in serum alkaline phosphatase, presumably due to ductal obstruction.

The reader is referred to more detailed references on the specific indications for and interpretation of gut function tests (Burrows and Merritt, 1992).

DIAGNOSTIC TOOLS

Radiologic Examination

Radiologic examination of the gastrointestinal tract and related organs in older dogs and cats continues to be an important clinical tool. Survey radiographs should be made of both the thorax and the abdomen, especially in animals presented with the complaint of vomiting. It is surprising how often an abnormality such as megaesophagus, aspiration pneumonia, or unsuspected metastatic disease may be found in thoracic radiographs made in animals with signs of chronic gastrointestinal disease. Signs of gastrointestinal disease in survey films are listed in Table 10–8.

If the patient has a history of vomiting, it may be prudent to consider an esophagram, a gastrogram, or a complete upper gastrointestinal series. However, an upper gastrointestinal series is of little diagnostic value in the patient with chronic

TABLE 10–8. HELPFUL FINDINGS IN ABDOMINAL SURVEY RADIOGRAPHS IN DOGS WITH GASTROINTESTINAL DISEASE

Ileus: May be either paralytic or obstructive.

Peritoneal effusion: Fluid accumulation in the abdominal cavity is uncommon in gastrointestinal disease. The most common causes are ascitic fluid, seen in hypoproteinemia and some types of liver disease, and the inflammatory exudate of peritonitis.

Radiopaque foreign objects: Will be visible on survey abdominal radiographs.

Abnormal soft tissue shadows and/or displacement of the viscera: Displacement of the viscera can often be used as an indirect indication of a mass in a contiguous organ or structure. A displaced stomach, for example, suggests a tumor in that region of the abdomen. Gastric dilatation-volvulus is an obvious radiographic diagnosis. Lateral displacement of the duodenum may be seen in chronic pancreatitis or pancreatic tumors.

Pneumoperitoneum: Free gas in the peritoneal cavity may result from gas-forming bacteria (usually a result of rupture of some portion of the alimentary tract), a penetrating wound in the abdominal wall, or recent abdominal surgery.

Thickened or irregular intestine: An irregular mucosa suggests severe inflammatory or neoplastic intestinal disease. The "apple core" intestine is virtually pathognomic for intestinal lymphosarcoma.

diarrhea, as most lesions responsible for diarrhea are too small to be seen on abdominal radiographs, and is contraindicated if endoscopy is to be performed; such duplication simply wastes the owner's money. An upper gastrointestinal series can define gross lesions such as intestinal obstruction, perforation, and severe inflammatory change and can be used in the evaluation of the vomiting patient, where it may reveal radiolucent foreign bodies or filling defects suggestive of neoplastic or ulcerative disease (Fig. 10–2). A barium enema may be of some use in detecting proximal colonic lesions but has been superseded by colonoscopy for the diagnosis of colitis.

Abdominal Ultrasonography

A thorough ultrasound examination of the abdomen currently is part of the routine evaluation of patients with a history and signs of gastrointestinal disease. However, ultrasound is more beneficial in the evaluation of parenchymal organs outside the gastrointestinal tract. Ultrasound examination can accurately measure intestinal wall thickness, especially of the ileum and the ileocolonic junction, and confirm or repudiate findings at physical examination. Mesenteric nodes also can be evaluated. It is usually difficult to accurately evaluate the stomach because of air and fluid interference with the image.

Endoscopy

Evaluation of the upper and lower portions of the gastrointestinal tract using a flexible fiberoptic or video endoscope has revolutionized the diagnosis and treatment of patients with gastrointestinal disease. Endoscopy is noninvasive and carries a lower risk than surgery, especially in high-risk patients, and permits the veterinarian to obtain multiple biopsy specimens. In some instances endoscopy may even be therapeutic, allowing, for example, the nonsurgical removal of esophageal or gastric foreign bodies or the dilation of esophageal strictures (Tams, 1990).

A variety of new or used endoscopes are available. Best are those with a working length of 120 mm or greater and a diameter not greater than 9 mm. The biopsy channel should also be at least 2.4 mm in diameter. For upper gastrointestinal endoscopy, the patient should be fasted for at least 12 hours, anesthetized, and placed in left lateral recumbency (Tams, 1990). The normal esophagus should be empty of anything but a small quantity of saliva. The stomach should contain nothing other than perhaps a small amount of bile-stained liquid. The gastric rugae should be uniform in color and can be readily identified if the stomach has not been overdistended with air. In most patients the endoscope can be passed through the pylorus to allow examination and biopsy of the duodenum and the proximal jejunum. If indicated, a sterile tube can be passed down

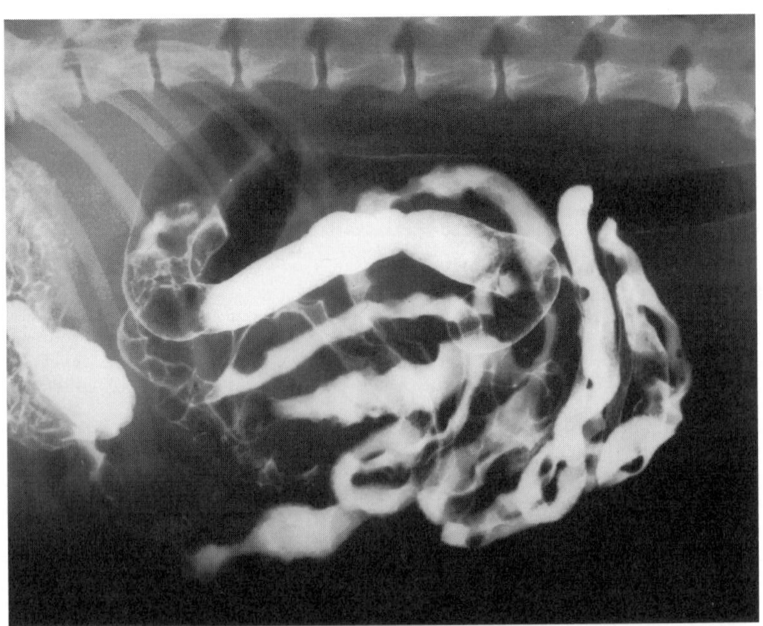

Figure 10–2. This upper gastrointestinal contrast study in a dog with a history of chronic vomiting revealed multiple filling defects compatible with lymphosarcoma (the so-called "apple core" intestine).

the biopsy channel and intestinal juice aspirated for later culture or microscopic examination (Burrows and Merritt, 1992).

Colonoscopy can be performed in a sedated animal using a rigid colonoscope or, if the entire colon must be evaluated, in an anesthetized patient using a flexible fiberoptic or video endoscope. In both instances it is critical that the colon be properly prepared because it is difficult to navigate the tip of an endoscope through a sea of feces. For rigid colonoscopy, the patient should be fasted for 48 hours and the colon prepared with plain water enemas both the night before and the morning of the procedure. The enemas should be repeated until the effluent is clear. For flexible colonoscopy, the patient should be fasted for at least 24 hours and preferably given plain water enemas the day before the procedure, again until the effluent is clear. The patient must also be given oral doses of colonic lavage solution (e.g., GoLYTELY or Colyte) at a dose of 80 ml/kg in two divided doses 1 to 2 hours apart (Burrows, 1989). In dogs the solution is best given by stomach tube and in cats by a nasoesophageal tube.

For rigid colonoscopy, the patient can be examined either standing or in left lateral recumbency. For flexible colonoscopy, the patient should be in left lateral recumbency. A rectal examination should be performed before the procedure to ensure that the distal rectum has no obstruction. The lubricated tip of the colonoscope is then inserted and advanced under direct observation. Normal colonic mucosa is pink with linear or circular folds. In the normal colon it is possible to see the network of submucosal vessels, which is an important criterion of normality. The endoscope is advanced with the mucosa under direct observation and the tip kept as much as possible in the center of the lumen. With practice it is possible to navigate both the splenic and the hepatic flexures and to evaluate the cecum and the ileocolonic junction. It is occasionally possible to pass the endoscope through the sphincter and examine the distal ileum. Biopsy specimens should be taken from representative areas as the endoscope is advanced.

Endoscopic Biopsy and Exploratory Laparotomy

In patients with chronic vomiting and/or diarrhea, a specific diagnosis can often be made only by examination of the histologic changes in the stomach and/or the intestine. Information about such changes is important, because it determines both the prognosis and the nature of subsequent therapy. For example, specific diagnosis of such diseases as intestinal lymphangiectasia, villus atrophy, gastric/intestinal tumors, and inflammatory bowel disease (i.e., eosinophilic gastroenteritis and lymphocytic-plasmacytic enteritis or colitis) can be made only by microscopic examination of an appropriate biopsy specimen. Laparotomy and open biopsy are viable alternatives when endoscopy equipment is unavailable or full-thickness biopsy specimens are needed. During laparotomy, biopsy specimens should always be taken, even if the gastrointestinal tract looks and feels normal, because the veterinarian's eyes and fingers are no substitute for a microscope.

DISORDERS OF DOGS

Esophagus

Megaesophagus

Megaesophagus is a relatively common disorder in older dogs. The cause is usually unknown. Megaesophagus is considered to be the result of one of a variety of nerve or muscle diseases that cause a loss of esophageal motor function (Table 10–9).

History and Clinical Signs. Regardless of the cause of megaesophagus, the esophageal muscles degenerate, resulting in a flaccid, atonic organ in

TABLE 10–9. CAUSES OF MEGAESOPHAGUS IN OLDER DOGS

Esophageal inflammatory disease
Esophagitis (thermal, chemical, reflux)
Granuloma (fungal, bacterial, parasitic)
Extraluminal esophageal compression
Thymoma
Other intrathoracic tumors
Hilar lymphadenopathy (tumor, fungal)
Intraluminal esophageal obstruction
Stricture
Foreign body
Tumor
Esophageal diverticulum
Neuromuscular dysfunction
Idiopathic megaesophagus
Myasthenia gravis
Polymyositis
Hyperadrenocorticism
Lead toxicity
Organophosphate toxicity
Systemic lupus erythematosis
Polyneuritis
Hypothyroidism (?)

which food and saliva accumulate to be almost effortlessly regurgitated at various times after eating. Regurgitated material is often in the form of a mucus-covered tube of food or large quantities of foamy mucus. Secondary signs are weight loss, polyphagia, weakness, dehydration, ballooning of the cervical esophagus, gurgling or burping sounds, coughing, and halitosis. The time from eating until regurgitation depends on the degree of dilation and the activity of the animal and can range from a few minutes to 24 hours or more.

Diagnosis. The fact that an animal has megaesophagus can usually be ascertained from the history and the changes on thoracic radiographs. A confirmatory esophagram or esophagoscopy can be performed if the diagnosis is in doubt. The differential diagnosis of the causes of acquired megaesophagus in older dogs should include disorders listed in Table 10–9. Elimination of specific disease often leads to the diagnosis of idiopathic megaesophagus. Some patients with megaesophagus may also have hypothyroidism, but thyroid replacement rarely, if ever, results in remission. Diagnostic tests that may help in the differential diagnosis are listed in Table 10–10.

TABLE 10–10. TESTS FOR THE DIAGNOSIS OF MEGAESOPHAGUS IN THE DOG

TEST	MAY BE ABNORMAL IN:
Hemogram	Infection, immune-mediated disease, endocrinopathy, lead toxicity
Blood chemistry	Hypoadrenocorticism
Creatinine phosphokinase	Muscle disease
Adrenocorticotropic hormone stimulation	Hypoadrenocorticism
Cholinesterase	Organophosphate toxicity
Acetylcholine receptor antibody and edrophonium (Tensilon) tests	Myasthenia gravis
Antinuclear antibody test	Immune-mediated disease
Survey thoracic radiographs	Mediastinal or pulmonary disease, megaesophagus, vascular ring anomaly, esophageal foreign body
T_3, T_4, and thyroid-stimulating hormone response	Hypothyroidism
Contrast esophagram	Obstructive disease, megaesophagus
Fluoroscopy	Esophageal motility disorders, megaesophagus
Esophagoscopy and biopsy	Obstructive disease, inflammation, tumors, megaesophagus
Electromyography and muscle biopsy	Muscle disease, polyneuropathy

T_3, Triiodothyronine; T_4, thyroxine.

Treatment. Treatment of megaesophagus must be directed, if at all possible, at relief of the underlying disease. If present, aspiration pneumonia should be treated with antimicrobial agents and adequate nutrition maintained. If the patient is very ill, I prefer to rehydrate and then anesthetize and perform bronchoscopy with pulmonary lavage for subsequent cytology and culture. I then aspirate all food debris and liquid from the esophagus and place a percutaneous endoscopic gastrostomy tube (Bright and Burrows, 1988). This approach ensures an accurate bacterial culture and sensitivity and provides adequate nutrition. The gastrostomy tube can also be used to place medications directly into the stomach, as they are unlikely to be absorbed if given orally. While awaiting the results of the bacterial culture and sensitivity testing, the animal should be placed on parenteral antimicrobial therapy (i.e., combination of intravenous cephalosporin and subcutaneous gentamycin or intramuscular enrofloxacin).

If the diagnosis is idiopathic megaesophagus, the prognosis is always guarded to grave. A few dogs will do well if they are frequently fed small volumes from a height, with all food and water removed at night. The choice of food must be found by trial and error. Some dogs do well with canned food blended with water. Most dogs, however, appear to do better with dry food. Because most dogs do not do well even on this regimen, frequent and recurrent bouts of aspiration pneumonia contribute to extreme medical management or euthanasia. A few dogs, especially those with dedicated owners, can be maintained with a long-term tube gastrostomy using an indwelling mushroom feeding tube. One Doberman pinscher in which idiopathic megaesophagus was diagnosed at the age of 10 lived for 3 more years while being maintained entirely via tube gastrostomy feedings.

Esophageal Foreign Bodies

Esophageal foreign bodies are occasionally diagnosed in older dogs. Bones are the most common esophageal foreign bodies and usually lodge at the thoracic inlet, the base of the heart, and just proximal to the lower esophageal sphincter.

History and Clinical Signs. Diligent questioning will usually reveal that the owners have fed the dog a chop bone or a similar sized object or that the dog had been playing with a small toy immediately before the onset of signs. Signs include anorexia, ptyalism, persistent gulping and swallowing, pacing, and lethargy.

Diagnosis and Treatment. Diagnosis is made from the thoracic radiographs or by esophagoscopy. Some foreign bodies can be removed via endoscopy or, in the occasional patient, pushed into the stomach, where, if digestible, they can be left to the ravages of the normal digestive processes. If nondigestible, they either can be left in the stomach in the hope that the dog will pass them or can be removed at elective gastrostomy. Endoscopy usually allows good visualization and manipulation of the foreign body as well as assessment of mucosal damage. Surgical removal is indicated if no endoscope is available or the owner refuses referral. Surgery should be performed immediately in long-standing cases when perforation or severe mucosal damage is suspected. Follow-up thoracic radiographs should always be made to assess for pneumomediastinum. Treatment for esophagitis should also be instigated if the esophagus is badly damaged.

Treatment includes resting the esophagus by placement of a percutaneous endoscopic or surgical gastrostomy feeding tube, suppression of acid secretion with H_2 receptor antagonists (e.g., cimetidine 5 mg/kg q 8 hr), and mucosal protection with a sucralfate slurry (1-g tablet ground up in 10 to 20 ml of tap water and given orally in divided doses every 6 to 8 hours for 5 to 6 days). Parenteral antimicrobial agents (e.g., cephalosporin and gentamycin) should be given if pneumomediastinum is present, and the patient must be monitored closely for signs of sepsis. Sequelae include intraluminal stricture, which may require later endoscopic dilation, bougienage, or surgical resection. Pulsion diverticula and esophageal rupture fortunately are uncommon complications.

Esophageal Tumors

Tumors of the esophagus are rare. Primary tumors include leiomyomas, carcinomas, and sarcomas. In one report, metastatic thyroid carcinoma was the most common esophageal tumor encountered (Ridgeway and Suter, 1979). Proximal gastric carcinomas can also involve the gastroesophageal junction and distal esophagus. Signs are usually those of a stricture with secondary dilatation and dysmotility (regurgitation, anorexia, fever, and cough). Little can be done either medically or surgically for such patients. Surgical resection may be considered as a palliative procedure with perhaps transplantation of a length of small intestine in place of the resected segment.

Esophagitis

Esophagitis can occur after ingestion of strong acid or alkaline solutions, after ingestion of hot liquids, after removal of an esophageal foreign body, or as a complication of the chronic reflux of acidic gastric contents into the esophagus. Reflux of acid gastric contents into the esophagus also occurs during general anesthesia, particularly in stressed or septic patients in which gastric acid secretion may be increased (Odonkor et al, 1981). Causes of reflux esophagitis include reduced lower esophageal sphincter (LES) pressure caused by neuromuscular disease and structural abnormalities, including hiatal hernia and neoplasia. Chronic vomiting is also a common cause. About one in seven dogs undergoing endoscopic evaluation for chronic vomiting at the University of Florida Veterinary Medical Teaching Hospital, for example, have signs of distal esophagitis. The most common cause in old dogs, however, appears to be a defective LES sphincter. Also, once esophagitis is present, the LES tends to become incompetent and perpetuate and exacerbate the problem.

History and Clinical Signs. Signs of esophagitis are often vague and include a history of regurgitation, dysphagia, inappetence, or anorexia. Weight loss and ptyalism are frequent complications, and the patient may appear dejected, dehydrated, and lethargic. Aerophagia with secondary gastric dilatation may also occur, and there may be a history of recent anesthesia.

Diagnosis and Treatment. Diagnosis is usually made by endoscopy with confirmatory biopsy. Radiographic diagnosis is difficult, but contrast studies may occasionally reveal reflux or an anatomic defect such as hiatal hernia. Esophagitis is best treated symptomatically by means of H_2 receptor antagonists (e.g., cimetidine 5 mg/kg q 8 hr) or, in severe cases, by H^+K^+ adenosine triphosphatase (ATPase) pump inhibition with omeprazole (0.7 to 1 mg/kg sid). A sucralfate slurry is also useful (1-g tablet ground up in 15 to 20 ml of tap water and given orally in equal divided doses every 8 hours). Metoclopramide (0.4 to 0.5 mg/kg q 8 hr) also increases LES tone and may be beneficial. In severe cases tube gastrostomy may be needed to rest the esophagus. Surgical treatment of hiatal hernia also may be indicated.

Stomach

Most old dogs with gastric disease are presented for evaluation of vomiting, which is a frequent but not invariable result of gastritis. Other causes of gastric disease and associated vomiting include dietary indiscretion, gastric foreign bodies, tumors, defective gastric mucosal immune mechanisms, abnormal motility, excess acid secretion, and, rarely, infectious agents. Vomiting can also occur as a result of abdominal, systemic, metabolic, and neurologic disorders, the incidence of which varies with the age of the animal (Table 10–11). Although old dogs can present with any type of gastric disease, gastritis, gastric ulcers, and gastric tumors are more commonly diagnosed. Gastric foreign bodies, gastric motility disorder (i.e., gastric dilatation volvulus), and gastric outlet obstruction also occur.

TABLE 10–11. MAJOR CAUSES OF VOMITING ACCORDING TO AGE IN THE DOG

Young Dogs
Diet: Sudden change, ingestion of foreign material, poor feeding practices, dietary indiscretion (garbage, bones, sticks, plastic, food wrappers)
Gastrointestinal parasites (roundworms)
Infectious diseases: Canine distemper, parvovirus infection, coronavirus infection
Motion sickness
Intestinal obstruction (foreign body, intussusception)
Toxicoses
Acute gastritis
Gastric foreign body
Adrenal insufficiency
Enteritis (viral, bacterial, parasitic)

Mature Dogs
Dietary indiscretion (garbage, bones, food wrappers)
Gastrointestinal parasites *(Physaloptera)*
Infectious diseases
Pancreatitis
Acute and chronic gastritis
Gastric foreign body
Enteritis or colitis
Gastric outlet obstruction
Gastric or small intestinal tumor
Adrenal insufficiency
Abdominal disorders (peritonitis, prostatitis, pyometra)
Ketoacidosis
Central nervous system disorders (encephalitis, trauma, vestibular disease)

Old Dogs
Chronic renal failure
Gastric or small intestinal tumors
Dietary indiscretion
Pancreatitis
Chronic gastritis
Inflammatory bowel disease
Enteritis or colitis
Abdominal disorders (prostatitis, pyometra)
Ketoacidosis
Central nervous system disorders
Gastric ulcers

Gastric Tumors

Primary gastric tumors are rare in the dog. Those seen include adenomatous polyps, adenomas, leiomyomas, adenocarcinomas, leiomyosarcomas, fibrosarcomas, and lymphosarcoma. Adenocarcinomas are the most common, accounting for 75 per cent of all gastric tumors. They are most likely to be found in the distal stomach or the pyloric region of older male dogs. Gastric tumors are characterized by chronic vomiting of gradually increasing severity, inappetence or anorexia, and loss of body weight and condition. Anemia, diarrhea, and hematemesis also may be present. The time from onset of signs to presentation may vary from as little as 2 to 3 weeks to as long as 12 months. Signs may be more subtle in some animals, with, for example, anorexia of sudden onset as the only presenting sign.

Diagnosis is made by contrast radiography, in which the patient may exhibit delayed gastric emptying, mucosal filling defects, a rigid gastric wall, or ulcers. Diagnosis is confirmed by surgical biopsy or by gastroscopy and biopsy. Some tumors ulcerate and resemble peptic ulcers, and therefore examination of a deep biopsy specimen is essential to diagnosis.

Treatment is by wide surgical excision if clinically feasible. Depending on the diagnosis, chemotherapy also may be possible in selected patients. The prognosis, however, is almost invariably grave to hopeless.

Gastric Ulcers

Ulcers are defined as circumscribed breaks in the surface of the gastrointestinal mucosa in regions bathed in acid and pepsin. They may be acute or chronic, superficial or deep; almost all superficial ulcers are acute. Ulceration of the gastric and duodenal mucosa is a relatively common finding in dogs suffering from a variety of severe diseases. Development of ulcers in such patients is believed to be a complication of protein-calorie malnutrition, with its associated decrease in cell-mediated immunity and epithelial cell turnover, and of stress and hypoxia, which increase acid secretion and decrease mucosal blood flow. Sepsis, especially peritonitis, is also associated with gastric ulceration, although the predisposing mechanisms are unclear (Odonkor et al, 1981). Gastric ulcers also have a strong correlation with liver disease and mast cell tumors (Murray et al, 1972).

Nonsteroidal anti-inflammatory drug (NSAID) (e.g., aspirin, flunixine, ibuprofen, naproxin, phenylbutazone, indomethacin, and piroxicam) administration is arguably the most common cause of ulcers in older dogs. All NSAIDs inhibit the action of cycloxygenase (Fig. 10–3), which is critical in the synthesis of mucosal prostaglandins, particularly prostaglandin $E_2\alpha$ ($PGE_2\alpha$). Prostaglandins play an important role in the maintenance of normal gastric mucosal blood flow. They also exert a tonic inhibition on acid secretion, stimulate mucus production, and help maintain epithelial cell integrity. Thus, a decrease in mucosal prostaglandin content will have a devastating effect on gastric mucosal defense mechanisms. When combined with corticosteroids, which inhibit prostacyclin and diminish gastric epithelial cell turnover, the effect of NSAIDs can be devastating, with ulcers the almost inevitable sequela. Because of their propensity to cause inflammation, NSAIDs should never be used routinely in dogs unless specifically indicated for the health and well-being of the patient. An example of such an indication might be the old dog with severe arthritis, but even then, NSAIDs should be introduced with caution and the owner counseled about potential side effects.

History and Clinical Signs. Signs of peptic ulceration are poorly defined. Chronic vomiting, with or without hematemesis, is probably the most frequent sign. Unlike humans, dogs do not secrete acid continuously, and blood in the vomitus does not, therefore, always appear digested. Melena and anemia also may be observed if bleeding is severe. Inappetence and anorexia are common. The history must also include specific questions about any medications the owner may be giving the dog. The differential diagnosis includes gastric adenocarcinoma, adrenal insufficiency, and renal failure. Animals that have received long-term NSAID and/or corticosteroid therapy for chronic joint disease should always be suspected of having a gastric ulcer.

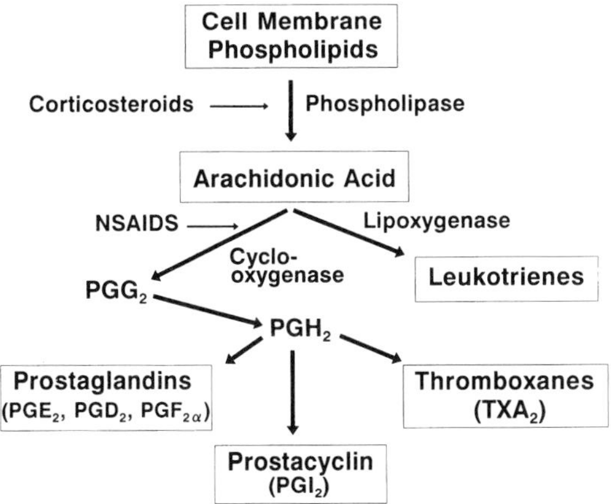

Figure 10–3. Action of nonsteroidal anti-inflammatory drugs (NSAIDs) and steroids on gastric mucosal prostaglandin synthesis.

Diagnosis and Treatment. Diagnosis is best made by gastroscopy, but contrast radiographic studies or exploratory laparotomy and biopsy are an acceptable alternative. Treatment is predicated on eliminating any underlying cause and reducing or neutralizing acid secretions. Most patients respond to treatment with a combination of H_2 receptor antagonists and sucralfate. If mucosal damage is sepsis related, higher doses of cimetidine (12 mg/kg q 8 hr) are indicated (Odonkor et al, 1981). Treatment with omeprazole is indicated in life-threatening situations, and exploratory laparotomy should be considered if the packed cell volume continues to decrease or perforation is suspected. If NSAID treatment is considered essential in such patients, it should be combined with the oral synthetic prostaglandin misoprostol (0.3 mg/kg q 8 hr), which replaces depleted mucosal prostaglandins. The prognosis is usually good if predisposing causes are eliminated.

Chronic Gastritis

It is arguable whether older dogs have an increased incidence of gastritis when compared with younger animals, but the incidence of gastritis in older dogs is still marked. Chronic gastritis is characterized by chronic persistent (occasionally sporadic) vomiting of variable frequency and character. Most cases are idiopathic, but chronic hypertrophic, eosinophilic, atrophic, and reflux gastritis are specific causes that can be diagnosed by appropriate techniques. A gastric foreign body and repetitive ingestion of foreign material are other causes. Because inflammation impairs motility and delays emptying, dogs with chronic gastritis may retain food in the stomach for long periods of time. Vomitus that contains any food more than 10 hours after ingestion strongly suggests delayed gastric emptying and the need to focus diagnostic studies on the proximal portion of the gastrointestinal tract.

Chronic Lymphocytic-Plasmacytic Gastritis. Most dogs with chronic gastritis fall into the idiopathic lymphocytic-plasmacytic category. Physical findings are usually unremarkable except for occasional mild dehydration; severely afflicted animals or those with long-standing disease may appear emaciated. The differential diagnosis includes all the causes of chronic vomiting in the dog (see Table 10–11). Hematologic and blood chemical changes are unremarkable; a few animals may have hypoproteinemia or anemia. Radiographs may occasionally reveal a thickened gastric wall. Gastroscopy reveals mucosal hyperemia and edema. Areas of gastric hemorrhage may be seen, particularly in the antrum; inflammation is diffuse in most patients, and histologic examination of a biopsy specimen is usually diagnostic. The mucosa is usually hypertrophic with an infiltrate of lymphocytes and plasma cells. A full-thickness gastric mucosal biopsy may be necessary for diagnosis in some patients, especially when the wall is thickened or infiltrated and the mucosa is relatively normal.

Treatment is predicated on inhibiting or neutralizing acid secretion so that it can no longer perpetuate inflammation by diffusing back through the disrupted mucosal barrier. When appropriate, acid–base and electrolyte abnormalities should also be identified and corrected. Foreign bodies must be removed and the gastritis treated with cimetidine (5 mg/kg orally q 8 hr). If vomiting and delayed emptying persist, then metoclopramide (0.4 to 0.5 mg/kg orally q 6 to 8 hr) should be used. A diet containing protein sources to which the patient has not been previously exposed also may be useful. If this approach fails, prednisone (1 mg/kg PO q 12 hr for 10 to 14 days and then tapered in 50–per cent decrements every 2 weeks) should be effective.

Chronic Hypertrophic Gastritis. Chronic hypertrophic gastritis is a rare disorder that appears either as a diffuse generalized mucosal hypertrophy or, more frequently, as a localized hypertrophy of the antral mucosa that may cause intermittent or chronic pyloric obstruction. The diffuse form has a predilection for boxers and basenjis, whereas the localized form has a predilection for miniature and toy breeds (i.e., Lhasa apso, Shih Tzu, Pekingese, and dachshund). The cause is unknown. The hypertrophic mucosa is inflamed and causes delayed emptying, chronic vomiting, anorexia, and lethargy. The localized form is associated with chronic vomiting and signs of gastric outlet obstruction. Hypokalemia and metabolic alkalosis may cause bizarre multifocal neurologic abnormalities. Diagnosis is made with either contrast radiography or endoscopy and mucosal biopsy. Resection of hypertrophic mucosa with an ample pyloroplasty is the treatment of choice. Cimetidine in conjunction with frequent small feedings of a low-fat diet is beneficial. The prognosis for the localized form is better than for the diffuse form. Neurologic abnormalities resolve as electrolyte and acid–base abnormalities improve.

Eosinophilic Gastritis. Eosinophilic gastritis is an uncommon disorder of unknown cause that is characterized by diffuse eosinophilic infiltration of any combination of the distal stomach, small bowel, or colon. Gastric infiltration is usually restricted to the mucosa but in a few patients may extend through the muscularis to the serosa. Mucosal involvement causes enlargement of the rugal folds. The diseased mucosa may become ulcerated, which leads to bleeding or leakage of plasma protein into the gastric lumen. Peripheral eosinophilia is a common but varied finding. Questioning of the owner may occasionally reveal a history of either urticaria or vomiting that may be associated with the ingestion of a specific diet. Mucosal protection and treatment with prednisone (1 to 2 mg/kg q 12 hr for 10 to 14 days, tapered over 3 to 6 weeks depending on severity) is usually effective in maintaining remission. Once the diagnosis is confirmed, occasional recurrences can be controlled by a repeat course of prednisone. Patients resistant to this therapeutic approach may need long-term, alternate-day prednisone therapy. Dietary adjustments, such as frequent feeding and hypoallergenic diets containing a protein to which the animal has not been previously exposed (usually lamb, mutton, rabbit, or cottage cheese), may be required. Azathioprine (1 mg/kg sid) in combination with prednisone may be effective in patients that are resistant to corticosteroid therapy alone.

Chronic Atrophic Gastritis. Atrophic gastritis is a rare disorder in which the gastric mucosa atrophies and loses its secretory function. The cause is unknown, but the condition occurs mainly in older dogs and is thought to be mediated through immune mechanisms. It may also be a sequela to chronic reflux gastritis in dogs. The predominant complaint is chronic intermittent vomiting. Mucosal degeneration is thought to result in achlorhydria, which may predispose the patient to bacterial overgrowth in the proximal small intestine. This can lead to malabsorption, chronic diarrhea, and loss of body weight and condition. Diagnosis is facilitated by endoscopy and mucosal biopsy. At endoscopy, the mucosa appears flattened, with loss of rugal folds and readily visualized submucosal vessels. (Care should be taken not to confuse this with gastric overdistention as a result of excessive air insufflation.) As with other types of gastric disease, an alternative approach to diagnosis is exploratory surgery with full-thickness biopsy. Treatment is symptomatic and based on frequent small feedings, prednisone, and cimetidine. Azathioprine has been used with limited success in a few patients. Antimicrobial agents such as tetracycline and tylosin are indicated to control secondary bacterial overgrowth and chronic diarrhea. Treatment with cimetidine may sound paradoxical, but the drug results in an increase in serum gastrin levels. Gastrin is trophic to the gastric mucosa, and mucosal growth is stimulated.

Reflux Gastritis. Reflux of bile and small intestinal contents into the stomach is a normal physiologic event in the fasting dog (Muller-Lissner et al, 1982). In some dogs, however, because of excessive biliary secretion, a defective pylorus, or ineffective gastric motility, the gastric mucosa is exposed to bile for long periods. Bile disrupts phospholipids in the apical lining of gastric mucosal cells, thereby disrupting the barrier and allowing acid influx and subsequent erosive gastritis. Aspirin also changes pyloric function in the dog, and aspirin-induced gastritis is believed to result from a combination of bile reflux, decreased prostaglandin synthesis, and direct mucosal damage. Reflux gastritis is manifested by chronic vomiting of bile-stained mucus after a prolonged (approximately 8- to 12-hour) fast. In dogs fed once daily in the evening, for example, vomiting may be an early morning event. Endoscopy may reveal bile-stained fluid in the stomach, erosive gastritis (especially in the antrum), and mucosal edema. Biopsy may confirm gastritis but not the underlying cause. Supportive treatment involves increasing the frequency of feeding to two or three times daily (especially first thing in the morning) to relieve signs; cimetidine (5 mg/kg orally q 8 hr) and metoclopramide (0.4 to 0.5 mg/kg orally q 6 to 8 hr) also are useful. The prognosis depends on the underlying cause.

Gastric Outlet Obstruction

Chronic vomiting as a result of occlusion of the pyloric or antral region of the stomach is a relatively common occurrence in the dog. The disorder occurs most frequently as a result of abnormal pyloric function or congenital or acquired pyloric stenosis. Less frequent causes are tumors of the pylorus and adjacent structures and chronic recurrent pancreatitis. Hypertrophic gastritis, a condition that is being diagnosed with increasing frequency, is another cause of gastric outlet obstruction. Acquired pyloric stenosis results from hypertrophy of the circular muscle of the pylorus and must always be differentiated from "pylorospasm," which is a poorly documented disorder that appears to be a stress-related failure of the pylorus to relax appropriately and occurs mainly in miniature and toy breeds.

History and Clinical Signs. Afflicted animals appear normal except for intermittent postprandial vomiting. The vomitus is characteristically undigested or partly digested and occasionally mucoid and may have an acid pH; bile is absent. The precise interrelationships between pyloric stenosis and pylorospasm are unclear. Signs of gastric outlet obstruction vary with the degree of obstruction. Vomiting is the predominant sign and may occur at any time after a meal. The time for complete emptying of a normal meal from the stomach in a dog fed once daily is 7 to 8 hours. Vomiting of all or part of a meal at periods more than 10 hours after ingestion suggests delayed gastric emptying and the probability of a gastric, pancreatic, or proximal duodenal lesion.

Diagnosis. Diagnosis is by contrast radiography or gastroscopy, with surgical confirmation an absolute necessity in most patients. In some dogs food may be present in the stomach at gastroscopy some 12 to 24 hours after the previous meal. This suggests delayed gastric emptying and, in an otherwise normal animal, supports the diagnosis of gastric outlet obstruction. Mucosal biopsy specimens are usually normal in animals with pyloric dysfunction. Chronic vomiting in outlet obstruction may result in hyponatremia, hypokalemia, hypochloremia, and metabolic alkalosis. A variety of neurologic abnormalities associated with the electrolyte abnormalities and the metabolic alkalosis occur in long-standing cases. These quickly reverse with appropriate fluid and electrolyte therapy. Animals with pylorospasm respond well to parasympatholytic agents such as propantheline bromide; barbiturates also may be useful as adjunctive therapy. Response to treatment serves to differentiate pylorospasm from pyloric hypertrophy. The only effective treatment for hypertrophic disease is pyloroplasty. In a few patients, outlet obstruction may be sufficiently severe that nutritional homeostasis cannot be sustained on any kind of diet, and enteral or parenteral feeding becomes essential.

Gastric Motility Disorders

Although primary gastric motility disorders are poorly documented because of the lack of appropriate diagnostic techniques, they appear to be an unusual but distinct clinical entity. It is probable that many patients with pylorospasm have underlying gastric atony. Impaired gastric motility also appears to develop in a few dogs that have had severe parvovirus type 2 infection. The syndrome is characterized by frequent eructation and chronic vomiting, usually of all or part of a meal 6 to 18 hours after ingestion. Radiographs may reveal an enlarged stomach. Diagnosis is difficult, because afflicted animals may exhibit normal emptying of liquid contrast material and may even appear to adequately empty contrast material mixed with a small quantity of dog food.

Gastroscopy reveals a large but otherwise apparently normal stomach; food or excessive amounts of gastric fluid may be present after an overnight fast. Mucosal biopsy specimens are normal or reveal only mild superficial gastritis, which is not compatible with the presenting complaint. Diagnosis is by exclusion of all other gastric diseases and complete evaluation of the history. A low-fat, highly digestible, blended or liquid diet along with increased frequency of feeding and metoclopramide (0.3 to 0.5 mg/kg orally q 6 to 8 hr) may be helpful. Pyloroplasty may be diagnostic and therapeutic. The prognosis is guarded.

Acute Gastric Dilatation-Volvulus

Acute gastric dilatation-volvulus (GDV) is a sudden and often fatal gastrointestinal disorder that affects many breeds but particularly the large, deep-chested breeds (i.e., German shepherd, Irish setter, Great Dane, St. Bernard, bloodhound, boxer, weimaraner, collie, Irish wolfhound, basset hound, and Doberman pinscher). It has been estimated that there are as many as 60,000 cases in the United States each year, with an overall mortality of about 20 per cent depending on the time from onset of signs to treatment. Dogs of all ages are afflicted, but there is a predilection for older intact female dogs. Gastric dilatation, which is the rapid distention of the stomach with food, fluid, and especially gas (from swallowed air and/or fermentation), may progress to volvulus. This occurs because the forces exerted on the distended canine stomach cause it to rotate either to the right or left (most often to the left, or clockwise) on an axis at right angles to a line between the esophageal and pyloric sphincters.

The cause is unknown and the subject of much debate. Risk factors are believed to include diet (bulky, dry cereal–based dog food, which may stretch the gastric ligaments), breed, stress, overeating, overdrinking, exercise, anesthesia, aerophagia, intragastric fermentation, and previous gastric "trauma." Postprandial exercise and excitement are additional frequently reported risk factors. This is not the whole picture, however, as is apparent from the many dogs belonging to knowledgeable breeders that still suffer from GDV despite all known precautions.

Acute gastric dilatation should be differentiated from GDV by survey radiographs made after a period of initial stabilization. Prolonged gastric distention markedly decreases the prognosis, because mucosal ischemic changes may be irreversible. Death from hypovolemic and cardiogenic shock may occur within a few hours of the onset of signs. Rapid gastric distention adversely affects the function of the lower esophageal sphincter and appears to impair gastric motility and emptying. It has been postulated that distention occludes the gastroesophageal junction, precluding emptying by either eructation or emesis. Distention decreases gastric motility by impairing normal contraction and by inhibiting reflex nerves. After dilatation, the gastric mucosa and, later, the gastric smooth muscle undergoes potentially irreversible ischemic necrosis. There is also an accumulation and sequestration of gastric secretions. The distended stomach occludes venous return from the rear limbs and caudal abdomen and precipitates hypovolemic and cardiogenic shock. Lactic acid and other metabolic byproducts accumulate in the hypoperfused hindlimbs and viscera to cause severe metabolic acidosis, especially after relief of dilatation. Signs of reperfusion injury, endotoxemia, disseminated intravascular coagulation, and fatal cardiac arrhythmias also may occur. Splenic torsion with infarction and necrosis is a common sequela.

History and Clinical Signs. The typical history is that of rapid ingestion of a large meal late at night in conjunction with consumption of large quantities of water followed by exercise. Dry (cereal-based) dog food has also been incriminated, as most large breed dogs are fed these diets for reasons of cost and ease of use. Abdominal distention is associated with progressive restlessness, unproductive retching, salivation, dyspnea, gastric tympany, and shock.

Diagnosis and Initial Treatment. Diagnosis is made from the clinical signs and confirmatory radiographs. Depending on the type and severity of the signs, treatment may consist of immediate gastric intubation and decompression, vigorous fluid therapy, and intravenous cimetidine (5 to 10 mg/kg q 6 hr) and lidocaine (1 mg/kg), which stabilizes the gastric mucosa as well as the myocardium. Free radical scavenger therapy is also becoming increasingly accepted. Gastrostomy or gastrocentesis also may facilitate decompression. After decompression, shock treatment should be maintained. When vital signs are stable, the dog should be taken to surgery for decompression and treatment of the volvulus. Contemporary surgical experience suggests that the incidence of recurrence may be reduced by gastropexy. Cardiac arrhythmias (usually premature ventricular contraction or ventricular tachycardia) frequently occur 2 to 3 days after surgical correction and should be treated appropriately. Follow-up management includes feeding of a meat-based, canned, highly digestible diet at least three times daily in conjunction with gastropexy; this is the best approach to the prevention of recurrence. Pyloroplasty does not influence the rate of recurrence.

Small Intestine

With the possible exception of some types of neoplasia, there are no specific age-related small intestinal diseases of older dogs. However, chronic inflammatory bowel disease is seen with sufficient frequency in older dogs to merit discussion.

Lymphocytic-Plasmacytic Enteritis

Lymphocytic-plasmacytic enteritis is characterized by infiltration of the mucosa with varying numbers of plasma cells and lymphocytes. It has been reported as a morphologic entity in young adult German shepherd dogs with relatively mild clinical disease (Hayden and Van Kruiningen, 1992) and as an hereditary enteropathy in basenji dogs with a relatively severe protein-losing enteropathy (Ochoa et al, 1984). The cause of lymphocytic-plasmacytic enteritis is unknown. It is most likely a nonspecific response to mucosal injury, as mucosal infiltration with lymphocytes and plasma cells has been documented in a variety of diseases, including small intestinal bacterial overgrowth, giardiasis, lymphangiectasia, regional enteritis, and intestinal lymphoma (DiBartola et al, 1982). The infiltrate may represent an immune-mediated inflammatory reaction directed against antigens from the intestinal lumen, most likely of bacterial or dietary origin (Rutgers et al, 1988). As yet, no direct evidence exists indicating a sensitivity to dietary protein as a cause of the infiltrates, but similar infiltrates in the colonic mucosa respond to changes in diet (Nelson et al, 1988).

History and Clinical Signs. Dogs with lymphocytic-plasmacytic enteritis present with a history of chronic small bowel diarrhea. There also may be a history of vomiting, which occasionally may be the sole complaint. The animal may be cachectic if mucosal damage is severe, and edema or ascites may be detected if the disease process is sufficiently advanced to cause protein-losing enteropathy. Thickened intestinal loops may occasionally be palpated.

Diagnosis. Major differential diagnoses include intestinal lymphoma, lymphangiectasia, fungal infection, chronic parasitism, and eosinophilic enteritis. The disease is suspected from the history and clinical signs and is confirmed by a small intestinal biopsy taken by endoscope or laparotomy. The hemogram is often normal in dogs with lymphocytic-plasmacytic enteritis, but indications of mild inflammation or blood loss exist. The serum chemistry tests are usually normal except for a mild to moderate increase in liver enzyme activity. Some patients with advanced disease may have panhypoproteinemia. Serum folate concentration may be increased, suggesting bacterial overgrowth, or normal to decreased, suggesting severe proximal small intestinal disease. Serum cobalamin activity is either normal or decreased, suggesting distal small intestinal disease (Burrows and Merritt, 1992).

Treatment. Treatment is symptomatic and usually consists of a combination of dietary, antimicrobial, and immunosuppression therapy.

DIETARY THERAPY. Animals appear to benefit from being fed a diet containing a protein to which they have not been previously exposed and that is also low in fat, with rice as the carbohydrate source (Table 10–12). Recurrence of signs after challenge with known allergens such as soya, beef, and gluten is essential to document the specific dietary sensitivity.

ANTIMICROBIAL THERAPY. On the premise that bacterial overgrowth may be the primary cause or at least a treatable complicating factor, antimicrobial therapy is always warranted. Oral oxytetracycline (10 to 20 mg/kg q 12 hr for 4 to 6 weeks) appears to be effective and has the advantage of being inexpensive. Other choices include metronidazole (10 to 20 mg/kg q 12 hr for 4 to 6 weeks) and tylosin (10 to 20 mg/kg q 12 hr for 4 to 6 weeks). Some owners find that they can reduce the antimicrobial dose to once daily and still bring about a remission of signs. Experimentation with various antimicrobial agents and/or diet combinations may be helpful in particular patients.

IMMUNOSUPPRESSION THERAPY. The initial drug of choice is prednisone (or prednisolone) at an initial dose of 1 to 2 mg/kg orally bid for 2 weeks and then tapered in 50–per cent decrements every 2 weeks if signs improve. If moderate to severe infiltrate or hypoproteinemia is pres-

TABLE 10–12. HOME-PREPARED DIETS FOR INTESTINAL DISEASE IN A DOG WEIGHING APPROXIMATELY 10 KG

HIGHLY DIGESTIBLE, LOW-FAT HYPOALLERGENIC DIETS (SINGLE-SOURCE PROTEIN)

Lamb	Venison	Rabbit
6 oz lean lamb	6 oz venison	6 oz rabbit
No corn oil	2 teaspoons corn oil	1 teaspoon corn oil

Add to:
- 10 oz boiled white rice
- 1 teaspoon dicalcium phosphate
- 1 teaspoon "lite" salt
- ½ capsule Centrum (Lederle Laboratories) adult multivitamins or ½ to 1 tablet of Vitaline Total Formula (Vitaline Formulas)

Supplies 675 to 700 kcal (20% to 34% protein, 46% to 48% carbohydrate, 19% to 22% fat)

HIGHLY DIGESTIBLE, MODERATE- AND HIGH-FAT DIETS

Chicken (Moderate Fat)	Beef (High Fat)
6 oz chicken	6 oz hamburger (lean)
8 oz boiled white rice	5 oz boiled white rice
2 teaspoons corn oil	No corn oil

Add to:
- 1 teaspoon dicalcium phosphate
- 1 teaspoon "lite" salt
- ½ capsule Centrum adult multivitamins

Supplies 680 kcal (33% protein, 30% fat [chicken]; 33% protein, 43% fat [beef])

Ingredients for each diet should be well mixed and cooked in a microwave oven or casserole before serving

ent, the concurrent use of azathioprine at a dose of 1 mg/kg sid for 2 to 4 weeks also is indicated. The owner should be advised about the possible side effect of drug-induced pancreatitis if azathioprine is used in combination with prednisone. The white blood cell count should be checked weekly and treatment stopped if the count falls below 4500 mm^3.

Supplemental Therapy. If weight loss and mucosal disease are severe, secondary vitamin deficiencies are probably present. Parenteral injection of cobalamin (750 μg/month) and oral folic acid administration (5 mg/day for 1 to 6 months) may be beneficial, as deficiencies of these vitamins may be due to impaired mucosal uptake.

Diarrhea in hypoproteinemic patients may be exacerbated by decreased plasma oncotic pressure (< 4.0 g/dl). Empirically, we have found that plasma transfusion in conjunction with other aggressive therapy can sometimes bring about a dramatic resolution of signs. Cimetidine or some other type of gastric mucosal protection also is beneficial, as the gastric mucosa almost always exhibits erosive gastritis in hypoproteinemic patients. Ascites, if present, should not be treated by paracentesis, because this procedure removes protein from the body and may exacerbate hypoproteinemia. Diuretic therapy using spironolactone is indicated if the ascites is sufficient to cause respiratory distress. Furosemide should be used only in emergency situations when rapid fluid loss is required. Diuretic therapy should be more aggressive in patients with concomitant congestive heart failure, and the use of prednisone should always be balanced against its possible negative effects in patients with azotemia resulting from chronic renal disease.

Eosinophilic Enteritis

Eosinophilic enteritis is a disease of the stomach, the small intestine, the large intestine, or a combination of these organs and has been described previously under eosinophilic gastritis. The disease is characterized by infiltration of the lamina propria and, less commonly, the deeper tissues with eosinophils and sometimes a mixture of other inflammatory cells. The cause is unknown, but the disease may arise secondary to dietary sensitivity or parasitism. Signs include vomiting and diarrhea, which may be intermittent and bloody. The disease may be confused with acute pancreatitis. Mesenteric lymph nodes are sometimes enlarged and can be detected on abdominal palpation or abdominal ultrasound. A peripheral eosinophilia may not necessarily be present. Diagnosis is made from biopsies of the small intestine. Treatment is the same as for lymphocytic-plasmacytic enteritis.

Canine Sprue or Villous Atrophy

Canine sprue, an uncommon enteropathy, represents an extreme example of chronic small intestinal disease in the dog (Batt et al, 1983). Dogs with this disorder present with a history of severe chronic diarrhea and weight loss, with older German shepherds being particularly sensitive. Low serum folate and cobalamin concentrations suggest extensive intestinal disease. Intestinal biopsy reveals partial villous atrophy and fusion, accompanied by a variable infiltrate of plasma cells and lymphocytes into the lamina propria. Treatment is nonspecific and consists of a highly digestible, low-fat diet (see Table 10–12); oxytetracycline (10 to 20 mg/kg q 8 hr); prednisone (0.5 to 1.0 mg/kg q 12 hr) proportional to the severity of the mucosal infiltrate; and vitamin and mineral supplementation. The prognosis is grave.

Small Intestinal Tumors

Leiomyosarcoma, leiomyoma, lymphosarcoma, and adenocarcinoma are the most common intestinal tumors of older dogs. Signs include vomiting, diarrhea, and weight loss and are related to malabsorption and protein-losing enteropathy secondary to infiltration of the intestinal wall. Bacterial overgrowth is a common sequela, especially if the tumor causes partial intestinal obstruction. Intestinal tumors are more common in older dogs, although lymphosarcoma occurs sporadically in dogs of almost any age. Survey abdominal and contrast radiographs may be helpful for diagnosis when an abdominal mass cannot be palpated. Exploratory laparotomy and intestinal and mesenteric node biopsy are confirmatory. Adenocarcinomas may cause signs of intermittent obstruction and may metastasize to the liver or pancreas and produce signs of secondary organ dysfunction. Pulmonary metastasis is rare. The prognosis is guarded with lymphosarcoma; the alimentary type usually responds poorly to treatment. Adenocarcinoma has a poor prognosis unless diagnosed very early, in which case resection of a localized lesion can produce marked clinical improvement for up to 18 months. Leiomyomas and leiomyosarcomas are often slow-growing tumors with a good prognosis after complete surgical excision.

Colon, Rectum, and Anus

Colonic and rectoanal disease is relatively uncommon in older dogs. Such animals do, however, occasionally suffer from colonic or rectal tumors and appear to have the same incidence of colonic inflammatory disease as younger dogs. The major large intestinal problem in older dogs is constipation, usually caused by colonic impaction.

Colonic Impaction

Impaction of the colon with a mixture of feces and ingested hair or foreign material such as bone or chewed wood is probably the most common cause of constipation in older dogs. Constipation is defined as infrequent defecation as a result of excessively hard or dry feces, with an associated increased straining to defecate and too small a fecal volume. Although dogs seem to be able to retain feces in the colon for days with no outwardly apparent adverse effects, the longer feces are retained, the harder and drier they become, with defecation becoming progressively more difficult until it is virtually impossible. This intractable constipation, or obstipation, is nearly always associated with a guarded prognosis, as changes in the colon wall may be irreversible.

Constipation is often confused with megacolon, defined as a condition of extreme dilatation of the colon. These terms are not synonymous, because dogs with megacolon are always constipated, whereas constipated animals do not necessarily have megacolon. The cause of primary megacolon is still unknown in dogs but may be due to a defect of smooth muscle function or possibly to defective innervation. Secondary megacolon can occur as a result of any lesion or disease that prevents normal defecation over a prolonged period and causes colonic distention with secondary colonic muscle degeneration. Contributing factors and specific therapy for colonic impaction with constipation are shown in Table 10–13.

History and Clinical Signs. Dogs with colonic impaction are usually presented with a history of tenesmus and dyschezia for a period of time ranging from days to weeks. In some dogs a small amount of liquid feces, often containing blood or mucus, may be passed with much effort. Such dogs may be presented with a spurious history of diarrhea.

Physical Findings and Diagnostic Studies. The constipated dog may be depressed and is often dehydrated. Abdominal palpation may reveal a hard tubular mass. When searching for potential causes, the clinician should always lift the tail and carefully examine and palpate the perineum for abnormalities. Digital rectal examination typically reveals an empty rectum with hard feces at the pelvic brim. If the rectum contains feces and the dog is frequently straining to defecate, a colonic motility defect should be suspected, as this implies that the marked colonic contraction, called a mass movement, is ineffective. Rectal examination occasionally reveals a rectal foreign body, prostatic enlargement, or a narrow pelvic canal. Rectal sacculation or dilatation also may be identified by rectal examination, even if obvious signs of perineal hernia are absent. Anal protrusion and some ventral breakdown of the pelvic diaphragm are to be expected in dogs with a long history of tenesmus. Abdominal survey radiographs confirm the presence of colonic dilatation and impaction and in some instances may reveal the cause.

TABLE 10–13. SPECIFIC TREATMENT OF COLONIC IMPACTION WITH CONSTIPATION AND DYSCHEZIA

CONTRIBUTING FACTORS	SPECIFIC THERAPY
Dietary	
Ingestion of hair, bones, and foreign material	Soften feces with enemas; remove bone fragments manually, if necessary; administer fecal softeners; prevent recurrence by grooming, dietary modification, and appropriate exercise
Environmental	
Hospitalization, litter box dirty or absent	Correct underlying cause; provide opportunity for defecation; administer enemas, suppositories, or laxatives, depending on severity
Painful Defecation	
Rectal foreign body	Remove
Anorectal disease	Clip hair; apply topical corticosteroids; treat myiasis
Tumors	Surgical correction or chemotherapy
Pseudocoprostasis	
Orthropedic disease	
Obstruction	
Healed pelvic fracture with narrow lumen	Surgical correction, if possible; fecal softeners
Intrapelvic tumor	Surgical correction, chemotherapy
Rectal lymphoma	Chemotherapy
Perineal hernia	
Neurogenic	
Spinal cord disease	Supportive care, colectomy
Idiopathic megacolon	Enemas, fecal softeners, and/or stimulant laxatives; colectomy
Pelvic nerve dysfunction	
Metabolic and Endocrine	
Hypokalemia	Treat underlying disorder; provide potassium supplementation
Hypercalcemia	
Hypothyroidism	
Drug-Induced	Change drugs or decrease dosage if possible
Barium	
Anticholingerics	
Narcotics	

Treatment. Treatment of colonic impaction includes removal of fecal concretions and correction of the underlying disorder. Most specific treatments are surgical and range from castration, in the case of prostatic enlargement or perineal hernia (along with hernia repair), to resection of colonic tumors or realignment of an old pelvic fracture. Breakdown and removal of fecal masses impacted in the colon should be accomplished as slowly and gently as possible. It is less traumatic for the dog if the feces are softened and removed over a 2- to 4-day period than if complete removal is attempted at one time. The severely constipated animal is often cachectic and dehydrated and may require corrective fluid and electrolyte therapy before any attempt is made to remove the impaction.

Impaction can be treated either with oral laxatives and enemas or by manual removal of material with the dog under general anesthesia after administration of enemas and laxatives. Simple impaction of relatively short duration is best treated by oral administration of a softening agent and a lubricant such as mineral oil. This can be given alone or in combination with dioctyl sodium sulfosuccinate (DSS), which is a wetting agent and colonic irritant. In severe cases, manual removal of the fecal concretions piece by piece with the aid of a small pair of whelping or sponge forceps is best. Once the underlying cause has been treated and the fecal concretions removed, attention should be directed toward prevention of recurrence. Nondigestible items should be eliminated from the diet, regular grooming instituted, and the opportunity provided for regular defecation. Prevention of recurrence may not be possible in dogs with secondary megacolon. In every case the therapeutic goal should be to have the dog form soft feces and defecate regularly. Fecal bulking and softening agents containing methylcellulose, psyllium hydrophilic mucilloid, bisacodyl, or DSS can be added to the diet. Fiber supplements in the form of bran are also useful. The best prophylaxis, however, is lactulose (0.5 to 3 ml/kg orally q 8 hr), a safe and nonabsorbable osmotic laxative; the dose can be titrated to produce the required fecal consistency.

Colonic and Rectal Tumors

Colonic and rectal tumors are relatively uncommon in dogs. Adenomatous polyps are the most common, accounting for 50 per cent of colonic lesions; lymphosarcoma and adenocarcinoma are the most common malignant tumors. Carcinomas, leiomyosarcomas, lymphosarcomas, carcinoid tumors, and anaplastic sarcomas also occur. Adenocarcinomas occur predominantly in dogs older than 9 years of age, are more frequent in males than in females, and have a high incidence in collies and German shepherd dogs. Adenocarcinomas are classified infiltrative, ulcerative, or proliferative, based on their gross characteristics. Infiltrating tumors spread within the rectal or colonic wall, causing fibrosis and stricture formation of variable length. The ulcerative type produces a typical malignant ulcer with a firm base and a raised edge, whereas the proliferative type has a wart-like appearance. Although slow growing, the tumor eventually spreads through the rectal wall, penetrates the lymphatics, and metastasizes to the local lymph nodes, the lungs, and the liver.

Colonic and rectal lymphosarcomas are uncommon and occur either as a discrete mass or as diffuse mural infiltration along the length of the organ. Carcinoid tumors, although rare, occur in the small and large intestines. These tumors are associated with diarrhea and gastrointestinal hemorrhage and, as a result of their secretion of serotonin, with systemic vasomotor effects. Adenomatous polyps are the most common benign tumors of the colon and the rectum, with most being found in the rectum. Although all breeds are affected, there appears to be a predilection in collies and West Highland white terriers.

History and Physical Findings. Dogs with large intestinal tumors usually have a history of dyschezia, hematochezia, tenesmus, and diarrhea and appear to be chronically ill and debilitated. Specific signs depend on the tumor location and type. Tenesmus tends to worsen as lesions develop, especially with proliferative or obstructive masses. Only a thin ribbon of feces may be passed with infiltrating adenocarcinomas, whereas hematochezia is a frequent complaint with ulcerating masses. Rectal examination reveals a painful, ring-like mass or stenotic area. Infiltrative lymphosarcomas of the large intestine cause a chronic unresponsive diarrhea such as that seen in chronic histoplasmosis. Dogs with colonic or rectal polyps are not as debilitated as dogs with malignant tumors. In these animals, tenesmus after defecation and perhaps a chronic, unresponsive bloody or mucoid diarrhea occur. If tenesmus is severe, the tumor may prolapse through the anus.

Diagnosis and Treatment. Rectal examination is sufficient to confirm the presence of a rectal mass, and biopsy is usually diagnostic. Colonic tumors are diagnosed by colonoscopy (Fig. 10–4). Colonoscopy may be difficult or impossible when the tumor causes rectal stenosis. Surgical resection of carcinomas and adenocarcinomas should be attempted. About 75 per cent of polyps are removed by surgical excision or electrocautery through the anus; they can be easily removed if the rectal mucosa is everted by gentle traction. Polyps located more proximally can be excised with an electrocautery snare passed through the colonoscope or, as a last resort, via a colectomy. The prognosis after removal is good.

Anal Tumors

The most common and clinically important tumor of the anal region is the perianal gland adenoma. Other benign neoplasms that are occasionally found include lipomas, melanomas, and leiomyomas. Malignant anal tumors (i.e., squamous cell carcinoma, malignant melanoma, perianal adenocarcinoma, and anal gland adenocarcinoma) are rare.

Perianal Gland Adenomas. Perianal gland adenomas arise from the perianal and circumanal glands of dogs and occur most often in intact males older than 6 years. The tumors are benign

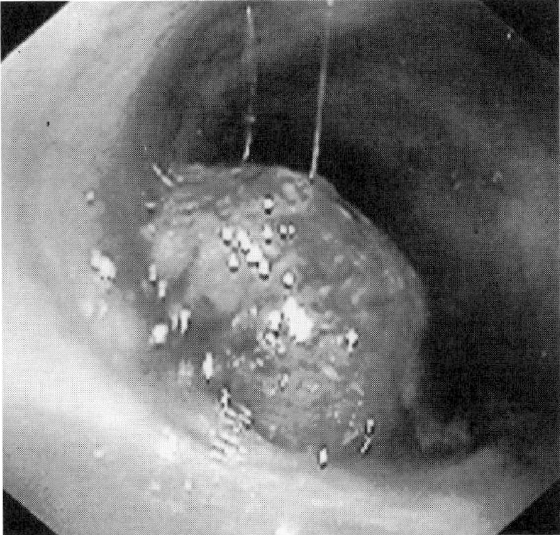

Figure 10–4. Endoscopic appearance of a rectal polyp in a 10-year-old mixed breed dog with a 2-year history of dyschezia and hematochezia. The tumor was resected, and the dog made an uneventful recovery.

but cause owner concern because of their tendency for ulceration and hemorrhage, their unsightliness, their interference with defecation, and the animal's excessive licking of the perineum. Perianal gland adenomas occur most often in the skin surrounding the anus but can be found anywhere on the perineum, tail base, or external genitalia. Diagnosis is confirmed by biopsy. The tumors are hormone sensitive, and their development can be impaired with estrogen therapy. Definitive treatment includes surgical excision and castration, although radiation therapy and cryosurgery are also highly effective. The prognosis is favorable with all forms of treatment.

Malignant Anal Tumors. Squamous cell carcinoma of a distinct cloacogenic type has been reported to occur in the anal canal of the dog. Squamous cell carcinoma of the cutaneous portion of the anus may also be encountered infrequently. The tumor initially appears as a small indurated ulcer and progresses to a cauliflower-like ulcerated mass with irregular edges. The tumor metastasizes readily, and early radical excision is essential if a cure is to be effected. The prognosis is fair if the tumor is excised early. These tumors are often associated with pseudohyperparathyroidism. A malignant melanoma occasionally occurs as a flat to round nodule on the anus, especially in breeds with heavily pigmented skin. An adenocarcinoma emanating from the apocrine cells in the anal glands occurs in aged female dogs. These tumors are an ectopic source of a parathyroid-like substance that causes signs of pseudohyperparathyroidism. All malignant anal tumors cause extensive local invasion and metastasize to iliac lymph nodes, liver, and lungs. The prognosis is almost always poor.

DISORDERS OF CATS

Esophagus and Stomach

Esophageal disease is rare in the cat. Tumors, especially carcinomas, used to be quite common but currently are seldom seen. When present, tumors cause signs associated with chronic esophageal obstruction and secondary megaesophagus (Fig. 10–5). As in dogs, most gastric diseases in the cat are associated with vomiting. Major causes of vomiting in the cat are shown in Table 10–14.

Gastric Tumors

Gastric tumors have a lower incidence in cats than in dogs. Lymphoma and adenocarcinoma are the primary tumor types. Signs vary and can range from sudden anorexia to acute or chronic vomiting of increasing incidence and severity. Cats with gastric tumors are usually thin and underweight, and with careful palpation a mass may sometimes be found in the cranial abdomen. The differential diagnosis of vomiting and weight loss includes hyperthyroidism, uremia and uremic gastritis, inflammatory bowel disease, megacolon, gastric outlet obstruction, drugs or toxins, and heartworm disease. Gastroscopy with endoscopic biopsy is helpful. Treatment is based on the tumor type and location. Gastric lymphoma can sometimes be placed into remission with chemotherapy. Surgical resection of adenocarcinoma can result in cessation of signs for a period of up to 12 months because adenocarcinoma in the cat is very slow growing.

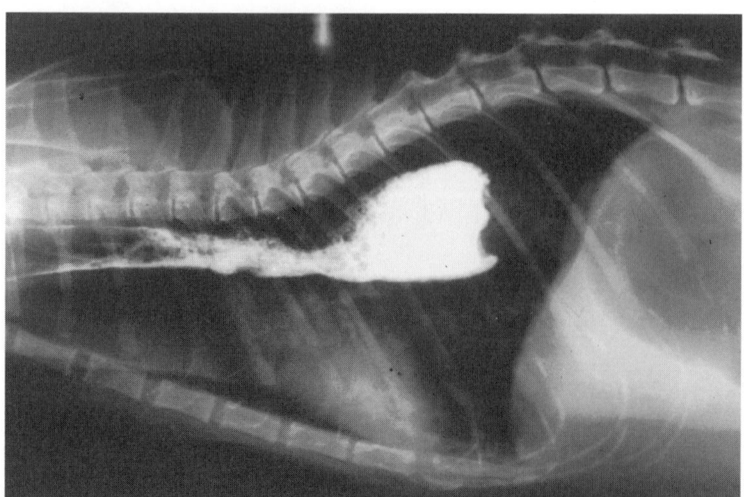

Figure 10–5. Radiographic appearance of an esophageal carcinoma with secondary megaesophagus in a 13-year-old cat.

TABLE 10–14. MAJOR CAUSES OF VOMITING ACCORDING TO AGE IN THE CAT

Young Cats
Diet: Sudden change, dietary indiscretion, overeating
Gastrointestinal parasites
Infectious diseases (parvovirus, feline infectious peritonitis, coronavirus)
Gastrointestinal foreign body (toys and string, hairballs)
Toxicoses
Gastritis
Enteritis
Ingestion of grass or other plants
Mature Cats
Gastrointestinal parasites
Pancreatitis
Gastric tumors
Gastritis
Enteritis
Intestinal tumors, obstruction
Toxicoses (drugs)
Gastric outlet obstruction
Inflammatory bowel disease
Tumors
Foreign body
Peritonitis
Liver disease
Heartworm disease
Hyperthyroidism (≥5 yrs of age)
Old Cats
Chronic renal failure
Gastric tumors
Hyperthyroidism
Pancreatitis
Enteritis
Inflammatory bowel disease
Megacolon
Feline infectious peritonitis
Gastric outlet obstruction
Drugs or toxins
Heartworm disease

Gastritis and Hairballs

Gastritis occurs in older cats but is usually part of the inflammatory bowel disease. The clinical signs, the diagnostic approach, and the treatment regimens are the same as for dogs except that the azathioprine dosage in cats is 0.3 mg/kg sid. Hairballs are a frequently diagnosed cause of chronic gagging and vomiting in the cat, particularly the long-haired breeds. Although minor pharyngeal irritation during grooming is common, accumulation of hair in the stomach and initiation of clinical signs as a primary disorder are not. Hair is normally emptied from the stomach by powerful interdigestive, distally propagated gastric contractions; its accumulation to form a hairball, therefore, strongly suggests an underlying defect in gastric motility. Often a gastric mucosal biopsy in cats with hairballs reveals plasmacytic-lymphocytic gastritis and concomitant lymphocytic-plasmacytic enteritis. Treatment with prednisone and possibly cimetidine for the underlying gastritis almost always results in recovery.

Small and Large Intestine

Inflammatory Bowel Disease

Inflammatory bowel disease (IBD) is characterized by the mucosal infiltration of excessive numbers of plasma cells, lymphocytes, eosinophils, and neutrophils. Lymphocytic-plasmacytic gastroenteritis is the most common diagnosis. Known causes of the inflammatory reaction are the same as outlined previously for dogs. As in dogs, IBD can involve the stomach, the small intestine, the colon, or a combination of these organs.

History and Clinical Signs. Cats with IBD typically present with chronic vomiting, both vomiting and diarrhea, or diarrhea alone. Associated signs include decreased appetite or ravenous appetite, weight loss, and lethargy. Signs are cyclic in many cats; vomiting bouts may last 2 to 4 days and then subside into a regular pattern. The vomitus may consist of partially digested food but most often contains only bile-stained mucus. Chronic small bowel diarrhea is another important sign, although bouts of large bowel disease occasionally predominate.

Physical Findings and Diagnosis. Cats with IBD vary tremendously in their physical appearance, being cachectic if the disease is severe and long-standing with malabsorption and perhaps protein-losing enteropathy. Other cats, sometimes even with severe intestinal disease, appear plump and robust. Abdominal palpation may reveal a thickened small intestine with perhaps enlarged mesenteric lymph nodes. Differential diagnosis includes hyperthyroidism, intestinal parasitism (especially giardiasis), lymphosarcoma, heartworm disease, bacterial overgrowth, intestinal adenocarcinoma, and exocrine pancreatic insufficiency secondary to chronic pancreatitis. Survey abdominal and contrast radiographs are usually normal. Abnormal findings on abdominal palpation allow the veterinarian to avoid radiographs but to perform exploratory surgery or endoscopic biopsy. An alternative approach, if a palpable mass can be fixed and brought to the abdominal wall, is to perform transabdominal fine-needle aspiration cytology. Biopsy is diagnostic for IBD.

Treatment. Prednisone is the drug of choice for treatment of IBD in cats. Mild to moderate cases often respond to prednisone at an initial dose of 1 to 2 mg/kg divided q 12 hr, followed by a gradual decrease in 50–per cent decrements every 2 to 4 weeks until an alternate daily dose of 2.5 to 5 mg is reached. Signs usually abate within 2 to 4 weeks, but treatment must be continued for at least an additional 4 weeks to minimize the chance of recurrence. Even old cats tolerate prednisone therapy very well with minimal or no side effects. If biopsy specimens reveal moderate to severe mucosal disease, prednisone should be given at a dose of 2 to 4 mg/kg divided twice daily for 2 to 4 weeks until signs resolve. If signs are severe, it is advisable to combine the prednisone with a once-daily dose of azathioprine (0.3 mg/kg) for 2 to 4 weeks. The white blood cell count should be checked weekly while the patient is on this regimen and the drug stopped or changed to an alternate-day regimen if the white blood cell count is <4500 mm^3.

In cats with chronic IBD-related diarrhea, metronidazole should be added to the treatment regimen at an initial dose of 10 mg/kg q 12 hr. This drug is well tolerated by most cats and should be continued for at least 4 weeks after prednisone therapy has ceased. Metronidazole can always be reintroduced if diarrhea recurs. Some owners have found that diarrhea can be controlled in their cats by administering as little as ¼ to ⅛ of a 250-mg metronidazole tablet once daily. If the owner has difficulty administering oral medication, methylprednisolone acetate injections can be given intramuscularly every 2 to 4 weeks at a dose of 20 to 40 mg. However, this does not appear to work as well as oral prednisone in most cats. Because dietary allergens may play a role in the pathogenesis of IBD, it is advisable, if possible, to change the diet to one containing a protein to which the cat has not been previously exposed. To minimize the risk of the animal becoming sensitized to the new diet, the diet should be instituted about 2 to 4 weeks after drug therapy has begun. Many cats, however, have been exposed to a wide range of protein sources, and this approach does not work as well as in dogs. Commercial rabbit- or lamb-based diets are available, but palatability is poor, and even a hungry cat may refuse to eat them. Poor treatment response of cats with IBD usually results from inadequate corticosteroid dosage, poor owner compliance, or, most often, treatment for only small intestinal disease when the cat has concomitant colitis. In these animals, sulfasalazine (20 mg/kg sid) should be initiated for a period of 7 to 10 days. If the cat stops eating, the drug should be withdrawn.

Intestinal Tumors

Cats suffer from a variety of enteric neoplasms, but three predominate: focal lymphoma, diffuse lymphoma, and adenocarcinoma. Signs of focal lymphoma depend on the location. The course is progressive and characterized by vomiting, diarrhea, and anorexia. Diagnosis is usually straightforward, and the prognosis is always guarded after surgery or chemotherapy. Diffuse lymphoma is characterized by mucosal infiltration of lymphocytes, particularly in Peyer's patches. Signs resemble those of IBD, and diagnosis is by biopsy. Afflicted cats usually test negative for feline leukemia virus (FeLV). Treatment with vincristine, cyclophosphamide, and prednisone is preferred. Adenocarcinoma is a relatively common tumor of the distal small intestine in the older cat. Signs include vomiting, anorexia, and diarrhea. Abdominal palpation may reveal small intestine on either side of a mass; mesenteric nodes may also be enlarged in advanced cases. Diagnosis can be made by aspiration cytology, but surgical excision with wide margins is preferred. The tumor is slow to metastasize, and the prognosis is fair. I have had cats live for up to 25 months before signs of recurrence. The prognosis, however, depends on the stage of the tumor at diagnosis.

Constipation, Obstipation, and Megacolon

Constipation is a relatively common complaint in the cat and should be differentiated from obstipation. Unlike constipation, obstipation is inevitably associated with a guarded or grave prognosis, as degenerative changes in the colon wall are usually irreversible. Dyschezia is usually associated with lesions in or near the anus. Afflicted animals may cry out as they attempt to defecate and may exhibit prolonged tenesmus. Constipation, which occurs when the colon becomes impacted with feces, is sometimes used synonymously with the term *megacolon,* a disorder of extreme dilatation of the colon. The two terms are not synonymous, however. Constipation is a sign of disease, whereas megacolon is a disorder of both structure and function. Megacolon may be either primary or secondary; the cause of primary megacolon is unknown, but in most patients it is probably attributable either to a defect in smooth muscle function or to disrupted colonic innervation. Secondary megacolon may occur as a sequel to any lesion or disease that prevents normal defecation for a prolonged period of time.

Constipation can occur in association with any disorder that impairs the passage of fecal material through the colon. Defects in muscle or nerve function, luminal obstruction, or suppression of the urge to defecate all delay fecal transit. This increased contact time allows the mucosa to remove additional electrolytes and water, resulting in harder and drier feces.

Colonic Impaction

Cause. Impaction of the colon with feces and ingested hair or foreign material is the most common cause of constipation and dyschezia in the cat. In some apparently susceptible animals, the disorder is a recurrent problem and may lead to secondary megacolon. A variety of circumstances and diseases predispose the cat to impaction and constipation. These can be divided into six main groups: dietary and environmental, painful, obstructive, neurogenic, metabolic and endocrine, and drug-induced (see Table 10–13). Obstructive and neurogenic causes are the most frequently diagnosed.

History and Clinical Signs. Cats with colonic impaction may be presented with a history of reduced frequency of defecation or failure to defecate for a period of time ranging from days to weeks. In some patients a small amount of liquid feces, often containing blood or mucus, may be passed with prolonged tenesmus. If defecation has been unobserved, the patient might also be presented only because it is lethargic, inappetent or anorectic, and vomiting intermittently (Fig. 10–6). Abdominal palpation reveals a hard, irregular, tubular colonic mass, which may fill the whole length of the colon. Rectal examination combined with abdominal palpation is useful in localizing the fecal mass and in identifying lesions such as rectal foreign bodies or a narrowed pelvic canal that may be the underlying causes.

Treatment. Treatment consists of several components: restoration of electrolyte and fluid balance; removal or amelioration, if possible, of any underlying cause; administration of laxatives or cathartics; and enemas. After successful treatment the possibility of recurrence is minimized by owner education, dietary manipulation, and, if necessary, long-term medication. A guide to treatment of the common causes of colonic impaction is given in Table 10–13. For practical purposes, constipated patients can be conveniently divided into two groups: the cat presented for initial evaluation and treatment of severe colonic impaction or obstipation and the cat with a long history of moderate constipation. Both may require long-term medical therapy.

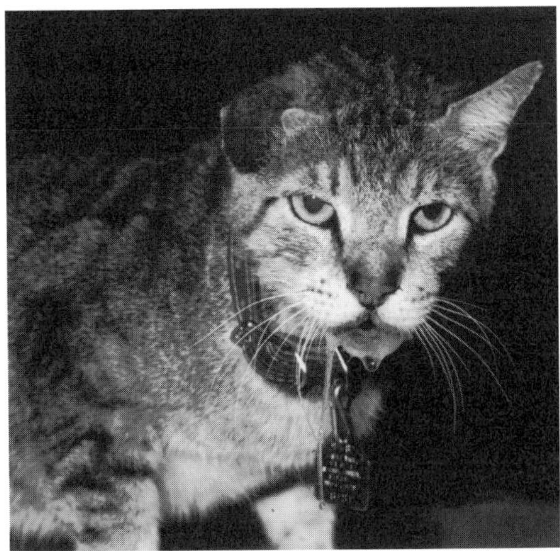

Figure 10–6. Ptyalism, probably associated with nausea after abdominal palpation, in a 10-year-old cat with severe megacolon.

Megacolon

Cause. Megacolon is more common in the cat than in the dog but is an uncommon cause of constipation in both species. It may be primary or secondary; the cause of primary megacolon is unknown but is possibly related to a primary defect in smooth muscle function. The muscle does not contract, and fecal material is retained in the colon and eventually causes severe constipation. Secondary megacolon may occur as a sequel to any lesion or disease that prevents normal defecation over a prolonged period. The colon distends to the point that the muscle degenerates to leave a large flaccid sac filled with rock-like fecal material.

History and Clinical Signs. Megacolon may occur at any age, although primary megacolon seems to have a higher prevalence in older cats. The patient is usually presented with a history of lethargy, loss of appetite, and failure to defecate over a long period of time. Ptyalism and intermittent vomiting are common complaints. The disorder is seemingly insidious in onset and progressive in nature, and recurrent episodes of constipation of increasing severity and frequency may occur before their significance is realized. Most cats with megacolon are depressed and have an unkempt appearance. The rectum is usu-

TABLE 10–15. SUMMARY OF THERAPEUTIC PRODUCTS AVAILABLE FOR MANAGEMENT OF GASTROINTESTINAL DISORDERS

THERAPEUTIC AGENT	DOSAGE AND ROUTE	COMMENTS
Antiemetic and Promotility Drugs		
Metoclopramide (Reglan)	0.3–0.4 mg/kg PO q 8 hr	For gastric motility disorders and reflux gastritis. Give 30 min before meals and at bedtime.
Chlorpromazine	0.5 mg/kg IM/IV q 4 hr	Potent antemetic in the severely vomiting patient. Can be used with metoclopramide.
Erythromycin	1–2 mg/kg PO q 8 hr	At this dose the drug binds with motilon receptors and stimulates gastric emptying.
Antimicrobial Agents		
Metronidazole	10–20 mg/kg PO q 8 hr	For management of small intestinal bacterial overgrowth in dogs and cats.
Oxytetracycline	10 mg/kg PO q 8–12 hr	For management of small intestinal bacterial overgrowth in dogs and cats.
Tylosin	10–20 mg/kg PO q 12 hr	For management of small intestinal bacterial overgrowth in dogs and cats.
H_2 Receptor Antagonists		
Cimetidine (Tagamet)	5–12 mg/kg PO/IV q 8 hr	Suppresses acid secretion and improves mucosal barrier. High dose indicated in septic patients.
Ranitidine (Zantac)	2 mg/kg PO/IV q 12 hr	Suppresses acid production.
Gastric Protectants		
Sucralfate (Carafate)	0.2–1.0 mg PO q 8 hr in dogs and cats. Can be made into a slurry by crushing a pill and mixing with 10–20 ml tapwater	Protects and enhances mucosal barrier. Requires pH <4 for maximum effect, but barrier protection occurs at neutral pH.
Misoprostol (Cytotec)	2–3 μg/kg PO q 6–12 hr	Synthetic prostaglandin protects mucosa when nonsteroidal anti-inflammatory drugs must be used.
Proton Pump Antagonists		
Omeprazole (Prilosec)	0.7–1.0 mg/kg PO sid	Blocks all acid secretion. Use in severe gastric ulceration. Four days required to reach peak blood levels.
Immunomodulating Agents		
Prednisone	0.5–2 mg/kg PO q 12 hr and then tapering by 50 per cent every 2 weeks	Initial control of lymphocytic-plasmacytic and eosinophilic gastroenteritis in dogs and cats.
Azathioprine	1 mg/kg q 24 hr (dog) 0.3 mg/kg q 24 hr (cat) Initial course should be 2 weeks	Adjunctive therapy in severe lymphocytic-plasmacytic gastroenteritis. Possible pancreatitis when used with prednisone. Monitor white blood cell count weekly in cat. Stop if <4500 mm^3.
Sulfasalazine	25–40 mg/kg PO q 8 hr (dog) 20 mg/kg PO q 12–24 hr (cat)	For the treatment of colitis in dogs and cats.
Laxatives		
Lactulose (Cephulac)	0.5–3 mg/kg PO q 8–12 hr in dog or cat	Use as a laxative. Start at lower dose and titrate to achieve appropriate fecal consistency. Overdose causes diarrhea.

ally empty and dilated on rectal examination, with a mass of hard feces felt at the pelvic inlet. Abdominal palpation confirms the presence of a large mass of feces in the colon. The entire length of the descending colon and even the ascending and transverse colon may be distended with large volumes of rock-like fecal material, which may be 4 to 5 cm in diameter in severe cases. Abdominal radiographs confirm the diagnosis (Fig. 10–7). Patients with long-standing megacolon may be hypokalemic and anemic. Leukocytosis with a left shift and toxic neutrophils also may be observed.

Treatment. Treatment of megacolon should

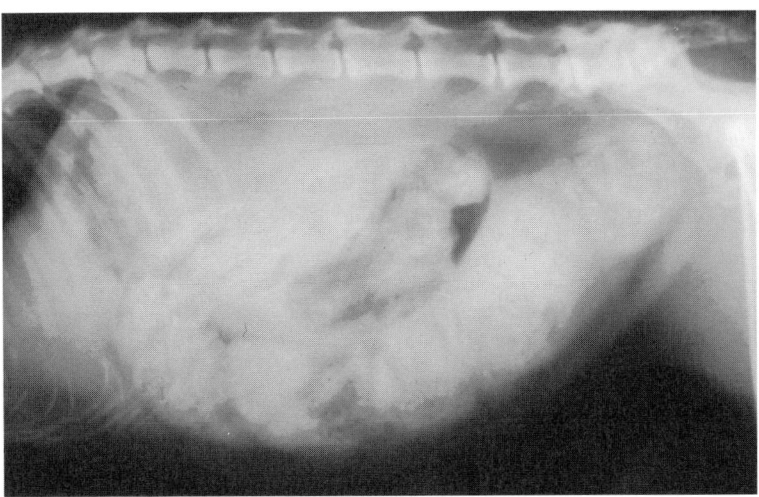

Figure 10–7. Survey abdominal radiographs of the cat shown in Figure 10–6. There is marked colonic distention with radioopaque fecal material.

initially proceed along the same lines as for colonic impaction until it becomes clear that degenerative changes in the colonic wall are irreversible and the organ cannot contract enough to move the material into the rectum. Preventive measures are needed for the duration of the animal's life. These include dietary modification and the regular administration of laxatives, of which lactulose is most effective. The initial dose is 1 to 3 ml/kg q 8 hr, but it may be increased by up to 10 times without harming the patient. The objective is to titrate the dose of lactulose against fecal consistency. Lactulose is not digested in the small intestine and is poorly metabolized by colonic bacteria to short-chain fatty acids. It thus remains in the colonic lumen and retains water by osmosis. If lactulose is used, the diet should consist of highly digestible commercial diets to reduce fecal bulk. If not, the diet should include laxative foods such as raw liver (not more than 20 per cent of the diet because of the tendency for hypervitaminosis) and bulking agents such as methylcellulose, canned pumpkin, and bran.

Subtotal Colectomy. Surgical resection of the atonic colon has been described (Rosin et al, 1988). The procedure is technically simple and provides a successful and realistic alternative to the stress of repeated enemas and long-term laxative therapy. The colon is removed from just above the ileocolonic junction to a point immediately proximal to the pubic brim. The ileum is then anastomosed to the terminal colon in an end-to-end or end-to-side fashion. Cats treated by subtotal colectomy usually maintain a soft or semisolid fecal consistency that is acceptable to owners. The need for enemas and laxatives is obviated, and most cats, unless there are other underlying disorders, go on to live normal lives. The prognosis is guarded for medical therapy and depends on the stage of the disease at first examination and the ability of the owner to persist with preventive and ongoing therapeutic measures.

References and Supplemental Reading

Batt RM, Bush BM, Peters TJ. Subcellular biochemical studies of a naturally occurring enteropathy in the dog resembling chronic tropical sprue in human beings. Am J Vet Res 44:1492–1496, 1983.

Benno Y, Mitsuoka T. Effect of age on intestinal microflora of beagle dogs. Microecol Ther 19:85–91, 1989.

Bright RM, Burrows CF. Percutaneous endoscopic tube gastroscopy in dogs. Am J Vet Res 49:629–633, 1988.

Burrows CF. Evaluation of a colonic lavage solution to prepare the canine colon for colonoscopy. J Am Vet Med Assoc 195:1719–1721, 1989.

Burrows CF, Merritt AM. Assessment of gastrointestinal function. In Anderson NV, ed. Veterinary Gastroenterology. 2nd ed. Philadelphia, Lea & Febiger, 1992, pp 16–42.

DiBartola SP, Rogers WA, Boyce JT, et al. Regional enteritis in two dogs. J Am Vet Med Assoc 181:904–908, 1982.

Hayden DW, Van Kruiningen HJ. Lymphocytic plasmacytic enteritis in German shepherd dogs. J Am Anim Hosp Assoc 18:898, 1992.

Muller-Lissner SA, Sonnenberg A, et al. Gastric emptying and post-prandial duodenal gastric reflux in pylorectomized dogs. Am J Physiol 247:G9–G13, 1982.

Murray M, Robinson P, McKeating FJ, et al. Peptic ulceration in the dog: A clinicopathological study. Vet Rec 91:441–447, 1972.

Nelson RW, Stookey LJ, Kazacos E. Nutritional management of idiopathic chronic colitis in the dog. J Vet Intern Med 2:133–137, 1988.

Ochoa R, Breitschwerdt EB, Lincoln KL. Immunoproliferative small intestinal disease (IPSID) in basenji dogs: Morphological observations. Am J Vet Res 45:482–490, 1984.

Odonkor P, Monat C, Himal HS. Prevention of sepsis-induced gastric lesions in dogs by cimetidine via inhibition of gastric secretion and by prostaglandin via cytoprotection. Gastroenterology 80:375–379, 1981.

Raphel V, Moreau H, et al. Dog gastric lipase: Stimulation of its secretion in vivo and cytolocalization in mucous pit cells. Gastroenterology 102:1535–1545, 1992.

Ridgeway RL, Suter PF. Clinical and radiographic signs in primary and metastatic esophageal neoplasms of the dog. J Am Vet Med Assoc 174:700–704, 1979.

Rosin E, Walshaw R, Melhatt C, et al. Subtotal colectomy for treatment of chronic constipation associated with idiopathic megacolon in cats: 38 cases (1979–1985). J Am Vet Med Assoc 193:850–853, 1988.

Rutgers HC, Batt RM, Kelly DF. Lymphocytic-plasmacytic enteritis associated with bacterial overgrowth in a dog. J Am Vet Med Assoc 192:1739–1742, 1988.

Tams T: Gastroscopy. In Tams T, ed. Small Animal Endoscopy. St Louis, CV Mosby, 1990, pp 89–166.

CHAPTER 11

The Liver and Exocrine Pancreas

DONNA S. DIMSKI

THE LIVER

Normal Aging Changes

Little is known about the effects of the normal aging process on hepatic structure and function in dogs and cats. Although fibrosis is commonly seen in the hepatic parenchyma of older animals, it does not have a marked effect on hepatic function (Mays et al, 1991). Normal function of the liver does not appear to change significantly as a result of age. Despite this, however, older dogs and cats are at greater risk for untoward drug effects (Kitani, 1986).

Effects of Liver Disease

The astute veterinarian often evaluates the older dog or cat with a "jaundiced eye" for liver disease, beginning with the case history and physical examination (Tables 11–1 and 11–2). Many animals with severe liver disease will be inappropriately depressed, stuporous, or even comatose (Fig. 11–1). In liver disease metabolic functions are disrupted, resulting in a multitude of clinical manifestations or death from the effects of metabolic disturbances (Table 11–3). Thus, effects of severe liver disease and treatment of these effects are similar for many different types of liver disease.

Hepatoencephalopathy. Hepatoencephalopathy (HE) is defined as the neurologic derangements that occur secondary to abnormal liver function, presumably because the dysfunctional liver cannot remove toxins absorbed from the gastrointestinal tract (Tyler, 1990a,b). The pathogenesis of HE is complex. Classically hyperammonemia is associated with HE. Toxic concentrations of ammonia disturb energy metabolism in the central nervous system (CNS), interfere with neurotransmission, disrupt the blood–brain barrier, and decrease concentrations of excitatory neurotransmitters (Cooper and Plum, 1987).

TABLE 11–1. HISTORICAL SIGNS ASSOCIATED WITH LIVER DISEASE

Depression	Polyuria
Lethargy	Polydipsia
Exercise intolerance	Bilirubinuria
Anorexia	Poor haircoat
"Picky" eater	Dermatopathies
Weight loss	Apparent blindness
Halitosis	Aggression
Vomiting	Abdominal docility
Hematemesis	Ataxia
Diarrhea	Stupor
Melena	Circling
Abdominal pain	Aimless wandering
Abdominal enlargement	Head pressing
Ascites	Abnormal vocalization
Petechiation	Coma
Easy bruising	

TABLE 11–2. PHYSICAL EXAMINATION FINDINGS ASSOCIATED WITH LIVER DISEASE

Depression	Hepatomegaly
Weight loss	Abdominal enlargement
Loss of muscle mass	Ascites
Icterus	Abdominal mass
Pale mucous membranes	Poor haircoat
Fever	Dermatopathies
Stupor	Petechiation
Blindness	Bruising
Gait abnormalities	Halitosis
Coma	Melena
Peripheral pitting edema	Excessive bleeding

However, neurotoxins other than ammonia are usually required for HE to develop. These other neurotoxins include inhibitory neurotransmitters (gamma-aminobutyric acid [GABA] and serotonin), mercaptans, and short-chain fatty acids (SCFAs) (Tyler, 1990b). Alterations in plasma amino acids may also worsen HE, because increases in aromatic amino acids and decreases in branched-chain amino acids promote the synthesis of inhibitory neurotransmitters in the CNS (Laflamme, 1988). Thus, hepatic failure leads to a multitude of biochemical derangements that contribute to HE.

HE is recognized clinically by the development of neurologic signs (Tyler, 1990a,b). Neurologic signs may be seen at any time, but are often more prominent after ingestion of a high-protein meal. Initial signs of HE include depression, lethargy, and mild behavior changes ranging from increased docility to aggression. Aimless pacing or circling, apparent blindness, and head pressing may ensue, followed by stupor, seizure activity, or coma. The diagnosis of HE is based on identification of liver disease, laboratory values supportive of hepatic failure, and response to treatment. Laboratory evaluation for HE should include hepatic function testing. Fasting ammonia and serum bile acid concentrations are usually markedly elevated in HE (Tyler, 1990a).

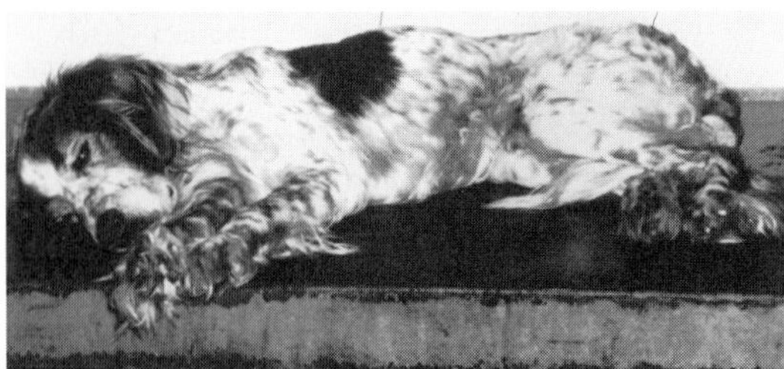

Figure 11–1. A 12-year-old English setter with coma secondary to hepatoencephalopathy.

TABLE 11–3. COMPLICATIONS ASSOCIATED WITH LIVER DISEASE

Hepatoencephalopathy
Ascites
Peripheral edema
Coagulopathies
Gastrointestinal ulceration
Infections
Endotoxemia

Treatment of HE is aimed at reducing the formation and absorption of toxic metabolites from the gastrointestinal (GI) tract—i.e., decreasing substrates for bacterial production of ammonia, mercaptans, SCFAs, and other substances and reducing GI bacterial flora (Table 11–4). In comatose or stuporous animals, evacuation of the colon with cleansing enemas, followed by a retention enema containing antimicrobials or lactulose, is recommended (Laflamme, 1988). If hypoglycemia is present, infusion of glucose-containing fluids should be instituted. Fluid therapy aimed at restoring normovolemia and correcting acid–base and electrolyte imbalances is integral to the emergency treatment of HE. Extended therapy includes dietary manipulation to reduce ingestion of protein and management of gastrointestinal flora to reduce bacterial synthesis of toxic metabolites. Diets should contain decreased quantities of a high-quality protein source that contains adequate amounts of branched-chain amino acids and arginine and decreased amounts of aromatic amino acids and methionine. In addition, diets should contain adequate calories, be easily digestible, and contain balanced amounts of vitamins and minerals. Although no commercially available diet is ideal, dietary formulations designed for renal failure are commonly employed (e.g., Prescription Diet Canine and Feline k/d, Hill's Pet Products). Home-made diets may also be used (Lewis et al, 1987). Commonly used oral antimicrobial agents include metronidazole and neomycin. Both antimicrobial agents have good activity against gram-negative organisms in the colon, which are the primary source of ammonia production. Lactulose is also used in the treatment of HE. Lactulose is degraded by colonic bacteria, resulting in acidification of the colon and osmotic diarrhea. Lactulose syrup can be administered orally in conscious animals or as a retention enema in severely ill animals.

Ascites and Edema. Liver disease frequently causes alterations in plasma proteins (hypoalbuminemia) and vascular hydrostatic pressures, resulting in ascites or edema. Diffuse liver disease

TABLE 11–4. THERAPEUTIC APPROACH TO HEPATOENCEPHALOPATHY

TREATMENT	DOSAGE	GOALS
Fluid therapy	To meet hydration needs	Maintain vascular volume Correct acid-base disturbances Correct electrolyte imbalances Correct hypoglycemia
Cleansing enemas	As needed	Remove ammonia from colon Decrease colonic bacteria
Therapeutic retention enemas	Lactulose, 300 g in 200 ml water Neomycin, 20 mg/kg in 200 ml water	
Dietary therapy	To meet energy needs (e.g., Prescription Diet Canine or Feline k/d, Hill's Pet Products)	Decrease protein Increase branched-chain amino acids Decrease aromatic amino acids Low sodium
Lactulose	1–2 ml per 5–10 kg q 8 hr	Alter gastrointestinal flora Alter colonic pH Osmotic laxative
Neomycin	20 mg/kg q 8 hr	Decrease gastrointestinal flora
Metronidazole	7.5 mg/kg q 8 hr	Decrease gastrointestinal flora

and fibrosis increase resistance to blood flow in the liver (portal hypertension), which can lead to acquired portosystemic shunts, increased lymph formation, increased plasma volume, and ascites/edema. Decreased return of blood volume to the systemic circulation also leads to retention of sodium and water. Decreased return of blood is perceived by the kidneys as hypovolemia, leading to activation of the renin-angiotensin-aldosterone system (RAAS). The RAAS induces vasoconstriction and increased aldosterone production, which increases plasma volume and promotes sodium and water retention, further aggravating portal hypertension. Liver-induced ascites can be diagnosed by physical examination and laboratory evaluation of peritoneal fluid, blood, and urine (Fig. 11–2). In liver disease ascitic fluid is usually a transudate or modified transudate, which is further substantiated by the presence of hypoalbuminemia. Edema may occur secondary to liver failure but is not as common as ascites. The same pathophysiologic mechanisms that trigger ascites may cause peripheral edema (i.e., distal legs, ventral abdomen and thorax, ventral neck region).

Treatment of ascites/edema is aimed at reducing sodium and water retention and managing portal hypertension and hypoalbuminemia (Fig. 11–3). Diuretics and a low-sodium diet are the mainstay of management of ascites/edema (Johnson, 1987a,b). Spironolactone, an aldosterone antagonist, is used to reduce ascites/edema without causing hypokalemia (Magne and Chiapella, 1986). A low-sodium diet (e.g., Prescription Diet Canine h/d or k/d, Hill's Pet Products) further reduces retention of sodium and water. If these measures are ineffective, furosemide may be substituted, although serum concentrations of electrolytes should be evaluated frequently.

Coagulopathy. Liver disease may interfere with production of coagulation factors, alter clearance of fibrin degradation products (FDPs), and impair platelet function (Table 11–5). Management of coagulopathy and bleeding is often required in severe liver disease, in which synthesis of some or all clotting factors may be impaired. Such impairment can be identified by coagulation parameters (e.g., prothrombin time, activated partial thromboplastin time, activated clotting time) or by identification of bleeding disorders (i.e., when coagulation factor activity decreases by 30 per cent of normal). Although decreased production of clotting factors may be relatively common, this abnormality alone is seldom sufficient to cause overt bleeding (Badylak, 1988). Because the liver is also a major site for degradation of FDPs, infectious organisms, and endotoxins, severe liver disease may also lead to disseminated intravascular coagulation (DIC) (Slappendel, 1989). Widespread thrombosis, fol-

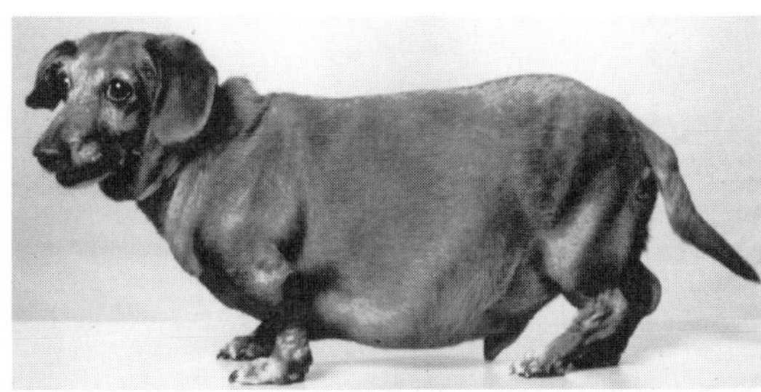

Figure 11–2. A 10-year-old dachshund with ascites secondary to liver disease.

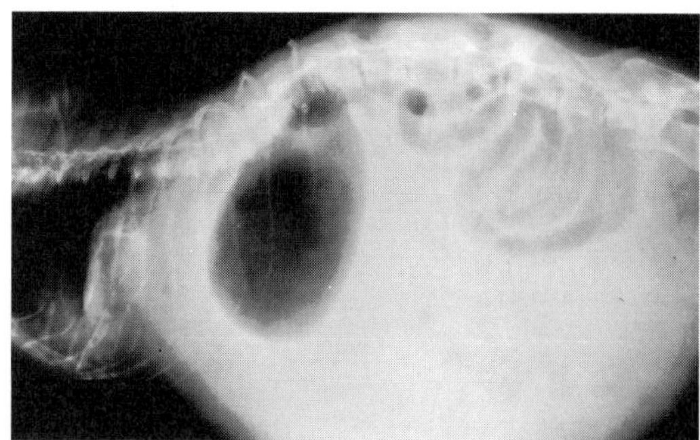

Figure 11–3. Lateral abdominal radiograph of a 14-year-old cat with severe ascites. Paracentesis for relief of respiratory compromise would be appropriate in this case.

lowed by bleeding, is commonly seen with DIC. Liver disease may also affect platelet number and function. Treatment of coagulopathies associated with liver disease is dependent on the underlying cause. It is difficult to promote production of coagulation factors in the severely diseased liver. If complete extrahepatic bile duct obstruction is suspected, administration of parenteral vitamin K_1 can be instituted (Center, 1986). Administration of fresh or fresh frozen plasma will temporarily correct coagulation factor deficiencies, but this therapy is feasible only for animals undergoing surgery or other procedures in which bleeding is likely. Therapy for DIC includes volume expansion with intravenous fluids, replacement of clotting factors with administration of fresh plasma, and inhibition of further thrombosis with heparin administration (Slappendel, 1989).

Gastrointestinal Bleeding and Ulceration. Gastrointestinal bleeding and ulceration often occur secondary to severe liver disease in older dogs and cats. Because the liver is responsible for the removal of gastrin and histamine from the circulation, severe liver disease may lead to increases in these substances, promoting gastric acid secretion and subsequent ulceration (Strombeck and Guilford, 1990). In addition, portal hypertension can decrease blood flow through the stomach, promoting ulcer formation. Treatment of gastrointestinal ulceration includes local protectants (sucralfate) and histamine receptor antagonists (e.g., ranitidine, famotidine) (Magne and Chiapella, 1986). Because cimetidine alters hepatic metabolism of drugs dependent on either hepatic blood flow or biotransformation, it should not be chosen as therapy for animals with liver disease (Center, 1986).

Infections and Endotoxemia. The normal liver serves as the clearinghouse for drugs, toxins, bacteria, and endotoxins absorbed via the GI tract. In severe liver disease, this function is impaired (Hardy, 1992). In chronic hepatic disease, acquired portosystemic shunts also allow portal blood to reach the systemic circulation, thus bypassing the liver altogether. This alteration in liver function may increase susceptibility to bacterial infections and endotoxemia. Parenteral administration of penicillins or cephalosporins in combination with an aminoglycoside has been advocated for the treatment or prophylaxis of sepsis and endotoxemia associated with severe liver disease (Magne and Chiapella, 1986). Antimicrobial agents to avoid include chlortetracycline, oxytetracycline, erythromycin, hetacillin, lincomycin, streptomycin, and sulfonamides, as these either are dependent on hepatic metabolism or may cause hepatotoxicity (Center, 1986).

Diagnostic Approach to Liver Disease

The diagnosis of liver disease is initiated by the veterinarian's suspicion that liver disease might

TABLE 11–5. CAUSES OF ABNORMAL BLEEDING PARAMETERS IN LIVER DISEASE

ABNORMAL BLEEDING PARAMETER	POSSIBLE CAUSE
Thrombocytopenia	Platelet sequestration in spleen Disseminated intravascular coagulopathy
Prolonged buccal mucosal bleeding time	Platelet function defect Von Willebrand's disease
Prolonged activated clotting time	Decreased production of clotting factors Disseminated intravascular coagulopathy
Prolonged activated partial thromboplastin time	Decreased production of clotting factors Disseminated intravascular coagulopathy
Prolonged prothrombin time	Decreased production of clotting factors Disseminated intravascular coagulopathy
Increased fibrin degradation products	Decreased hepatic clearance Disseminated intravascular coagulopathy
Decreased coagulation factor activities	Decreased production of clotting factors

TABLE 11–6. DIAGNOSTIC APPROACH TO LIVER DISEASE

DIAGNOSTIC PROCEDURE	GOALS
Complete blood cell count	Identify anemia Identify inflammation
Serum biochemistry panel	Identify hepatocellular damage Identify cholestasis Assess for severe liver dysfunction Rule out other organ system involvement
Urinalysis	Identify bilirubinuria or crystals Rule out renal disease Assess hydration status
Serum bile acids	Assess functional state of liver
Abdominal radiographs	Define liver size Evaluate other abdominal organs Identify some hepatic structural changes
Abdominal ultrasonography	Assess intrahepatic and biliary structure Evaluate relative density of liver parenchyma Identify shunts, nodules, other changes
Hepatic fine-needle aspiration cytology	Identify diffuse infiltrative hepatic diseases
Liver biopsy	Identify and classify hepatic disease Develop rational therapeutic plan Assess response to therapy

be present, followed by a case history and physical examination. The initial work-up for the older dog or cat with suspected liver disease should begin with a minimal data base (complete blood cell [CBC] count, serum chemistry profile, urinalysis). This may be followed by a liver function test, radiographic and/or ultrasonographic studies, hepatic fine-needle aspiration, and, ultimately, liver biopsy (Table 11–6). The CBC count is evaluated for anemia, thrombocytopenia, and other morphologic changes. The urinalysis is evaluated for evidence of dilute urine or bilirubinuria. Mild to moderate bilirubinuria is normal in healthy dogs, especially males; however, any degree of bilirubinuria in cats is abnormal and should be investigated (Meyer and Center, 1986). The serum chemistry profile identifies abnormalities in liver enzyme activities and, to a lesser extent, liver function (Table 11–7). Liver enzyme activities are used to classify changes as indicative of either hepatocellular damage or cholestasis. Serum alanine aminotransferase (ALT) and aspartate aminotransferase (AST) activities will increase in response to hepatocellular damage. Alkaline phosphatase (ALP) and gamma-glutamyl transferase (GGT) activities increase in cholesta-

TABLE 11–7. SERUM CHEMICAL ABNORMALITIES ASSOCIATED WITH LIVER DISEASE

ABNORMALITY	HEPATIC CAUSES	NONHEPATIC CAUSES
Hypoglycemia	Severe liver dysfunction Hepatic neoplasia	Septicemia Insulinoma Others
Hypoalbuminemia	Severe liver dysfunction	Renal loss Gastrointestinal loss Inflammatory losses Severe malnutrition
Low blood urea nitrogen	Decreased hepatic production	Anorexia Malnutrition Low protein diet
Increased ALT activity	Hepatocellular damage	Muscle degeneration (rare)
Increased AST activity	Hepatocellular damage	Muscle damage
Increased ALP activity	Cholestasis	Steroid induction (dogs) Growth
Increased GGT activity	Cholestasis	Steroid induction (dogs)
Increased total bilirubin concentration	Intrahepatic cholestasis Extrahepatic cholestasis	Hemolysis

ALP, Alkaline phosphatase; ALT, alanine aminotransferase; AST, aspartate aminotransferase; GGT, gamma-glutamyl transferase.

sis (Center et al, 1986). In cats, any increase in serum ALP is indicative of cholestasis. Hyperbilirubinemia may also occur with cholestasis secondary to extrahepatic bacterial infections (Taboada and Meyer, 1989).

Liver Function Tests. If liver disease is suspected on the basis of history, physical examination, and minimal data base, then assessment of liver function is recommended. Liver function tests are unnecessary in older dogs and cats with cholestasis and hyperbilirubinemia, as hyperbilirubinemia is indicative of impaired hepatic function (Meyer and Center, 1986). Evaluation of serum bile acids is the most widely recommended and practical method of assessing liver function in older dogs and cats. After a 12-hour fast, 1 ml of serum is obtained, and the animal is fed several tablespoons of a high-protein diet (e.g., Prescription Diet Canine p/d, Hill's Pet Products); a second 1-ml serum sample is collected 2 hours after feeding. Serum is analyzed for total bile acid concentration by either radioimmunoassay or spectrophotometry (Bunch et al, 1984). Fasting and postprandial bile acid concentrations will be increased with primary or cholestatic liver disease (Center et al, 1991).

Diagnostic Imaging Studies. Abdominal radiographs occasionally are helpful in diagnosing liver disease. Liver size can be assessed subjectively by evaluating the position of the caudal portion of the liver and gastric gas shadow. Abdominal radiographs may also be used to identify cholelithiasis (Meyer and Center, 1986). Radiographic contrast studies can be used to identify disorders of the hepatic vasculature or biliary system. Mesenteric or splenic portography is usually performed in animals suspected of having a congenital portosystemic shunt and therefore is rarely performed in older animals. Hepatic ultrasonography is very useful in identifying dilated bile ducts, enlargement of the gallbladder, differences in echogenicity within the hepatic parenchyma that would suggest diffuse infiltrative diseases (e.g., hepatic lipidosis or cirrhosis), or nodular changes (e.g., primary or metastatic neoplasia) (Biller et al, 1992).

Hepatic Cytology. Fine-needle aspiration of the liver is a relatively safe and accurate method of obtaining cells from the liver for diagnosis of hepatic disease. Liver aspirates may be obtained from a conscious dog or cat placed in either dorsal or right lateral recumbency (Fig. 11–4). The abdomen is clipped and scrubbed, and a 1.5-inch, 22-gauge needle is advanced into the liver parenchyma. Gentle aspiration with a 12-ml syringe

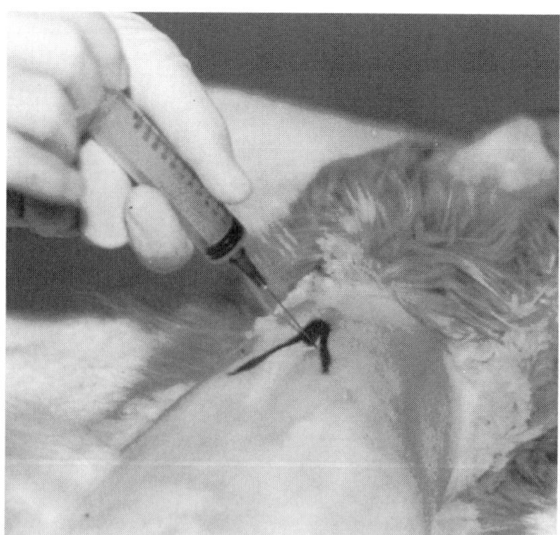

Figure 11–4. Hepatic fine-needle aspiration in a cat. The needle enters the liver from the left side, between the xiphoid process and the costal arch (as marked on the cat).

will usually yield adequate numbers of cells for cytologic interpretation. Smears of the sample are made, and the slide is stained with Wright-Giemsa or Diff-Quick stain (Fig. 11–5). Fine-needle aspiration cytology of the liver is most useful for diffuse, infiltrative diseases such as hepatic lipidosis and lymphosarcoma. Other abnormalities detected include retention of bile pigment, steroid hepatopathy, and other neoplasms affecting the liver. Although easy to perform, cytology cannot totally replace hepatic biopsy in the diagnosis of some liver diseases.

Hepatic Biopsy. Liver biopsy is the single most important diagnostic test for liver disease. Although laboratory and diagnostic imaging studies can confirm the presence of hepatic disease, a biopsy is required for definitive differentiation of types of liver disease. Evaluation before liver biopsy should include determination of coagulation parameters and, if needed, suitability for anesthesia. Liver biopsy may be performed in many ways: percutaneous biopsy via a transabdominal or transthoracic approach; ultrasonography-guided transabdominal percutaneous liver biopsy; or keyhole, laparoscopic, and modified laparoscopic (using a sterile otoscope) techniques (Strombeck and Guilford, 1990). Laparotomy and surgical biopsy can also be performed, with the advantage of being able to visualize the entire liver and extrahepatic biliary system (Bunch et al, 1985). Histologic evaluation of any liver biopsy specimen should be performed by a veterinary pathologist well versed in hepatic diseases.

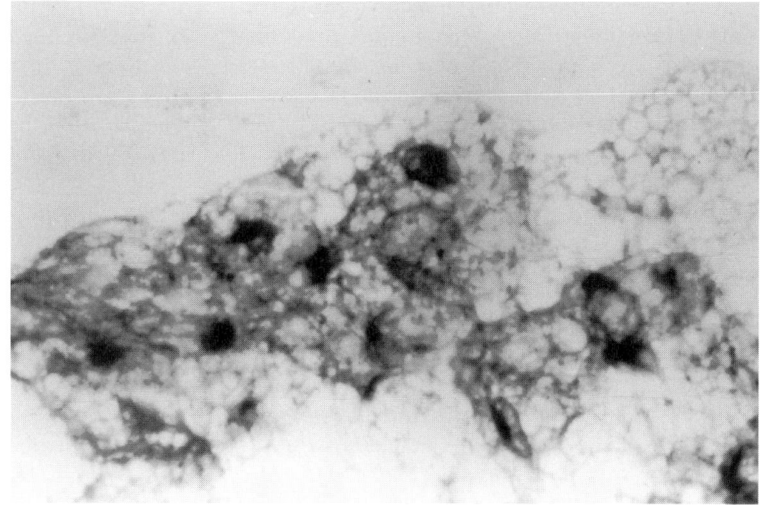

Figure 11–5. Cytologic specimen of a hepatic fine-needle aspirate from a cat with idiopathic hepatic lipidosis syndrome. Note the widespread vacuolization in all hepatocytes. (Wright-Giemsa stain; × 1000).

HEPATOBILIARY DISEASES OF THE DOG

Chronic Inflammatory Hepatopathies

Chronic hepatitis can be caused by infections, drugs, or retention of copper, or it can occur as an idiopathic process. The pathologic process involved in chronic hepatitis often begins with necrosis, followed by infiltration of the liver with lymphocytes or macrophages, which may lead to hepatic fibrosis and cirrhosis. When chronic changes of fibrosis and infiltration of inflammatory cells are accompanied by more acute changes of necrosis, the term *chronic active hepatitis* is often used. Both acute and chronic hepatitis can be caused by viral and bacterial infection. Viral diseases such as infectious canine hepatitis and the probable viral agent of canine acidophil hepatitis can lead to chronic hepatitis (Strombeck and Guilford, 1990). Canine leptospirosis can cause both acute and chronic hepatitis in dogs (Baldwin and Atkins, 1987). Although these diseases tend to cause hepatic necrosis in their early stages, they may result in the same type of chronic injury seen with other chronic hepatopathies.

Drugs can induce chronic hepatitis. Although almost any drug has the capacity to produce an idiosyncratic reaction in any given individual, some drugs are more likely than others to be associated with chronic hepatic inflammation. For example, the anticonvulsants primidone and phenobarbital are associated with chronic hepatic disease in dogs (Dayrell-Hart et al, 1991). Administration of diethylcarbamazine-oxibendazole has also been associated with periportal hepatitis and hepatic vacuolar change (Hardy et al, 1989). It is interesting to note that adverse drug reactions occur more frequently in elderly people than in younger people (Kitani, 1986), and this may also apply to older dogs and cats.

Abnormal hepatic retention of dietary copper and copper hepatopathy are known to occur with a genetic predisposition in Bedlington terriers, and a breed-related increased incidence is seen in West Highland white terriers and Doberman pinschers (Johnson et al, 1980; Thornburg et al, 1984, 1990). In Bedlington terriers the disease is caused by a defect in biliary excretion of copper (Owen and McCall, 1983; Hultgren et al, 1986). Doberman pinschers can exhibit a form of chronic active hepatitis that is currently believed to occur secondary to copper accumulation in hepatocytes (Franklin and Saunders, 1988; van den Ingh et al, 1988). As copper accumulates in hepatocytes, necrosis, inflammation, and fibrosis occur, leading to eventual liver failure. Copper retention in hepatocytes occurs in many cholestatic liver diseases, regardless of cause; therefore, it is often difficult to differentiate primary or secondary copper retention when liver disease is advanced (Thornburg et al, 1986). Primary copper hepatopathy as the inciting cause of liver disease should be considered in those breeds known to have an increased incidence of copper retention. The diagnosis is confirmed by liver biopsy revealing copper-containing granules in excess of what might be considered normal for the degree of cholestasis and fibrosis seen (Thornburg et al, 1984).

Although chronic hepatitis can occur secondary to infections, drugs, or copper accumulation, many cases of chronic hepatitis are idiopathic. It is theorized that idiopathic hepatitis is immune mediated. Dogs with chronic hepatitis of any cause usually have a slowly progressive onset of disease characterized by depression, weight loss, anorexia, and polyuria/polydipsia. Most dogs are not examined until the hepatic disease is advanced. There are no pathognomonic physical examination signs of chronic hepatitis in dogs. Laboratory evaluation of dogs with chronic hepatitis can vary depending on the stage of illness. Initially, affected dogs will have marked increases in ALT and AST activities, with little evidence of cholestasis or liver function changes. As the disease progresses, cholestasis develops, with resultant increases in ALP activity and bilirubin concentration. Liver function progressively decreases, first seen in serum bile acid concentrations and later obvious in albumin, urea nitrogen, glucose, and coagulation factor concentrations. Studies using radioactive copper can also be performed to assess copper uptake in the gut. Measurement of radioactive copper in the feces after intravenous radiolabeled copper can identify affected dogs (Brewer et al, 1992b). Liver biopsy is the only method available for the diagnosis of chronic hepatitis. The histopathologic findings required for a diagnosis of chronic active hepatitis include piecemeal necrosis, bridging necrosis (i.e., the presence of inflammatory cells bridging the limiting plate between lobules), and active cirrhosis (Hardy, 1986). Specimens should also be stained to detect copper, although the presence of excess copper in a liver with severe cholestasis and cirrhosis could be secondary, not primary, copper hepatopathy. Collagen and other stains may also be useful in determining the extent of disease in chronic active hepatitis. If enough liver tissue is obtained, then copper concentrations within the liver should be determined.

Therapy for chronic hepatitis is aimed at the primary inciting event. For example, withdrawal of possible hepatotoxic drugs to correct the liver dysfunction or antimicrobial agents for bacterial infections. In addition, supportive therapies for complications associated with hepatic disease are employed. Some of the drugs used in the treatment of chronic hepatitis are presented in Table 11–8. Therapy for copper-associated hepatopathy includes reduction in dietary copper and chelation therapy. Currently drugs used for copper chelation are D-penicillamine and tetramine chelators (Allen et al, 1987). D-Penicillamine is effective at reducing hepatic copper concentrations, although the rate of hepatic "decoppering" is slow (Brewer et al, 1992a). Trientine is as effective as D-penicillamine at reducing hepatic copper concentrations and is currently being investigated in dogs (Allen et al, 1987; Twedt et al, 1988). It is likely that Bedlington terriers, West Highland white terriers, and possibly Doberman pinschers will benefit from copper chelation or oral zinc therapy as part of their therapeutic plan.

Other therapies that can be considered in dogs with idiopathic chronic active hepatitis include corticosteroids and antifibrotic drugs. In a retrospective study of 151 dogs with chronic hepatitis, dogs in which corticosteroids were used at recommended doses had increased survival times compared with untreated dogs (Strombeck et al, 1988). Corticosteroids have immunosuppressive, anti-inflammatory, and antifibrotic effects at the dosage used. It is imperative that infectious causes of hepatitis be ruled out (based on hepatic biopsy) before corticosteroid therapy is instituted (Magne and Chiapella, 1986). Other antifibrotic agents such as colchicine can be used to prevent or treat hepatic fibrosis and cirrhosis. Use of antifibrotic agents is discussed with other aspects of hepatic cirrhosis.

Hepatic Fibrosis and Cirrhosis

The liver can respond to severe damage and necrosis by either regeneration or fibrosis, de-

TABLE 11–8. DRUGS USED IN THE MANAGEMENT OF CHRONIC HEPATITIS IN OLDER DOGS

DRUG	DOSAGE	INDICATIONS
D-Penicillamine	10–15 mg/kg q 12 hr	Copper chelation Antifibrotic
Trientine	15–30 mg/kg q 12 hr	Copper chelation
Zinc acetate	25–50 mg elemental zinc q 12 hr	Decrease copper absorption
Prednisone	0.5–2.0 mg/kg q 24–48 hr	Immunosuppressive Anti-inflammatory Antifibrotic
Azathioprine	1.0 mg/kg q 24–48 hr	Immunosuppressive

pending on the severity of the challenge and the degree of damage to the supporting connective tissue structure. Loss of hepatocytes and connective tissue integrity caused by any disease can lead to hepatic fibrosis; thus, identification of hepatic fibrosis is not pathognomonic for any particular liver disease. When hepatic fibrosis is severe and leads to formation of small or large regenerative nodules limited by fibrous tissue, the term *cirrhosis* is used (Fig. 11–6). Hepatic cirrhosis is most often considered an end-stage lesion, responding to whatever the inciting disease process. Because this condition is advanced, most affected dogs have other clinical and laboratory evidence of impaired hepatic function. As cirrhosis progresses, portal hypertension develops, and many dogs with cirrhosis have ascites and acquired portosystemic shunts (Johnson, 1987a). Most chronic hepatopathies will progress slowly, and fibrosis occurs in concert with the progression of necrosis and inflammation. Radiographic evaluation may reveal a small liver, and ultrasonography shows an increase in hepatic echogenicity and possibly the presence of acquired portosystemic shunts. Liver biopsy is required for the diagnosis of hepatic fibrosis and cirrhosis (Strombeck and Guilford, 1990).

Treatment of hepatic fibrosis is aimed at the underlying disease process and managing the complications of liver failure. Inhibition of collagen formation and lysis of excess hepatic fibrous tissue are additional goals of therapy for hepatic cirrhosis. Several drugs are currently used for this purpose, with limited information available in dogs. Colchicine is an antimitotic drug that inhibits the microtubular apparatus and the transcellular movement of collagen (Magne and Chiapella, 1986). When used for treatment of hepatic fibrosis in affected dogs, it has produced improvement in clinical signs for several months (Boer et al, 1984). However, colchicine has been used in a limited number of dogs. Other drugs being studied for the treatment of hepatic fibrosis include D-penicillamine, which inhibits collagen polymerization secondary to its copper-chelating effects, and oral zinc, which inhibits copper absorption in the intestine (Chvapil, 1976).

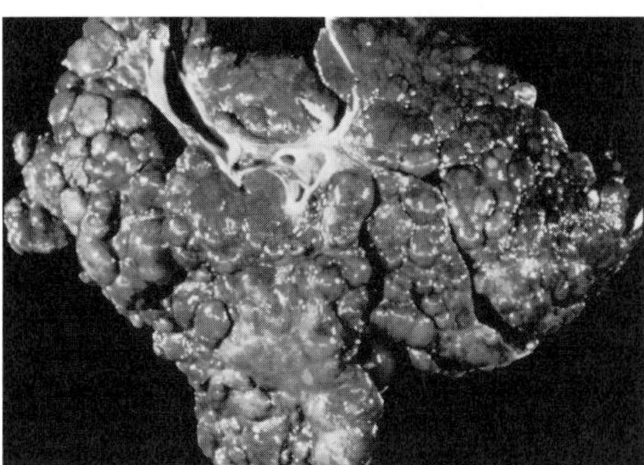

Figure 11–6. Severe hepatic cirrhosis in a dog.

Chronic Infiltrative Hepatopathies

Alterations in hepatic structure and function can occur when hepatocytes are infiltrated with fat, glycogen, amyloid, or other substances. Although hepatic lipidosis is a common morphologic finding in dogs with diabetes mellitus, it seldom becomes a clinical problem associated with liver dysfunction. Other, less common infiltrative disorders include amyloid deposition and hemochromatosis (Strombeck and Guilford, 1990). Exogenous glucocorticoids and spontaneous hyperadrenocorticism often lead to steroid hepatopathy in older dogs. Impairment of liver function can occur with severe steroid hepatopathy, but most dogs do not develop signs referable to hepatic dysfunction (Rogers and Ruebner, 1977).

Laboratory evaluation of dogs with steroid hepatopathy will usually reveal a marked increase in ALP and GGT activity, occasionally up to a 60-fold increase over normal values (Badylak and Van Vleet, 1981). Values for hepatocellular enzyme activities (ALT and AST) will usually be elevated, but not to the magnitude of ALP and GGT. Serum bilirubin concentrations are usually normal, which supports the idea that ALP activity increase is secondary to steroid induction, not cholestasis. Liver function tests, if performed, may demonstrate mild increases in fasting and postprandial serum bile acid concentration (Strombeck and Guilford, 1990). Liver biopsy is seldom performed, but expected changes of increased hepatic vacuolization are seen on histopathologic evaluation.

Vascular Diseases of the Liver

The most common vascular disease of the liver in older dogs is acquired portosystemic shunts. However, congenital portosystemic shunts have been initially diagnosed in dogs as old as 10 years (Johnson et al, 1989). Acquired portosystemic shunting occurs secondary to portal hypertension (Fig. 11–7). As portal pressures increase, small vessels routing the portal circulation to the sys-

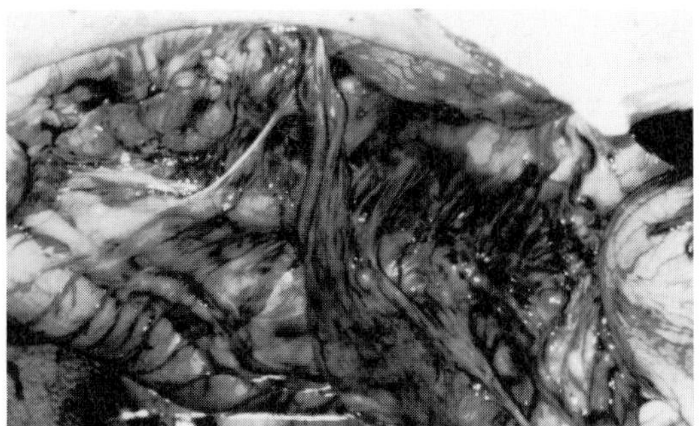

Figure 11–7. Multiple acquired portosystemic shunts in a dog. This dog had chronic active hepatitis and severe portal hypertension.

temic circulation increase in size and volume capacity, thus providing a "pop-off valve" for the increased portal pressures. Cocker spaniels are known to have veno-occlusive disease in the liver that leads to portal hypertension and acquired portosystemic shunts at a young age (Rand et al, 1988). However, most cases of acquired portosystemic shunting occur in older animals with advanced liver disease, hepatic fibrosis or cirrhosis, and portal hypertension. Specific diagnosis of acquired portosystemic shunts requires mesenteric venography revealing several small, tortuous anomalous vessels from the portal vein to a systemic vein, with minimal hepatic uptake of contrast dye. If surgical exploration is performed, these shunts may be visualized on the dorsal side of the liver.

Treatment of acquired portosystemic shunts is aimed primarily at the associated hepatoencephalopathy. Although surgical attenuation of congenital portosystemic shunts can be highly successful, attenuation of acquired portosystemic shunts is contraindicated, because this would result in extremely elevated portal pressures, shock, and death. Banding of the caudal vena cava has been used with some success to treat dogs with multiple portosystemic shunts (Strombeck and Guilford, 1990). However, this procedure will work only in dogs without significant liver disease or portal hypertension; therefore, the use of this surgical procedure is limited to multiple shunts that are likely congenital in nature (Strombeck and Guilford, 1990).

Other vascular disorders of the liver include arteriovenous (AV) fistulas and portal vein thrombosis. In dogs AV fistulas may be congenital or acquired; acquired AV fistulas are usually the result of trauma (Hosgood, 1989). The clinical signs associated with hepatic AV fistulas in dogs include ascites and hepatoencephalopathy. Diagnosis is based on radiographic dye studies, and surgical resection of the affected liver lobe usually results in resolution of clinical signs. Portal vein thrombosis resulting in altered laboratory parameters indicative of cholestasis, hepatocellular damage, and impaired liver function has also been reported in dogs (Willard et al, 1989). Thrombosis was diagnosed based on mesenteric venography, and no treatment was attempted (Willard et al, 1989).

Hepatobiliary Neoplasia

In older dogs the most common primary neoplasm of the liver is hepatocellular carcinoma, followed by hepatocellular adenoma, bile duct adenoma and carcinoma, and hepatic carcinoids (Magne, 1984). Many types of carcinomas, adenocarcinomas, and sarcomas can metastasize to the liver (Fig. 11–8). Hepatocellular carcinomas can occur as a large mass arising from a single liver lobe; multiple neoplastic nodules (resembling metastatic disease); or diffuse, infiltrative disease. This tumor metastasizes rapidly to regional lymph nodes, lung, peritoneum, and other abdominal organs. The historical and physical examination findings of hepatocellular carcinoma are often nonspecific; hepatomegaly or an abdominal mass may be detected. Laboratory eval-

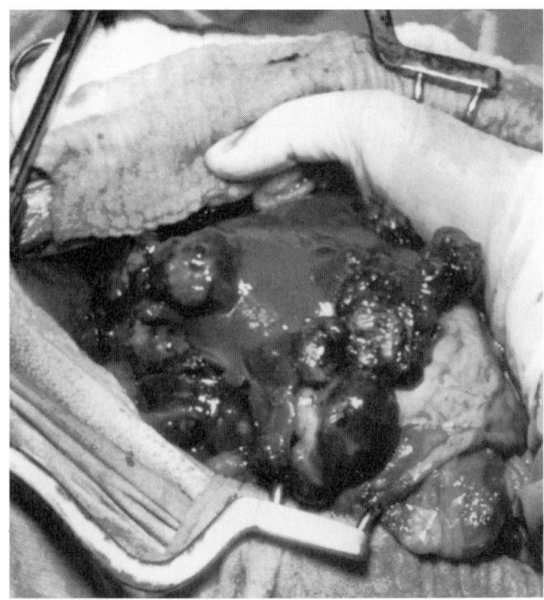

Figure 11–8. Surgical exploration of an 11-year-old Siberian husky with metastatic neoplasia in the liver. Multiple nodules are seen over the liver surface. Histopathologic evaluation identified the metastases as hemangiosarcoma.

uation usually shows mild to moderate increases in liver enzyme activities, with some dogs displaying abnormal liver function based on serum bile acid evaluation (Magne, 1984). Hypoglycemia occurs in some dogs with hepatocellular carcinoma and other hepatic neoplasms. A laboratory test that shows promise in the diagnosis of hepatic tumors (primarily hepatocellular carcinoma) is evaluation of serum alpha-fetoprotein concentrations. Alpha-fetoprotein levels are normally high before birth but decrease to minimal concentrations shortly after birth. Humans and dogs with hepatocellular carcinoma have increased concentrations of serum alpha-fetoprotein, presumably because the neoplastic hepatic tissue synthesizes detectable quantities of this protein (Lowseth et al, 1991).

Abdominal radiographs and ultrasonography are useful in the identification of hepatomegaly and abnormal hepatic echogenicity associated with neoplasia. Diagnosis of hepatocellular carcinoma requires a liver biopsy. Treatment of hepatocellular carcinoma is primarily surgical. Massive and nodular forms of hepatocellular carcinoma are often amenable to surgical resection of the affected lobe or lobes, with the average survival time being 308 days (Kosovsky et al, 1989). If metastasis has occurred, then surgery will not be helpful. Chemotherapy for hepatocellular carcinoma has not been well studied, but survival times in both humans and dogs are poor (Magne, 1984).

Diseases of the Gallbladder

Diseases of the gallbladder (i.e., cholecystitis, cholelithiasis) are uncommon in older dogs. Cholecystitis often leads to vague signs of vomiting, fever, and abdominal pain, thus making the diagnosis more difficult (Church and Matthiesen, 1988). The usual cause of cholecystitis is thought to be bacterial (i.e., ascending bacteria from the gastrointestinal tract or hematogenous bacteria) or chemical (i.e., activation of refluxed pancreatic enzymes) (Strombeck and Guilford, 1990). When cholecystitis becomes severe, necrosis and gallbladder rupture, with subsequent peritonitis, may occur (Church and Matthiesen, 1988). Cholecystitis is diagnosed on the basis of patient history, physical examination, laboratory and diagnostic imaging studies, and surgical exploration. Abdominal ultrasonography may identify increased gallbladder wall thickness; dilated, tortuous bile ducts; and concurrent cholelithiasis. Antimicrobial therapy, based on bacterial culture and sensitivity test results, is the optimal treatment of cholecystitis. Severe cases of cholecystitis (e.g., emphysematous or necrotic cholecystitis) may be treated surgically with cholecystectomy (Church and Matthiesen, 1988).

Choleliths are also uncommon in older dogs. Choleliths are usually composed of cholesterol, bile acids, pigments, calcium, and protein (Strombeck and Guilford, 1990); diet and cholecystitis are predisposing causes. The clinical signs and diagnostic approach to cholelithiasis are similar to those for cholecystitis. Treatment of cholelithiasis may be surgical or medical. Cholecystectomy can be performed and will prevent recurrence. Medical therapy includes antimicrobial agents for concurrent cholecystitis and medical alteration of bile acids such that cholesterol solubility increases. Agents such as chenodeoxycholic acid and ursodeoxycholic acid have been used for the medical dissolution of choleliths in humans, but little experience is available on the use of these drugs in older dogs.

HEPATOBILIARY DISEASES OF THE CAT

Cholangiohepatitis Complex

Cholangiohepatitis is an inflammatory disease of the liver and biliary system. Primary forms of cholangiohepatitis recognized in older cats include suppurative (neutrophilic infiltration) and chronic lymphocytic (infiltration of the liver and biliary system with lymphocytes and plasma cells) cholangiohepatitis. Bacterial infection with either aerobic or anaerobic enteric bacteria is suspected as the cause of suppurative cholangiohepatitis (Hirsch and Doige, 1983). Cats with suppurative cholangiohepatitis usually have an acute onset of anorexia, fever, vomiting, and overt icterus (Hirsch and Doige, 1983). Antimicrobial agents are the mainstay of medical therapy for suppurative cholangiohepatitis (Table 11–9). Ideally, the choice of antimicrobial agent is based on the results of bacterial identification and sensitivity testing; however, this is usually not possible, as most cats do not undergo exploratory laparotomy or liver biopsy. To obtain good therapeutic levels at the site of infection, it is important to select an antimicrobial agent that is excreted in bile. Because coliforms are suspected as the primary pathogens, antimicrobial choices include ampicillin, chloramphenicol, and metronidazole (Zawie and Shaker, 1989). The prognosis for suppurative cholangiohepatitis is usually good, and most cats

TABLE 11–9. DRUGS USED IN THE MANAGEMENT OF CHOLANGIOHEPATITIS IN OLDER CATS

DRUG	DOSAGE	INDICATIONS
Ampicillin	20 mg/kg q 6–8 hr	Suppurative cholangiohepatitis
Chloramphenicol	50 mg/kg q 12 hr	Suppurative cholangiohepatitis
Metronidazole	7.5 mg/kg q 8 hr	Suppurative cholangiohepatitis
Prednisone	2–4 mg/kg q 24–48 hr	Lymphocytic cholangiohepatitis

respond quickly to antimicrobial therapy and supportive care.

Lymphocytic cholangiohepatitis is a chronic form of progressive liver disease in cats. The clinical presentation of cats with lymphocytic cholangiohepatitis differs somewhat from the suppurative form. Cats with lymphocytic cholangiohepatitis tend to be younger, with ages ranging from 3 to 10 years (Lucke and Davies, 1984). The onset of disease is usually more insidious, with the primary complaints being weight loss, anorexia, ascites, and icterus (Lucke and Davies, 1984). Icterus is often present on physical examination, but usually there are few other signs referable to liver disease. Laboratory evaluation is indicative of cholestasis. The diagnosis of lymphocytic cholangiohepatitis is based on histopathologic evaluation of a liver biopsy. Lesions vary from mild to severe, with all cats having a primarily nonsuppurative inflammation surrounding the intrahepatic and extrahepatic bile duct (Lucke and Davies, 1984). Other findings may include a scattering of polymorphonuclear cells, hepatic fibrosis, sclerosis of the biliary system, and duplication or hypertrophy of the intrahepatic bile ducts (Lucke and Davies, 1984). The treatment of lymphocytic cholangiohepatitis is unclear. Because the disease is characterized by infiltration of the biliary system and hepatic parenchyma with lymphocytes and plasma cells, an immunologic mechanism is suspected as the cause of the disease, and immunosuppressive therapy is used (Lucke and Davies, 1984). Corticosteroids, used at immunosuppressive doses, are the mainstay of treatment of lymphocytic cholangiohepatitis (see Table 11–9). The prognosis for cats with lymphocytic cholangiohepatitis varies. Cats may live for months to years, occasionally experiencing bouts of clinical disease alternating with periods of remission. A factor that may influence the prognosis for cats with lymphocytic cholangiohepatitis is the presence of concurrent diseases. Lymphocytic cholangiohepatitis has been associated with concurrent diseases of the pancreas, intestinal tract, and kidneys. As could be expected, cats with concurrent involvement of other organs do not have as favorable a prognosis as those that only have involvement of the liver and biliary tree.

Pyogranulomatous Hepatitis (Feline Infectious Peritonitis)

Feline infectious peritonitis virus (FIPV) can induce a multisystemic disease process that may affect the liver by inducing a pyogranulomatous hepatitis. Both effusive and noneffusive forms of FIP may affect the liver (Fig. 11–9). Common clinical signs seen with pyogranulomatous hepatitis are anorexia, weight loss, fever, depression, icterus, and abdominal distention secondary to fluid accumulation. Laboratory evaluation of cats with FIPV-induced liver disease may reveal leukocytosis, anemia, and hyperglobulinemia. In addition, increased serum activities of ALT, AST, and ALP and increased bilirubin concentrations may be present. There is no pathognomonic pattern of biochemical changes indicative of FIPV-induced liver disease. Ultrasonography may confirm the effusion, outline evidence of mild gallbladder enlargement, and define nodular involvement of the liver secondary to the pyogranulomatous inflammation. Alternatively, fine-

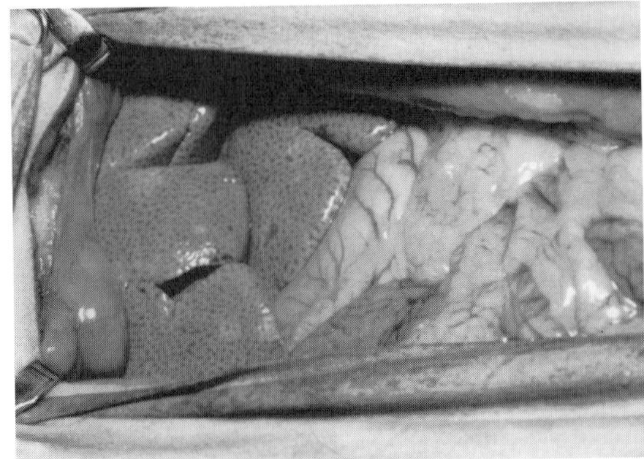

Figure 11–9. Hepatic disease associated with feline infectious peritonitis in a 13-year-old cat. Note the lighter colored granulomas in the liver.

needle aspiration cytology of the liver may reveal pyogranulomatous inflammation. Liver biopsy is the most reliable method to confirm FIP of the liver. There is no specific treatment for FIPV-induced liver disease in cats. Supportive measures, as previously outlined, can be used along with good nutrition and nursing care. Immunosuppressive therapy has been used to reduce the intense inflammatory response to FIPV, but the response rate is low.

Idiopathic Hepatic Lipidosis

Idiopathic hepatic lipidosis (IHL) is characterized by progressive infiltration of hepatocytes with fat and concomitant hepatic dysfunction (Fig. 11–10). The usual clinical findings include a period of anorexia in a previously obese cat, obvious weight loss, muscle wasting, icterus, and vomiting (Thornburg, 1982) (Fig. 11–11). Icterus is usually seen in the later stages of disease, and some cats have palpable hepatomegaly. Laboratory evaluation will show evidence of cholestatic liver disease, and serum ALP activity will increase before serum bilirubin concentrations begin to rise. Ultrasonography shows a fine, diffuse increase in echogenicity (Biller et al, 1992). Cytologic evaluation of fine-needle aspirates shows hepatocytes with marked vacuolar change (Meyer and French, 1989). Histologic evaluation of a liver biopsy specimen will demonstrate marked macro- or microvesicular vacuolar change in most hepatocytes, with evidence of bile stasis. Oil-red-O staining confirms the content of the vacuoles as lipid (Center, 1986). Because the metabolic cause of IHL is not known, treatment is empirical and is aimed at restoring nutritional status. Enteral nutritional support by nasoesophageal, pharyngostomy, or gastrostomy tube feeding is advocated (Biourge et al, 1990) (Fig. 11–12).

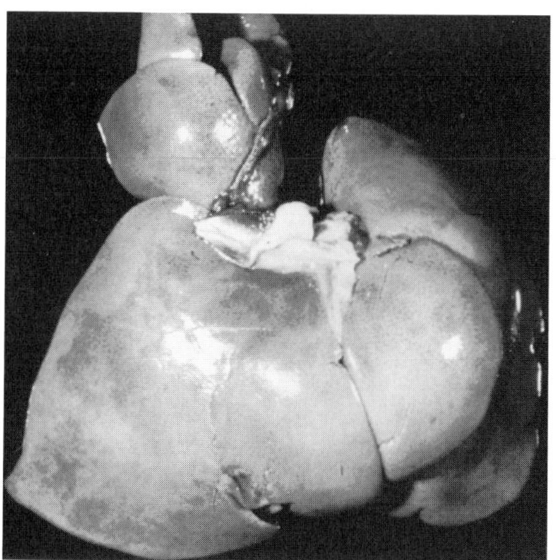

Figure 11–10. Liver from a cat with idiopathic hepatic lipidosis. Note the abnormally light color and the large size.

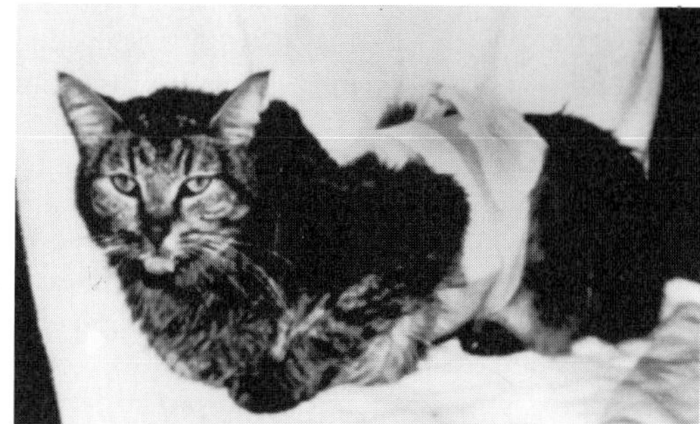

Figure 11–11. A 10-year-old cat with severe idiopathic hepatic lipidosis syndrome. Note the emaciation, unkempt appearance, and ptyalism. A tube gastrostomy has just been placed.

Hepatobiliary Neoplasia

Primary neoplasia of the liver and biliary system is rare in older cats. In a series of 21 cats with nonhematopoietic tumors of the liver, 9 cats had bile duct adenoma, 6 cats had bile duct adenocarcinoma, 2 cats had hepatocellular carcinoma, 1 cat had a neuroendocrine carcinoma, and 3 cats had hemangiosarcoma (Post and Patnaik, 1992). Metastatic neoplasia, primarily lymphosarcoma, is more common in cats than primary hepatic neoplasia (Center, 1986). Other metastatic neoplasias seen in cats include myeloproliferative diseases and mast cell tumors (Center, 1986). Clinical signs may include anorexia,

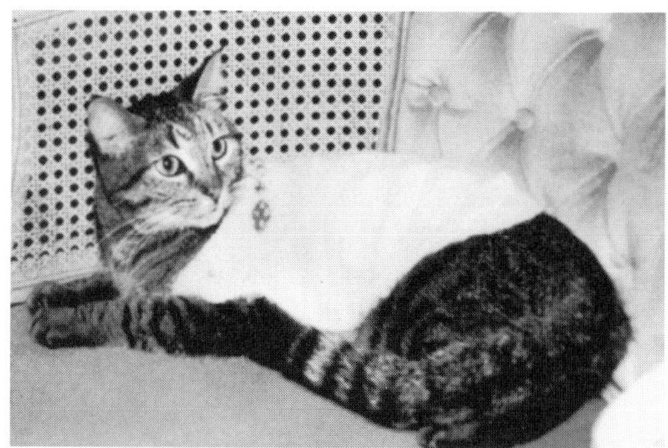

Figure 11–12. Same cat as in Figure 11–11, 6 weeks after initiation of tube feeding. The tube is still in place and was removed 2 weeks after the photograph was made.

lethargy, hepatomegaly, and icterus (Post and Patnaik, 1992). If biliary obstruction is complete, clinical signs of extrahepatic bile duct obstruction will also be observed. Diagnosis is made by a combination of laboratory findings, radiographic and ultrasonographic evaluation, cytologic evaluation, and biopsy. Fine-needle aspiration and cytologic evaluation can be particularly helpful with diffuse metastatic neoplasia such as lymphosarcoma, mastocytosis, or myeloproliferative disorders (Meyer and French, 1989). Treatment of primary hepatobiliary neoplasia is primarily surgical; however, too few cases have been evaluated to identify an optimal treatment or prognosis. Treatment of metastatic neoplasia is aimed at the primary tumor.

Diseases of the Gallbladder

Extrahepatic bile duct obstruction can occur in older cats, usually secondary to cholelithiasis, inspissated bile, or parasitic infection. Choleliths reported in cats contain cholesterol, bilirubin derivatives, and calcium (Neer, 1992). Occasionally, bile sludging secondary to increased mucosal uptake of bile fluid can result in overt inspissation of bile with biliary obstruction. Both conditions result in anorexia, vomiting, fever, icterus, and acholic (depigmented) stools in severely affected cats (Zawie and Shaker, 1989). Cats of any age may be affected with parasitic infection of the biliary tree with flukes. The most common fluke infections are with *Platynosomum* spp., found primarily in Florida and Hawaii (Zawie and Shaker, 1989; Neer, 1992). Clinical signs of fluke infestation are similar to those of other causes of extrahepatic biliary obstruction. Diagnosis of flukes is made by routine fecal sedimentation or use of formalin-ether sedimentation techniques to identify ova (Neer, 1992). Occasionally ova may be detected in abdominal fluid or liver cysts (Thornbrugh et al, 1990). Optimal treatment of liver flukes is not known, although praziquantel (20 to 30 mg/kg in a single dose or daily for 3 days) and nitroscanate are currently recommended (Neer, 1992). Cats with severe liver disease secondary to biliary tract obstruction may have a guarded prognosis.

THE EXOCRINE PANCREAS

Normal Aging Changes

In older dogs and cats, it is likely that pancreatic structure and function do not significantly change with age. However, the pancreas may be less likely to withstand stresses such as drastic diet changes, systemic illness, or pancreatitis. Thus, the older dog or cat may develop exocrine pancreatic insufficiency secondary to severe stress and demands on pancreatic function.

The Dog

Exocrine Pancreatic Diseases

Pancreatitis. Pancreatitis is caused by the activation of pancreatic digestion enzymes within the pancreas itself, resulting in severe inflammation, necrosis, and metabolic abnormalities. Acute pancreatitis may occur in a milder edematous form or a severe hemorrhagic form (Schaer, 1991). Repeated bouts of pancreatitis often lead to chronic pancreatitis, with fibrosis and subsequent exocrine pancreatic insufficiency and/or diabetes mellitus (Matthiesen and Rosin, 1986). Affected dogs usually present with sudden onset of vomiting, anorexia, and depression. Physical examination may reveal abdominal pain and fever. Chronic pancreatitis occurs in dogs that are predisposed to repeated bouts of acute pancreatitis, such as dogs receiving long-term immunosuppressive therapy or a high-fat diet or dogs with persistent hyperlipemia. Exacerbations of chronic pancreatitis resemble acute pancreatitis. Some dogs with chronic pancreatitis may be asymptomatic, with clinical signs developing only as severe pancreatic fibrosis ensues.

Diagnosis of pancreatitis includes evaluation of laboratory values and diagnostic imaging of the cranial abdomen. The most common laboratory findings include neutrophilia, azotemia, and increased activities of ALT, AST, and ALP (Schaer, 1979). The most specific tests available for the diagnosis of pancreatitis in dogs are serum amylase and lipase activity tests. Serum trypsin-like immunoreactivity increases with acute pancreatitis in some dogs, but this test lacks the degree of sensitivity needed for a reliable test (Strombeck and Guilford, 1990). Abdominal radiographs may show loss of abdominal detail, lateral displacement of the duodenum, and abdominal and/or pleural effusion (Schaer, 1979). Ultrasonography of the cranial abdomen may also be useful, identifying cholestasis, pancreatic mass formation (secondary to peripancreatic fat necrosis), pancreatic pseudocysts, and abscesses in the region of the pancreas (Schaer, 1991).

Therapy for pancreatitis is aimed at maintaining fluid balance and restricting oral intake (Table 11–10). For dogs with moderate to severe

TABLE 11–10. THERAPIES FOR ACUTE PANCREATITIS IN OLDER DOGS

TREATMENT	GOALS
Nothing per os	Decrease pancreatic secretions
Intravenous fluid therapy	Replace gastrointestinal losses Maintain vascular volume Increase blood flow to pancreas
Dietary change	Decrease need for fat digestion Increase availability of carbohydrates for energy
Analgesic agents Meperidine Butorphanol	Relieve peritonitis-associated pain
Broad-spectrum antimicrobials	Minimize risk of bacterial infection
Peritoneal lavage	Reduce enzymatic effects in peritoneal cavity
Surgical debridement	Remove devitalized pancreas and fat Resect pancreatic abscesses Divert obstructed biliary system

pancreatitis, intravenous fluid therapy at doses calculated to meet rehydration and maintenance needs and compensate for ongoing losses should be provided. The goals of fluid therapy are to maintain normal blood pressure, replace losses induced by vomiting or exudation into body cavities, and maintain blood flow through the devitalized pancreas (Mulvaney et al, 1982). Food should be withheld until the dog has not vomited for 24 hours; then water is provided in small amounts, followed by small amounts of a bland diet. If no vomiting occurs, a bland diet (i.e., containing minimal fat and fiber, with moderate quantities of easily digestible carbohydrates and proteins) can be fed for several days before shifting gradually to an appropriate diet. Other therapies used for pancreatitis include analgesic (meperidine or butorphanol) and antimicrobial agents (ampicillin or a cephalosporin). Although pancreatitis itself is seldom a bacterial disease, the devitalized pancreas and peripancreatic fat, along with the localized peritonitis, can create a site for bacterial replication. Severe pancreatitis may also require the use of peritoneal lavage to reduce the caustic effect of pancreatic enzymes within the abdominal cavity (Mulvaney et al, 1982).

Complications of severe pancreatitis can include pancreatic and peripancreatic mass formation (with the mass composed of necrotic pancreatic and omental tissue), pancreatic abscess formation, and biliary obstruction (Edwards et al, 1990). Surgical intervention necessary for treatment of pancreatic masses or abscesses is often unsuccessful, and most dogs with these conditions die. Occasionally, severe extrahepatic bile duct obstruction induced by fibrosing pancreatitis will also necessitate surgical intervention for a biliary diversion procedure (Matthiesen and Rosin, 1986).

Exocrine Pancreatic Insufficiency. In older dogs, exocrine pancreatic insufficiency (EPI) is usually seen secondary to severe chronic pancreatitis. When more than 85 per cent of enzyme production is lost, clinical signs of EPI become obvious (Strombeck and Guilford, 1990). Clinical signs include severe small bowel diarrhea with steatorrhea, weight loss, and polyphagia. Dogs that continue to have pancreatitis in combination with EPI may have vomiting and a decreased appetite. Physical examination may reveal signs of weight loss and diarrhea. The preferred laboratory test for the diagnosis of EPI in dogs is the serum trypsin-like immunoreactivity (TLI) test (Williams and Batt, 1988). Decreased TLI concentrations in a fasted dog indicate that pancreatic function is impaired.

Exogenous pancreatic enzymes and dietary therapy are used to treat EPI in dogs (Simpson et al, 1989). Dogs with EPI should be fed an easily digestible, low-fat diet in amounts sufficient to provide 120 per cent of their calculated energy requirements to compensate for decreased digestion capabilities (Pidgeon, 1982). Additional supplemental vitamins may be given either orally or parenterally, as vitamin absorption may be impaired in dogs with EPI. Some dogs may also require antimicrobial therapy, as intestinal bacterial overgrowth is common in dogs with EPI (Simpson et al, 1990).

Exocrine Pancreatic Neoplasia. Pancreatic adenocarcinoma may arise from the pancreatic acinar cells, disrupting normal pancreatic structure and function. Dogs with pancreatic adenocarcinoma may have clinical signs of acute pancreatitis and will not respond to conventional therapy. Pancreatic adenocarcinoma frequently metastasizes to regional lymph nodes, stomach, duodenum, and liver (Strombeck and Guilford, 1990). Diagnosis requires a surgical biopsy. Surgical resection of the tumor is difficult. Chemotherapy for pancreatic adenocarcinoma can be attempted, but the prognosis is poor.

The Cat

Exocrine Pancreatic Diseases

Pancreatitis. Although older cats may develop either acute or chronic pancreatitis, these conditions are seldom diagnosed. Cats with acute pancreatitis have clinical signs of fever and abdominal pain, with less vomiting than seen in dogs (Kitchell et al, 1986). Laboratory evaluation of cats with pancreatitis often reveals azotemia, leukocytosis, and hyperglycemia (Schaer, 1979). Measurement of serum amylase and lipase activities is less helpful in cats than in dogs for identifying acute pancreatitis. Most diagnoses of pancreatitis in older cats are based on nebulous findings (Fig. 11–13). Chronic pancreatitis is somewhat more common in older cats. Infiltration of the pancreas with lymphocytes and plasma cells may accompany lymphocytic cholangiohepatitis, inflammatory bowel disease, and/or chronic renal failure (Owens et al, 1975). Cats with chronic pancreatitis may also be asymptomatic or exhibit vague signs of anorexia, weight loss, and vomiting. As with acute pancreatitis, evaluation of serum amylase and lipase activities is often unrewarding. Diagnosis may require a surgical biopsy.

The optimal therapy for pancreatitis in older cats is unknown. Food restriction, as used for pancreatitis in dogs, can result in hepatic lipidosis if continued too long. Short-term fasting followed by feeding a low-fat, bland diet may be a reasonable choice. If lymphocytic infiltration is found in concert with cholangiohepatitis or inflammatory bowel disease, then immunosuppressive therapy may be used. Unfortunately, information on treatment of pancreatitis in cats is quite limited.

Exocrine Pancreatic Insufficiency. Cats affected with EPI may develop diarrhea and weight loss, although most cats display a good appetite. Diagnosis of EPI is based on ruling out other causes of weight loss in older cats (e.g., hyperthyroidism, diabetes mellitus, liver disease, or chronic renal failure) and tests of pancreatic function. Evaluation of serum TLI is not currently performed in cats, because the assay is species specific (Williams et al, 1990). Measurement of fecal proteolytic activity using azocasein hydrolysis or radial enzyme diffusion is the best method for diagnosing EPI (Williams et al, 1990). Response to therapy using pancreatic enzyme powder may be used as both a diagnostic and therapeutic trial, but improvement may be seen with diseases other than EPI. Treatment of EPI is similar to that used in older dogs.

Exocrine Pancreatic Neoplasia. Benign nodular hyperplasia, adenoma, and pancreatic adenocarcinoma have all been reported in cats (Owens et al, 1975). Nodular hyperplasia and adenoma usually do not cause disease and are an incidental necropsy finding. In cats with adenocarcinoma of the pancreas, a palpable cranial abdominal mass may be the only significant finding (Owens et al, 1975). Surgical resection of the mass may be attempted, but the overall prognosis is very poor.

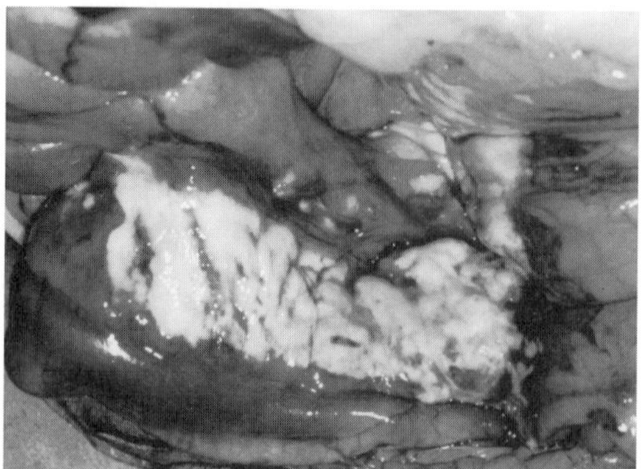

Figure 11–13. Surgical exploration of a 12-year-old cat with acute pancreatitis. Note the severe fat saponification and inflammation of the duodenum.

References and Supplemental Reading

Allen K, Twedt D, Hunsaker H. Tetramine cupruretic agents: A comparison in dogs. Am J Vet Res 48:28, 1987.
Badylak S. Coagulation disorders and liver disease. Vet Clin North Am 18:87, 1988.
Badylak S, Van Vleet J. Sequential morphologic and clinicopathologic alterations in dogs with experimentally induced glucocorticoid hepatopathy. Am J Vet Res 42:1310, 1981.
Baldwin C, Atkins C. Leptospirosis in dogs. Compend Contin Educ Pract Vet 9:499, 1987.
Biller D, Kantrowitz B, Miyabayashi T. Ultrasonography of diffuse liver disease. J Vet Intern Med 6:71, 1992.
Biourge V, MacDonald M, King L. Feline hepatic lipidosis: Pathogenesis and nutritional management. Compend Contin Educ Pract Vet 12:1244, 1990.
Boer H, Nelson R, Long G. Colchicine therapy for hepatic fibrosis in a dog. J Am Anim Hosp Assoc 185:303, 1984.
Brewer G, Dick R, Schall W, et al. Use of zinc acetate to

treat copper toxicosis in dogs. J Am Vet Med Assoc 201:564, 1992a.

Brewer G, Schall W, Dick R, et al: Use of 64-copper measurements to diagnose canine copper toxicosis. J Vet Intern Med 6:41, 1992b.

Bunch S, Center S, Baldwin B, et al. Radioimmunoassay of conjugated bile acids in canine and feline sera. Am J Vet Res 45:2051, 1984.

Bunch S, Polak D, Hornbuckle W. A modified laparoscopic approach for liver biopsy in dogs. J Am Vet Med Assoc 187:1032, 1985.

Center S. Feline liver disorders and their management. Compend Contin Educ Pract Vet 8:889, 1986.

Center S, Baldwin B, Dillingham S, et al. Diagnostic value of serum gamma-glutamyl transferase and alkaline phosphatase activities in hepatobiliary disease in the cat. J Am Vet Med Assoc 188:507, 1986.

Center S, ManWarren T, Slater M, et al. Evaluation of twelve-hour preprandial and two-hour postprandial serum bile acids concentrations for diagnosis of hepatobiliary disease in dogs. J Am Vet Med Assoc 199:217, 1991.

Church E, Matthiesen D. Surgical treatment of 23 dogs with necrotizing cholecystitis. J Am Anim Hosp Assoc 24:305, 1988.

Chvapil M. Pharmacology of fibrosis: definitions, limits, and perspectives. Life Sci 16:1345, 1976.

Cooper A, Plum F. Biochemistry and physiology of brain ammonia. Physiol Rev 67:440, 1987.

Dayrell-Hart B, Steinberg S, VanWinkle T, et al. Hepatotoxicity of phenobarbital in dogs: 18 cases (1985–1989). J Am Vet Med Assoc 199:1060, 1991.

Edwards D, Bauer M, Walker M, et al. Pancreatic masses in seven dogs following acute pancreatitis. J Am Anim Hosp Assoc 26:189, 1990.

Franklin J, Saunders G. Chronic active hepatitis in Doberman pinschers. Compend Contin Educ Pract Vet 10:1247, 1988.

Hardy R. Chronic hepatitis in dogs: A syndrome. Compend Contin Educ Pract Vet 8:904, 1986.

Hardy R. Hepatic encephalopathy. In Kirk R, Bonagura J, eds. Current Veterinary Therapy XI. Philadelphia, WB Saunders, 1992, p 639.

Hardy R, O'Brien T, Adams L, et al. Periportal hepatitis associated with the use of a heartworm-hookworm preventative (diethylcarbamazine-oxibendazole) in 13 dogs. J Am Anim Hosp Assoc 25:419, 1989.

Hirsch V, Doige C. Suppurative cholangitis in cats. J Am Vet Med Assoc 182:1223, 1983.

Hosgood G. Arteriovenous fistulas: Pathophysiology, diagnosis, and treatment. Compend Contin Educ Pract Vet 11:625, 1989.

Hultgren B, Stevens J, Hardy R. Inherited, chronic, progressive hepatic degeneration in Bedlington terriers with increased liver copper concentrations: Clinical and pathologic observations and comparison with other copper-associated liver diseases. Am J Vet Res 47:365, 1986.

Johnson G, Sternlieb I, Twedt D, et al. Inheritance of copper toxicosis in Bedlington terriers. Am J Vet Res 41:1865, 1980.

Johnson S. Portal hypertension. Part I. Pathophysiology and clinical consequences. Compend Contin Educ Pract Vet 9:741, 1987a.

Johnson S. Portal hypertension. Part II. Clinical assessment and treatment. Compend Contin Educ Pract Vet 9:917, 1987b.

Johnson S, Crisp S, Smeak D, et al. Hepatic encephalopathy in two aged dogs secondary to a presumed congenital portal-azygous shunt. J Am Anim Hosp Assoc 25:129, 1989.

Kitani K. Hepatic drug metabolism in the elderly. Hepatology 6:316, 1986.

Kitchell B, Strombeck D, Cullen J, et al. Clinical and pathologic changes in experimentally induced acute pancreatitis in cats. Am J Vet Res 47:1170, 1986.

Kosovsky J, Manfra-Marretta S, Matthiesen D, et al. Results of partial hepatectomy in 18 dogs with hepatocellular carcinoma. J Am Anim Hosp Assoc 25:203, 1989.

Laflamme D. Dietary management of canine hepatic encephalopathy. Compend Contin Educ Pract Vet 10:1258, 1988.

Lewis L, Morris M, Hand M. Small Animal Clinical Nutrition. Topeka, KS, Mark Morris Associates, 1987.

Lowseth L, Gillett N, Chang I-Y, et al. Detection of serum alpha-fetoprotein in dogs with hepatic tumors. J Am Vet Med Assoc 199:735, 1991.

Lucke V, Davies J. Progressive lymphocytic cholangitis in the cat. J Sm Anim Pract 25:249, 1984.

Magne M. Primary epithelial hepatic tumors in the dog. Compend Contin Educ Pract Vet 6:506, 1984.

Magne M, Chiapella A. Medical management of canine chronic hepatitis. Compend Contin Educ Pract Vet 8:915, 1986.

Matthiesen D, Rosin E. Common bile duct obstruction secondary to chronic fibrosing pancreatitis: Treatment by use of cholecystoduodenostomy in the dog. J Am Vet Med Assoc 189:1443, 1986.

Mays P, McAnulty R, Laurent G. Age-related changes in total protein and collagen metabolism in rat liver. Hepatology 14:1224, 1991.

Meyer D, Center S. Approach to the diagnosis of liver disorders in dogs and cats. Compend Contin Educ Pract Vet 8:880, 1986.

Meyer D, French T. The liver. In Cowell R, Tyler R, eds. Diagnostic Cytology of the Dog and Cat. Goleta, CA, American Veterinary Publications, 1989, p 189.

Mulvaney M, Feinberg C, Tilson D. Clinical characterization of acute necrotizing pancreatitis. Compend Contin Educ Pract Vet 4:394, 1982.

Neer T. A review of disorders of the gallbladder and extrahepatic biliary tract in the dog and cat. J Vet Intern Med 6:186, 1992.

Owen C, McCall J. Identification of the carrier of the Bedlington terrier copper disease. Am J Vet Res 44:694, 1983.

Owens J, Drazner F, Gilbertson S. Pancreatic disease in the cat. J Am Anim Hosp Assoc 11:83, 1975.

Pidgeon G. Effect of diet on exocrine pancreatic insufficiency in dogs. J Am Vet Med Assoc 181:232, 1982.

Post G, Patnaik A. Nonhematopoietic hepatic neoplasms in cats: 21 cases (1983–1988). J Am Vet Med Assoc 201:1080, 1992.

Rand J, Best S, Mathews K. Portosystemic vascular shunts in a family of American cocker spaniels. J Am Anim Hosp Assoc 24:265, 1988.

Rogers W, Ruebner B. A retrospective study of probable glucocorticoid-induced hepatopathy in dogs. J Am Vet Med Assoc 170:603, 1977.

Schaer M. A clinicopathologic survey of acute pancreatitis in 30 dogs and 5 cats. J Am Anim Hosp Assoc 15:681, 1979.

Schaer M. Acute pancreatitis in dogs. Compend Contin Educ Pract Vet 13:1769, 1991.

Simpson K, Batt R, Jones D, et al. Effects of exocrine pancreatic insufficiency and replacement therapy on the bacterial flora of the duodenum in dogs. Am J Vet Res 51:203, 1990.

Simpson K, Batt R, McLean L, et al. Circulating concentrations of trypsin-like immunoreactivity and activities of lipase and amylase after pancreatic duct ligation in dogs. Am J Vet Res 50:629, 1989.

Slappendel R. Disseminated intravascular coagulation. In Kirk RW, ed. Current Veterinary Therapy X. Philadelphia, WB Saunders, 1989, p 451.

Strombeck D, Guilford W. Small Animal Gastroenterology. Davis, CA, Stonegate Publishing, 1990.

Strombeck D, Miller L, Harrold D. Effects of corticosteroid treatment on survival time in dogs with chronic hepatitis: 151 cases (1977–1985). J Am Vet Med Assoc 193:1109, 1988.

Taboada J, Meyer D. Cholestasis associated with extrahepatic bacterial infection in five dogs. J Vet Intern Med 3:216, 1989.

Thornbrugh J, Edwards N, Jordan H. *Metametorchis* infection in a domestic cat. J Am Anim Hosp Assoc 26:494, 1990.

Thornburg L. Fatty liver syndrome in cats. J Am Anim Hosp Assoc 18:397, 1982.

Thornburg L, Rottinghaus G, Gage H. Chronic liver disease associated with high hepatic copper concentration in a dog. J Am Vet Med Assoc 188:1190, 1986.

Thornburg L, Rottinghaus G, Koch J, et al. High liver copper levels in two Doberman pinschers with subacute hepatitis. J Am Anim Hosp Assoc 20:1003, 1984.

Thornburg L, Rottinghaus G, McGowan M, et al. Hepatic copper concentrations in purebred and mixed-breed dogs. Vet Pathol 27:81, 1990.

Twedt D, Hunsaker H, Allen K. Use of 2,3,2-tetramine as a hepatic copper chelating agent for treatment of copper hepatotoxicosis in Bedlington Terriers. J Am Vet Med Assoc 192:52, 1988.

Tyler J. Hepatoencephalopathy. Part I. Clinical signs and diagnosis. Compend Contin Educ Pract Vet 12:1069, 1990a.

Tyler J. Hepatoencephalopathy. Part II. Pathophysiology and treatment. Compend Contin Educ Pract Vet 12:1260, 1990b.

van den Ingh T, Rothuizen J, Ruurdje C. Chronic active hepatitis with cirrhosis in the Doberman pinscher. Vet Q 10:84, 1988.

Willard M, Bailey M, Hauptman J, et al. Obstructed portal venous flow and portal vein thrombosis in a dog. J Am Vet Med Assoc 194:1449, 1989.

Williams D, Batt R. Sensitivity and specificity of radioimmunoassay of serum trypsin-like immunoreactivity for the diagnosis of canine exocrine pancreatic insufficiency. J Am Vet Med Assoc 192:195, 1988.

Williams D, Reed S, Perry L. Fecal proteolytic activity in clinically normal cats and in a cat with exocrine pancreatic insufficiency. J Am Vet Med Assoc 197:210, 1990.

Zawie D, Shaker E. Diseases of the liver. In Sherding R, ed. The Cat: Diseases and Clinical Management. New York, Churchill Livingstone, 1989, p 1015.

CHAPTER 12

The Skin

SANDRA R. MERCHANT

No skin disease is found exclusively in the older animal. However, the aging process tends to predispose dogs and cats to various skin diseases. Impaired immunity, structural changes in the skin, and internal diseases with cutaneous manifestations can increase the frequency of certain skin diseases in the aged animal.

As a general rule, decreased immune surveillance is believed to play a role in susceptibility to neoplasia. Endocrinopathies such as hypothyroidism, hyperthyroidism, diabetes mellitus, and hyperadrenocorticism are seen more often in older animals. Adult-onset demodicosis may also be associated with the aging process by way of its link to an underlying disease process (e.g., neoplasia, endocrinopathy). Many internal diseases that occur in aged animals may have specific or nonspecific cutaneous manifestations. A catabolic or cachectic state occurring in an animal for any number of reasons may be reflected in the skin and haircoat by seborrhea and a dull, dry, brittle, sparse haircoat.

SENILE CHANGES OF THE SKIN

Senile changes of human skin have been well described, but little information is available on skin changes of older dogs and cats. The most comprehensive information is found in a study of the histopathologic changes seen in the skin of 14 dogs ranging in age from 12 to 17 years (Baker, 1967). Few histologic changes were observed except in extreme age (17 years). Epidermal and follicular hyperkeratosis was evident. Many follicles did not contain hair shafts, appeared flask shaped, and were lined by a single layer of flattened epidermal cells. Atrophy of the epidermis and dermis was seen in extreme age. The epidermal cells were flattened, with pyknotic nuclei, and the viable epidermis was often only one cell thick. The dermis was almost cell free (Baker, 1967). With advancing age, collagen bundles became granular and fragmented, and in extreme cases the dermis presented an eosinophilic hyaline appearance. Apparent decrease in reticulin tissue was noted. Pigmented areas had a marked increase in dermal pigmentation.

Variable changes were seen in the glands of the skin. In some animals, cystic dilation and/or hyperplasia of the apocrine glands were seen. Some apocrine glands contained large yellow refractile granules located in the secretory cells. The individual cells of the circumanal glands were reduced in size and contained pyknotic nuclei. The arrector pili muscles were more eosinophilic and fragmented, with vacuolization within individual fibers. In extreme age, all traces of these muscles sometimes disappeared. Changes in cutaneous blood vessels were not evident. Clinically, the hair of some dogs became dull and lusterless, with areas of alopecia and callus formation over pressure points. Increased numbers of white hairs on the muzzle and body were frequently noted. The footpads were sometimes hyperkeratinized and the claws malformed and brittle.

PATIENT EVALUATION

Dermatologic History. When geriatric dogs or cats are presented because the owner has noted a skin problem, a thorough dermatologic history and examination are important parts of the minimum data base. The dermatologic history is the most important part of the evaluation of the skin and hair. The use of a dermatology history questionnaire that can be filled out by the owner before the examination will provide an effective format for the veterinarian to quickly gather information. In this way a standard dermatologic history is taken on all cases and important questions are not forgotten (August, 1986; Muller et al, 1989; Smith, 1988) (Fig. 12–1).

Dermatologic Examination. The veterinarian who performs a thorough dermatologic examination will gain valuable information and be able to efficiently choose the specialized diagnostic tests needed to define the skin disease. Because recheck dermatologic examinations are often necessary, recording the examination findings and test results at each visit is important to document the progression or regression of the disease. Having a standard figure in the medical record can be helpful in systematically recording location and severity of lesions (Fig. 12–2).

NUTRITIONAL DISORDERS

Nutrition plays an important role in the development and maintenance of healthy skin and haircoat. Dogs and cats require amino acids, fatty acids, glucose precursors, vitamins, and minerals for normal growth and maintenance. Deficiencies of any of these nutrients can result in abnormal keratinization of skin and hair, as well as changes in sebaceous and epidermal lipids. The resulting clinical picture is one of an animal with a poor, dry haircoat and scaly skin. Nutrient excess or imbalance can also cause skin disease. Nutrient imbalances are most likely to occur in dogs and cats consuming poor-quality pet foods, improperly prepared homemade diets, or excessively supplemented diets and in animals with metabolic disorders. Animals that consume high-quality, commercially prepared pet foods are unlikely to become nutrient deficient and experience skin disease of nutritional origin. Many drugs can significantly depress food intake (Roe and Campbell, 1984). Nonabsorbable antimicrobial agents and cholestyramine may impair fat and fat-soluble vitamin absorption, which in turn may depress calcium and magnesium absorption (Buffington, 1987). Anticonvulsant drugs may inhibit calcium and folate absorption.

ENDOCRINOPATHIES

Canine Hypothyroidism

A myriad of clinical signs are associated with hypothyroidism. Primary hypothyroidism is a result of either lymphocytic thyroiditis or idiopathic thyroidal atrophy. Thyroid biopsy specimens taken during acute stages of lymphocytic thyroiditis show infiltration of lymphocytes and plasma cells. Idiopathic thyroidal atrophy is characterized by loss of normal thyroid parenchyma without evidence of inflammatory infiltrate and replacement with adipose tissue.

Clinical Features and Diagnosis. Clinical signs of hypothyroidism are usually insidious in nature, with signs being attributed simply to the aging process or completely overlooked. Early dermatologic manifestations of hypothyroidism include dryness (Fig. 12–3), scaliness, and excessive shedding. Failure of hair regrowth secondary to cessation of the anagen hair phase leads to progressive symmetric alopecia. Hair loss is most often bilateral and symmetric, especially in the flanks, ventral neck (Fig. 12–4), abdomen, dorsal tail, and pressure points. The tail may become alopecic, with a "rat-tail" appearance (Fig. 12–5). The skin may be hyperpigmented and occasionally thickened secondary to myxedema. Focal accumulations of mucin may lead to vesicular mucinosis. Pruritus may be associated with secondary dermatologic diseases as seborrhea oleosa (Fig. 12–6), seborrhea sicca, seborrheic dermatitis (Fig. 12–7), *Malassezia* dermatitis, and staphylococcal pyoderma. Some animals may present for the clinical complaint of recurrent staphylococcal pyoderma, and in very rare cases, hypertrichosis may be seen.

Confirmation of hypothyroidism involves assessment of thyroid gland function. Measurement of basal serum thyroid hormone concentration is the most widely available and practiced method of diagnosing hypothyroidism in the dog (Belshaw and Rijnberk, 1979). Measurement of basal T_4 (thyroxine) concentration should be viewed as a screening test. A T_4 concentration that is well within the normal range should rule out hypothyroidism. However, the use of basal T_4 concentration becomes problematic when the value is borderline. Overdiagnosis often occurs by erroneous interpretation of borderline low thyroid hormone levels. Numerous factors can

DERMATOLOGY HISTORY

NAME ______ CASE NO.

STREET ______

CITY, STATE, ZIP ______

PHONE. BUS ______ HOME ______

SPECIES ______ BREED ______ SEX ______

ANIMAL'S NAME ______ DATE OF BIRTH ______

COLOR-IDENTIFYING MARK ______

DATE:	CLINICIAN:	STUDENT:

CHIEF COMPLAINT(S) ______

Date (age) Problem First Noticed ______ Onset: Sudden ______ Slow ______

Is there a seasonal influence? No ______ Summer ______ Fall ______ Winter ______

Where did problem begin? ______

What did it look like then? ______

Does animal itch? Yes ______ No ______ When? Constant ______ Sporadic ______ Night ______

Is there any exposure to other animals (neighbors, etc?) ______

Do other animals or people have skin problems, rash? ______

Describe animal's indoor environment, time (%): ______

Describe animal's outdoor environment, time (%): ______

What does animal sleep on? ______

What diagnostic tests have been performed? ______

What local treatment has been used? success? ______

What systemic treatment has been used? success? ______

Does owner have an idea of the cause? What makes it worse? ______

When did owner last see fleas? ______ Describe flea control ______

Animal's diet ______

Reproductive history: age of neutering? ______ Date, duration of last estrus ______

Breeding history (male or female) ______

Medical History: Previous diseases, treatments, results: ______

Is animal on any medication at present? ______

What other facts does owner think would be helpful? ______

Figure 12–1. Dermatology history form used at the Veterinary Teaching Hospital and Clinics, Louisiana State University School of Veterinary Medicine.

NAME ______ CASE NO.
STREET ______
CITY, STATE, ZIP ______
PHONE. BUS ______ HOME ______
SPECIES ______ BREED ______ SEX
ANIMAL'S NAME ______ DATE OF BIRTH
COLOR-IDENTIFYING MARK

DATE:	CLINICIAN:	STUDENT:

PRURITUS?

PARASITES?

PRIMARY LESIONS (Circle)

Macule	Patch	Papule	Plaque
Vesicle	Bulla	Pustule	Wheal
Nodule	Tumor		

SECONDARY LESIONS (Circle)

Scale	Epidermal collarette	Scar	Ulcer
Erosion	Crust	Excoriation	Fissure
Comedone	Cyst	Abscess	Hypopigmentation
Hyperpigmentation	Erythema	Hyperkeratosis	Callus
Alopecia	Lichenification		

CONFIGURATION OF LESIONS (Circle)

Regional Linear Annular (Target) Grouped Irregular

QUALITY OF HAIR COAT

Epilation: + −
Pelage is: Dry,
Brittle, Dull, Oily

OTHER FACTORS

Footpads
Nails
Hyperhidrosis

LABORATORY TESTS

Scotch Tape: ______ Wood's Light + −
Skin Scraping: ______
KOH Digestion: ______
Direct Smear: ______
Fungal Culture: ______
Bacterial Culture: ______
Sensitivity: ______
Allergy: ______
Endocrine: ______
Immune:
D.I.T.: ______
I.I.T.: ______
ANA: ______
Other: ______
Biopsy: Site(s) ______ Path As. No. ______
RESULTS: ______

DISTRIBUTION OF LESIONS

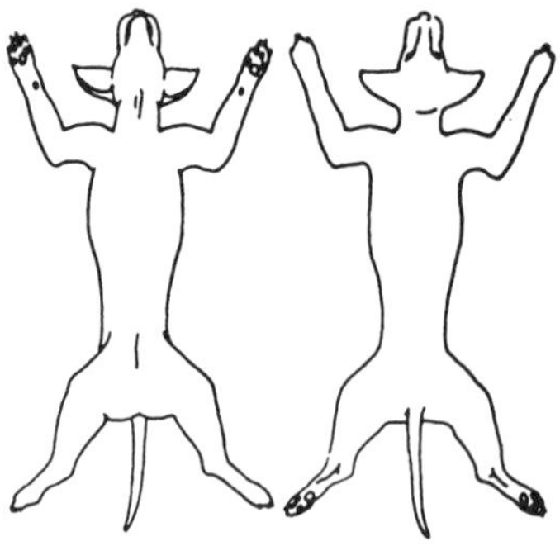

Ventral Dorsal

DIFFERENTIAL DIAGNOSIS:

COMMENTS:

SIGNED BY ATTENDING CLINICIAN

Medical Records—White
Clinician—Canary

Figure 12–2. Dermatology examination form used at the Veterinary Teaching Hospital and Clinics, Louisiana State University School of Veterinary Medicine.

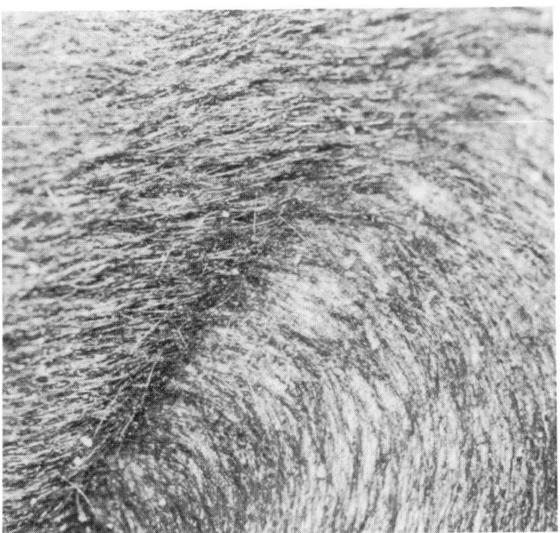

Figure 12–3. Dry, scaling skin and haircoat of a dog with hypothyroidism.

influence thyroid hormone concentration (Table 12–1). The most commonly used provocative function test is the thyroid-stimulating hormone (TSH) stimulation test. Laboratories vary in their recommendations for sampling techniques and should be consulted before a TSH stimulation test is performed.

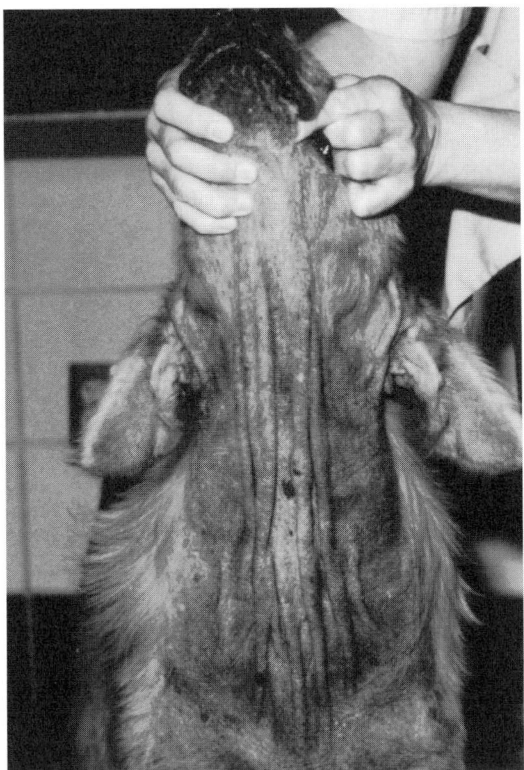

Figure 12–4. Extreme hyperpigmentation on the ventral cervical region of a hypothyroid golden retriever dog.

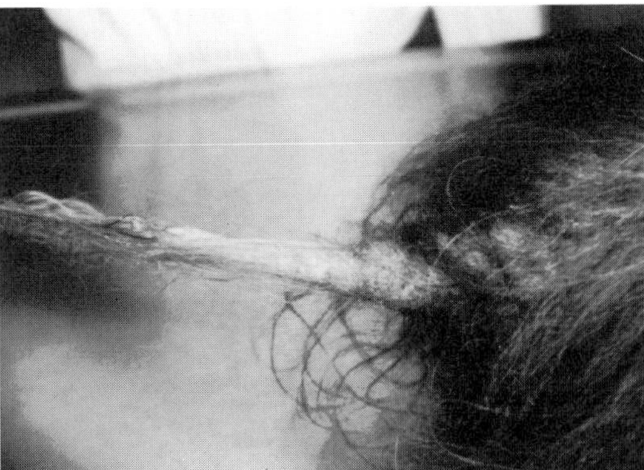

Figure 12–5. Hair loss on the tail of a dog with hypothyroidism.

Other diagnostic tests used to determine thyroid function are thyrotropin-releasing hormone (TRH) stimulation and determination of free T_3 (triiodothyronine) and free T_4. Injection of TRH causes an increase in TSH with a resultant release of T_4 and T_3. However, two problems affect the usefulness of this test. First, the increases in serum T_4 and T_3 are small and somewhat variable, and second, the influence of nonthyroidal factors on this response has not been determined. Measurement of free T_3 and free T_4 provides an accurate test for the amount of active thyroid hormone present. Theoretically, free hormone concentrations should not be greatly affected in nonthyroidal illnesses, but unfortunately, this is not the case. Free thyroid hormone concentrations may also be adversely affected in the euthyroid sick syndrome. However, evaluating free T_4 in conjunction with total T_4 reduces the false-positive diagnosis of hypothyroidism by approximately 15 per cent (Feldman and Nelson, 1987). Measurement of endogenous TSH is a very useful test in human medicine, but a valid assay for canine TSH has yet to be developed.

In some situations a therapeutic trial with T_4 supplementation is warranted. However, response to therapy is nonspecific. Because of its anabolic nature, thyroid hormone supplementation can create a positive effect in some dogs without thyroid dysfunction. Activity level should increase within 10 days, but complete hair regrowth may take as long as 4 to 6 months. Thyroid hormone will cause increased hair growth to some extent in most dogs, regardless of their thyroid status. If clinical signs resolve completely and recur when the drug is stopped, then the dog is probably hypothyroid.

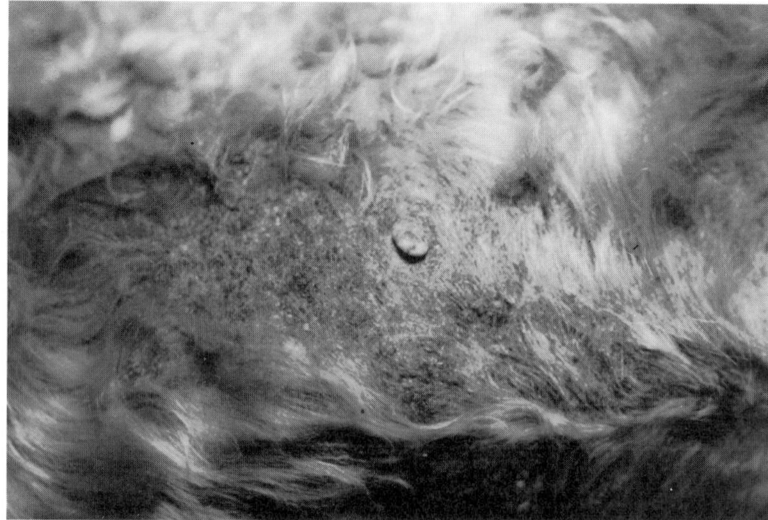

Figure 12–6. Seborrhea oleosa on the ventral abdomen of a hypothyroid cocker spaniel.

Therapy. Lifelong therapy should be initiated once hypothyroidism has been diagnosed. Synthetic levothyroxine (0.01 mg/lb every 12 hours) is the initial therapy of choice. The plasma half-life of levothyroxine is probably between 12 and 16 hours, with peak plasma concentration occurring 4 to 12 hours after administration. Clinical signs should begin to improve in a few weeks. After 6 weeks of treatment, T_4 concentration should be measured before and 6 hours after pill administration. Ideally, both concentrations of T_4 should be within the normal range, although it is acceptable to have the pre–pill administration value within the normal range and the post–pill administration value slightly above the normal range, if the dog is not showing signs of hyperthyroidism. If the pre-pill T_4 value is low and the post-pill T_4 value is within the normal range, supplementation should be adjusted upward and pre- and post-pill T_4 values reevaluated in 6 weeks. The opposite holds for T_4 values that are too high. If T_4 values continue to be low, a problem with pill administration should be ruled out. A change to a different brand of T_4 is recommended to rule out poor bioavailability. When the dog is stable, it may be possible to change from twice-daily to once-daily supplementation. A dose of 0.01 mg/lb is administered once daily, and after 6 weeks T_4 values before and 8 to 10 hours after administration are evaluated. Because of the variable nature of metabolism of T_4 in the dog, some dogs do well on once-daily supplementation. Once the dog is stabilized, pre- and post-pill T_4 values should be measured every 6 to 12 months for the remainder of the dog's life, with the dose adjusted accordingly.

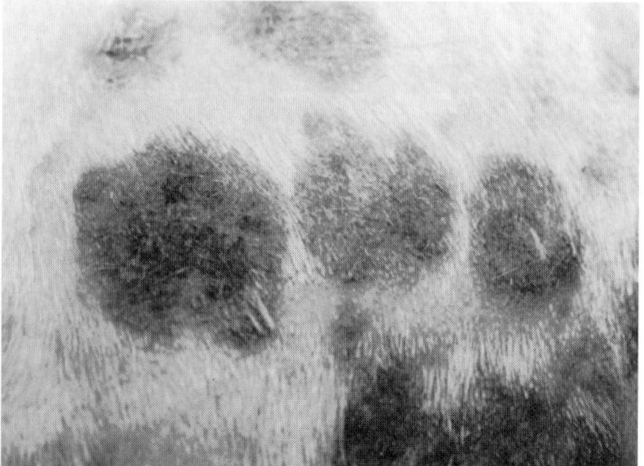

Figure 12–7. Plaques of seborrheic dermatitis on the ventral thorax and abdomen of a hypothyroid cocker spaniel.

Canine Hyperadrenocorticism

Hyperadrenocorticism refers to the constellation of clinical and biochemical abnormalities resulting from prolonged exposure to excess endogenous or exogenous glucocorticoids. Glucocorticoid administration is by far the most common cause of hyperadrenocorticism.

Clinical Features and Diagnosis. Spontaneous hyperadrenocorticism is a disease of middle-age to older dogs. Common clinical complaints include polyuria; polydipsia; polyphagia; weight gain; behavior changes, including lethargy and reluctance to exercise; panting; and skin disease. Dermatologic signs may be quite striking. Classic changes include hair loss, which is usually bilateral and symmetric (Fig. 12–8), but focal

TABLE 12–1. NONTHYROIDAL FACTORS THAT CAN INFLUENCE BASAL T_4 CONCENTRATION

Factor	Effect
Age:	Increased T_4 concentration in neonates, decreased T_4 with age in adult dogs.
Breed:	Tendency for increased T_4 in small breed dogs, decreased T_4 in large breed dogs, and increased serum T_4 in greyhounds.
Obesity:	Increased T_4.
Hypoproteinemia:	Increased T_4 as a result of decreased plasma protein binding.
Drugs:	Glucocorticoids, anticonvulsants, some antimicrobial agents (penicillin, trimethoprim-sulfamethoxazole), androgens, phenylbutazone, quinidine, propylthiouracil, salicylates, sulfonylureas, and dopamine all decrease T_4; insulin increases T_4 (Beale, 1990a; Feldman and Nelson, 1987; Ferguson, 1984, 1988; Hall et al, 1992; Wenzel, 1981).
Euthyroid sick syndrome:	Acute and chronic illnesses lower T_4; these include renal disease, liver disease, diabetes mellitus, infectious disease, gastrointestinal dysfunction, hyperadrenocorticism, and demodicosis.

hair loss may also occur. Other changes include hyperpigmentation; seborrhea sicca; comedones and thin skin, especially on the ventral abdomen (Fig. 12–9); telangiectasia; increased prominence of surgical scars; lack of hair regrowth after shaving; and adult-onset generalized demodicosis. One dramatic manifestation seen in 5 per cent of dogs is calcinosis cutis (Fig. 12–10) (White et al, 1989). Adult dogs that have never had bacterial skin disease may show a marked predisposition to recurrent staphylococcal skin infections (Fig. 12–11).

A presumptive diagnosis of canine hyperadrenocorticism is based on history, physical examination findings, and supportive laboratory abnormalities (Table 12–2). A complete evaluation of the skin disease should include a skin scraping for *Demodex* mites, dermatophyte fungal culture, and cytologic examination. Bacterial culture and sensitivity testing should be performed if a pustular disease is present. Immunosuppressed animals are potentially predisposed to demodicosis and infectious skin disease. A skin biopsy may be helpful in differentiating an endocrine-induced alopecia from other causes of hair loss.

Therapy. Treatment depends on the cause of the hyperadrenocorticism. In general, treatment modalities include medical, surgical, and/or radiation therapy. Medical management is aimed at decreasing cortisol production by the adrenal cortex. Drugs used for this purpose include mitotane (Lysodren), ketoconazole, aminoglutethimide, metyrapone, and L-deprenyl (Bruyette et al, 1993). The most commonly used drug is mitotane. L-Deprenyl has been used successfully to treat canine pituitary-dependent hyperadrenocorticism; 71 per cent of the dogs in one study were treated successfully with no untoward effects or laboratory abnormalities (Bruyette et al,

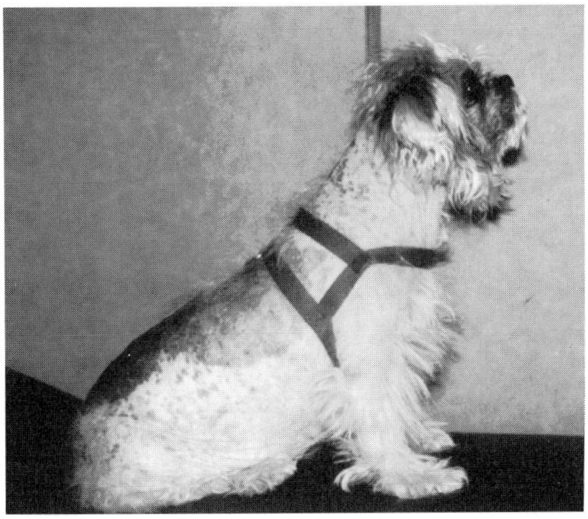

Figure 12–8. Truncal hair loss in a dog with pituitary dependent hyperadrenocorticism. (Courtesy of Joy Barbet, DVM, Archer, FL.)

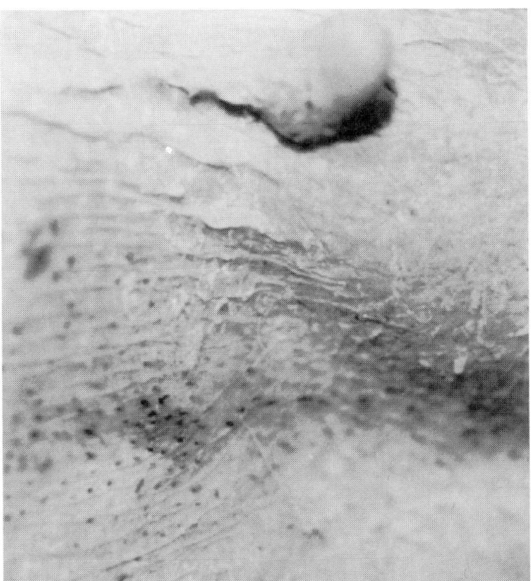

Figure 12–9. Thin, "crepe paper" skin with comedones on the ventral surface of a dog with pituitary dependent hyperadrenocorticism.

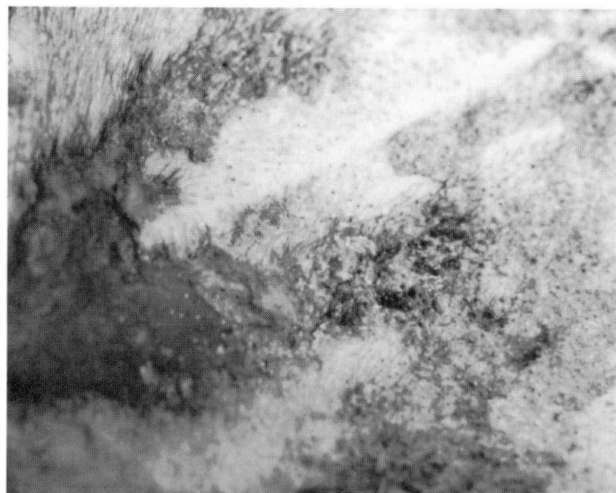

Figure 12–10. Plaques and ulcerated plaques of calcinosis cutis on the ventrum of a dog with iatrogenic hyperadrenocorticism.

1993). Surgery remains the treatment of choice for an adrenal tumor; approximately 50 per cent of the tumors are benign adenomas, and the animal is cured by adrenalectomy.

Feline Hyperadrenocorticism

Hyperadrenocorticism is a relatively rare disease in the cat compared with the dog. The average age at onset in the cat is 10.4 years (Zerbe and MacDonald, 1993). Polyuria, polydipsia, polyphagia, and a pendulous abdomen with hepatomegaly and muscle wasting and weight gain are the most common signs noted. Dermatologic abnormalities include truncal and abdominal alopecia, unkempt haircoat, thin skin, comedones, hyperpigmentation bruising, and abscesses. In some cats excessively fragile skin leads to tearing with normal manipulation or handling (Helton-Rhodes et al, 1992; Zerbe and MacDonald, 1993). Approximately 81 per cent of cats with hyperadrenocorticism have overt diabetes mellitus.

Diagnosis of hyperadrenocorticism is difficult in cats. Diagnostic test results are often inconsistent, and testing has not been standardized. The adrenocorticotropic hormone (ACTH) stimula-

TABLE 12–2. HEMATOLOGIC, SERUM BIOCHEMICAL, AND URINE ABNORMALITIES CONSISTENT WITH CANINE HYPERADRENOCORTICISM

Hematologic Abnormalities
Mature leukocytosis
Neutrophilia
Lymphopenia
Eosinopenia*
Erythrocytosis
Nucleated red blood cells
Serum Biochemical Abnormalities
Increased alkaline phosphatase*
Increased alanine aminotransferase (serum glutamic-pyruvic transaminase)
Increased fasting cholesterol and lipemia
Increased fasting blood glucose
Decreased blood urea nitrogen
Urinalysis
Specific gravity <1.015 (often <1.008)
Urinary tract infection (bacteriuria may be noted without inflammation)
Glucosuria if concomitant diabetes mellitus

*Most commonly seen abnormalities.

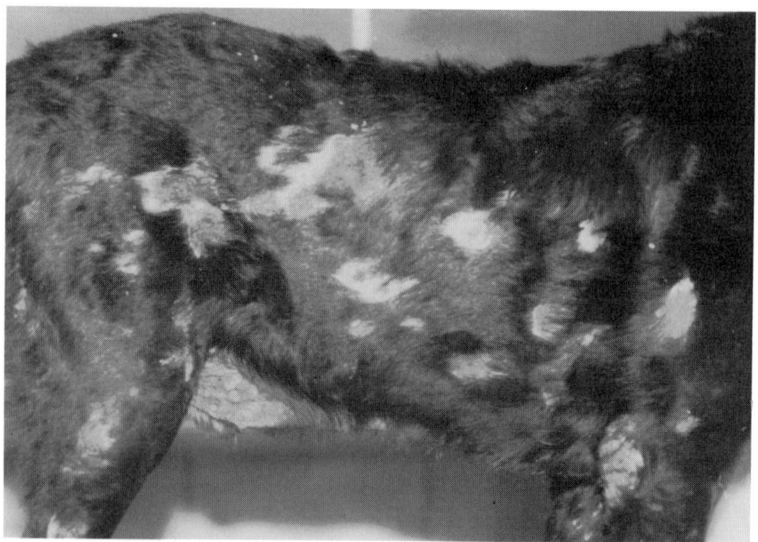

Figure 12–11. Multiple staphylococcal epidermal collarettes on the lateral thorax and abdomen of a dog with pituitary-dependent hyperadrenocorticism.

tion test is probably the best test (Peterson and Kemppainen, 1993).

Mitotane, ketoconazole, cobalt irradiation, metyrapone, and bilateral adrenalectomy have all been used for the treatment of feline pituitary-dependent hyperadrenocorticism. Bilateral adrenalectomy followed by mineralocorticoid and glucocorticoid replacement therapy appears to be the most successful treatment. Cats do not appear to experience the complications of surgical intervention reported in dogs. Treatment for an adrenal tumor consists of surgical excision (Nelson and Feldman, 1991). In cats exhibiting extremely fragile skin that tears easily during manipulation, metyrapone should be initiated at 65 mg/kg every 12 hours until cortisol levels are normal and skin lesions have healed (Daley et al, 1993). Ketoconazole at a dose of 5 to 10 mg/kg every 8 hours may be used if the response to metyrapone is not adequate (Zerbe and MacDonald, 1993).

Feline Hyperthyroidism

Hyperthyroidism is the most common endocrine disorder of middle-age to old cats. Approximately one half of cats have an unkempt haircoat, with excessive shedding and matting of the hair (Peterson and Ferguson, 1989). Changes in hair texture, partial hair loss, and increased nail growth also are features of feline hyperthyroidism. In cats with areas of complete alopecia, behavioral changes associated with excessive grooming have been documented (Peterson et al, 1983).

Diabetes Mellitus

Dermatologic lesions associated with diabetes mellitus are uncommon. The most common dermatologic manifestations are pyoderma, seborrheic skin disease, demodicosis, thin skin, alopecia, and xanthomatosis (Muller et al, 1989; White, 1989). Necrolytic migratory erythema (also known as hepatocutaneous syndrome, superficial necrolytic dermatitis, or metabolic epidermal necrosis) has been seen in dogs with diabetes mellitus.

SKIN TUMORS

Papilloma

Cutaneous papillomas that occur in older dogs and cats are not caused by a virus, unlike the cutaneous papillomas that occur in younger dogs.

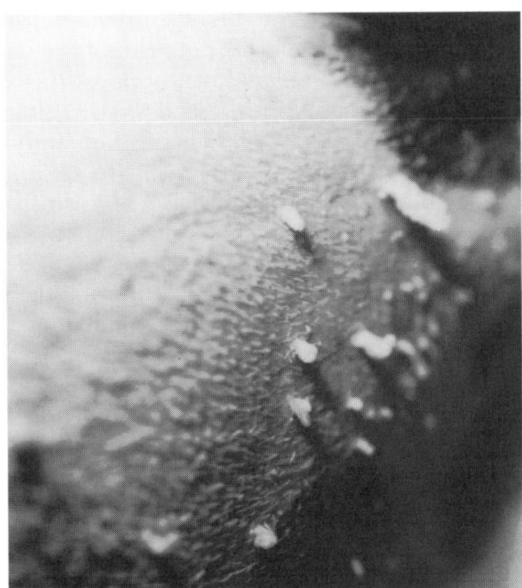

Figure 12–12. Multiple fibropapillomas on the abdomen of a dog. (Courtesy of Carol Foil, DVM, Louisiana State University, Baton Rouge, LA.)

Clinical Features and Diagnosis. In dogs, papillomas are more common in males and in cocker spaniels and Kerry blue terriers (Muller et al, 1989). There is no breed or sex predilection in cats. Cutaneous papillomas in dogs and cats are usually solitary but may be multiple, occurring most commonly on the head, eyelids, feet, and genitalia (Susaneck and Withrow, 1989). They tend to be less than 0.5 cm in diameter, pedunculated or cauliflower-like, well circumscribed, and alopecic and vary from firm to soft (Fig. 12–12). Although these masses are benign, they may be traumatized and may rarely transform into squamous cell carcinoma (Watrach et al, 1970). Diagnosis is by excisional biopsy. Histologically, papillomas are divided into two types. The most common type is the squamous papilloma, which is characterized by papillated epidermal hyperplasia and papillomatosis, with ballooning degeneration and basophilic intranuclear inclusion bodies as variable findings. The fibropapilloma is characterized by a fibroma-like proliferation of collagen with a hyperplastic epidermis.

Therapy. Clinical management of cutaneous papillomas may include surgical excision, cryosurgery, electrosurgery, or observation without treatment. Immune-modulating drugs have no documented value.

Basal Cell Tumors

Basal cell tumors in veterinary medicine comprise a large group of neoplasms in the dog and cat that are derived from basal epithelial cells of the epidermis and adnexa. Some authors reserve the term *basal cell tumor* for neoplasms that do not have any adnexal features and are completely benign (Gross et al, 1992). These same authors use the term *basal cell carcinoma* to describe tumors of low-grade malignancy that arise from small, pluripotential epithelial cells within the basal cell layer of the epidermis and adnexa. The pluripotential nature of the basaloid epithelial cell is manifested by limited differentiation toward hair follicles, sebaceous glands, and sweat glands in some basal cell carcinomas. In the older literature, basal cell and adnexa-derived tumors, when placed in a single category, represented 3 to 12 per cent of all skin tumors in dogs and 15 to 18 per cent of all skin tumors in cats.

Clinical Features and Diagnosis. Basal cell tumors in cats can occur anywhere on the body but show a predilection for the head and neck. Siamese and long-haired cats may be predisposed, and the average age at onset is 7 to 10 years (Gross et al, 1992). The tumors are solitary, well-circumscribed, firm, hairless, dome-shaped, elevated masses usually less than 2.5 cm in diameter and freely movable over underlying structures. Basal cell tumors in dogs are usually solitary and are found most frequently on the head, neck, and shoulders (Madewell and Theilen, 1987). Basal cell tumors on the head are frequently located on the skin of the commissures of the lips, periocular tissue, pinna, and cheek. They are usually less than 2.5 cm in diameter but can become as large as 10 cm or more. They are well circumscribed, encapsulated, and hairless, with a white, glistening surface. They can also be pigmented, appearing brown or black.

Diagnosis is made by excisional biopsy. Following Gross et al's (1992) classification scheme, a benign feline basal cell tumor is a well-circumscribed dermal nodule that generally has a fairly broad zone of connection to the overlying epidermis. Ulceration is common. The neoplasm is composed of small basaloid epithelial cells arranged in tightly packed lobules and trabeculae. Basal cell carcinomas can be subdivided into solid basal cell carcinomas, keratinizing basal cell carcinomas (basosquamous carcinoma), and clear cell basal cell carcinomas. The solid basal cell carcinoma is a circumscribed, irregular dermal mass composed of multiple epithelial cell aggregates of varying size and shape. The boundaries of the neoplasm are not well demarcated from the adjacent dermis. The keratinizing basal cell carcinoma is an irregular dermal mass comprising epithelial cell aggregates that vary considerably in size and shape; a plaque-like configuration is common. The center of many epithelial islands displays abrupt squamous differentiation and keratinization. The clear cell basal cell carcinoma is structurally identical to the solid basal cell carcinoma. The cells are large and polygonal and have a characteristic water-clear, fine granular cytoplasm that gives the tumor its name.

In traditional classification of basal cell tumors, histopathologic analysis reveals basal cells with prominent oval nuclei and relatively little cytoplasm. The cells are usually small and uniform in size and lack intercellular bridges. Some basal cell tumors contain abundant amounts of melanin. They are subclassified as solid, cystic, ribbon, or medusoid, based on their histologic appearance (Pulley and Stannard, 1990).

Therapy. The treatment of choice for basal cell tumors is surgical excision. Cryosurgery is an alternative approach.

Squamous Cell Carcinoma: Bowen's Disease

Multicentric squamous cell carcinoma in situ (Bowen's disease) has been reported in cats (Miller et al, 1992; Turrel and Gross, 1991) and in dogs (Gross and Brimacomb, 1986; Gross et al, 1992).

Clinical Features and Diagnosis. In cats, no breed predilection exists, and the median age at onset ranges from 11.5 to 13.5 years. This tumor is not solar induced. The lesions are located predominantly on the head, digits, neck, thorax, shoulders, and ventral abdomen. In some cases the skin becomes pigmented and then ulcerates in the center of the lesion. Lesions expand peripherally, and some lesions are greater than 4 cm in diameter. The tumors may also appear as raised, red, crusted lesions that subsequently ulcerate and may intermittently bleed. In dogs, multifocal intraepidermal carcinoma that histologically resembled Bowen's disease is plaque-like, nodular or verrucous, and sometimes covered with dark brown or black scale. The lesions are seen on the glabrous skin of the abdomen and on the feet near the carpal and tarsal pads. The mucous membranes of the mouth and genitalia may be affected. Lesions begin in sun-exposed, glabrous skin and progress to hairy skin and mucous membranes (Gross and Brimacomb, 1986).

Diagnosis is made by excisional biopsy. Unlike solar-associated squamous cell carcinoma, the neoplastic epidermal cells do not penetrate the basement membrane into the surrounding dermis (carcinoma in situ) except late in the course of the disease. The lesions are characterized microscopically by proliferation of dysplastic, highly disordered keratinocytes that replace normal epidermis and sometimes the follicular infundibula.

Therapy. Successful treatment consists of radiation therapy with strontium 90 to a total dose of 150 Gy. Lesions heal in 4 to 6 weeks with no recurrence, although new lesions requiring radiation therapy often develop at other sites. Successful surgical excision and spontaneous remission do occur. Strontium 90 plesiotherapy results in partial regression of plaques but does not cure large, thick plaques.

Sebaceous Gland Tumors

Sebaceous gland tumors are epithelial growths arising from sebaceous gland cells; their cause is unknown. They are a common skin tumor in dogs, accounting for 6 to 35 per cent of all skin tumors (Susaneck and Withrow, 1989). They are rare in cats. Sebaceous gland tumors can be histologically classified as nodular hyperplasia, sebaceous adenoma, sebaceous epithelioma, sebaceous nevus, or sebaceous adenocarcinoma.

Clinical Features and Diagnosis. These tumors occur in dogs and cats; average age at diagnosis is 9 to 10 years. No sex or breed predilection exists in cats. However, in dogs, the cocker spaniel, Kerry blue terrier, Boston terrier, poodle, beagle, dachshund, Norwegian elkhound, and basset hound are predisposed (Muller et al, 1989). These tumors can affect any area of the body but are found most often on the head, neck, legs, dorsal and lateral aspect of the trunk, and anus. They may occur singly or at multiple sites.

Nodular sebaceous hyperplasia usually consists of single or multiple, 2- to 10-mm-diameter, firm, elevated, well-circumscribed, alopecic, shiny, dome-shaped or papillated, pink to yellowish masses with a waxy to pearly quality (Fig. 12–13). Sebaceous adenomas are solitary or multiple and tend to be larger (up to 2 to 3 cm in diameter) and less lobulated. The overlying skin is alopecic and sometimes ulcerated. Sebaceous epitheliomas are clinically similar to basal cell tumors; they are usually solitary, firm, nodular or plaque-like masses ranging from several millimeters to several centimeters in diameter. Surface ulceration is frequent. Sebaceous nevi appear as alopecic, scaly plaques less than 2 cm in diameter and with irregular or papillated surfaces. Sebaceous adenocarcinomas are usually solitary, firm, poorly circumscribed nodules less than 4 cm in diameter. Alopecia and ulceration are common.

Diagnosis is made by excisional biopsy. Sebaceous hyperplasia displays greatly enlarged sebaceous glands composed of numerous lobules grouped around centrally located sebaceous ducts. Sebaceous adenomas typically comprise multiple large lobules of sebaceous cells that

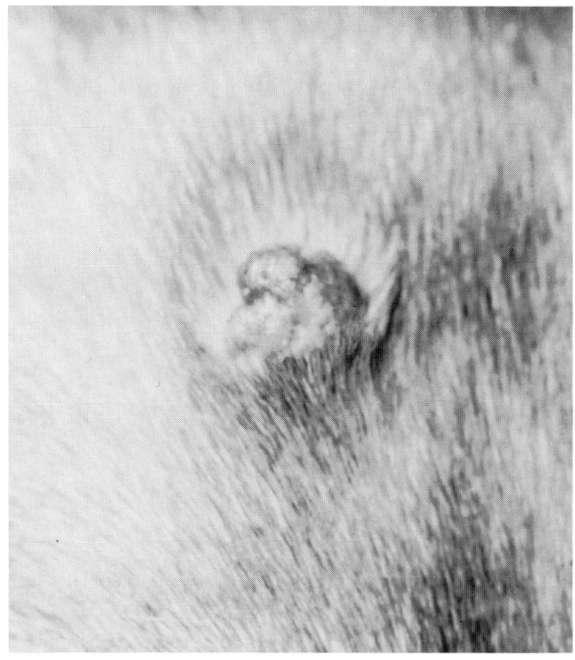

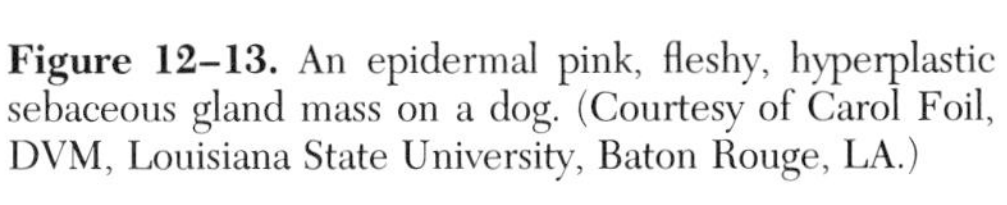

Figure 12–13. An epidermal pink, fleshy, hyperplastic sebaceous gland mass on a dog. (Courtesy of Carol Foil, DVM, Louisiana State University, Baton Rouge, LA.)

show normal maturation. In contrast to sebaceous hyperplasia, the lobules are not oriented around ducts or follicular infundibula. Sebaceous nevus is a plaque-like lesion covered by hyperplastic, hyperkeratotic epidermis that has a papillated configuration (Gross et al, 1992). Sebaceous glands are large, numerous, and randomly distributed through the superficial dermis. Sebaceous epitheliomas are composed of multiple lobules of basaloid epithelial cells. Sebaceous adenocarcinoma is an irregular, circumscribed, multilobular dermal neoplasm composed of islands of pleomorphic polygonal cells with atypia.

Therapy. Surgical excision, cryotherapy, electrosurgery, or observation without treatment are clinical management options for sebaceous nodular hyperplasia, sebaceous adenoma, sebaceous epithelioma, and sebaceous nevus. Sebaceous adenocarcinomas should be completely surgically excised.

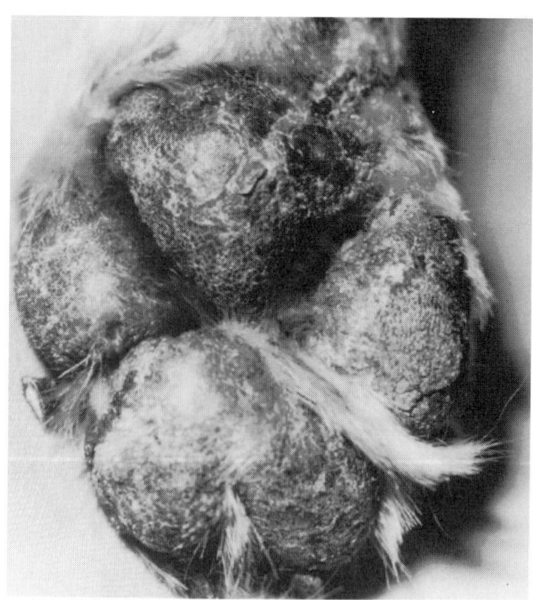

Figure 12–14. Small, round, pigmented melanoma on the central pad (upper right corner) of a dog. (Courtesy of Carol Foil, DVM, Louisiana State University, Baton Rouge, LA.)

Melanocytic Tumors

Benign and malignant melanomas together make up 5 to 9 per cent of all skin tumors in dogs (Aronsohn and Carpenter, 1990; Madewell and Theilen, 1987). Melanoma is rare in the cat, accounting for less than 2 per cent of all feline tumors (Gross et al, 1992; Patnaik and Mooney, 1988).

Clinical Features and Diagnosis. Melanomas occur in both dogs and cats, with an average age at diagnosis of 9 years. In cats, no breed or sex predilection exists. In dogs, Scottish terriers, Boston terriers, Airedale terriers, cocker and springer spaniels, boxers, Irish setters, Irish terriers, chow chows, Chihuahuas, and Doberman pinschers are predisposed; males are affected more commonly than females (Muller et al, 1989). In dogs, tumors are usually solitary, dome shaped, and pigmented and have a uniform, smooth appearance (Fig. 12–14). The overlying epidermis is usually intact and hairless, and the tumors vary from 0.5 cm to several centimeters in diameter (Goldschmidt and Shofer, 1992). Some melanomas lack pigmentation and have a pale to dark red color. Melanomas occur most commonly on the face, trunk, feet, and scrotum (Muller et al, 1989). At mucocutaneous junctions the tumor appears as a pedunculated, pigmented, glistening nodule or mass measuring 1 to 4 cm in diameter (Madewell and Theilen, 1987). In cats, melanomas are hyperpigmented and occur most commonly on the head, especially the ears. They vary in color from gray to black and range in size from 0.3 to 2 cm in diameter.

Malignant melanomas in dogs are usually rapidly growing and larger than 2 cm in diameter; ulceration is common. Most malignant melanomas are sessile, but occasionally they are polypoid or plaque-like. Eyelids, digits, and the trunk are common sites in dogs. In cats, malignant melanomas usually present as ulcerated, solitary, elevated, alopecic intradermal masses, often red to red-brown in color. They range from 0.3 to 2.5 cm in diameter. The face and digits are preferential sites in cats (Goldschmidt and Shofer, 1992; Gross et al, 1992).

Diagnosis is made by excisional biopsy. Differentiating benign from malignant lesions can be challenging. Important criteria that suggest malignancy in the dog are metastasis, a mitotic index greater than or equal to 3 mitoses per 10 high power fields, nuclear and nucleolar pleomorphism, and location of the melanoma. Malignant melanomas often arise from the mucocutaneous junction, oral cavity, and subungual area. Because melanomas are rare in cats, specific criteria for differentiating benign from malignant tumors have not been established (Goldschmidt and Shofer, 1992).

Therapy. Wide surgical excision is the treatment of choice. Malignant melanomas often recur and metastasize via lymphatic and hematogenous routes. Regional lymph node and lung metastases are common findings. Other metastasis sites include the brain, heart, liver, kidney, and spleen. Local recurrence is most frequently encountered with dermal tumors that are inva-

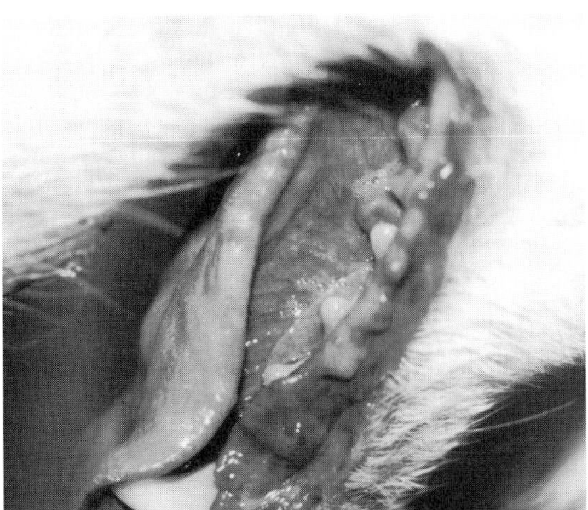

Figure 12–15. Ulceration at the mucocutaneous junction of the mouth in an 8-year-old Samoyed with cutaneous epitheliotrophic lymphoma.

sive and arising at mucocutaneous junctions. Prognosis for dogs is not influenced by age, sex, location, size, presence or absence of ulceration, or histologic cell type or other histologic features (Aronsohn and Carpenter, 1990). Feline malignant melanoma often recurs at the surgical site (67 per cent) (Goldschmidt and Shofer, 1992). Metastasis to regional lymph nodes occurs in 50 per cent of cases. Metastatic lesions can be found in any organ but are especially common in the lungs. Cryotherapy appears to have no benefit over conventional surgery. Malignant melanomas are generally radioresistant, and chemotherapy has not been successful.

Cutaneous Lymphosarcoma

Cutaneous lymphosarcoma is characterized by an infiltration of neoplastic lymphoid cells. Primary cutaneous lymphosarcoma can be classified as either epitheliotrophic (i.e., tumor cells accumulating in the epidermal or adnexal epithelium) or nonepitheliotrophic. Epitheliotrophic lymphosarcoma includes cutaneous T-cell lymphoma, cutaneous lymphoma, cutaneous lymphosarcoma, mycosis fungoides, and lymphoproliferative disease resembling pagetoid reticulosis. Cutaneous lymphosarcoma and leukemia resembling Sézary's syndrome have also been reported in the dog and cat (Schick et al, 1989; Thrall et al, 1984). In humans, nonepitheliotrophic lymphosarcoma is presumed to be of B-cell origin, and epitheliotrophic lymphosarcoma is presumed to be of T-cell origin. Epitheliotrophic lymphosarcomas in cats and one case in the dog were of T-cell origin (Caciolo et al, 1984; DeBoer et al, 1990).

Clinical Features and Diagnosis. Clinical features of epitheliotrophic lymphosarcoma are highly varied. In dogs, different stages occur as the lymphosarcoma progresses. The first stage includes macular, erythematous lesions with scale. The lymphosarcoma then progresses to a plaque stage consisting of firm, raised, pink to reddish purple brown papules that coalesce to form smooth solid erythematous scaling plaques. The tumor stage occurs thereafter. These tumors are firm and sessile and may be brightly erythematous. The tumors may either regress spontaneously or enlarge, ulcerate, and become infected. Some lymphosarcomas in dogs do not always have distinct stages. In a retrospective study, 80 per cent of such cases had patchy to generalized erythema, 61.5 per cent had plaques and scaling, 57.7 per cent had nodules, 42.3 per cent had ulcerations, and 38.5 per cent had pruritus and crusting. Mucosal lesions were seen in 38.5 per cent of the cases (Beale and Bolon, 1992) (Figs. 12–15 and 12–16). Peripheral lymphadenopathy is present in 30.8 per cent of the cases. Mucosal lesions may be the only clinical signs of epitheliotrophic lymphosarcoma.

Nonepitheliotrophic lymphosarcoma in dogs is similar to the epitheliotrophic form but may appear as nodular, possibly solitary, masses of varying size. Ulceration, erythema, scaling, and alopecia are common. An unusual presentation includes multiple, firm, raised, erythematous, serpiginous or branching cutaneous tracts that are bilaterally symmetric (Beale et al, 1990b). In cats, cutaneous lymphosarcoma (epitheliotrophic

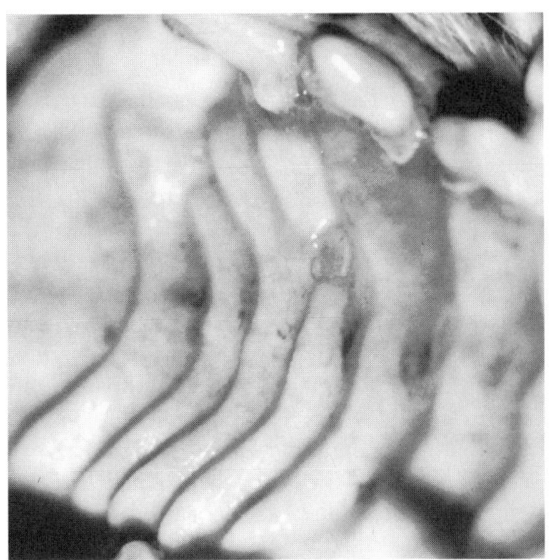

Figure 12–16. Ulceration on the hard palate of the dog shown in Figure 12–15.

and nonepitheliotrophic) can present in the patch, plaque, or tumor stage. The tumor often begins as a single plaque, with additional plaques appearing as the tumor progresses. Tumor progression is more common in cats than in dogs (Goldschmidt and Shofer, 1992). Lesions also appear to be more pruritic in cats, leading to self-trauma and ulceration. Solitary nodules are more common in cats.

Diagnosis is made by excisional biopsy of the skin and/or mucosa. Nonepitheliotrophic lymphosarcoma is characterized by a nodular to diffuse infiltration of homogeneous neoplastic lymphocytes in the dermis and subcutis. Neoplastic lymphocytes are infrequently noted within the epidermis, and dermal adnexa are usually effaced by tumor cells. Epitheliotrophic lymphosarcoma is characterized by progressive accumulation of neoplastic cells within the epidermis and adnexal epithelium. The histopathology findings vary depending on the lymphosarcoma stage. Early exfoliative lesions in dogs are characterized by small numbers of intraepithelial lymphocytes that are not overtly neoplastic (Gross et al, 1992). In the plaque and nodule stages, lymphocytes increase in number and appear more malignant, being characterized by large, pale nuclei with a convoluted contour. The skin of cats tends to retain morphologically well differentiated lymphocytes even in advanced stages (Gross et al, 1992). In the plaque and nodule stages, the epidermis becomes thickened and contains infiltrating lymphocytes. Groups of neoplastic lymphocytes in the epidermis are termed *Pautrier's microabscess.* The dermis contains similar neoplastic lymphocytes that frequently obscure the dermoepidermal junction. This phenomenon is referred to as a *lichenoid band* (i.e., cells hugging the dermoepidermal junction). As the disease progresses, the lymphocytes form dense infiltrates in the superficial dermis (plaque stage) or extend into the deep dermis and panniculus (tumor stage).

Therapy. Most cases of cutaneous lymphosarcoma in dogs and cats progress, resulting in additional cutaneous lesions and metastasis to regional lymph nodes and internal organs. Treatment trials in animals have used several systemic chemotherapeutic agents, including prednisolone, prednisone, vincristine, cyclophosphamide, polyethylene glycol (PEG) L-asparaginase, mechlorethamine, and methotrexate, but results have been poor (McKeever et al, 1982; Moriello et al, 1992; Zenoble and George, 1980). Many therapies are palliative, designed to control the erythema and scaling, but do not lengthen the survival time of the patient. In addition, mechlorethamine (topical nitrogen mustard) can be a potent contact sensitizer and is itself potentially carcinogenic. Isotretinoin at a dosage of 1 to 2 mg/kg has been used and is well tolerated in dogs and cats. This therapy is only palliative; cure is not achieved, but the length and quality of life in treated animals are improved (Kwochka, 1989). In dogs, response to isotretinoin may be dose dependent, and a higher dose (3 mg/kg) may produce a better response (Power and Ihrke, 1990). Etretinate at 0.75 to 1.0 mg/kg/day has been used, with equivocal clinical response. The average time from onset of clinical signs to diagnosis is 6.5 months, with the average time from diagnosis until euthanasia or natural death being 4.5 months (Walton, 1986).

TESTICULAR TUMORS

Dermatologic manifestations of testicular tumors (i.e., Sertoli cell tumors, interstitial cell tumors, and seminomas) are uncommon in the dog. Dermatologic manifestations occur most commonly in the male feminization syndrome (mostly with Sertoli cell tumors), but may also occur with other testicular tumors (Muller et al, 1989).

Clinical Features and Diagnosis. Testicular tumors usually occur in middle-age to older dogs, with the average age at diagnosis being 9 years for Sertoli cell tumors, 11.5 years for interstitial cell tumors, and 10 years for seminomas (Postorino, 1989). Breeds predisposed to testicular tumors include boxers, Shetland sheepdogs, weimaraners, German shepherd dogs, Cairn terriers, Pekingese, and collies (Feldman and Nelson, 1987; Madewell and Theilen, 1987; Muller et al, 1989). Male dogs with feminization syndrome display dermatologic signs of bilaterally symmetric alopecia that is nonpruritic. The alopecia usually begins in the perineal and genital regions and spreads to the ventral abdomen, thorax, flank, and neck (Fig. 12–17). In chronic cases, generalized truncal alopecia may be seen. The haircoat may be dull and dry. Hyperpigmentation is variable but is usually present. Other signs include gynecomastia, lactation, pendulous prepuce, attraction from other male dogs, decreased libido, and standing in a female posture to urinate (Feldman and Nelson, 1987; Rosser, 1993). Signs caused by excess androgens include tail gland hyperplasia, perianal gland hyperplasia or neoplasia, and benign prostatic hypertrophy (Rosser, 1993). Other dermatologic manifestations of testicular tumors include seborrhea, ceruminous oti-

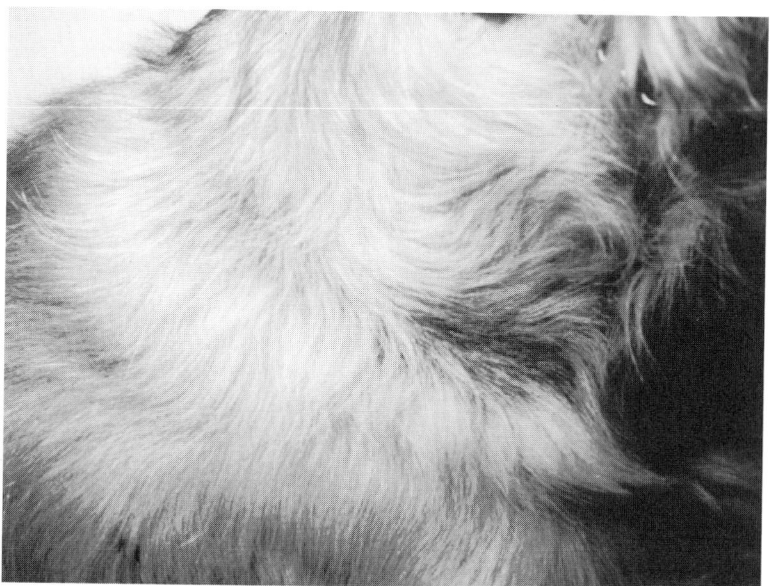

Figure 12–17. Neck alopecia in a golden retriever with a Sertoli cell tumor.

tis externa, macular melanosis of the inguinal and perianal skin, and a linear erythematous or melanotic macular change along the ventral aspect of the prepuce and extending to the scrotum (Fig. 12–18) (Griffin and Rosenkrantz, 1986; Miller, 1989). Occasionally a dog will be quite pruritic and have a papular eruption (White, 1989).

Clinical suspicion of testicular tumor is based on the presence of a combination of physical examination findings. Testicular examination may reveal testicular dyssymmetry, with the nontumorous testicle being soft and atrophic as a result of excess sex hormone production from the tumorous testicle. Occasionally there is no palpable testicular abnormality. Castration and submission of both testicles for histopathologic evaluation should be the first diagnostic recommendation to the owner. If tumor is present, histologic examination of the testicle will confirm the type of tumor. If the owner requests other diagnostic tests before electing for castration, serum samples can be submitted to measure estradiol, progesterone, and testosterone levels. In most cases, one of these hormones will be elevated (Rosser,

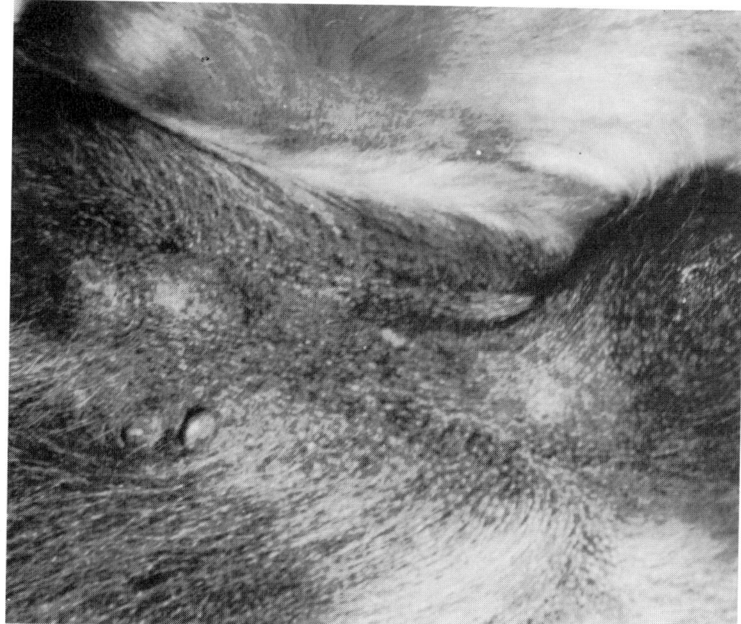

Figure 12–18. Linear preputial erythema in a dog with a Sertoli cell tumor.

1993). However, normal hormone values do not rule out a testicular tumor. Skin biopsies can support the presence of a hormonally related skin disease, but the changes are not specific for testicular tumors. Histologic skin changes include orthokeratotic hyperkeratosis, epidermal atrophy with or without melanosis, follicular keratosis, follicular dilatation, follicular atrophy, predominance of telogen hair follicles, and sebaceous gland atrophy.

Therapy. Castration is the treatment of choice. Dogs that have blood dyscrasia or bone marrow hypoplasia as the result of an estrogen-secreting testicular tumor will require additional adjunctive treatment. Advanced bone marrow suppression carries a grave prognosis for recovery. Cutaneous improvement will be seen within 3 months after castration. If metastatic disease occurs, chemotherapy or radiation therapy may be attempted. Sertoli cell tumors are somewhat responsive to cyclophosphamide, vinblastine, or methotrexate therapy, whereas seminomas are radiosensitive and also responsive to cyclophosphamide and vincristine (Feldman and Nelson, 1987; Postorino, 1989). The prognosis for patients with metastatic testicular neoplasia is guarded to poor.

PHEOCHROMOCYTOMA

Pheochromocytomas are uncommon endocrine tumors arising from the adrenal medulla. Clinical signs result from excessive production of catecholamines and local invasive spread of the tumor.

Clinical Features and Diagnosis. Pheochromocytomas occur most often in older dogs; there is no breed or sex predilection. Because of episodic secretion of tumor catecholamine, signs may be subtle or not evident. Respiratory signs are common and are characterized by episodic panting or dyspnea and increased bronchovesicular sounds. Other signs include episodic weakness, polyuria, polydipsia, muscle tremors, anorexia, weight loss, emaciation, cardiac arrhythmias, systolic murmur, lethargy, and depression. The dermatologic manifestation is intermittent flushing of the pinna (Wheeler, 1986).

There are no consistent abnormalities encountered in laboratory evaluation of dogs with pheochromocytomas. Hypertension may be present intermittently. Abdominal radiographs will identify an adrenal mass in about 35 per cent of cases. Vena caval venography should be performed in all suspect cases, because tumor thrombus invading the posterior vena cava is common. Ultrasonography is superior to abdominal radiography when examining the adrenal glands in dogs. Determination of the urinary excretion of catecholamines or their metabolites is most reliable in the diagnosis of pheochromocytoma.

Therapy. Therapy for pheochromocytoma consists of surgical excision. Medical therapy is needed before surgery to stabilize the cardiovascular and metabolic status of the patient, as well as to control blood pressure and cardiac arrhythmias. Surgical success is dependent on the invasive nature of the adrenal tumor. Most tumors are associated with only one adrenal gland.

PARASITIC DERMATOSIS

Demodicosis

Demodectic mange of the dog is caused by *Demodex canis.* Demodectic mange of the cat is caused by *Demodex cati* and another as-yet-unnamed species of *Demodex.* Two types of canine demodicosis are generally recognized: localized and generalized. It is important to differentiate between localized and generalized, because therapeutic intervention and prognosis are very different. Localized demodicosis is found more often in the juvenile animal, whereas generalized demodicosis is found in both the juvenile and the adult. Adult-onset canine generalized demodicosis is most likely caused by suppression of the immune system. Several factors have been suggested as initiating canine generalized demodicosis; these include administration of immuno-

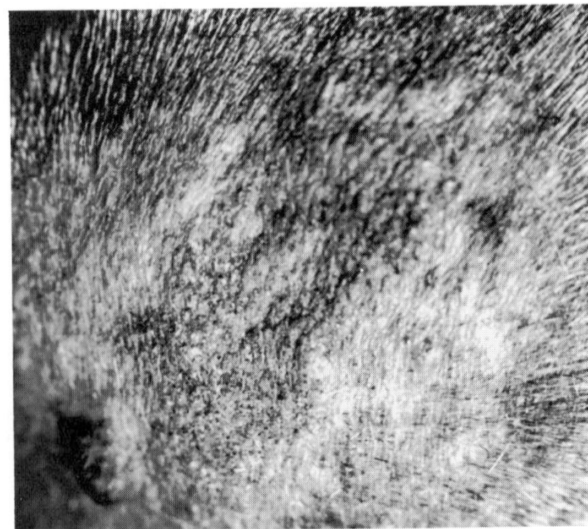

Figure 12–19. Area of alopecia, erythema, and follicular plugging (comedones) associated with demodicosis on a dog.

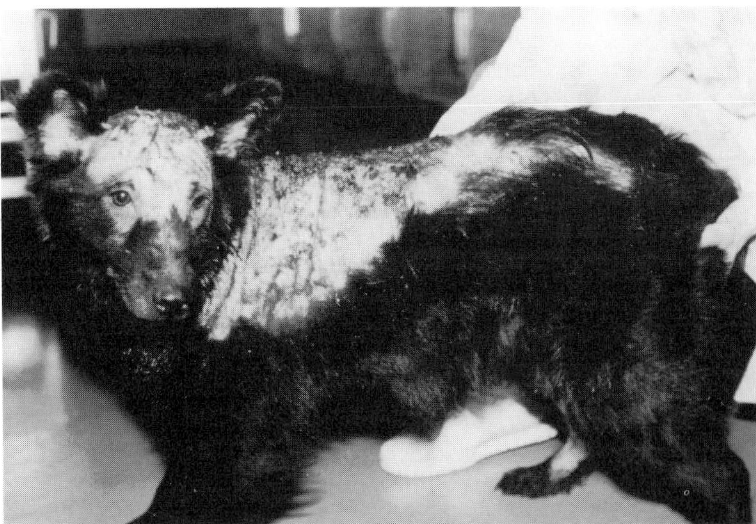

Figure 12–20. Chow chow dog with generalized demodicosis that began on the head and progressed caudally down the back.

suppressive drugs and serious systemic disease, including hyperadrenocorticism, hypothyroidism, diabetes mellitus, blastomycosis and other deep mycoses, lymphosarcoma, hemangiosarcoma, and mammary adenocarcinoma.

Because most cases of feline demodectic mange occur in adults, immunosuppression caused by an underlying disease has been proposed as the initiating factor. Generalized demodicosis has been seen in cats with diabetes mellitus, respiratory infection, feline leukemia virus infection (FeLV), systemic lupus erythematosus, toxoplasmosis, feline endocrine alopecia, feline immunodeficiency virus (FIV), hyperadrenocorticism, feline infectious peritonitis (FIP), and neoplasia. Immunosuppressive drugs (glucocorticoids and progestational compounds) should also be considered as potential initiating factors (Batey and Thompson, 1981; Chalmer et al, 1989; Kwochka, 1993; Medleau et al, 1988; Scott, 1980; Stogdale and Moore, 1982; White et al, 1987; Zerbe et al, 1987).

Localized demodicosis is usually seen as circumscribed patches of alopecia with various degrees of follicular plugging, erythema, scaling, and hyperpigmentation (Fig. 12–19). The lesions tend to be seen on the head, neck, and forelimbs. Generalized demodicosis can be seen on any area of the body, many times beginning cranially and progressing caudally (Fig. 12–20). Generalized patches of alopecia or diffuse alopecia with erythema, scaling, crusting, and follicular plugging are seen (Fig. 12–21). Secondary bacterial infection may be superficial and characterized by pustules or papules or deep and characterized by furunculosis, which can progress to painful cellu-

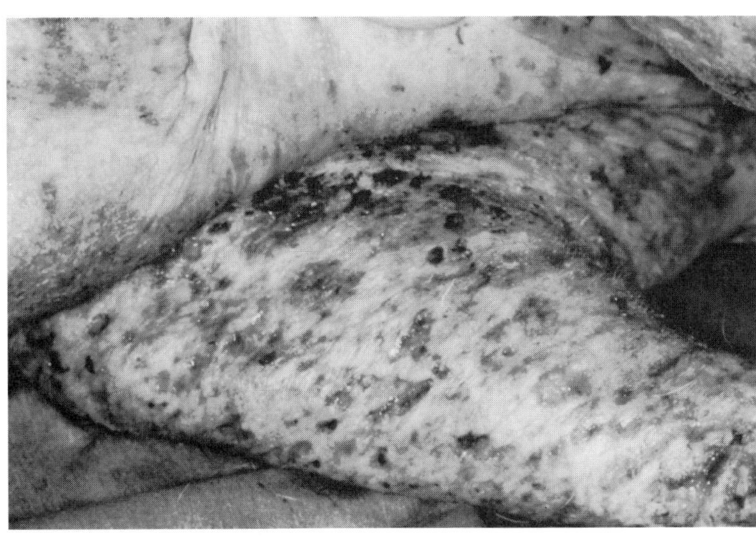

Figure 12–21. Deep bacterial furunculosis and cellulitis associated with adult-onset generalized demodicosis in a Dalmatian dog.

litis. Pruritus and peripheral lymphadenopathy are seen most often in dogs with demodicosis complicated by a secondary bacterial infection. In some cases infections are confined to the feet. Such cases should be considered generalized for therapeutic purposes, because the treatment and prognosis are more closely aligned with those for generalized demodicosis than those for localized demodicosis (Fig. 12–22).

Localized demodicosis in cats can be seen as a single area of alopecia and scaling of the eyelids, periocular area, head, and neck (Fig. 12–23). Localized ceruminous otitis externa also occurs (Scott, 1980). Signs of generalized demodicosis secondary to *Demodex cati* infestation include multifocal to generalized patches of alopecia with variable scaling; macules; papules; erythema; hyperpigmentation; crusting; and symmetric alopecia of the head, neck, legs, and trunk. Pruritus, when present, may be intermittent or mild. Clinical signs associated with the unnamed species of *Demodex* include more severe pruritus; mild erythema; broken hairs; and alopecia of the hindlimbs, flank, and ventral abdomen. In some cats, mild clinical signs and patterns of involvement have been such that the condition could mimic psychogenic alopecia (Scott, 1980).

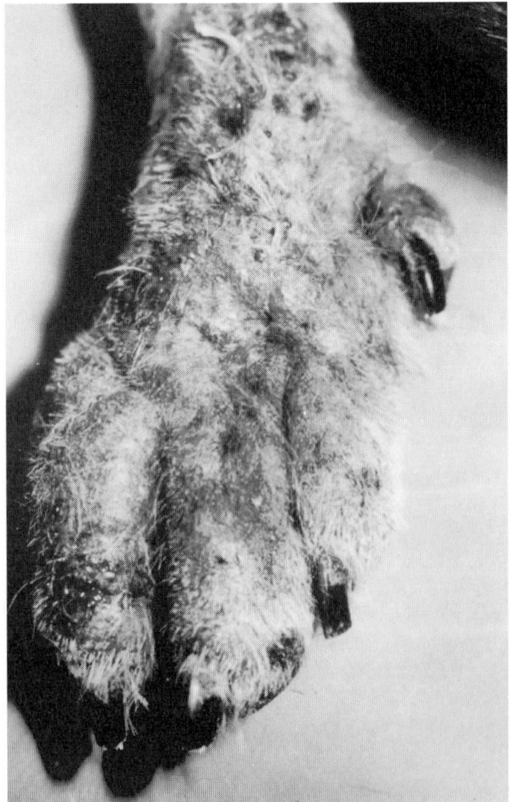

Figure 12–22. Chronic demodicosis on the foot with erythema alopecia, hyperpigmentation, and a secondary deep bacterial infection.

Differential diagnosis for demodicosis includes any other reason for hair follicle infection or infestation (folliculitis). The most important differential diagnoses include bacterial infection and dermatophytosis. All animals with significant skin disease should undergo skin scraping for *Demodex* mites, which are best found with concentrated deep skin scrapings performed with a *dull* No. 10 scapel blade (Fig. 12–24). A minimum of three to five areas should be scraped to differentiate localized from generalized demodicosis. Sites that should be scraped include lesions, the lip area, and interdigital spaces. Skin biopsy may have to be performed (especially in the Chinese shar pei) to make the diagnosis. A substantial number of live adult mites or immature forms and eggs are needed to confirm the diagnosis. In cats, one species of *Demodex* mites lives in the stratum corneum, whereas the other occupies hair follicles; therefore, both superficial skin scrapings over large areas and deep, concentrated skin scrapings must be performed. Careful examination of the skin scraping slide is necessary, as the stratum corneum mite is more transparent and easily overlooked (Fig. 12–25).

When a diagnosis of adult-onset generalized demodicosis has been made, the veterinarian should begin a thorough search for any predisposing factors or underlying immunosuppressive or serious metabolic disease (Kwochka, 1993). In all cases of generalized demodicosis and adult-onset localized demodicosis in dogs, a complete medical evaluation should be performed. A thorough physical examination, complete blood cell count, serum chemistry panel, fecal flotation, heartworm test, and urinalysis are the minimum evaluations required. A low-dose dexamethasone suppression test or TSH response test should be considered in a dog with any evidence of an endocrinopathy. Any animal with deep pustular disease associated with the demodicosis should undergo a bacterial culture and sensitivity test.

Diagnosis of localized demodicosis in older dogs and cats is cause for concern. It is prudent to look for underlying factors that may predispose the animal to the onset of the disease. Amitraz liquid concentrate is efficacious for localized demodicosis but should be reserved for generalized demodicosis. Topical therapies that may be used once daily on localized lesions include 1 per cent rotenone ointment or benzoyl peroxide gel. Pustular localized demodicosis should be treated with an appropriate antimicrobial for 2 weeks

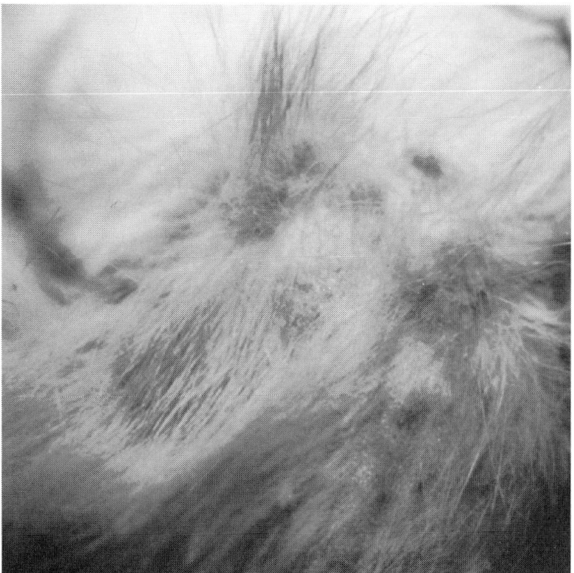

Figure 12–23. Excoriation with alopecia and erythema on the neck of a cat infested with superficial *Demodex* mites.

after resolution of the infection. Treatment of adult-onset generalized demodicosis is lengthy and expensive. The only drug approved by the U.S. Food and Drug Administration for treatment of generalized demodicosis is amitraz, approved for biweekly use at a concentration of 0.025 per cent, but weekly amitraz dips appear to be more efficacious than dips every 2 weeks (Kwochka et al, 1985). To achieve maximal results with amitraz dips, the veterinarian should follow the guidelines in Table 12–3.

Alternative Therapeutic Protocol for Use of Amitraz. In one clinical trial, application of a 12.5 per cent amitraz solution diluted to a 0.125 per cent solution (1 ml of concentrate solution per 100 ml of water) applied daily to half of the body on an alternating basis showed an overall resolution rate of 79 per cent (Medleau and Willemse, 1991). The average duration of treatment was 3.7 months. Dogs that previously did not respond to amitraz therapy had a resolution rate of 75 per cent with the daily amitraz treatment. No serious toxic reactions were seen. Follow-up periods varied from 4 to 12 months.

Alternative Therapeutic Options. In two independent studies, milbemycin oxime was used to treat cases of generalized demodicosis. Initial doses used in the first study varied from 0.5 to 0.82 mg/kg given daily for a minimum of 30 days. If the dogs were still positive after 90 days, the

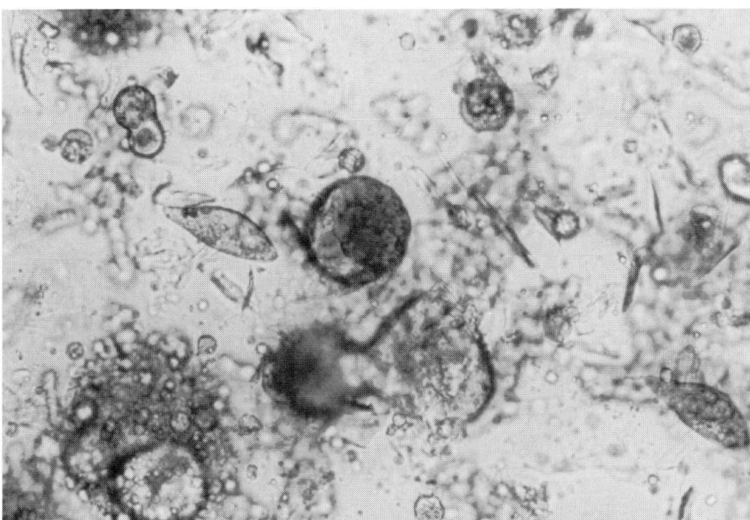

Figure 12–24. Skin scraping displaying *Demodex* mite eggs with red blood cells in the background.

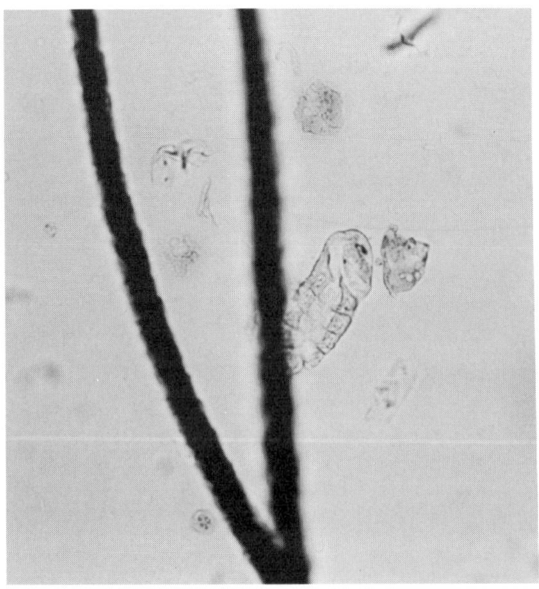

Figure 12–25. Superficial stratum corneum *Demodex* mite of the cat.

dose was increased to 1.0 to 1.14 mg/kg. Skin scrapings were evaluated every 30 days. After a negative skin scraping, dogs were treated for an additional 30 days. Remission (i.e., negative skin scraping results) was achieved in 83 per cent of dogs in one study; 16 per cent remained in remission for 12 months, 25 per cent remained in remission for 6 months, and 42 per cent relapsed (Reedy and Garfield, 1992). In a second study, remission was achieved in 82 per cent; 14 per cent relapsed shortly after the drug was discontinued, 28.6 per cent were in remission for 1 to 4 months, 21.5 per cent were in remission for 5 to 8 months, 7 per cent were in remission for 9 to 12 months, and 28.6 per cent were still in remission after 12 months (Miller and Scott, 1991).

Ivermectin has shown limited efficacy. Subcutaneous doses of 400 μg/kg given weekly for a total of 8 to 10 treatments showed no tangible benefit (Paradis, 1989; Scott and Walton, 1985). Another study reported efficacy at 600 μg/kg given weekly for five treatments in eight dogs with generalized demodicosis (Gravino et al, 1985). Yet another study used ivermectin on one dog at a dose of 600 μg/kg orally once daily; a negative skin scraping was obtained after 7 months of therapy. Therapy with 300 μg/kg of ivermectin was continued daily because of owner request (Paradis and Laperriere, 1992).

A 3 per cent aqueous trichlorfon solution used as a whole-body dip every 4 days has been effective, but no firm conclusions can be drawn because of the low number of animals treated (Kwochka, 1993).

Feline Generalized Demodicosis

Several treatment regimens have been used to treat feline generalized demodicosis, but no widely accepted successful treatment regimen exists. Treatments include weekly dips of lime sulfur, phosmet, or fenchlorphos (Medleau et al, 1988); 0.0125 per cent amitraz (half-strength) (Cowan and Campbell, 1988); carbaryl shampoo; malathion dips; and one part rotenone in three parts mineral oil for the ears (Muller et al, 1989). One author (Kwochka, 1993) recommends 2 per cent lime sulfur dips for six to eight treatments as the initial therapy, followed by malathion diluted to 0.25 ounce per gallon of water and applied weekly. Amitraz is another choice, with 0.0125 per cent dips performed weekly. If the cat tolerates the 0.0125 per cent amitraz well but is not cured after 8 to 10 dips, then a 0.025 per cent dip is applied weekly (Kwochka, 1993). Amitraz, fenchlorphos, and malathion are not approved for use in the cat. Organophosphate toxicity is a concern when fenchlorphos and malathion are used. Side effects of amitraz therapy in the cat are anorexia, depression, diarrhea, hypersalivation, and hiding under furniture (Cowan and Campbell, 1988; Gunaratnam et al, 1983). Generalized demodicosis in cats seems to be more responsive to therapy than that in dogs,

TABLE 12–3. GUIDELINES IN TREATMENT OF CANINE GENERALIZED DEMODICOSIS

1. A total-body clip is necessary, and the haircoat must be kept very short throughout the entire treatment period. This usually requires clipping the haircoat every 3 to 4 weeks.
2. Bathe the dog 12 to 24 hours before an amitraz dip in follicular-flushing benzoyl peroxide shampoo. If the bath is given immediately before the dip, towel dry the animal completely so as not to dilute the amitraz dip.
3. Train in-hospital personnel to use amitraz dip appropriately. The dipping procedure should consist of a good 10 to 15 minutes of dip contact time, with the person performing the dip continually gathering and repouring dip that has dripped off of the haircoat. The animal should be standing in the dip pooling in the bottom of the bathtub or dipping area. Most owners will not dip appropriately or for the appropriate length of time.
4. The amitraz dip must be made fresh and the solution used immediately, as the dipping solution quickly loses its efficacy and degrades to compounds potentially more toxic. For this reason, once the bottle of amitraz has been opened, the entire bottle should be used immediately.
5. Allow the animal to drip dry without toweling.
6. Monitor for any side effects. All dogs, if clipped and dipped appropriately, will have some degree of side effects after the first amitraz dip. These may be mild and will usually disappear with subsequent dips. The most common side effect is sedation or lethargy. This is usually transitory and lasts for 24 to 48 hours. Other side effects include anorexia, vomiting, diarrhea, pruritus, seizures, ataxia, hyperexcitability, personality change, hypothermia, appetite stimulation, bloat, polyuria, edema, erythema, and other various degrees of skin irritation. Yohimbine will reverse the side effects of amitraz therapy and can be given subcutaneously to effect (intravenously if acute probems are seen). The pretreatment dose is 0.03 mg/kg, and the post-treatment dose is 0.01 mg/kg. The subcutaneous dose will usually last for 4 to 6 hours.
7. The dog should be kept dry between applications. Powdered products should be used instead of liquid solution between dips (e.g., flea powders versus flea sprays).
8. Aggressively treat any secondary bacterial infection.
9. Monitor therapeutic success with serial skin scrapings every 2 to 4 weeks and record total mite counts. Note number of mites that are live, dead, mature (adults and nymphs), immature (larvae and eggs). Continue to skin scrape the five sites scraped for the original diagnosis. When one site is negative for two serial skin scrapings, delete that site and add another affected site to the areas monitored.
10. A positive therapeutic response initially consists of a decreased number of immature forms and eventually a decreased number of mature and live adults.
11. Continue amitraz dips for 1 month (two to four treatments) after the first negative skin scraping. Rescrape 1 month after the last dip. Follow through with skin scrapings every few months for 12 months.
12. If clinical or skin scraping improvement is not seen after 4 to 8 amitraz dips, increase dip solution to once-weekly (0.025 or 0.05 per cent) strength.
13. Additional therapy that may be used along with the amitraz dips consists of rotenone (Goodwinol) shampoo (in addition to benzoyl peroxide shampoo) before the dip and/or 400 IU of vitamin E given four times daily.
14. If scrapings of the feet or lips continue to test positive, daily application of 1 ml of amitraz in 29 ml of propylene glycol or mineral oil to the lesions may be helpful. This solution should be made weekly (if dipping weekly) or every other week (if dipping biweekly). Be sure to decrease the amount of water used to dilute the dip if the 1 ml of amitraz was removed from the amitraz bottle to make the painting solution.
15. If the animal is clinically normal but scrapings of the skin still test positive after 8 to 10 amitraz dips, consider a maintenance dip protocol or change to a different treatment.
16. A maintenance amitraz dip protocol will vary with the individual animal. Most dogs will have to be dipped every 2 to 4 weeks for the rest of their lives to remain asymptomatic. Unfortunately, long-haired dogs should remain closely clipped.
17. If the animal is still symptomatic after the amitraz dipping procedure described in step 12, consider a different treatment or a different dipping protocol.
18. All intact female dogs with adult-onset generalized demodicosis should be spayed once the mite counts have decreased significantly, as the stress of estrus may trigger a relapse of the disease. If amitraz dipping is done on a biweekly schedule, the spay should be done during the nondipping week. If the animal is being dipped weekly, do not dip with amitraz during the week of the spaying.

which may be a reflection of the more superficial location of the mites in many cases.

MISCELLANEOUS DISORDERS

Necrolytic Migratory Erythema

Necrolytic migratory erythema (diabetic dermatopathy, hepatocutaneous syndrome, superficial necrolytic dermatitis, or metabolic epidermal necrosis) may occur in dogs (average age at diagnosis, 10 years) with diabetes mellitus or glucagon-secreting tumors of the pancreas, but it is more often associated with hepatic disease. Either sex may be affected, but an almost 2:1 male-to-female ratio has been reported (Angarano, 1993).

Clinical Features and Diagnosis. Necrolytic migratory erythema is an ulcerative dermatosis, displaying erythema, crusts, and alopecia in the perioral and periocular areas (Fig. 12–26), legs, feet, and external genitalia area (Fig. 12–27). The footpads are usually hyperkeratotic (Fig. 12–28)

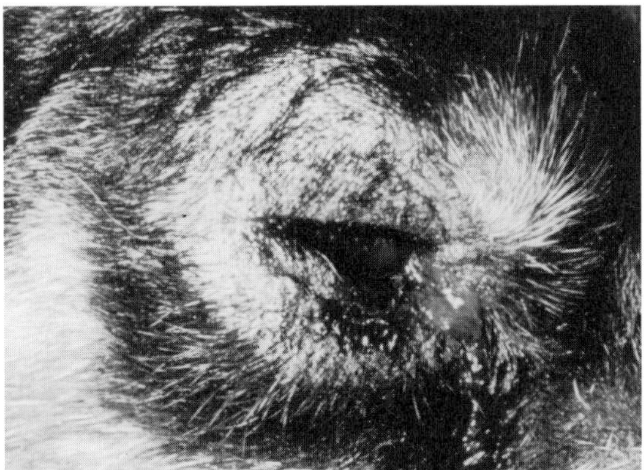

Figure 12–26. Periocular crusting on a miniature pinscher with necrolytic migratory erythema.

and may be fissured and ulcerated. Lesions often follow a waxing and waning course and may be mildly pruritic or painful. Cutaneous signs may precede evidence of internal disease by weeks to months (Angarano, 1993). The disease should be suspected on the basis of the history and physical examination findings and typically involves a middle-age or older dog with a progressive crusting dermatitis affecting the face, distal extremities, and external genitalia. Skin biopsies of affected dogs reveal a unique combination of diffuse parakeratotic hyperkeratosis, epidermal necrosis, marked superficial epidermal edema, irregular epidermal hyperplasia, and mild superficial perivascular dermatitis. The epidermal edema is intercellular and intracellular and localized to the upper half of the epidermis (Fig. 12–29). Severe edema may result in intraepidermal clefts and vesicles.

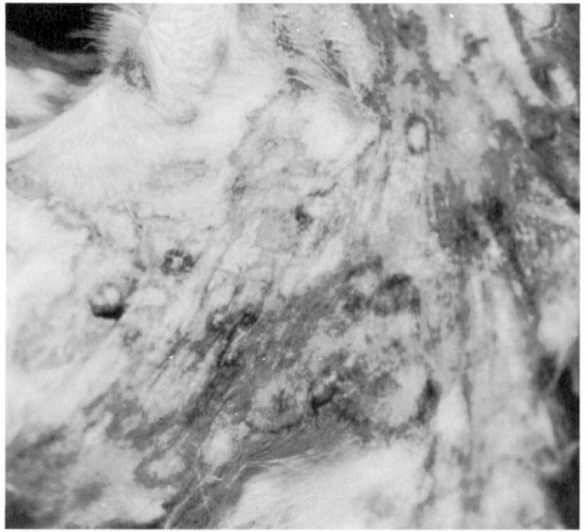

Figure 12–27. Circular ulcerations on the groin of a dog with necrolytic migratory erythema. (Courtesy of Carol Foil, DVM, Louisiana State University, Baton Rouge, LA.)

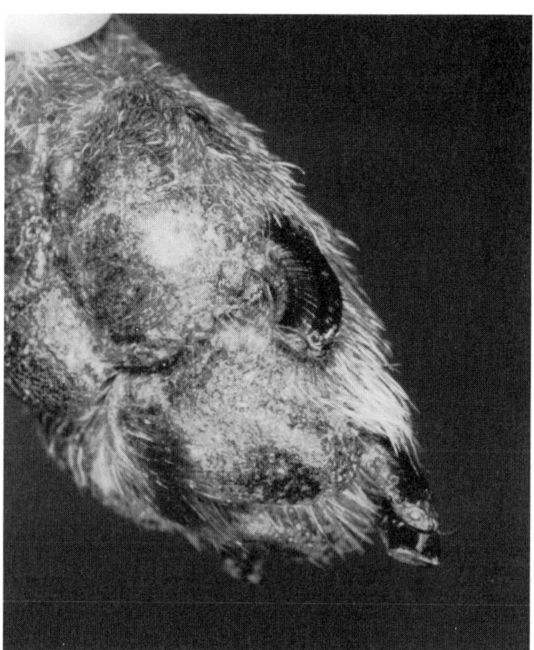

Figure 12–28. Footpad crusting on a miniature pinscher with necrolytic migratory erythema.

Clinicopathologic abnormalities vary depending on the inciting organ system and progression of the disease. Hematologic abnormalities include anemia and neutrophilic leukocytosis. Serum biochemical abnormalities include increased liver enzyme, total bilirubin, and bile acid levels. Hypoalbuminemia and hyperglycemia are common findings. Glucagon concentrations are increased in some cases.

Therapy. Treatment is aimed at correcting the underlying metabolic disease. If the dog is diabetic, insulin therapy is indicated, although glucose regulation is difficult. Surgical excision of a glucagon-secreting tumor of pancreatic alpha cells may be possible. Unfortunately, however, most cases are associated with irreversible chronic liver disease and cirrhosis, making treatment usually unrewarding. Therapy for the cutaneous manifestations is symptomatic. Antimicrobial and/or antifungal agents should be used to treat secondary infections. Hydrotherapy and shampoo therapy can help remove crusts and lessen the pruritus and pain. Glucocorticoid therapy has been associated with improvement in cutaneous signs, but should be used with caution, as it may worsen the underlying metabolic disease.

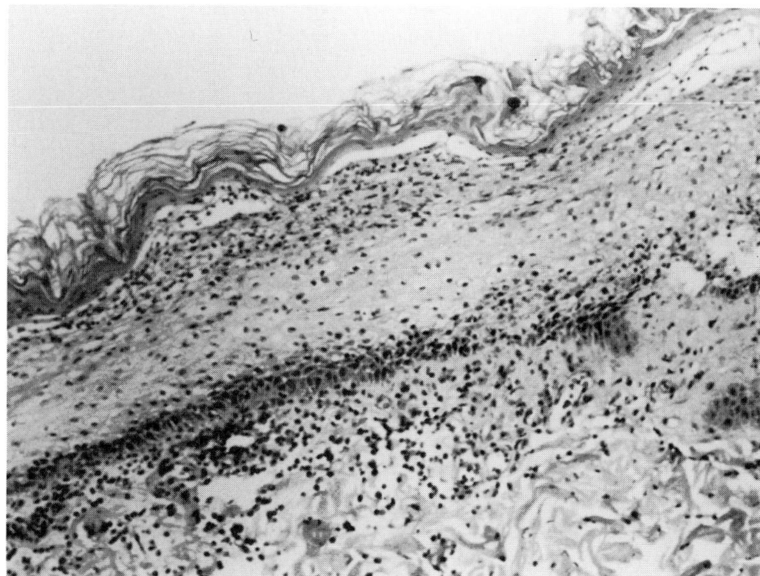

Figure 12–29. Epidermis displaying intracellular and intercellular edema in the stratum granulosum and stratum spinosum, characteristic of necrolytic migratory erythema (×400).

Nodular Dermatofibrosis

Nodular dermatofibrosis is a syndrome in the German shepherd dog that was first reported in Switzerland (Suter et al, 1983). Pedigree analysis suggests that the syndrome is inherited as an autosomal dominant trait (Lium and Moe, 1985). Renal abnormalities (e.g., cysts, adenomas, and adenocarcinomas) and an increased frequency of uterine leiomyomas are associated with the cutaneous nodular disease.

Clinical Features and Diagnosis. Nodular dermatofibrosis occurs in German shepherd or German shepherd mix dogs ranging from 3 to 11 years of age (Atlee et al, 1991). No sex predilection has been noted. Multiple collagenous nevi initially appear on the extremities and later on the head and trunk (Fig. 12–30). Nevi may precede signs of renal disease by up to 3 to 5 years (Muller et al, 1989). The nevi are usually firm, well circumscribed, and 0.5 to 5 cm in diameter. The nodules may be pigmented, haired, alopecic, pitted, or ulcerated. Lesions usually cause no signs unless ulcerated or in an area that hinders locomotion. With time, nodules can proliferate and become locally infiltrative. Clinical signs of

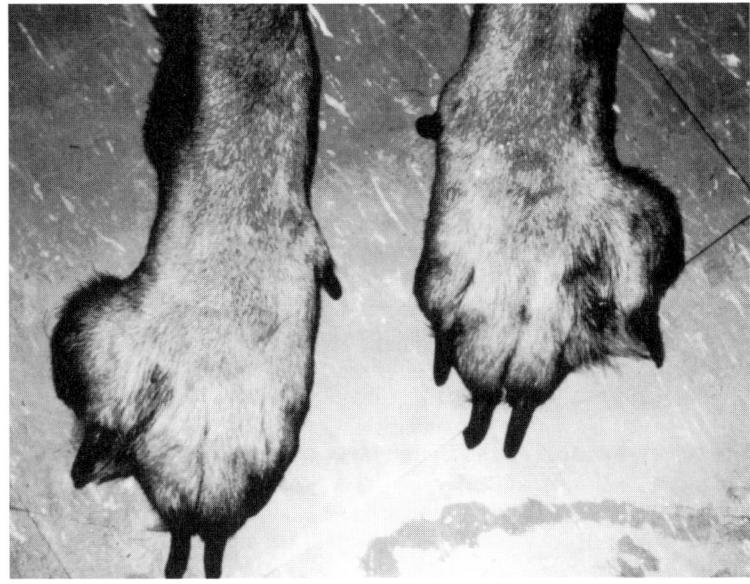

Figure 12–30. Nodules on the legs of a German shepherd dog with dermatofibrosis. (Courtesy of Carol Foil, DVM, Louisiana State University, Baton Rouge, LA.)

renal failure may not be present in affected dogs. Dogs that present with impaired renal function may have anorexia, polydipsia, vomiting, diarrhea, weight loss, abdominal distention, weakness, and uremia (Cosenza and Seely, 1986; Lium and Moe, 1985).

A German shepherd dog that presents with multiple cutaneous nodules should arouse clinical suspicion of nodular dermatofibrosis. A diagnostic work-up should include a hemogram, serum chemistry panel, urinalysis, abdominal radiographs and/or ultrasonography, and dermal nodule biopsy. Hematologic, serum chemistry, and urinalysis abnormalities will vary depending on the degree of renal impairment. Radiographs may reveal renomegaly, and ultrasound may document numerous renal cortical cysts of varying size. Skin biopsy reveals a subcutaneous nodule composed of irregular bundles of dense collagen fibers with few fibrocytes, and secondary inflammation with infiltrates of neutrophils and plasma cells is seen in some nodules. Uterine biopsies show interlacing bundles of smooth muscle fibers with characteristic cigar-shaped nuclei (Lium and Moe, 1985). Renal adenomas show parenchymal compression associated with multilobular cystic masses; cellular atypia and mitotic activity are absent. The adenocarcinomatous lesions range from multifocal hyperplasia to malignant renal tubular epithelial cell proliferations. Necropsy findings may include metastatic disease of lymph and blood vessels in regional lymph nodes, liver, and lungs (Lium and Moe, 1985).

Therapy. Treatment of dermal nodules may not be necessary, depending on their location and severity. Some nodules are surgically excised if they are ulcerated, infected, or in a location that hinders locomotion. Although progression of the disease is usually slow, long-term prognosis is guarded to poor owing to induced renal failure and metastatic disease.

Erythema Multiforme

Erythema multiforme is a cutaneous reaction pattern of multifactorial causes and is rarely seen in dogs and cats. An immunologic basis for the syndrome has been hypothesized, but most documented cases of erythema multiforme are associated with drug hypersensitivity; neoplasia and infection are less common causes (Gross et al, 1992). Erythema multiforme has been seen in older dogs without a history of drug hypersensitivity or concurrent disease.

Clinical Features and Diagnosis. No breed or sex predilection exists for old dogs with erythema multiforme. Lesions are acute in onset and appear as erythematous macules and papules. Crusting occurs as the lesions spread peripherally and form arciform patterns. Epidermal collarettes and annular target lesions with central clearing are seen at some stages of the syndrome. Widespread ulcers may evolve from urticarial or plaque-like lesions. The lesions are exudative, tend to be more proliferative than other subsets of erythema multiforme, and often involve the face and ears. Occult leukemias, pancreatic endocrine tumors, and *Pneumocystis* pneumonia have been identified in several affected dogs. Diagnosis is made by histopathologic examination of a skin biopsy. It is best to biopsy areas of erythema without crusting or ulceration, because an intact epidermis is necessary for the diagnosis. Individual cell necrosis of epidermal cells is the most characteristic histologic lesion of erythema multiforme. Acanthosis is present, and lymphocytes may closely surround the necrotic epidermal cells. Superficial follicular epidermal necrosis may be prominent.

Therapy. A search for an underlying disease is warranted, because there is no specific treatment for the skin disease. Correction of the underlying disease can possibly reverse the cutaneous signs. Symptomatic treatment of ulcerative skin disease and secondary bacterial infections (i.e., hydrotherapy, antibacterial shampoos, and antimicrobial agents) is indicated.

References

Angarano DW. Metabolic epidermal necrosis. In Griffin CE, Kwochka KW, MacDonald JM, eds. Current Veterinary Dermatology; The Science and Art of Therapy. St. Louis, Mosby–Year Book, 1993, p 303.

Aronsohn MG, Carpenter JL. Distal extremity melanocytic nevi and malignant melanomas in dog. J Am Anim Hosp Assoc 26:605, 1990.

Atlee BA, DeBoer DJ, Ihrke PJ. Nodular dermatofibrosis in German shepherd dogs as a marker for renal cystadenocarcinoma. J Am Anim Hosp Assoc 27:481, 1991.

August JR. Taking a dermatologic history. Compend Contin Educ Pract Vet 8:510, 1986.

Baker KP. Senile changes of dog skin. J Small Anim Pract 8:49, 1967.

Batey RG, Thompson RCA. Demodectic mange in a cat. Aust Vet J 57:49, 1981.

Beale KM, Bolon B. Canine cutaneous lymphosarcoma: Epitheliotrophic and non-epitheliotrophic, a retrospective study. Proc World Congress Vet Dermatol 2:94, 1992.

Beale KM, Dill-Macky E, Meyer DJ. An unusual presentation of cutaneous lymphoma in two dogs. J Am Anim Hosp Assoc 26:429, 1990.

Beale KM. Techniques for evaluating thyroid function in the dog. Vet Clin North Am 20:1429, 1990a.

Belshaw BE, Rijnberk A. Radioimmunoassay of plasma thyroxine and triiodothyronine in the diagnosis of primary hypothyroidism in dogs. J Am Anim Hosp Assoc 15:17, 1979.

Bruyette DS, Ruehl WW, Smidberg TL. L-Deprenyl therapy of canine pituitary dependent hyperadrenocorticism. Proc Am Coll Vet Intern Med Forum 11:927, 1993.

Buffington CA. Nutrition and the skin. Proc Ann Kal Kan Symp 11:11, 1987.

Caciolo PL, Nesbitt GH, Patnaik AK. Cutaneous lymphosarcoma in the cat: A report of nine cases. J Am Anim Hosp Assoc 20:491, 1984.

Chalmer S, Schick RO, Jeffers J. Demodicosis in two cats seropositive for feline immunodeficiency virus. J Am Vet Med Assoc 194:256, 1989.

Cosenza SF, Seely JC. Generalized nodular dermatofibrosis and renal cystadenocarcinomas in a German shepherd dog. J Am Vet Med Assoc 189:1587, 1986.

Cowan LA, Campbell K. Generalized demodicosis in a cat responsive to amitraz. J Am Vet Med Assoc 192:1442, 1988.

Daley CA, Zerbe CA, Schick RO, et al. Use of metyrapone to treat pituitary-dependent hyperadrenocorticism in a cat with large cutaneous wounds. J Am Vet Med Assoc 202:956, 1993.

DeBoer DJ, Turrel JM, Moore PF. Mycosis fungoides in a dog: Demonstration of T cell specificity and response to radiotherapy. J Am Anim Hosp Assoc 26:566, 1990.

Feldman EC, Nelson RW. Canine and Feline Endocrinology and Reproduction. Philadelphia, WB Saunders, 1987.

Ferguson DC. Thyroid function tests in the dog. Vet Clin North Am 14:783, 1984.

Ferguson DC. The effect of nonthyroidal factors on thyroid function tests in dogs. Compend Cont Educ Pract Vet 10:1365, 1988.

Goldschmidt MH, Shofer FS. Skin Tumors of the Dog and Cat. Oxford, Pergamon Press, 1992.

Gravino AE, Caprariis DE, Agresti A. Treatment of demodectic mange natural infestations of dogs with ivermectin. Acta Med Vet 31:185, 1985.

Griffin CE, Rosenkrantz W. Linear preputial erythema. Proc Ann Members Meeting Am Acad Vet Dermatol/Am Coll Vet Dermatol 35, 1986.

Gross TL, Brimacomb BH. Multifocal intraepidermal carcinoma in a dog histologically resembling Bowen's disease. Am J Dermatopathol 8:509, 1986.

Gross TL, Ihrke PJ, Walder EJ. Veterinary Dermatopathology: A Macroscopic and Microscopic Evaluation of Canine and Feline Skin Disease. St. Louis, Mosby–Year Book, 1992.

Gunaratnam P, Wilkinson GT, Seawright AA. A study of amitraz toxicity in cats. Aust Vet J 60:278, 1983.

Hall IA, et al. Effect of trimethoprim/sulfamethoxazole on thyroid function in dogs with pyoderma. J Am Vet Med Assoc 202:1959, 1993.

Helton-Rhodes K, Wallace M, Baer K. Cutaneous manifestations of feline hyperadrenocorticism. Proc World Congress Vet Dermatol 2:109, 1992.

Kwochka KW. Demodicosis. In Griffin CE, Kowchka KW, MacDonald JM, eds. Current Veterinary Dermatology; The Science and Art of Therapy. St. Louis, Mosby–Year Book, 1993, p 72.

Kwochka KW. Retinoids in dermatology. In Kirk RW, ed. Current Veterinary Therapy X. Philadelphia, WB Saunders, 1989, p 553.

Kwochka KW, Kunkle G, O'Neill CS. The efficacy of amitraz for generalized demodicosis in dogs: A study of two concentrations and frequencies of application. Compend Contin Educ Pract Vet 7:8, 1985.

Lium G, Moe I. Hereditary multifocal renal cystadenocarcinomas and nodular dermatofibrosis in the German shepherd dog: Macroscopic and histopathologic changes. Vet Pathol 22:447, 1985.

Madewell BR, Theilen GH. Tumors of the skin and subcutaneous tissues. In Theilen GH, Madewell BR, eds. Veterinary Cancer Medicine. Philadelphia, Lea & Febiger, 1987, p 233.

McKeever PJ, Grindem CB, Stevens JB. Canine cutaneous lymphoma. J Am Vet Med Assoc 180:531, 1982.

Medleau L, Brown CA, Brown SA. Demodicosis in cats. J Am Anim Hosp Assoc 24:85, 1988.

Medleau L, Willemse T. Efficacy of daily amitraz therapy for generalized demodicosis in dogs: Two independent studies. Proc Ann Members Meeting Am Acad Vet Dermatol/Am Coll Vet Dermatol 7:41, 1991.

Miller WH. Sex hormone–related dermatoses in dogs. In Kirk RW, ed. Current Veterinary Therapy X. Philadelphia, WB Saunders, 1989, p 595.

Miller WH, Affolter VK, Scott DW, et al. Multicentric squamous cell carcinomas in situ resembling Bowen's disease in five cats. Vet Dermatol 3:117, 1992.

Miller WH, Scott DW. Milbemycin in the treatment of generalized demodicosis in the dog. Proc Ann Meeting Am Acad Vet Dermatol/Am Coll Vet Dermatol 7:44, 1991.

Moriello KA, MacEwen EG, Schultz KT. PEG L-asparaginase in the treatment of canine mycosis fungoides and sterile granulomatous dermatitis. Proc World Congress Vet Dermatol 2:97, 1992.

Muller GH, Kirk RW, Scott DW. Small Animal Dermatology. Philadelphia, WB Saunders, 1989.

Nelson RW, Feldman EC. Hyperadrenocorticism. In August JR, ed. Consultation in Feline Internal Medicine. Philadelphia, WB Saunders, 1991, p 267.

Paradis M. Ivermectin in small animal dermatology. In Kirk RW, ed. Current Veterinary Therapy X. Philadelphia, WB Saunders, 1989, p 560.

Paradis M, Laperriere E. Efficacy of daily ivermectin treatment in a dog with amitraz-resistant, generalized demodicosis. Vet Dermatol 3:85, 1992.

Patnaik AK, Mooney S. Feline melanoma: A comparative study of ocular, oral and dermal neoplasms. Vet Pathol 25:105, 1988.

Peterson ME, Ferguson DC. Thyroid disease. In Ettinger SJ, ed. Textbook of Veterinary Internal Medicine. Philadelphia, WB Saunders, 1989, p 1632.

Peterson ME, Kemppainen RJ. Dose-response relation between plasma concentrations of corticotropin and cortisol after administration of incremental doses of cosyntropin for corticotropin stimulation testing in cat. Am J Vet Res 54:300, 1993.

Peterson ME, Kintzer PP, Cavanagh PG. Feline hyperthyroidism: Pretreatment clinical and laboratory evaluation of 131 cases. J Am Vet Med Assoc 183:103, 1983.

Postorino NC. Tumors of the male reproductive tract. In Withrow SJ, MacEwen EG, eds. Clinical Veterinary Oncology. Philadelphia, JB Lippincott, 1989, p 305.

Power HT, Ihrke PJ. Synthetic retinoids in veterinary dermatology. Vet Clin North Am 20:1525, 1990.

Pulley LT, Stannard AA. Skin and soft tissue. In Moulton JE, ed. Tumors in Domestic Animals. Berkeley, CA, University of California Press, 1990, p 23.

Reedy LM, Garfield RA. Results of a clinical study with an oral antiparasitic agent in generalized demodicosis. Ann Meeting Am Acad Vet Dermatol/Am Coll Vet Dermatol 8:43, 1992.

Roe DA, Campbell TC, eds. Drugs and Nutrients: The Interactive Effects. New York, Marcel Dekker, 1984.

Rosser EJ. Sex hormones. In Griffin CE, Kwochka KW,

MacDonald JM, eds. Current Veterinary Dermatology; The Science and Art of Therapy. St. Louis, Mosby–Year Book, 1993, p 292.

Schick RO, Murphy G, Goldschmidt MH. Sézary syndrome in a cat. Proc Ann Members Meeting Am Acad Vet Dermatol/Am Coll Vet Dermatol 5:57, 1989.

Scott DW. Feline dermatology 1900–1978: A monograph. J Am Anim Hosp Assoc 16:331, 1980.

Scott DW, Walton DK. Experience with the use of amitraz and ivermectin for the treatment of generalized demodicosis in dogs. J Am Anim Hosp Assoc 21:535, 1985.

Smith EK. Planning the workup for dermatologic patients. Vet Med 83:35, 1988.

Stogdale L, Moore DJ. Feline demodicosis. J Am Anim Hosp Assoc 18:427, 1982.

Susaneck SJ, Withrow SJ. Tumors of the skin and subcutaneous tissues. In Withrow SJ, MacEwen EG, eds. Clinical Veterinary Oncology. Philadelphia, JB Lippincott, 1989, p 139.

Sutter M, Lott-Stoltz G, Wild P. Generalized nodular dermatofibrosis and renal cystadenocarcinomas in a German shepherd dog. Vet Pathol 20:632, 1983.

Thrall MA, Macy DW, Snyder SP. Cutaneous lymphosarcoma and leukemia in a dog resembling Sézary syndrome in man. Vet Pathol 21:182, 1984.

Turrel JM, Gross TL. Diagnosis and treatment of multicentric squamous cell carcinoma in situ (Bowen's disease) of cats. Proc Vet Cancer Soc 11:84, 1991.

Walton DK. Canine epidermotrophic lymphoma. In Kirk RW, ed. Current Veterinary Therapy IX. Philadelphia, WB Saunders, 1986, p 609.

Watrach AM, Small E, Case MT. Canine papillomas; progression of an oral papilloma to a carcinoma. J Natl Cancer Inst 45:915, 1970.

Wenzel KW. Pharmacologic interference with *in vitro* tests of thyroid function. Metabolism 30:717, 1981.

Wheeler SL. Canine pheochromocytoma. In Kirk RW, ed. Current Veterinary Therapy IX. Philadelphia, WB Saunders, 1986, p 987.

White SD. The skin as a sensor of internal medical disorders. In Ettinger SJ, ed. Textbook of Veterinary Internal Medicine. Philadelphia, WB Saunders, 1989, p 5.

White SD, Carpenter JL, Moore FM. Generalized demodicosis associated with diabetes mellitus in two cats. J Am Vet Med Assoc 191:448, 1987.

White SD, Ceragioli KL, Bullock LP. Cutaneous markers of canine hyperadrenocorticism. Compend Contin Educ Pract Vet 11:446, 1989.

Zenoble RD, George JW. Mycosis fungoides-like disease in a dog. J Am Anim Hosp Assoc 16:203, 1980.

Zerbe CA, MacDonald JM. Canine and feline Cushing's syndrome. In Griffin CE, Kwochka KW, MacDonald JM, eds. Current Veterinary Dermatology; The Science and Art of Therapy. St. Louis, Mosby–Year Book, 1993, p 273.

Zerbe CA, Nachreiner RF, Dunstan RW. Hyperadrenocorticism in a cat. J Am Vet Med Assoc 190:559, 1987.

CHAPTER 13

The Ear

A. J. VENKER-VAN HAAGEN
and I. VAN DER GAAG

Ear diseases occur at all ages in dogs and cats. In geriatric patients, ear diseases are generally characterized by chronicity and the development of tumors. Loss of hearing is an almost exclusively geriatric problem in dogs and cats, and several studies have helped delineate the degenerative changes in the cochlea associated with this loss (Knowles et al, 1989; Schuknecht et al, 1965).

Another aspect of dealing with the geriatric patient is that there is often an accumulation of other hampering dysfunctions, resulting in different treatment decisions than would be made for the ear problem alone.

The aim of this chapter is to provide effective support for the veterinarian confronted with common diseases of the ear in older dogs and cats, using our own experience and that of others.

MANAGEMENT OF EAR DISEASE

Management of ear diseases starts, as in all other diseases, with the taking of the history. In older dogs and cats the history of ear disease might well be short and plainly indicative of an acute problem with a circumscribed localization, but in a specialist practice receiving referral patients, the history usually reflects a life of both minor and severe diseases and many years of ups and downs. The ear should be seen as only a part of the older animal's body, and the veterinarian should obtain a general history before focusing on the problems of the ear. The history and the diagnosis together will lead to well-balanced advice for treatment.

The history is begun by asking the owner about the reason for the visit to the veterinarian. When the problem is clear and has been written down and then read back to the owner to avoid misunderstanding, questions can be directed toward understanding of the owner's relationship with the animal and the circumstances of the animal's life, including domestic relations involving the animal. The history of current diseases and medications is then examined, followed by a review of past diseases of the ears, including vestibular disease and hearing. Then the scope of the history is widened to include skin diseases and other diseases with or without a possible relation to the present problems. The history is written out and then summarized for the owner. Further information may be added during the subsequent clinical examination.

The clinical examination of the older patient should be thorough. The veterinarian's general impression of the patient will guide the way in which the animal is handled during the examination. The owner is usually proud that the animal has reached such an age, but fears at the same time the discovery of some fatal disorder. The veterinarian can help break the tension during the examination by making clear remarks about positive findings.

The general clinical examination begins with a general impression of the animal's alertness, its mobility, its relative weight, the coat, and any immediately obvious abnormalities. The general examination includes examination of respiratory movements, body temperature, pulse rate, skin and coat, mucous membranes, and lymph nodes and is supplemented by auscultation of heart and lung sounds. Neurologic examination may be indicated when the ear disease involves the vestibular system, the facial nerve, or other cranial nerves.

The examination of the ear starts with inspection of the externally visible parts of the ear and the adjacent structures. The pinna is the most important part and differs considerably in appearance from dog to dog. In cats the pinna is often scarred if the animal has had an adventurous outdoor life. The convex part of the pinna should be covered with hair. The concave part in most dogs and cats is haired at the tip but hairless or nearly so at the base.

Palpation of the pinna gives information about the temperature of the skin, the flexibility of the cartilage, induration (ossification) of the cartilage, or thickening of the structures of the pinna. The orifice of the ear canal is bounded by the tragus laterally and the base of the pinna medially, rostrally, and caudally. The orifice must be visible, and although variably filled by hair, it should be clean. In most dogs and cats the first part of the ear canal can be inspected without the use of an otoscope. The orifice may be narrowed by acute inflammation or proliferation of the skin or obstructed by excessive hair. Ceruminous or purulent material and epithelial lesions may give an impression of the severity of the ear problems. Palpation of the ear canal and the adjacent structures is very important in many chronic hypertrophic diseases, abscesses, and tumors.

Almost all ear diseases are extremely painful, and palpation of the ear canal and adjacent structures should be done with considerateness. Palpation will give information about the severity and extent of the disease, and in chronic proliferative otitis externa, in which there is hypertrophy of all structures of the skin lining the ear canal, it is the only way to assess the involvement of the structures. Further examination of the ear canal and the tympanic membrane requires the use of an otoscope. Before the otoscope is introduced, purulent or hemorrhagic exudate should be collected for microbiologic culture.

Otoscopic examination of the ear canal and the tympanic membrane is an essential part of the examination of the ear canal. In the dog and the cat, examination is almost always possible without sedation or anesthesia. The key to success is gentle handling of the patient and avoidance of pressure on the lining of the ear canal, which is very sensitive. If a dog is not cooperative, an experienced assistant can restrain it in a sternal position; a cat can be taken under the arm and its head stabilized. The veterinarian then grasps the tip of the pinna and pulls it firmly in a lateroventral direction. The ear canal is thereby formed into a long, straight canal, with the axis of the vertical and horizontal parts coming into line. The otoscope is then introduced under visual guidance, following the lumen of the ear canal and avoiding as much as possible any touching of the wall. To complete the examination the pinna and the ear canal are maneuvered under visual control so that the otoscope, passively following the movements, will illuminate the different parts of the ear canal and the tympanic membrane.

In most cases of external ear canal disease, the ear canal will be filled with cerumen or exudate. Cleaning of the ear canal is the most important part of management of otitis externa and is essential in both diagnosis and treatment (Venker-van Haagen, 1983). The cleaning must be complete and yet not irritating to the lining. The most effective way is with a forceful stream of water. This is best done using the Haeberle flusher (Haeberle G mbH Comp & Co, Stuttgart, Germany) designed for the cleaning or caloric testing of the human ear. The instrument is connected permanently to a cold water supply pipe; the water in the reservoir is electrically heated and thermostatically controlled. The instrument produces a forceful stream of water at supply line pressure, and the thermostat is set to body temperature. The dog or cat is held in the same way, and its ear kept in the same position used for otoscopic examination. The hand which held the otoscope now takes the handle of the flusher to introduce the stream of water into the canal. When the returning water is clean the animal is allowed to shake its head. This results in a dry ear canal and a dry tympanic membrane. The procedure can be repeated if necessary. Dogs and cats do not like the procedure, but they can be calmed by an experienced assistant. When an ear-flushing instrument is not available, the ear canal should be cleaned with water or 0.9 per cent sodium chloride solution under anesthesia. This method of cleaning and then drying by suction is clearly more complex, time consuming, and costly and therefore is often not repeated when it should be.

When the ear canal is clean and the lumen is sufficiently wide, the tympanic membrane can be inspected. The tympanic membrane is a transparent round membrane, but it appears to be oval because it is seen through the otoscope at a 60-degree angle, with the ventral part being farther away from the viewer than the dorsal part. The pars tensa, the tensed part, is transparent and slightly blue or gray with radial striping. The dorsal part, the pars flaccida, is pink and bulges slightly when pressure in the middle ear is increased. The manubrium of the malleus is a solid white structure in the pars tensa, bordered by small, bright red blood vessels. Changes in the tympanic membrane are usually caused by inflammatory changes in either the external ear canal or the middle ear. A small perforation has the appearance of a dark spot, but when there is a large perforation or tear, the structures in the middle ear cavity become visible. The transparent tympanic membrane is sometimes slightly more milky in older dogs, indicating thickening or an increase in nontransparent material in the layers of the membrane.

External otitis caused by mite infestation is rare in older dogs and cats. Otoscopic examination usually reveals the mites, but in case of doubt, microscopic examination of cerumen is helpful. Microbiologic culture of material is useful when there is purulent or hemorrhagic exudate.

Anesthesia is needed when manipulation of instruments in the ear canal is necessary for further diagnosis or treatment. For example, it may not be possible to remove a foreign body without risk of injury to the tympanic membrane unless the animal is anesthetized, and anesthesia is always required when chronic middle ear disease necessitates thorough flushing of the middle ear under visual control or when a biopsy in the ear canal is required.

Radiology is helpful when the chronicity of a process involving the middle or inner ear makes it likely that there are periosteal or osseous changes, but interpretation of radiographs of this area can be difficult. Positioning of the patient is very important, and the necessary manipulation makes the use of anesthesia indispensable. Computer tomography gives far better resolution in this area, and because processes involving this area usually have serious consequences and can even be life threatening, the greater requirements of time and expense of computer tomography are justified.

EAR DISEASES IN THE DOG AND CAT

Diseases of the Pinna

Lesions of the pinna may be part of more generalized skin diseases (Roth, 1988). They can be bacterial, fungal, parasitic, immune mediated, or vascular (drug mediated) in origin (Muller et al, 1983). These disorders are not age dependent, and hence older dogs and cats are not excluded. Bacterial folliculitis of the pinna with focal areas of alopecia has been described in dogs, and dermatophytosis of the pinna with focal alopecia and extensive crust formation can be found in cats (Angarano, 1988). Pruritus and crusting of the margins of the pinna can be caused by *Sarcoptes* mites in dogs and *Notoedres* mites in cats (Wisselink, 1986).

Trauma. Trauma to the pinna can occur at any age. A tear in the pinna is usually the result of a fight with another dog or cat. The cat's claw and the dog's canine teeth are the sharp instruments causing this trauma. The resulting bleeding is impressive, and the veterinarian must act immediately to induce primary wound healing.

In dogs it is often possible to place several sutures without local or general anesthesia. A small, fresh tear (up to 1 cm in length) can be sutured after cleaning and removal of some of the hair. The skin on the concave side of the pinna is apposed and sutured with interrupted sutures, starting at the edge of the pinna. Then the skin on the convex side is apposed and sutured in the same way. The cartilage is not included in these sutures. Bleeding stops during suturing, but a resistant artery may have to be ligated separately. The use of thermocauterization should be avoided.

Most cats will not submit to suturing without severe resistance, and hence they, as well as dogs with larger lacerations, should be anesthetized. A general clinical examination is indicated to detect other blood loss, as well as shock and other possible complications of trauma. The pinna is then prepared for surgery by clipping the hair and cleaning the skin with 0.9 per cent sodium chloride solution and disinfectant. Unless the tympanic membrane is known to be intact, the disinfectant should be prevented from reaching it.

Fine interrupted sutures with atraumatic, delayed-solubility material are used to join skin to skin, omitting the cartilage, first on the concave side and then on the convex side, always placing the first suture at the edge of the pinna. Starting at the edge of the pinna prevents the formation of very obvious irregularities at the edge. The use of delayed-solubility suture material is preferred, because these sutures do not have to be removed. In all cases the wound should be considered to be contaminated, and a short period of systemic antimicrobial treatment is often indicated. When the wound is not fresh and inflammation is apparent, surgical correction is postponed and the inflammation treated first. Surgical correction then begins with refreshening of the wound edges.

Othematoma. Othematomas occur at all ages. The bleeding occurs between the cartilaginous layers of the pinna and is usually considered to result from trauma, such as shaking the head or scratching the ear. Kuwashara (1986) has suggested an immune-mediated disease as an underlying cause. Surgical intervention is necessary, because without treatment the pinna will shrivel, and subsequent ossification of the cartilage will cause continuous irritation. Also, shriveling of the pinna may cause obstruction of the external orifice and thus induce chronic otitis externa. The purpose of surgery is to remove the blood clot and press the layers of the pinna together long enough to effectuate reunion of the layers. A reliable method consists of suturing through all layers of the pinna, placing sutures over the entire surface of the pinna. Interrupted mattress sutures of chromic catgut are excellent for this purpose because of the elasticity of the material and its dissolution in 2 weeks. The layers are reunited during that period, and the sutures can simply be wiped off.

Abscesses. In cats, abscesses of the pinna are usually caused by a penetrating wound inflicted by the claw of another cat. The cat is usually depressed and febrile, and the ear is obviously painful. The skin over the abscess should be opened and the pus removed by gentle compression, followed by flushing with 0.9 per cent sodium chloride solution. A systemic antimicrobial agent should be administered for 10 days. In some older cats both pinnas are shriveled as a consequence of multiple abscesses. The shriveled pinna can cause occlusion of the external orifice of the ear canal, and continuous otitis externa may be the result. Ossification of the pinna usually causes continuous irritation to the cat, and amputation of the pinna results in remarkable relief. Abscesses of the pinna are rare in dogs but are treated in the same way as in cats. Healing of the pinna can be slow and painful, and hence an analgesic agent should be given in addition to antimicrobial therapy. Also, in the dog a shriveled pinna can cause considerable irritation and chronic otitis externa. When there are also complications in the external ear canal, such as ossification of the cartilage or chronic proliferation of the skin, removal of the pinna and the ear canal in one procedure can be the best solution (Venker-van Haagen, 1989). This situation occurs in cats and in older dogs. This surgery may seem radical but there is no reason to exclude older dogs from radical surgery when the alternative is continuous distress and pain.

Tumors of the Pinna. Tumors of the pinna occur at all ages in dogs and cats. A survey of our cases of tumors removed from 116 pinnas in dogs revealed 72 histiocytomas, 22 mast cell tumors, 15 sebaceous gland adenomas, 4 fibromas, 2 unspecified sarcomas, and 1 hemangiopericytoma. Previously published information (van der Gaag, 1986) is included in these numbers. The average age of dogs with histiocytomas was 4.5 years (range, 4 months to 14 years); dogs with mast cell tumors, 8.2 years (range, 3 to 15 years); and dogs with sebaceous gland adenomas, 5.8 years (range, 1 to 13 years). Breeds most frequently represented in histiocytomas were retrievers (15) and boxers (9); in mast cell tumors, boxers (9) and rottweilers (3); and in sebaceous gland adenomas, cocker spaniels (8). Histiocytomas can be removed by partial resection of the pinna. In almost all other cases amputation of the pinna is necessary to prevent further extension of the tumor and eventual metastasis. Mast cell tumors should be excised with a wide margin of surrounding tissue. In many cases the pinna and the ear canal must be removed together.

In the cat squamous cell carcinoma is the most important tumor of the pinna, but four cases of rhabdomyosarcoma have been described (Roth, 1990). White cats seem to be especially susceptible to the development of squamous cell carcinoma, but it also occurs in colored cats (Angarano, 1988). In our experience older cats have been overrepresented. In 15 cats with squamous cell carcinoma of the pinna, the average age was 12.8 years (range, 7 to 18 years) (Fig. 13–1). The tumor first resembles a nonhealing granulomatous inflammation at the edge of the pinna and is easily misdiagnosed as an inflammatory lesion, not only because of its slow progression, but also because it is frequently bilateral. In the course of the tumor's development, hemorrhage from the defect at the edge of the pinna becomes a more

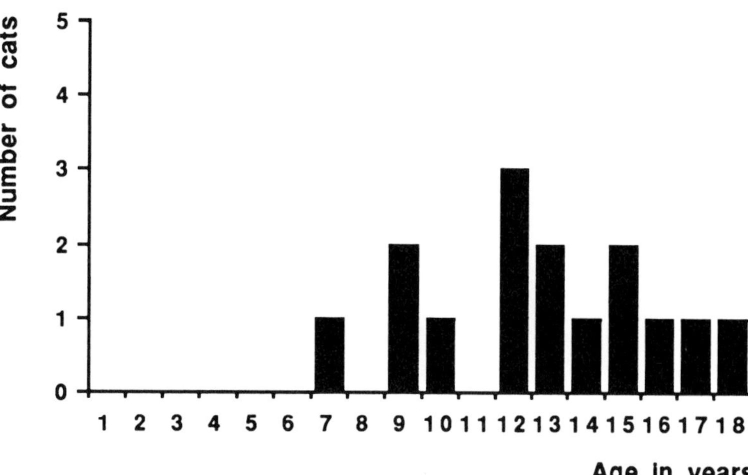

Figure 13–1. Age distribution of 15 cats in which the pinnas were removed because of squamous cell carcinoma. (Courtesy of the Department of Veterinary Pathology, University of Utrecht, Utrecht, The Netherlands.)

frequent nuisance. Cytologic examination of material collected by fine needle aspiration biopsy or histologic examination of surgical biopsy material will reveal the diagnosis. Unilateral or bilateral amputation of the pinna is an effective therapy, especially because metastasis seldom occurs in an early stage.

In the cat amputation of the pinna is a simple procedure. Under general anesthesia the pinna is removed by cutting along its base with scissors. There is remarkably little bleeding, and any bleeding that does occur is controlled by ligation of the vessels. The skin of the two sides of the pinna is joined over the cartilage, beginning with three or four sutures placed at equal distances over the curved wound. The closure is completed by many more sutures, taking care to cover the entire cartilage. The use of delayed-solubility suture material is preferred, as these sutures remain up to four weeks before falling out spontaneously. Unilateral or bilateral pinna amputation changes the appearance of the cat considerably, but the cat will live in comfort in and around the house, where previously the effects of the bleeding of the pinna had been most distressing (Fig. 13–2).

In the dog the principles of the surgical technique are similar, but there is considerable bleeding. In dogs we prefer to begin the surgery with an incision of the skin along the base of the pinna on the convex side. The arteries and veins are freed one by one and ligated separately. When this has been completed the pinna is removed by cutting the cartilage and the skin on the concave side, using scissors. From this point on the surgery is similar to that in the cat.

Diseases of the External Ear Canal

The characteristic diseases of the external ear canal in older dogs and cats are caused by chronic alterations resulting from previous unsuccessfully treated inflammation (Grono, 1980). Histologic findings in more severe cases reveal that all components of the ear canal are affected (Fig. 13–3). There is proliferation of the epithelial lining, sebaceous glands, and ceruminal glands; the connective tissue is increased in mass; and the cartilage is ossified (Fig. 13–4). A more specific finding in the ear canals of older cats is the cystic change of the ceruminal glands (Fig. 13–5). The narrowed lumen of the ear canal often becomes obstructed by abundant cerumen of abnormal

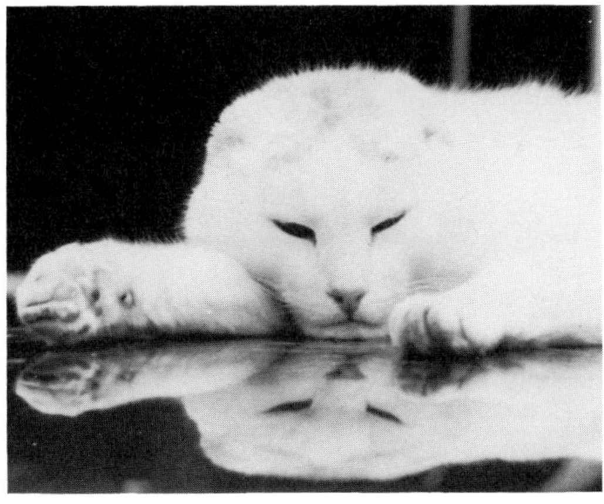

Figure 13–2. Bilateral pinna amputation changes the appearance of the cat considerably, but the cat lives in comfort.

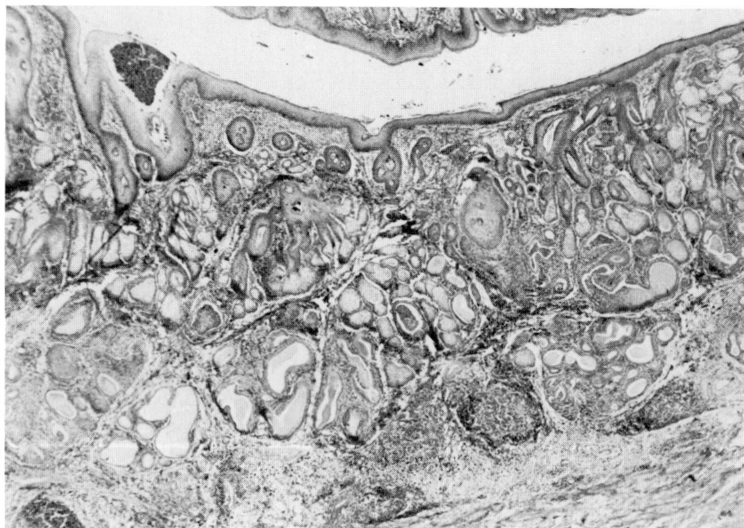

Figure 13–3. Chronic proliferative otitis externa with hyperplasia of the sebaceous and ceruminal glands, dilatation of the ceruminal glands, round cell infiltration and macrophages containing ceroid pigment in the connective tissue, and follicular proliferation in the basal area in a 4-year-old male cocker spaniel (H & E stain, ×46).

consistency and composition, resulting in irritation, inflammation, and increasing alterations in all components. The vicious cycle can be interrupted by flushing the ear canal to clean it and then applying corticosteroids and broad-spectrum antimicrobial agents in a liquid ointment that comes into contact with the entire epithelium of the ear canal. The ointment should be applied once or twice a week for the remainder of life, and the flushing can be restricted to once every 3 to 4 months, thus avoiding unnecessary irritation of the tissues. In these cases the owner will comply more readily with the regimen if the ointment has a water base instead of an oil base.

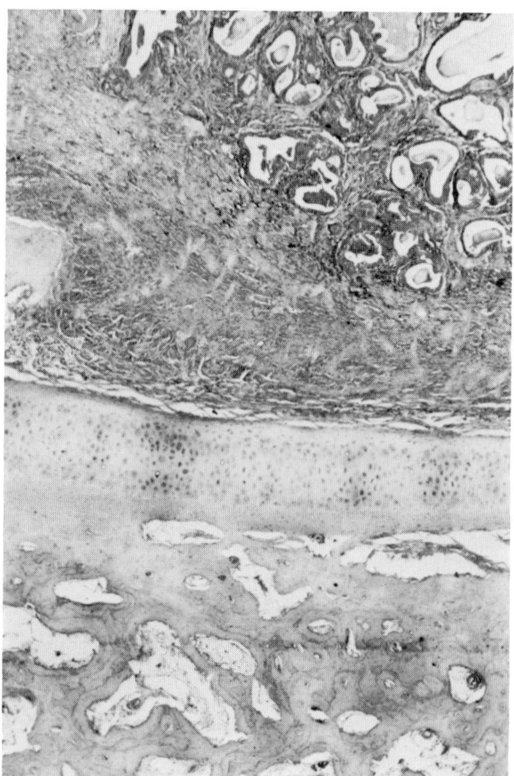

Figure 13–4. Chronic proliferative otitis externa with bone formation in the tissue around the cartilage of the ear canal in a 4-year-old male cocker spaniel (H & E stain, ×52).

In advanced proliferative otitis externa, the lumen of the ear canal is so narrow that the previously described strategy of continuous local treatment is impracticable (Fig. 13–6). The pain caused by the continuous inflammation and ossification of the ear canal justifies radical surgical removal of the canal. In most cases a total ablation of both ear canals is required. The effect of the surgery is very satisfactory, and complications such as fistulas are amazingly rare. The loss of hearing theoretically caused by the abolishment of air conduction of sound in the ear canal is not a concern, as such conduction had long been blocked by the chronic proliferative disease of the ear canal. The surgery itself, especially in dogs, is a serious intervention. The procedure takes at least 1½ hours for one ear, and the anesthesia should be deep; analgesic agents should be administered after surgery. The ablation of one ear canal at a time is better for the dog. Surgery on the second ear is delayed until wound healing is complete, usually 4 to 5 weeks. The pain caused by the advanced proliferative disease justifies the surgery, even in older dogs and cats, as long as anesthesia is an acceptable risk.

In our survey of unilateral or bilateral total

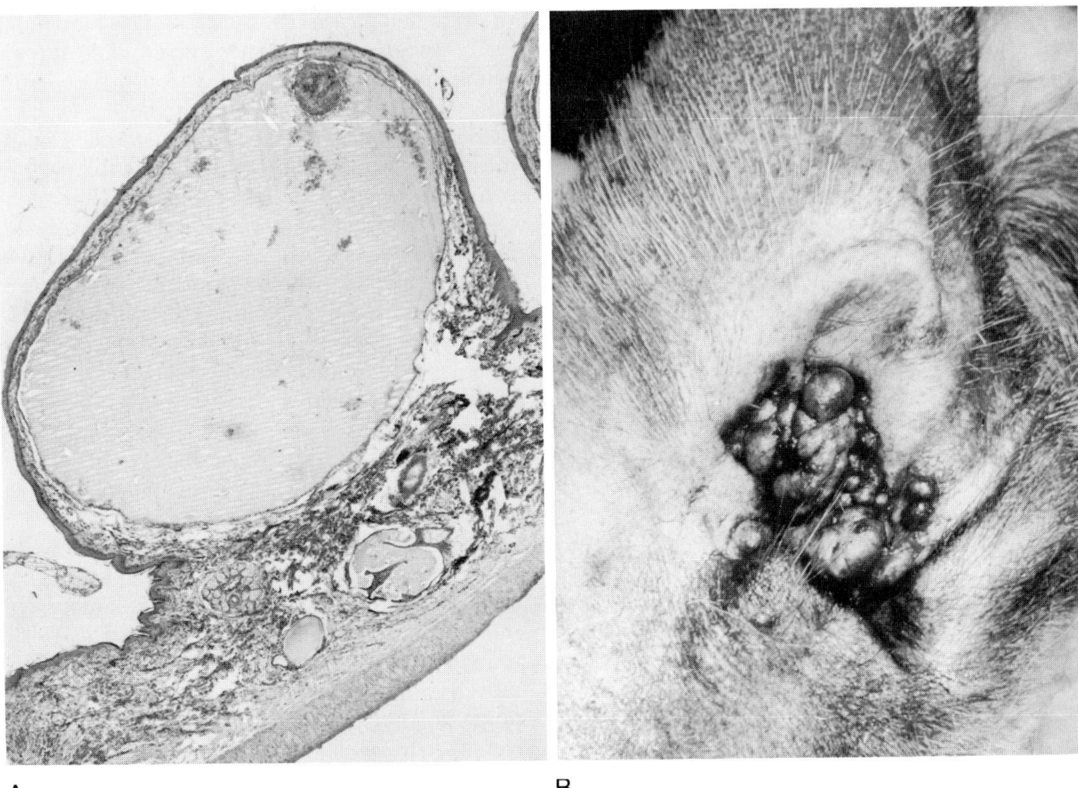

Figure 13–5. *A*, Large cyst of the ceruminal glands lined by flattened epithelium and containing cerumen and some inflammatory cells in a 5-year-old neutered male Persian cat. *B*, Multiple cysts of the ceruminal glands appear as black nodules at the base of the pinna in a cat.

ablation of the ear canal for chronic proliferative otitis externa in 262 dogs, the average age was 6.2 years (range, 1 to 15 years). In 10 dogs the age was unknown (Fig. 13–7). In 53 cats the average age was 6.7 years (range, 1 to 14 years) (Fig. 13–8). The dogs included 121 American cocker spaniels (short-nosed type), 25 terriers (various terrier breeds), 21 German shepherd dogs, 14 poodles (all sizes), 10 rottweilers, 10 Bouviers des Flandres, 8 English bulldogs, 5 retrievers, 5 Great Danes, 5 Irish setters, 4 Newfoundland dogs, 3 German pointers, 2 boxers, and 15 mixed and singly represented breeds. In 14 dogs the breed was unknown.

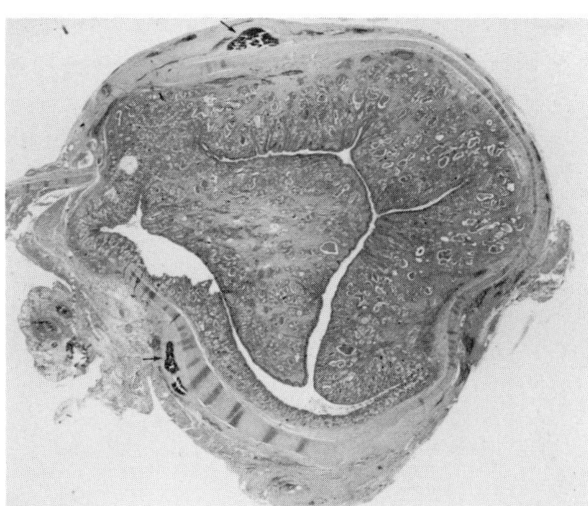

Figure 13–6. Chronic diffuse polypoid otitis externa causing narrowing of the lumen of the ear canal in a 2-year-old female cocker spaniel. There is a partly normal area in the wall of the ear canal and local calcification (*arrow*) (H & E stain, ×4).

The surgical technique is as follows. The patient is placed in the lateral recumbent position. Two incisions are made in the skin over the vertical part of the ear canal, one extending from the intertragic incisure to the ventral limit of the vertical ear canal (determined by palpation) and the second from the tragohelicine incisure to the same ventral point. The resulting triangular flap of skin is dissected, and the vertical part of the ear canal is freed from the subcutaneous and muscular tissues at the caudal, lateral, and rostral sides. The cartilage and skin of the medial wall of the ear canal are separated from the cartilage and skin of the base of the pinna on the inner (con-

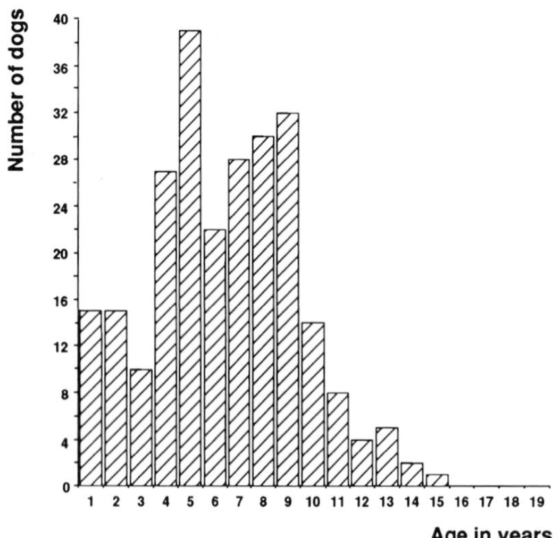

Figure 13–7. Age distribution of 252 dogs in which the ear canal was removed because of chronic proliferative otitis externa. (Courtesy of the Department of Veterinary Pathology, University of Utrecht, Utrecht, The Netherlands.)

cave) side by use of strong scissors. All proliferative tissue is included with portions to be removed. The medial side of the vertical part of the ear canal and all sides of the horizontal part of the ear canal are then carefully freed from the subcutaneous and muscular tissue.

Appropriate care must be taken to avoid the facial nerve, which emerges from the stylomastoid foramen and passes around the horizontal part of the ear canal at the caudal and lateral sides. In some cases the facial nerve is embedded in the inflammatory tissues surrounding the ear canal and must be separated from it very carefully. The cartilaginous part of the ear canal is then separated from the osseous external acoustic meatus with pointed scissors. This is followed by complete removal of all of the skin lining the osseous external ear canal and the tympanic membrane, using a small curette. The next step is the remodeling of the pinna according to its most natural way of folding. The base of the pinna is then sutured together, and the wound is closed after a Penrose drain is placed in the space left by the ear canal. The drain is left in place for 5 days, analgesics are administered for 5 days, and broad-spectrum antimicrobial agents are administered for at least 2 weeks (Venker-van Haagen, 1992).

In dogs a solitary, round polyp may be found in the ear canal. Histologic examination reveals inflammatory tissue covered with squamous epithelium and containing all components usually found in chronic otitis externa. The polyp is removed surgically. We have found this type of polyp in 31 dogs with an average age of 7 years (range, 1 to 15 years). In four dogs the age was unknown (Fig. 13–9). In some cases the polyps contained mainly connective tissue, sometimes many macrophages and even foreign body giant cells, and in one case there was bone formation (Fig. 13–10).

Tumors of the External Ear Canal. In dogs the development of a tumor in the ear canal is

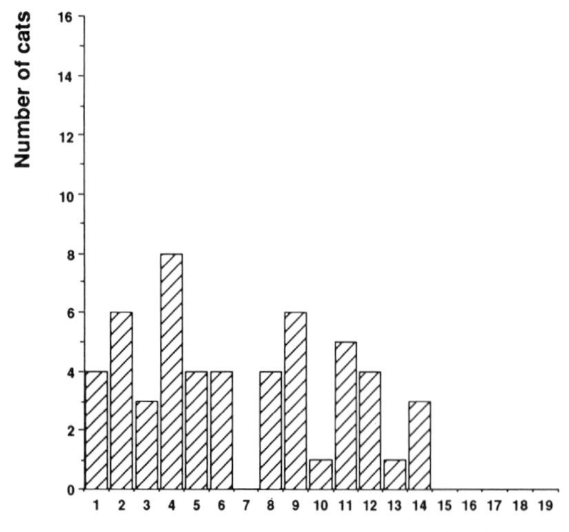

Figure 13–8. Age distribution of 53 cats in which the ear canal was removed because of chronic otitis externa. (Courtesy of the Department of Veterinary Pathology, University of Utrecht, Utrecht, The Netherlands.)

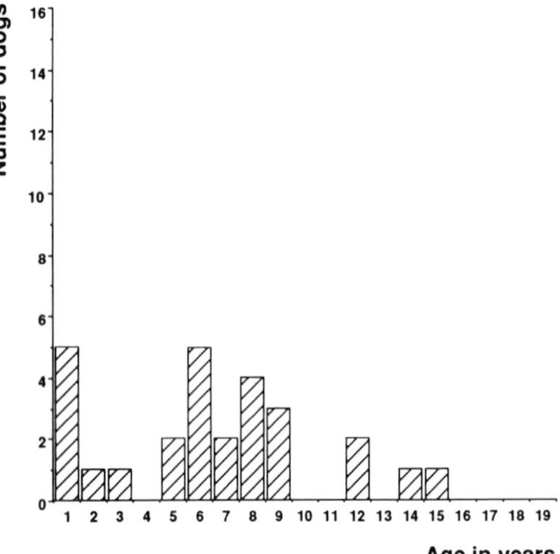

Figure 13–9. Age distribution of 27 dogs in which the ear canal was removed because of polyps. (Courtesy of the Department of Veterinary Pathology, University of Utrecht, Utrecht, The Netherlands.)

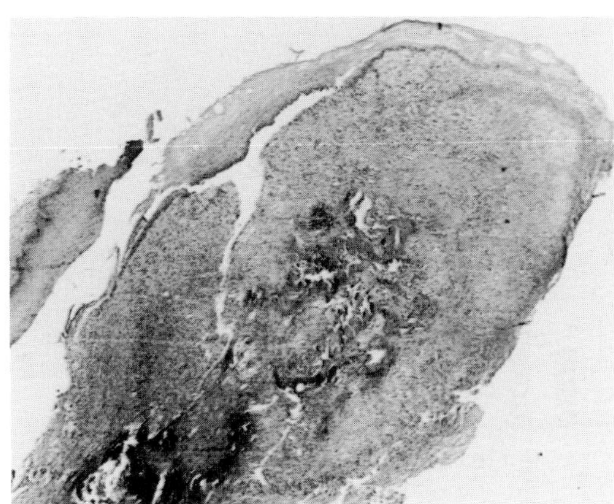

Figure 13–10. Polyp of the ear canal covered with squamous cell epithelium and consisting of connective tissue with calcification and bone formation in a 12-year-old spayed female cocker spaniel (H & E stain, ×36).

not exclusively a geriatric problem, but older dogs are well represented. The tumors found in specimens from total ear canal ablation in 36 dogs consisted of 14 ceruminal gland adenomas, 11 papillomas (Fig. 13–11), 6 ceruminal gland carcinomas, and 5 squamous cell carcinomas. The average age of the dogs with adenomas was 9.6 years (range, 8 to 13 years), and the dogs with other tumors ranged from young to old (Fig. 13–12). Previously published information (van der Gaag, 1986) is included in these numbers.

Tumors in the external ear canal occur more often in older than in younger cats (Fig. 13–13). The clinical signs are dominated by a purulent discharge, and the tumor can be diagnosed by otoscopic inspection. Tumors are usually unilateral but can be bilateral. Total ablation of the ear canal is indicated and should be performed at an early stage if possible. Various tumors occur in the ear canal, and sometimes more than one type is found in one ear canal. Of 29 ceruminal gland tumors, 14 were adenomas and 15 were carcinomas. The average age of cats with adenomas was 9 years (range, 4 to 17 years), and the average age of those with carcinomas was 11.2 years (range, 4 to 15 years). The age distribution is

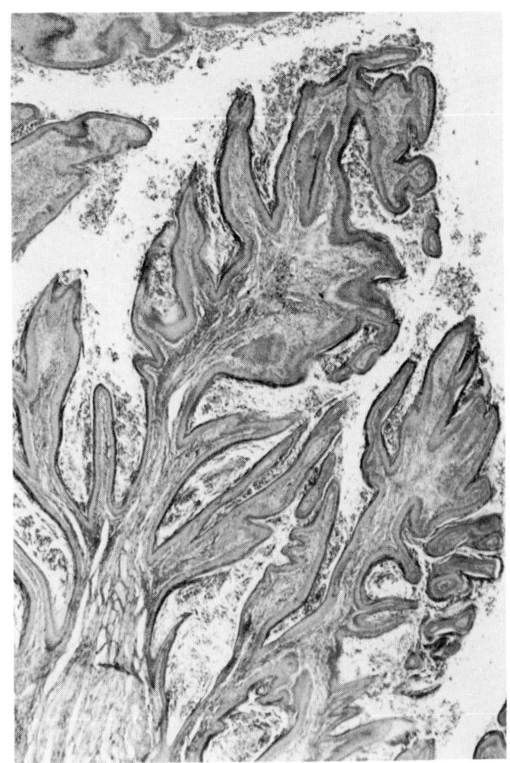

Figure 13–11. Multiple papillomas in the ear canal of a 6-year-old female mixed-breed shepherd dog (H & E stain, ×42).

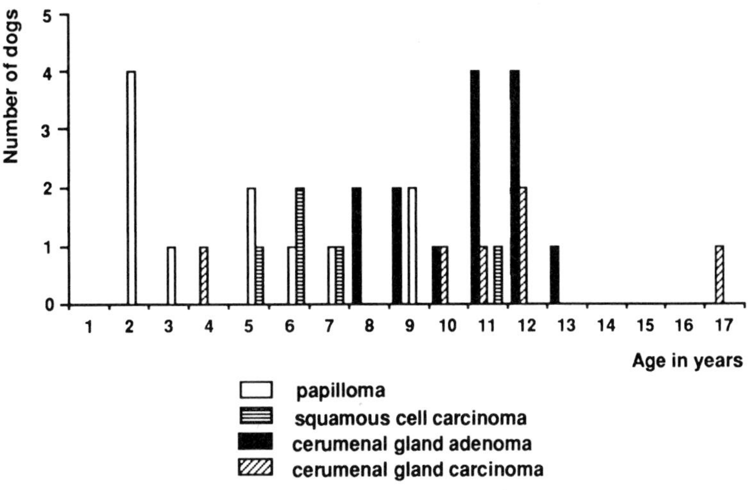

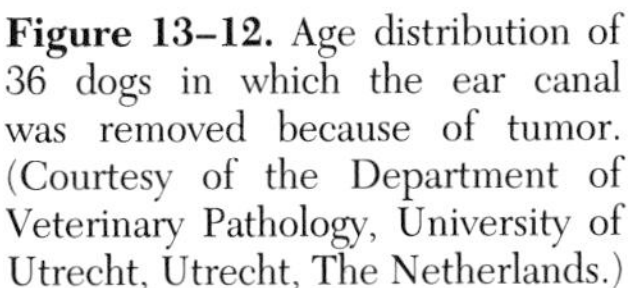

Figure 13–12. Age distribution of 36 dogs in which the ear canal was removed because of tumor. (Courtesy of the Department of Veterinary Pathology, University of Utrecht, Utrecht, The Netherlands.)

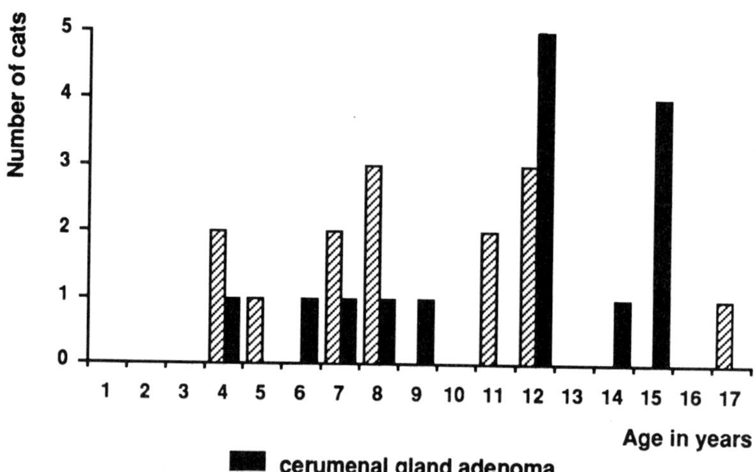

Figure 13–13. Age distribution of 29 cats in which the ear canal was removed because of tumor. (Courtesy of the Department of Veterinary Pathology, University of Utrecht, Utrecht, The Netherlands.)

similar to that described by Scott (1980). Other tumors found occasionally were sebaceous gland adenoma (Fig. 13–14), papilloma, and rhabdomyoma. A mast cell tumor has also been reported (Rogers, 1988). Because each tumor damages the ear canal and causes pain and continuous secondary inflammation, surgical removal is always indicated. Malignant tumors are especially threatening, because they will finally invade the tissues around the ear canal. The prognosis is then grave, because there is no way to remove the rapidly spreading tumor completely. Hence, total ablation of the ear canal is always indicated when a tumor is found in the ear canal of the cat, as long as the tumor is still confined within the cartilaginous wall and there is a reasonable chance that the cat can undergo an hour-long procedure under anesthesia.

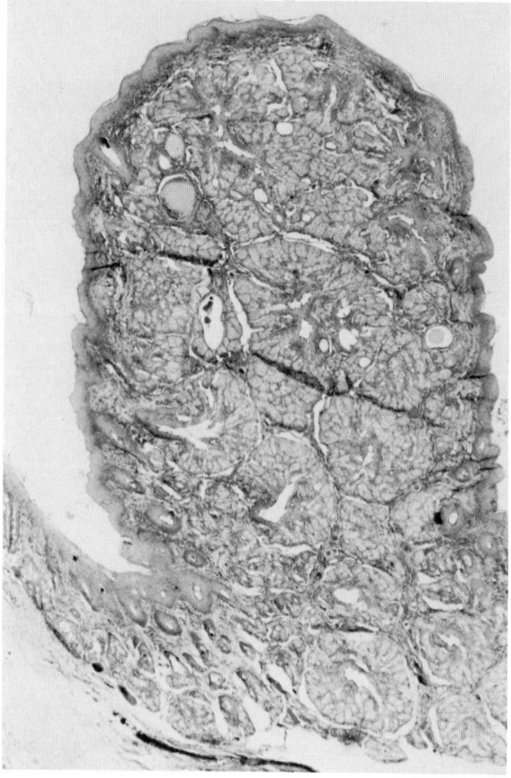

Figure 13–14. Sebaceous gland adenoma of the ear canal in a 10-year-old male European shorthair cat (H & E stain, ×36).

Diseases of the Tympanic Membrane and the Middle Ear

The tympanic membrane is composed of three layers: the epidermis, which is the continuation of the epidermis of the external ear canal; the lamina propria, or fibrous and vascular layer; and the mucosa, which is the continuation of the mucosa of the middle ear. The pathology of the tympanic membrane is usually related to the pathology of the external ear canal or that of the middle ear. Chronic irritation results in thickening of the tympanic membrane, recognized by the veterinarian as a loss of transparency. This may be seen, for example, after a long-standing ceruminal plug has been removed, and it is usually temporary. Middle ear disease is diagnosed more often in cats than in dogs. In cats reddening of the tympanic membrane is a common sign of middle ear disease. In dogs spontaneous rupture of the tympanic membrane is rare, and in one study it did not occur in experimentally induced purulent middle ear disease (Tojo et al, 1985). Ruptured tympanic membranes were found in chronic external ear disease, but the iatrogenic origin of the lesions was not excluded (Little et al, 1991). When the tympanic membrane is ruptured accidentally or experimentally and no middle ear disease occurs, the perforation heals in 1 to 3 weeks, depending on its size (Venker-van Haagen, 1983; Johnson et al, 1990; Steiss et al, 1992). In cats the most common cause of rupture is a polyp in the middle ear that grows through the tympanic membrane into the external ear canal. After removal of the polyp, the tympanic membrane is healed and transparent within 4 weeks, at least in cases in which the middle ear disease is cured.

Middle ear disease is apparently not an exclusively geriatric problem. In a study of 42 dogs with chronic middle ear disease, the majority of the dogs were found to be younger than 6 years of age (Little et al, 1991). A survey of the age distribution of 64 cats with middle ear polyps that were removed surgically does not exclude older cats (Fig. 13–15). This is in agreement with the findings of others (Faulkner and Budsberg, 1990).

Otitis media without proliferative disease of the external ear canal is diagnosed by endoscopic examination. The tympanic membrane is nontransparent and usually red or ruptured. The discharge from the middle ear is mucopurulent in acute inflammation but more dry and white in chronic inflammation. When external ear canal disease obscures the tympanic membrane from view, radiographs may reveal middle ear involvement.

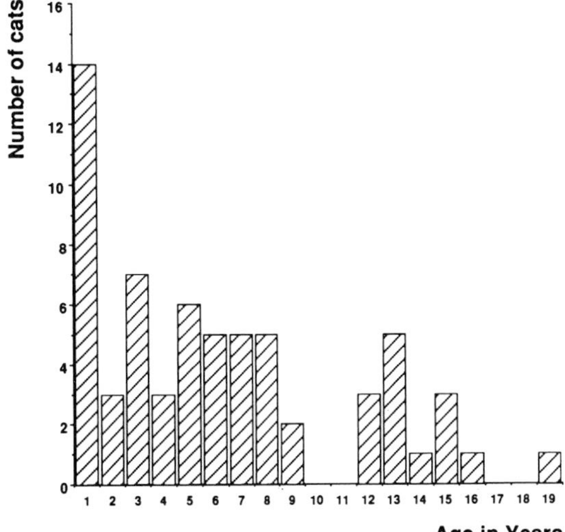

Figure 13–15. Age distribution of 64 cats in which middle ear polyps were removed. (Courtesy of the Department of Veterinary Pathology, University of Utrecht, Utrecht, The Netherlands.)

When the tympanic membrane is intact, treatment of otitis media consists of systemic broad-spectrum antimicrobial therapy for at least 2 weeks. The inflammation is resolved when the tympanic membrane appears to be normally colored and transparent. When the tympanic membrane is ruptured and the disease is apparently chronic, the middle ear cavity should be flushed with 0.9 per cent sodium chloride solution at body temperature. The procedure is performed under anesthesia and with otoscopic guidance. Systemic broad-spectrum antimicrobial treatment is given for 2 weeks. The tympanic membrane is closed within 4 weeks when the middle ear disease is cured.

Primary middle ear tumors are rare in dogs and cats. Squamous cell carcinomas have been described in older cats (Indrieri and Taylor, 1984; Fiorito, 1986). In our experience a keratoma (Schuknecht, 1974) or epidermoid cholesteatoma (Shanmugaraknam, 1991) was found in the tympanic bulla of an 7-year-old English cocker spaniel. This tumor was a cystic lesion lined by stratified squamous epithelium and filled with laminated masses of keratin (Fig. 13–16). It may be associated with chronic inflammatory reaction, hemorrhage, granulomatous reaction to keratin or cholesterol, and pressure necrosis of adjacent bone. Its occurrence is associated with otitis media (Shanmugaraknam, 1991). Tumor is suspected when the external ear canal is narrowed near the osseous external meatus and the discharge is hemorrhagic. Clinical signs include pain on the affected side and frequently vestibular dysfunction. Radiographs may reveal densities in and around the tympanic bulla, but the findings do not always enable differentiation between chronic inflammatory disease and tumor. Computer tomography is very helpful to detect lesions in the tympanic bulla and the petrosal bone but is not yet widely available. In our experience the destruction already caused by the tumor by the time of diagnosis precludes any attempt at surgery.

The Labyrinth

The labyrinth contains both the sensory cells for hearing and those for equilibrium. In labyrinthitis and ototoxicity both of these functions are impaired. When the sensory cells are destroyed, they are not replaced, and hence the hearing loss is permanent. The loss of function of the semicircular canals and utricle may be partially compen-

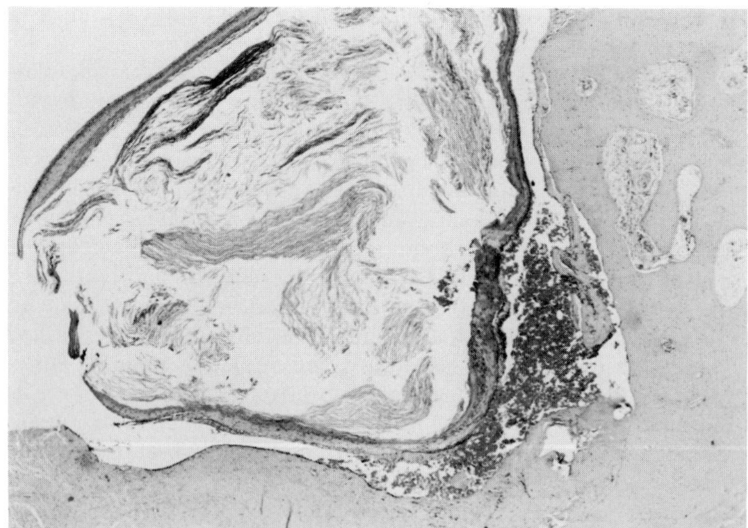

Figure 13–16. A laminated mass of keratin in a cavity lined by squamous cell epithelium: keratoma or epidermoid cholesteatoma in the middle ear of a 7-year-old spayed female cocker spaniel (H & E stain, ×36).

sated for by the central nervous system (Gacek et al, 1989, 1992). In the older dog or cat with vestibular dysfunction, the loss of sight can be especially disabling, for it represents the loss of one of the sensory inputs used to compensate for the loss of vestibular function. The combined dysfunction may result in diminished compensation for loss of equilibrium.

The loss of vestibular function as a result of middle ear disease, trauma, or ototoxicity can occur in dogs and cats of all ages. In a review of 83 dogs with peripheral vestibular dysfunction (Schunk and Averill, 1983), 33 were found to have idiopathic vestibular disease. The age at onset ranged from 2 to 17 years (average, 12.5 years). The older dog is apparently more susceptible to this disease than the younger dog. The clinical signs are ataxia alone or ataxia and head tilt, and sometimes vomiting in the acute state. The pathogenesis of the disease is unknown, and recovery varies from total to compensatory at various levels. In a review of idiopathic vestibular syndrome in 75 cats (Burke et al, 1985), only 33 had undergone clinical examination to exclude middle ear disease. In 26 of these the otoscopic findings were abnormal. Middle ear disease was therefore not excluded as the cause for the vestibular dysfunction in these cats, and the occurrence of the idiopathic vestibular syndrome was not adequately documented in the study.

Loss of hearing in older dogs and cats is well recognized. Social communication with a companion animal that has impaired hearing is difficult. When other sensory organs also diminish in function, the animal may be trapped in isolation. The cause of hearing loss was investigated in a 19-year-old cat and a 20-year-old dog (Schuknecht et al, 1965) and in four dogs with hearing impairment and five completely deaf dogs between 8 and 17 years of age (Knowles et al, 1989). In both reports there was a loss of spiral ganglion cells in the cochleas. In the first study the organ of Corti was also studied and reported to be degenerated.

Hearing in older dogs and cats can be tested most effectively by using brain stem auditory evoked responses. This noninvasive test should be used to measure the threshold for hearing by using stimuli of 0 to 70 dB hearing level (HL) (Sims, 1988; Venker-van Haagen et al, 1989). The histories provided by owners of older dogs and cats examined for hearing deficits in this clinic suggest a progressive elevation of the threshold rather than acute total hearing loss. Systematic testing of older dogs and cats has not yet been reported. Pathologic findings do not suggest a possible means of treatment. In explaining the nature of the hearing impairment in the older companion animal, the veterinarian can play an important role in maintaining a good relationship between owner and pet.

References and Supplemental Reading

Angarano DW. Diseases of the pinna. Vet Clin North Am [Small Anim Pract] 18:869, 1988.

Burke EE, Moise NS, de Lahunta A, Erb HN. Review of idiopathic feline vestibular syndrome in 75 cats. J Am Vet Med Assoc 187:941, 1985.

Faulkner JE, Budsberg SC. Results of ventral bulla osteotomy for treatment of middle ear polyps in cats. J Am Anim Hosp Assoc 26:496, 1990.

Fiorito DA. Oral and peripheral vestibular signs in a cat with squamous cell carcinoma. J Am Vet Med Assoc 188:71, 1986.

Gacek RR, Lyon MJ, Schoonmaker J. Morphologic correlates of vestibular compensation in the cat. Acta Otolaryngol [Suppl] (Stockh) 462:1, 1989.

Gacek RR, Schoonmaker J, Lyon MJ. Ultrastructural changes in contralateral superior vestibulo-ocular neurons one year after vestibular neurectomy in the cat. Acta Otolaryngol [Suppl] (Stockh) 495:1, 1992.

Grono L. Otitis externa. In Kirk RW, ed. Current Veterinary Therapy VII. Philadelphia, WB Saunders, 1980, p 461.

Indrieri RJ, Taylor RF. Vestibular dysfunction caused by squamous cell carcinoma involving the middle ear and inner ear in two cats. J Am Vet Med Assoc 184:471, 1984.

Johnson AP, Smallman LA, Kent SE. The mechanism of healing of tympanic membrane perforations. Acta Otolaryngol (Stockh) 109:406, 1990.

Knowles K, Blauch B, Leipold H, Cash W, Hewett J. Reduction of spiral ganglion neurons in the aged canine with hearing loss. J Vet Med Assoc 36:188, 1989.

Kuwashara J. Canine and feline aural hematoma: Clinical, experimental and clinicopathological observations. Am J Vet Res 47:2300, 1986.

Little CJL, Lane JG, Pearson GR. Inflammatory middle ear disease of the dog: The pathology of otitis media. Vet Rec 128:293, 1991.

Muller GH, Kirk RW, Scott DW. Small Animal Dermatology. 3rd ed. Philadelphia, WB Saunders, 1983, p 484.

Rogers KS. Tumors of the ear canal. Vet Clin North Am [Small Anim Pract] 18:86C, 1988.

Roth L. Pathologic changes in otitis externa. Vet Clin North Am [Small Anim Pract] 18:755, 1988.

Roth L. Rhabdomyoma of the ear pinna in four cats. J Comp Pathol 103:237, 1990.

Schuknecht HF. Pathology of the Ear. Cambridge, MA, Harvard University Press, 1974, p 461.

Schuknecht HF, Igarashi M, Gacek RR. The pathological types of cochleo-saccular degeneration. Acta Otolaryng 59:154, 1965.

Schunk KL, Averill DR. Peripheral vestibular syndrome in the dog: A review of 83 cases. J Am Vet Med Assoc 182:1354, 1983.

Scott DW. External ear disorders. J Am Anim Hosp Assoc 16:426, 1980.

Shanmugaraknam K. Histological typing of tumors of the upper respiratory tract and ear. In WHO International Histological Classification of Tumours. 2nd ed. Berlin, Springer-Verlag, 1991, pp 80, 186.

Sims MH. Electrodiagnostic evaluation of auditory function. Vet Clin North Am [Small Anim Pract] 18:913, 1988.

Steiss JE, Boosinger TR, Wright JC, et al. Healing of experimentally perforated tympanic membranes demonstrated by electrodiagnostic testing and histopathology. J Am Anim Hosp Assoc 28:307, 1992.

Tojo M, Matsuda H, Fuhui K, et al. Experimental induction of secretory and purulent otitis media by surgical obstruction of the eustachian tube in dogs. J Small Anim Pract 26:81, 1985.

Van der Gaag I. The pathology of external ear canal in dogs and cats. Vet Q 8:307, 1986.

Venker-van Haagen AJ. Management of ear diseases. In Kirk RW, ed. Current Veterinary Therapy VIII. Philadelphia, WB Saunders, 1983, p 47.

Venker-van Haagen AJ. Diseases and surgery of the ear. In Sherding RG, ed. The Cat. Diseases and Clinical Management. New York, Churchill Livingstone, 1989, p 1631.

Venker-van Haagen AJ. Total ablation of the external ear canal. In Sluijs FJ, ed. Atlas of Small Animal Surgery. University of Utrecht, Wetenschappelijke uitgeverij Bunge, 1992, p 14.

Venker-van Haagen AJ, Siemelink RJG, Smoorenburg GF. Auditory brainstem responses in the normal beagle. Vet Q 11:129, 1989.

Wisselink MA. The external ear in skin diseases of dogs and cats: A diagnostic challenge. Vet Q 8:307, 1986.

CHAPTER 14

The Hematopoietic System, Lymph Nodes, and Spleen

SHARON M. DIAL

The components of the hemolymphatic system include the bone marrow, lymph nodes, spleen, and other lymphoid tissue. These organs produce peripheral blood cells and resident tissue cells that participate in primary and secondary immune function, hemostasis, and delivery of oxygen to tissue. The bone marrow is responsible for providing the majority of the peripheral blood elements (e.g., granulocytes, monocytes, erythrocytes, and platelets) and serves as the initial source of lymphoid cells. The thymus, lymph nodes, and spleen serve as secondary sites of lymphocyte production and are primarily responsible for maintaining the integrity of the immune system. Along with its role as a secondary lymphoid organ, the spleen removes senescent or abnormal erythrocytes, stores blood, and, when necessary, participates in hematopoiesis. Age is not a primary factor in the function of these organs, but many diseases seen in the geriatric dog and cat result in secondary functional changes in the hemolymphatic organs. Several excellent references are available for general evaluation of the hemolymphatic system in dogs and cats (Ettinger, 1989; Jain, 1986).

PHYSICAL EXAMINATION

The hemolymphatic system has the advantage of being readily accessible for evaluation. Clinical findings that indicate disease involving the hemolymphatic system vary and include pale mucous membranes, hyperpnea, tachycardia, lymphadenopathy, and splenomegaly (Table 14–1). In most cases evaluation of the hemolymphatic system requires specific laboratory procedures along with the physical assessment of the dog and cat. Peripheral blood for analysis is easily obtained in most species. A complete blood cell (CBC) count and morphologic evaluation of circulating cells provide an excellent basis for assessment of hematopoietic capability. When necessary, a bone marrow aspirate can provide a direct assessment of function, with specific emphasis on cellular morphology. A core biopsy of bone marrow is necessary for confirmation of bone marrow conditions that require evaluation of the architecture of the organ (e.g., hypoplasia, aplasia, and fibrosis). The lymph nodes and spleen are evaluated by both physical examination and cytology or histopathology.

TABLE 14–1. COMMON CLINICAL SIGNS ASSOCIATED WITH DISEASE OF THE HEMOLYMPHATIC SYSTEM, LYMPH NODES, AND SPLEEN

DISEASE	CLINICAL SIGNS
Hematopoietic system (bone marrow)	
Anemia	Pale mucous membranes, exercise intolerance, mild systolic murmur, lethargy, weakness, sudden collapse.
Polycythemia	
Absolute	Brick-red mucous membranes, retinal hemorrhage or detachment, increased tortuosity of retinal blood vessels, seizures, generalized hemorrhagic tendencies.
Relative	Dehydration, cyanosis.
Neutropenia	Recurrent infections, fever.
Myeloproliferative disorders	Lethargy, anorexia, weight loss, fever, signs associated with anemia and neutropenia, splenomegaly ± hepatomegaly or lymphadenopathy.
Thrombocytopenia	Petechiae or ecchymoses, melena, epistaxis, episcleral and gingival hemorrhage, hematuria, signs associated with anemia and neutropenia.
Lymph nodes	Lethargy, weight loss, lymphadenopathy, fever, recurrent infections, edema, dysphagia, respiratory distress, tenesmus.
Spleen	Weakness, lethargy, fever, pale mucous membranes, shock, splenomegaly ± lymphadenopathy, anorexia, vomiting, abdominal distention, polyuria/polydipsia, clinical signs associated with anemia and neutropenia.

THE HEMATOPOIETIC SYSTEM

The CBC count is the standard method for initial evaluation not only of the bone marrow, but also of many other organ systems, including the lymph nodes and spleen. In the case of splenomegaly or lymphadenopathy, a CBC count can assist in determining whether the process involves inflammation or neoplasia. A CBC count consists of a packed cell volume (PCV) and/or hematocrit, red blood cell (RBC) count, hemoglobin concentration, RBC indices, total white blood cell count with differential, platelet count, and morphologic assessment of the peripheral blood elements including the platelets. The CBC count should also include a plasma protein value, but not all laboratories provide this value.

A CBC count consists of three parts: the erythrogram (PCV, RBC count, hemoglobin concentration, mean corpuscular volume [MCV], mean corpuscular hemoglobin concentration [MCHC], mean corpuscular hemoglobin [MCH], RBC morphology, and reticulocyte count, if needed), the leukogram (WBC count, differential, and WBC morphology), and the platelet count. Evaluation of hematology data from healthy beagle dogs age birth to 16 years showed no significant changes after the first year (Lowseth et al, 1990). Studies evaluating hematologic changes with age in the healthy cat have included only cats up to 1 year of age.

Anemia

The primary abnormalities associated with the erythrogram are anemia, erythrocytosis, and RBC morphologic changes. Causes of anemia in the geriatric dog and cat include blood loss, immune-mediated or parasitic RBC destruction, suppression of erythropoiesis by inflammation, drugs, extra marrow neoplasia, myelodysplasia, myelophthisis, and myeloproliferative disease. Initial assessment of anemia in any dog or cat requires determination of degree of regeneration. In most cases, anemias that are the result of RBC loss or destruction will exhibit a regenerative response characterized by a significant reticulocyte count and, in some instances, an increased MCV. Nonregenerative anemias are usually the result of suppressed erythropoiesis owing to either primary (marrow) or secondary (extramarrow) causes and are characterized by inadequate reticulocyte counts and normal MCV. There are several methods used to determine degree of regeneration. The absolute reticulocyte count can be determined by multiplying the percentage of reticulocytes by the RBC count. With this method, an absolute reticulocyte count of 60,000 cells/μl is considered evidence of bone marrow response. A corrected reticulocyte count can be determined by the following formula:

$$\text{Corrected reticulocyte count (\%)} = \text{Observed reticulocyte count (\%)} \times \frac{\text{Patient PCV}}{\text{Normal PCV}^*}$$

A corrected reticulocyte count of greater than 1 per cent in the cat or greater than 1.5 per cent

*Normal PCV for dogs = 45; for cats = 37.

in the dog is considered regenerative. The dog is thought to have a more pronounced regenerative response than the cat, and therefore a higher corrected count is required for an anemia to be classified as regenerative. Although the presence or absence of an appropriate reticulocytosis is the primary criterion for classification of anemias, it is important to remember that 2 to 5 days are required for regeneration to be evident after an acute episode of blood loss. A nonregenerative anemia with clinical findings consistent with acute disease or trauma suggests acute blood loss or destruction. Further characterization of an anemia requires evaluation of the RBC indices (primarily MCV and MCHC) and RBC morphology. Most regenerative anemias are macrocytic and hypochromic. Reticulocytes produced in response to anemia are usually larger and have a lower concentration of hemoglobin, which is reflected in an increased MCV and decreased MCHC. Nonregenerative anemias are usually normocytic and normochromic. Iron deficiency anemia is a microcytic hypochromic anemia that can be either regenerative or nonregenerative depending on the duration of iron deficiency and extent of iron depletion. Figure 14–1 illustrates a systematic approach to the anemias seen in geriatric patients.

Regenerative Anemias

Regenerative anemias are either hemolytic or hemorrhagic (i.e., extravascular or intravascular). In both cases there is a loss of erythrocytes that stimulates a responsive bone marrow to release young RBCs (reticulocytes or polychromatophilic cells). Again, about 2 to 5 days are required before evidence of regeneration is seen in the peripheral blood (Jain, 1986). As a result, acute hemorrhage or hemolysis appears nonregenerative initially (normocytic and normochromic) and then becomes macrocytic and hypochromic as the young RBCs are released from the bone marrow.

Hemolytic Anemias. Hemolytic anemia can result from immune-mediated or parasitic causes, oxidant injury, or fragmentation. Hemolytic anemias are common in both dogs and cats; however, each species is predisposed to specific causes. Primary immune-mediated hemolytic anemia is common in the dog but has not been well documented in the cat (Cain et al, 1988; Jain, 1986). Secondary immune-mediated hemolytic anemia associated with infectious disease is more common in the cat (Cain et al, 1988). Hemolytic anemia associated with oxidant injury is also more common in the cat as a result of the increased susceptibility of feline hemoglobin to oxidation (Gaunt et al, 1983).

Immune-Mediated Hemolytic Anemia. Primary immune-mediated anemia in which no underlying disorder can be found is the most common cause of hemolytic anemia in the dog. The antibodies involved in primary immune-mediated anemia may be directed toward innate RBC antigens; however, true autoimmune hemolytic anemia is thought to be uncommon (Jonas et al, 1987). The RBC is most likely an "innocent bystander," with absorption of an antigen (hapten) or immune complex on the membrane resulting in immune removal of the erythrocyte. Immune-mediated hemolytic disease associated with drugs has been reported in humans with some frequency (Petz, 1985), but has rarely been reported in dogs and cats (Weiser, 1989). Immune-mediated hemolytic anemia predominantly affects middle-age to older dogs, and there may be a predilection for females (Harvey, 1980). The pathophysiology of the disorder involves removal of antibody-coated erythrocytes, or of part of their membrane, by the mononuclear phagocyte system (i.e., extravascular hemolysis). Intravascular hemolysis resulting from complement fixation–induced RBC lysis occurs rarely (Harvey, 1980). Partial phagocytosis of RBCs results in the formation of spherocytes, a hallmark of hemolytic anemia.

The antibodies involved in immune-mediated hemolytic anemia are most often of the immunoglobulin G (IgG) or M (IgM) isotype (Jain, 1986). Agglutination is commonly associated with IgM antibodies and may be severe enough to be detected in the collection tube and on the peripheral blood film. It is important to differentiate agglutination from excess rouleaux formation by diluting a drop of blood in 5 ml of normal saline solution, centrifuging, and resuspending the pellet in fresh saline solution. This technique should remove the excess protein that causes rouleaux but not the antibodies responsible for agglutination.

Coombs' test is routinely used to diagnose immune-mediated hemolytic anemia. The test is negative in about 30 per cent of dogs with immune-mediated disease and therefore is best used to support rather than rule out a diagnosis of immune-mediated disease (Hohenhaus, 1992). Dogs with positive Coombs' test results may require a longer hospital stay but do not appear to differ in survival time from dogs with negative Coombs' test results (Hohenhaus, 1992). Occasionally, IgM-type cold agglutinins may cause in-

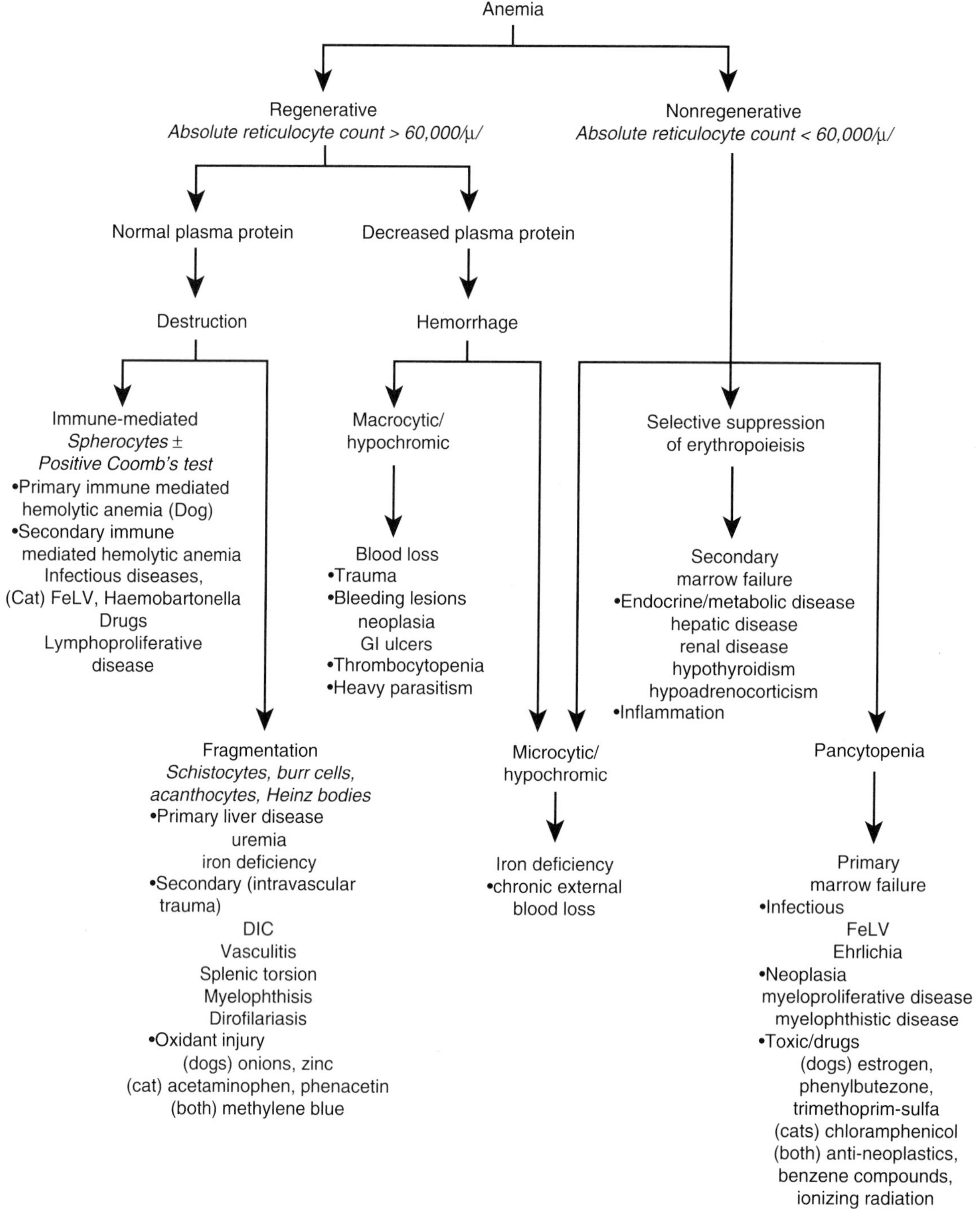

Figure 14–1. A systematic approach to anemias in dogs and cats.

travascular agglutination within small vessels of extremities (especially the ears), resulting in cyanosis and necrosis. One often overlooked diagnostic test that may contribute additional information in support of immune-mediated RBC injury is the saline fragility test. This assay has been used to document immune-mediated hemolytic anemia in which the presence of spherocytes is questionable (Weiser, 1989).

In most cases immune-mediated anemias are regenerative by the time the patient is seen in an acute crisis. A nonregenerative form of immune-mediated anemia has been reported (Jonas et al, 1987). In these cases the primary immune response is directed toward immature RBCs (e.g., polychromatophilic RBCs, metarubricytes, and rubricytes). The bone marrow is hypercellular, often with erythroid predominance and erythrophagia by marrow macrophages.

Immune-mediated hemolytic anemia is rarely reported in cats and is usually associated with either feline leukemia virus infection or haemobartonellosis. In these cases the hemolytic anemia is due to RBC acquisition of antigen from the infectious agent (Madewell and Feldman, 1980). One case of propylthiouracil-associated immune hemolytic anemia with development of antinuclear antibodies has been reported in the cat (Peterson, 1984).

Hemoparasite-induced Hemolytic Anemia. Hemoparasite-induced hemolytic anemia is not necessarily a geriatric problem but should be considered in older patients as well as younger ones. The hemotrophic parasites responsible for anemia in the cat are *Haemobartonella felis* and *Cytauxzoon felis*. *Haemobartonella canis*, *Babesia canis*, and *Babesia gibsoni* are the hemotropic parasites that are clinically relevant in dogs.

Hemolytic anemia associated with hemotropic parasites is by far most common in the cat, with *H. felis* being the most common parasite seen. The clinical signs that characterize feline haemobartonellosis include anorexia, depression, weakness, pale mucous membranes, jaundice, splenomegaly, and fever (MacWilliams, 1987). These signs are all related to the often severe anemia present in clinical cases of haemobartonellosis. *Haemobartonella* spp. can be either primary or secondary pathogens in both cats and dogs (Jain, 1986). When haemobartonellosis occurs as a secondary pathogen, the clinical signs of the primary disease may be difficult to separate from those caused by *Haemobartonella*.

H. felis is a pleomorphic organism that can be seen as a coccoid body, rod, or ring form. Although both mature and immature RBCs are parasitized, polychromatophilic cells have the highest incidence of parasitism. Fresh blood is best for evaluation for parasites, because the organism can detach from RBCs in vitro and be difficult to find on stored blood. Ethylenediaminetetra-acetic acid (EDTA) can also enhance detachment of the organism. Fluorescent immunocytologic and acridine orange staining methods are more sensitive than Romanowsky stains in detecting the organism (Jain, 1986).

H. felis is ubiquitous in the cat population. The incidence of carriers is not known but is considered to be large (Grindem et al, 1990). In many cases clinical haemobartonellosis in older cats occurs in association with a concurrent disease (e.g., feline leukemia virus infection, feline immunodeficiency virus infection, and neoplasia) or after splenectomy. Feline haemobartonellosis is a common cause of Coombs'-positive hemolytic anemia in cats (Zulty and Kociba, 1990). Definitive diagnosis is based on identification of the parasite on a peripheral blood film. However, haemobartonellosis should not be ruled out simply because the organism was not found on one blood film. The parasitemia is cyclic, and the number of organisms can be few, which makes identification difficult.

Canine haemobartonellosis is seen primarily in splenectomized dogs. The organism can be found in many nonsplenectomized dogs but is usually not pathogenic in these cases (MacWilliams, 1987). Nonsplenectomized dogs have developed clinical haemobartonellosis, usually in conjunction with an underlying primary disorder such as splenic disease, immunosuppression, or infestation with other hematopoietic parasites (MacWilliams, 1987). The clinical signs associated with canine haemobartonellosis are pale mucous membranes and listlessness. As with any secondary pathogen, the clinical signs of the underlying primary disease are difficult to separate from those caused by the secondary parasitic disease. *H. canis* differs in morphology from *H. felis* in that it occurs as chains (sometimes branching) rather than as single cocci or rods (Hoskins, 1991). The organism itself does not appear to cause membrane changes, and thus the hemolytic anemia is thought to be due primarily to immune-mediated mechanisms (Jain, 1986). Spherocytes and a positive Coombs' test are found with canine haemobartonellosis, supporting the mechanism of immune injury (Bellamy, 1978).

Dogs and cats that are kept as blood donors should be screened to detect *Haemobartonella* carriers. Older debilitated patients that receive blood from carriers are likely to develop clinical anemia.

C. felis is a protozoal parasite that is responsible for an acute lethal disease. Anemia, icterus, petechial and ecchymotic hemorrhages, pericardial effusion, splenomegaly, and lymphadenopathy are characteristic findings in cytauxzoonosis. The disease is relatively rare and is found primarily in Missouri, Texas, Arkansas, Georgia, Louisiana, and Oklahoma (Wrightman et al, 1977).

The primary canine hemotropic parasitic disease is babesiosis. Although the majority of cases occur in young animals (peracute disease), immune suppression or splenectomy can predispose dogs to acute or chronic babesiosis. *B. canis* is the species most prevalent in the United States. The organism is an intracellular piroplasm transmitted primarily by the brown dog tick *Rhipicephalus sanguineus.* The common hematologic changes noted with babesiosis include moderate to severe anemia, thrombocytopenia with or without evidence of disseminated intravascular coagulation (DIC), and hemoglobinemia. Erythrocyte morphology changes include anisocytosis, macrocytosis, polychromasia, reticulocytosis, metarubricytosis, poikilocytosis, and spherocytosis. If DIC is present, schistocytes may be present as well. The anemia is usually regenerative and is due to erythrophagocytosis and intravascular hemolysis by replicating trophozoites (MacWilliams, 1987). However, coinfection with *Ehrlichia canis* can result in a nonregenerative anemia (Taboada and Merchant, 1991). Diagnosis of babesiosis, like other hemoparasitic diseases, is based on demonstration of the organism in erythrocytes. In addition, a serologic test is available for diagnosis of babesiosis in dogs. Feline babesiosis (*Babesia felis*) has not been reported in the United States and appears to be a disease of young cats (i.e., less than 2 years of age).

Oxidant Injury Hemolytic Anemia. Oxidant injury to RBCs results in irreversible denaturation of hemoglobin, which precipitates to form Heinz bodies and binds to the inner surface of the RBC membrane. Binding of the denatured hemoglobin to the membrane causes a change in the cell shape and decreased flexibility, increasing removal of the affected RBCs from circulation by the mononuclear phagocyte system, especially the spleen (Harvey and Rackear, 1985). Heinz bodies are characterized with Romanowksy stain (Wright's stain) as pale refractile inclusions that may or may not protrude from the RBC. They are more readily seen with new methylene blue stain and appear as distinctive blue inclusions. In some instances oxidative injury causes eccentrocyte formation by RBC membrane fusion. (Eccentrocytes are RBCs with eccentric pale areas [Harvey and Rackear, 1985].)

The hemolysis associated with oxidant injury is usually extravascular, although severe cases may involve intravascular hemolysis. Oxidant agents that have been associated with Heinz body hemolytic anemia in the dog are onions, methylene blue, and benzocaine (Harvey et al 1979; Harvey and Rackear, 1985; Jain, 1986). The most common agents associated with Heinz body anemia in the cat are acetaminophen (and phenacetin), methylene blue, D-methionine, phenazopyridine, and propylene glycol (Christopher, 1989; Christopher et al 1989; Harvey and Kornick, 1976; Hjelle, 1986; Jain, 1986; Maede, 1987). Acetaminophen toxicity has been well characterized in the cat and dog (Gaunt et al, 1983; Harvey et al, 1986; Hjelle, 1986). Ingestion of as little as one half of a 325-mg tablet will cause clinical toxicity in cats. In addition to Heinz body anemia, oxidant injury can result in increased methemoglobin formation, further reducing the oxygen carrying capacity of the RBCs.

Feline hemoglobin is more susceptible to injury because of the increased numbers of exposed sulfhydryl groups that can be oxidized (Christopher et al, 1989). As a result, healthy cats can have a small number of Heinz bodies. Cats with various chronic illnesses can demonstrate a significant increase in Heinz bodies that is not associated with overt hemolytic disease. However, these Heinz bodies may contribute to the mild anemia seen in these chronic diseases (Christopher et al, 1989). Many of these diseases (e.g., hyperthyroidism, diabetes mellitus, chronic renal failure, and neoplasia) are common in the geriatric patient. Along with increased susceptibility of feline hemoglobin to oxidant injury, the feline spleen may have less ability to remove abnormal RBCs (Jain, 1986).

Depression of normal splenic function can cause an increase in circulating Heinz bodies in the dog. Dogs receiving prednisolone will often have numerous small Heinz bodies that, as in the ill cat, do not appear to be associated with hemolytic disease (Jain, 1986). In general, the Heinz bodies seen with significant oxidant injury are large enough to protrude beyond the RBCs' normal membrane profile and are easily seen with Romanowsky stains, whereas the Heinz bodies associated with illness or decreased splenic function are small and primarily evident with new methylene blue stain.

Fragmentation-Induced Hemolytic Anemia. Fragmentation hemolysis is a mild to moderate regenerative anemia associated with specific RBC morphology changes. Primary fragmentation hemolysis is associated with changes in the RBC membrane (e.g., iron deficiency or liver disease), whereas secondary fragmentation hemolysis is due to vascular changes that result in intravascular trauma (i.e., microangiopathic hemolysis) (Harvey, 1980). Iron deficiency and severe liver disease are both associated with decreased RBC membrane elasticity and increased membrane fragility (Weiser and Kociba, 1983a). The RBCs have a tendency to fragment, because they cannot traverse the small capillary beds as easily as cells with normal elasticity. Hemangiosarcoma (or other vascular tumors), DIC, vasculitis, splenic torsion, dirofilariasis, vena cava syndromes, and severe inflammation of a vascular organ (e.g., lungs or intestine) can result in microangiopathic hemolysis. Splenic torsion and vena caval syndromes are disorders associated with severe anemia resulting from fragmentation. In both disorders hemoglobinemia and hemoglobinuria occur because of extensive intravascular fragmentation (Weiser, 1989). Fibrin deposition in small vessels causes a shearing effect as RBCs try to circulate through the vascular bed (La Rue and Feldman, 1985). The fragmented RBCs have been described as schistocytes, acanthocytes, spur cells, apple-stem cells, and helmet cells. Microspherocytes can also be seen. Specific morphologic changes have been associated with certain disorders: acanthocytes with hemangiosarcoma, spur cells with severe liver disease, and apple-stem cells with iron deficiency. The anemia can be regenerative or nonregenerative depending on the primary cause of fragmentation. The fragmentation anemia seen with hemangiosarcoma is usually regenerative as a response to internal blood loss, whereas the anemia seen with acute DIC, severe liver disease, severe inflammatory disease, and other types of neoplasia is usually nonregenerative. Iron deficiency can be either regenerative or nonregenerative depending on the duration of illness.

Hemorrhagic Anemia. Trauma, hemorrhagic lesions (neoplasms, gastrointestinal ulcers, or foreign bodies), parasitism (external or internal), hemostatic abnormalities (thrombocytopenia or decreased coagulation factor activity), and iatrogenic blood loss can all result in blood loss anemia. Trauma is a common cause of blood loss anemia in dogs and cats of all ages. If no external evidence or history of trauma is present, then blood loss due to neoplasia or other bleeding lesions should be a primary differential diagnosis in the geriatric patient. Hemorrhagic lesions in the gastrointestinal and urinary tract can result in significant external blood loss that, with chronicity, can result in a microcytic, hypochromic iron deficiency anemia (Harvey et al, 1982; Weiser et al, 1983a). Internal blood loss from thoracic or abdominal lesions will not progress to iron deficiency, because the iron is reabsorbed rather than lost from the body.

Older animals with chronic inflammatory or neoplastic disease cannot always respond adequately to blood loss because of underlying bone marrow suppression from the primary disease. In these cases hemorrhage may be associated with a poor regenerative response. The reticulocyte count is increased above normal, but the corrected reticulocyte count is still less than 1 per cent. The release of reticulocytes indicates that the marrow is attempting to respond, but because of the underlying disease, the reticulocyte count is not appropriate for the degree of anemia.

The changes in hematologic values associated with blood loss anemia include decreases in PCV, RBC count, hemoglobin concentration, and total protein concentration. These changes are not evident within the first 12 hours, because the compensatory fluid shift from the extravascular compartment to the intravascular compartment occurs over time (Jain, 1986). As mentioned before, reticulocytosis, macrocytosis, and hypochromasia do not occur until at least 2 to 5 days after blood loss. Chronic blood loss will be regenerative until iron stores are depleted.

Hypoproteinemia is variable with blood loss anemias. Acute external blood loss is characterized by hypoproteinemia after fluid shifts from the extravascular space to the intravascular space. Chronic external blood loss may or may not be associated with hypoproteinemia. Chronic hemorrhage from a gastric lesion can result in loss of significant amounts of iron, whereas protein loss may be minimal. Chronic blood loss caused by parasitism, however, is characterized by significant hypoproteinemia (Jain, 1986). With hemorrhage into body cavities, the protein is usually reclaimed, and hypoproteinemia does not develop.

Iron deficiency anemia is more common in young animals as the result of dietary deficiency (in nursing kittens) or gastrointestinal or external parasitism (in kittens and puppies) (Weiser and Kociba, 1983a). Adult and geriatric dogs and cats are less commonly affected by iron deficiency anemia caused by parasitism. In subtropical or tropical locations, however, parasitism may be severe enough to cause clinical anemia (Harvey et al, 1982). In the geriatric dog or cat without evidence of parasitism, iron deficiency anemia should initiate a search for occult chronic external blood loss from a gastrointestinal or urinary tract lesion.

Although chronic hemorrhage occurs in the cat, iron deficiency does not appear to be recognized in this species to any appreciable extent. Iron deficiency in the adult cat was not well characterized until Fulton and coworkers (1988) reported a 17-year-old castrated male domestic shorthair with focal intestinal lymphoma. The authors suggested several reasons for the apparent low incidence of iron deficiency in the adult cat. Hypochromasia, a hallmark of iron deficiency, is not readily detected on feline blood film preparations, and the small MCV of feline microcytes may preclude their detection by standard electronic hematology instrumentation with fixed threshold values. Cats also have greater gastrointestinal iron absorption capacity than other species. In the geriatric patient there may be a decrease in iron absorption capacity, which would account for the development of overt iron deficiency anemia. This has not been evaluated in the cat, but geriatric dogs have significantly decreased levels of total serum iron (Lowseth et al, 1990). Transferrin, the principal carrier of iron in the blood, is decreased in geriatric dogs because of their decreased activity and subsequent decrease in oxygen demand at the tissue level. This causes decreased iron availability for incorporation into heme and may predispose the geriatric patient to iron deficiency due to chronic blood loss.

Nonregenerative Anemias

Nonregenerative anemias are due to lack of bone marrow response to decreased erythrocyte mass, as well as to acute blood loss. The causes of deficient bone marrow response may be primary or secondary. Primary causes of bone marrow suppression include drug toxicities, infectious agents, bone marrow aplasia, myelofibrosis, myelophthisis, and myeloproliferative disorders. Drugs associated with bone marrow suppression are estrogen, phenylbutazone, anticancer drugs, and various antimicrobial agents. Infectious agents that have been associated with bone marrow suppression are feline leukemia virus and *E. canis.* Secondary causes of bone marrow suppression include renal disease, liver disease, endocrine disorders, inflammation, and extramarrow neoplasia. Bone marrow cellularity in primary disorders is usually hypoplastic but in secondary disorders is normal or even increased as a result of granulocytic hyperplasia, as seen in inflammatory diseases. The most common causes of bone marrow failure are secondary, and many of the disorders associated with secondary bone marrow failure are common in the geriatric patient. With many of these disorders, especially in the geriatric patient, the owner may not recognize the signs associated with anemia, such as decreased activity or exercise intolerance. The anemia is usually a secondary finding.

In many cases bone marrow evaluation is necessary to determine whether a nonregenerative anemia is due to primary or secondary bone marrow failure. A bone marrow aspiration biopsy is indicated whenever an abnormality is found on examination of peripheral blood that suggests a pathologic change in the bone marrow. Neutropenia, thrombocytopenia, and nonregenerative anemia, separately or in concert, may indicate generalized bone marrow failure. With primary bone marrow failure, there usually are decreased numbers of all hematopoietic cell lines in peripheral blood, but this observation is not always true. Pure red cell aplasia characterized by a marked nonregenerative anemia with normal production and release of myeloid elements and platelets has been reported in both dogs and cats (Weiss, 1986b). Unexplained proliferation of any hematopoietic cell line (e.g., persistent thrombocytosis, polycythemia, and increased immature cells [nucleated RBCs without polychromasia and metamyelocytes and myelocytes without an orderly left shift]) indicates possible proliferative marrow disease.

Primary Bone Marrow Failure. Non-neoplastic causes of primary bone marrow failure that should be considered in the geriatric patient fall into two broad categories: toxic and infectious (Grindem, 1989). Antimicrobials, analgesics, hormones, and antineoplastics have all been associated with bone marrow hypoplasia. Drugs can cause idiosyncratic reactions in which bone marrow hypoplasia occurs without predictability (e.g., chloramphenicol, trimethoprim-sulfadiazine, cephalosporins, and estrogen) or as an anticipated side effect (e.g., antineoplastic drugs). Table 14–2 lists various drugs that have been associated with bone marrow hypoplasia in dogs and cats. Bone marrow toxicities usually result in pancytopenia (aplastic anemia) rather than pure red cell aplasia. Recovery of normal hematologic values usually occurs on withdrawal of the drug and may be rapid or prolonged depending on the severity of the bone marrow hypoplasia.

Estrogen is a bone marrow–toxic agent with an unusual chronology of events. Estrogen toxicity occurs primarily in dogs; cats are apparently resistant to the bone marrow suppressive effects of

TABLE 14–2. DRUGS ASSOCIATED WITH PRIMARY BONE MARROW FAILURE

IDIOSYNCRATIC REACTIONS	ANTICIPATED REACTIONS
Estrogen	Cyclophosphamide
Griseofulvin (cats)	Doxorubicin
Phenylbutazone	Cytosine arabinoside
Organic arsenicals (thiacetarsamide)	Methotrexate
	Azathioprine
Cephalosporin	Dimethyl myleran
Trimethoprim-sulfonamide	6-Thioguanine
	Chloramphenicol (cats)

estrogen. Diethylstilbestrol and estradiol cyclopentylpropionate are associated with significant bone marrow toxicity, but this effect is inconsistent among individuals. Estradiol cyclopentylpropionate is more consistent in producing toxic effects. Estrogen-producing Sertoli cell tumors are also associated with bone marrow hypoplasia/aplasia in male dogs. In the acute stage of toxicity, a marked granulocytosis occurs with granulocytic hyperplasia, erythroid hypoplasia, and megakaryocytic hypoplasia. A profound pancytopenia with marked bone marrow aplasia develops within 2 to 5 days of estrogen administration. A nonregenerative blood loss anemia may occur as a result of thrombocytopenia.

Prognosis for estrogen toxicity is fair to guarded. Recovery occurs more readily in younger animals and may be protracted in the geriatric patient (Jain, 1986; Lipschitz, 1984; Mauch, 1982). Marrow recovery depends on the severity of the toxic insult and cannot be reliably predicted. The use of estrogen compounds for treatment of urinary incontinence, perianal adenomas, or reproductive problems is discouraged in the geriatric patient.

Feline leukemia virus, feline panleukopenia virus, and *E. canis* are infectious agents commonly associated with marrow failure. In the geriatric patient, feline panleukopenia is rarely seen. Feline leukemia virus and *E. canis* infections, however, are seen with some frequency in older animals. Feline leukemia virus has a multiplicity of clinical presentations. In most cases the nonregenerative anemia associated with feline leukemia virus infection is due to suppression of erythropoiesis and not to marrow hypoplasia or infiltration (Weiser and Kociba, 1983b). Feline leukemia virus–infected cats have a significant decrease in burst forming unit–erythroid (BFU-E) and colony forming unit–erythroid (CFU-E) numbers, even in the presence of increased serum erythropoietin (EPo) (Wardrop et al, 1986). Granulocyte-macrophage progenitors may be normal or increased in these cases, suggesting that some strains of feline leukemia virus have a selective effect on erythropoiesis. Severe nonregenerative anemia with increased numbers of nucleated erythrocytes and no polychromasia may be seen with infiltration of the bone marrow with neoplastic cells. Although feline leukemia virus is most often associated with lymphoid malignancies, the virus can induce malignant transformation of pluripotential hematopoietic stem cells, which give rise to cells of all hematopoietic cell lines. Greater than 50 per cent of cats with anemia will be feline leukemia virus positive, and thus it is important to include screening tests for feline leukemia virus infection in the diagnostic work-up for anemia in the cat (Cotter, 1979; Weiser, 1989).

Chronic canine ehrlichiosis may manifest as a mild disease with occasional recrudescence of the signs associated with acute disease or severe disease with pancytopenia resulting from bone marrow hypoplasia (Woody and Hoskins, 1991). The determining factor is thought to be the inability of severely affected animals to mount an appropriate cell-mediated immune response. Severe bone marrow hypoplasia is not the most common presentation of ehrlichiosis. In most cases the clinicopathologic changes are thrombocytopenia and nonregenerative anemia with or without neutropenia. The bone marrow in these cases is hypercellular; megakaryocytosis, granulocytic hyperplasia with or without erythroid hypoplasia, and plasmacytosis are common cytologic findings. Immune-mediated mechanisms are responsible for the thrombocytopenia and may contribute to the neutropenia as well (Latimer and Meyer, 1989). The clinical signs become evident 2 to 4 months after infection and include anorexia, depression, emaciation, pyrexia, pallor, generalized lymphadenopathy, splenomegaly, and bleeding as a result of thrombocytopenia. Chronic ehrlichiosis may result in a persistent lymphocytosis (up to 10,000 cells/μl) that has been confused with chronic lymphocytic leukemia. Demonstration of *Ehrlichia* spp. organisms in peripheral blood is not common. In most cases, canine ehrlichiosis is diagnosed by clinical presentation and serology.

Myelodysplasia and myeloproliferative disease may be a continuum of the same process: stem cell injury (Weiser, 1989). Neoplastic causes of bone marrow failure can be due either to hematopoietic neoplasms or to metastatic neoplasms of extramarrow origin. Extramarrow neoplasia with a propensity for metastasis to bone marrow seldom results in complete bone marrow suppression. The metastases are usually focal and do not replace enough of the marrow to cause pancytopenia. These neoplasms will result in anemia of inflammatory disease (AID). Neoplasms of hematopoietic and lymphoid tissue commonly cause primary marrow failure. Replacement of normal functional hematopoietic tissue by leukemic cells will cause significant neutropenia, thrombocytopenia, and anemia because of the tendency of leukemic cells to cause widespread myelophthisis.

Secondary Bone Marrow Failure. Chronic renal disease is associated with a moderate to severe nonregenerative anemia. There are several factors that may contribute to the anemia of renal failure: lack of EPo production by the renal capillary endothelium in response to hypoxia, suppression of erythropoiesis by various uremic toxins (parathyroid hormone [PTH], methylguanidine, and spermine), decreased erythrocyte life span, and increase RBC loss through bleeding (Petrites-Murphy et al, 1989). Depressed EPo production appears to be the primary factor involved in development of a nonregenerative anemia in animals with chronic renal failure (King et al, 1992). EPo levels are low or within normal range in the majority of anemic individuals with chronic renal failure. The exact role of factors other than EPo in the genesis of the anemia of renal failure is poorly understood. Increased levels of serum phosphorus and PTH may have a negative effect on the action of EPo by decreasing production in response to anemia, decreasing function of EPo in stimulating erythropoiesis, and effecting metabolism of EPo (Petrites-Murphy et al, 1989).

Recombinant human EPo has been used in humans, dogs, and cats to successfully treat the anemia of renal failure. In the cases reported, normalization of PCV led to increased quality of life in the treated individuals (Cowgill, 1991). The use of androgenic steroids in the anemia of chronic renal disease is controversial. Androgenic steroids promote erythropoiesis primarily through EPo and may be not effective in increasing erythrogenesis in disorders associated with decreased capacity to produce EPo, such as chronic renal failure.

Androgens, corticosteroids, growth hormone, and thyroxine have a facilitative effect on erythropoiesis. Estrogen, on the other hand, inhibits erythropoiesis. A mild normocytic-normochromic nonregenerative anemia is associated with hypothyroidism, hypoadrenocorticism, and anterior pituitary insufficiency (Weiss and Armstrong, 1984). Hormones affect erythropoiesis primarily by increasing metabolism and oxygen consumption, thereby increasing EPo production. In addition, androgens, growth hormone, thyroxine, and corticosteroids enhance the responsiveness of the erythron to EPo (Jain, 1986). Correction of the underlying endocrine abnormality will result in restoration of normal erythropoiesis.

Anemia associated with liver disease is poorly understood. Such anemia is commonly nonregenerative but may show variable degrees of reticulocytosis. This suggests that the marrow is attempting to produce an appropriate response, but cannot. Several factors may be involved: decreased RBC survival, blood loss as a result of coagulopathies and thrombocytopenia, fragmentation hemolysis caused by microangiopathy or altered membrane fragility, and impaired bone marrow response (Weiss and Armstrong, 1984). Decreased RBC survival has been documented in liver disease; however, the exact mechanism is unknown at this time. Changes in membrane lipids that alter membrane flexibility and increase RBC fragility are thought to be a likely cause. Morphologic evidence of membrane changes can be seen on peripheral blood films as significant poikilocytosis, including spur cell formation. Decreased response by the marrow may be due to impaired mobilization of hepatic iron or inadequate erythropoietin activity. With inflammatory hepatic disease, the anemia may be due to effects of inflammation on erythropoiesis rather than a specific aspect of hepatic dysfunction.

AID and extramarrow neoplasia will be discussed together because they may share mechanisms, and inflammation is often a significant component of neoplastic lesions. The pathogenesis of AID has been extensively studied. Currently, both suppression of erythropoiesis and decreased RBC life span are thought to be of primary importance in AID. The anemia is usually mild to moderate and causes no serious consequence. Reduced levels of serum iron, decreased total serum transferrin, decreased per cent transferrin saturation, and increased bone marrow and hepatic nonheme iron are consistent findings in AID (Couto, 1993). The decreased availability of iron for heme synthesis is one factor that contributes to decreased erythropoiesis. Serum inhibitors of erythropoiesis have been found in several studies of AID, malignancy, and chronic renal failure (Weiss, 1986a). The identity of the inhibitors has not been elucidated; possibilities include interferon, prostaglandin E_1, and interleukins. The decreased RBC life span may be due to an accelerated form of normal senescent destruction in which there is increased RBC surface immunoglobulin, which promotes erythrophagocytosis (Weiss and McClay, 1988). Further studies have indicated that activated neutrophils play a role in altering the antigenic nature of RBC membranes (Weiss et al, 1991). Anemia of inflammation can be seen in concert with other types of anemia; in such cases the degree of anemia will be moderate to severe. Blood loss, RBC fragmentation, and other causes of regenerative anemia may be present; bone marrow response is poor in these cases.

Anemia is the most common hematologic abnormality associated with neoplastic disease (Couto, 1993). Chronic inflammation, bleeding, hemolysis (both immune mediated and microangiopathic), hypersplenism, and tumor cachexia all contribute to the anemia seen with neoplasia (Madewell and Feldman, 1980). Anemia associated with nonhematopoietic neoplasia is seldom due to marrow infiltration.

Pure red cell aplasia is defined as a severe nonregenerative anemia with normal leukocyte and platelet numbers. Several authors have provided convincing evidence that pure red cell aplasia is immune mediated in origin. The immune response is directed toward the committed erythroid stem cell. Bone marrow evaluation reveals normal granulocytic and megakaryocytic activity with severe erythroid aplasia (Harvey, 1980; Jonas et al, 1987; Weiss, 1986b; Zoumbos et al, 1985). The primary indicator of immune-mediated pure red cell aplasia is its steroid responsiveness.

Erythrocytosis (Polycythemia)

An increase in PCV caused by loss of plasma volume (dehydration or hemoconcentration) is termed *relative erythrocytosis* and is the most common cause of erythrocytosis in geriatric dogs and cats. Absolute erythrocytosis is due to either an appropriate or an inappropriate increase in erythropoiesis. Appropriate absolute erythrocytosis occurs in response to increased EPo production and is secondary to disorders that result in hypoxia (e.g., severe respiratory disease, renal hypoxia, and cardiac disease) or in an increase in EPo or EPo-like activity. As discussed previously, corticosteroids and thyroid hormone increase metabolism and oxygen consumption, thereby increasing EPo production and potentiating the effect of EPo on bone marrow stem cells. Neoplasms have been shown to produce EPo-like substances (Couto et al, 1989; Peterson and Zanjani, 1981).

Inappropriate absolute erythrocytosis or polycythemia vera is caused by uncontrolled EPo-independent erythropoiesis and is an uncommon myeloproliferative disorder. In addition to increased RBC mass, animals with polycythemia vera may have leukocytosis and thrombocytosis. A diagnosis of polycythemia vera can be made only after causes of appropriate erythrocytosis are eliminated. Causes of hypoxia (systemic or renal), neoplasia, and underlying endocrine disorders must be ruled out, and either serum or urine EPo concentrations must be shown to be normal or low before polycythemia vera can be considered as a diagnosis.

Leukocyte Abnormalities

The primary functions of peripheral blood leukocytes include nonspecific (neutrophils, eosinophils, basophils, and monocytes) and specific (lymphocytes) host defense. The leukogram provides a relatively simple method of evaluating an animal's response to disease. Although the changes found on the leukogram are seldom pathognomonic for a specific disease, the leukogram can assist in developing a differential diagnosis as well as a prognosis. Sequential leukograms are extremely useful in following the course of a disease and monitoring response to therapy. Marked changes in specific leukocyte numbers and morphology can occur very rapidly in disease states. The peripheral blood leukocyte pool is in constant state of flux. During a healthy state, the normal dynamics of cell turnover maintain a fairly consistent pool of circulating leukocytes with normal morphology. During disease processes, absolute leukocyte counts may increase above (leukocytosis) or decrease below (leukopenia) their established reference ranges. There are no leukocyte changes unique to the geriatric dog or cat. Excellent reviews (Ettinger, 1989; Jain, 1986) of normal and altered leukocyte responses are available. General differential diagnoses for leukocytosis or leukopenia in the dog and cat are summarized in Table 14–3.

Leukocytosis

Leukocytosis may be caused by an increase in any of the specific peripheral blood leukocytes. The most common leukocytosis is neutrophilia. The neutrophil's primary function is phagocytosis and killing of microorganisms such as bacteria. The performance of this function requires several processes: margination, adhesion, emigration, chemotaxis, phagocytosis, and killing. The total

TABLE 14–3. LEUKOCYTE ABNORMALITIES

LEUKOPENIA		
Neutropenia	Lymphopenia	Eosinopenia
Consumption/destruction	Metabolic	Corticosteroids
Inflammation or infection	Endogenous or exogenous corticosteroids	
Immune-mediated	Loss	
Drugs	Chylothorax	
Hypersplenism	Lymphangiectasia	
Decreased production	Decreased production	
Infectious (FeLV, FIV, *Ehrlichia canis*)	Antineoplastic drugs	
Toxicity (antineoplastic drugs, antibiotics, estrogen)	Radiation therapy	
Myelophthisis	Infectious (viral)	
Leukemia		
Myelofibrosis		
Myelodysplasia		
Testicular tumors (estrogen)		
Immune-mediated (T-lymphocyte suppression of granulopoiesis)		
Margination		
Sepsis		
Endotoxemia		
LEUKOCYTOSIS		
Neutrophilia	Lymphocytosis	Monocytosis
Inflammation	Antigenic stimulation	Inflammation
Infectious	Inflammation	Infectious
Necrosis	Immune-mediated	Necrosis
Neoplasia	Neoplasia	Neoplasia
Immune-mediated	Lymphoid leukemia	Physiologic
Myeloid leukemia	Physiologic	Corticosteroids
Physiologic	Epinephrine (cats)	Myelomonocytic leukemia
Epinephrine (cats)	Basophilia	Mastocytemia
Endogenous or exogenous corticosteroids	Inflammation	Inflammation
Eosinophilia	Parasitism	Mast cell tumor (systemic)
Inflammation	Allergies	
Parasitism	Basophilic leukemia	
Allergies		
Hypereosinophilic syndrome		
Eosinophilic leukemia		
Systemic mastocytoma		

FeLV, Feline leukemia virus; FIV, feline immunodeficiency virus.

number of leukocytes in the body can be divided into five compartments: three in the bone marrow (proliferative, maturation, and storage pools) and two within the vasculature (marginal and circulating pools). The circulating pool is sampled during venipuncture.

Peripheral neutrophilia in the geriatric dog and cat can result from several mechanisms: acute shift from the marginal pool to the circulating pool; acute shift from the storage pool into the circulating pool; increased proliferation, with increases in all the subsequent pools; and decreased emigration from the circulating pool.

The most common cause of neutrophilia is acute shift from the marginal pool into the circulating pool. Physiologic neutrophilia results from endogenous epinephrine release, which causes a shift of neutrophils from the marginal pool. Lymphocytosis, erythrocytosis, and thrombocytosis may accompany the neutrophilia. Although this phenomenon is usually seen in young cats and dogs, it should still be considered as a differential diagnosis, especially in excitable geriatric dogs and cats. The epinephrine-induced shift of leukocytes into the circulating pool is caused by decreased neutrophil adherence and increased blood flow; there is no increase in the total peripheral blood leukocyte pool.

Unlike physiologic neutrophilia, corticosteroid-induced neutrophilia is caused by an absolute increase in the total blood leukocyte pool and is accompanied by lymphopenia and eosinopenia. In dogs, a monocytosis may be present in the corticosteroid response. Corticosteroids decrease emigration of neutrophils from the circulation, decrease neutrophil adherence, and increase release of neutrophils from the bone marrow storage pool. The neutrophil count may return to normal values with chronic corticosteroid administration. The neutrophil count will return to previous values about 72 to 96 hours after withdrawal of exogenous corticosteroids. Because corticosteroids reduce neutrophil adherence and emigration into tissue, they are immunosuppressive and predispose patients to infections.

Neutrophilia with a left shift (i.e., an increase in circulating immature neutrophils [e.g., band neutrophils, metamyelocytes, and myelocytes]), is indicative of inflammation or infection. Although stress can cause a mature neutrophilia, the presence of band neutrophils is specific for an inflammatory response. A marked leukocytosis (total leukocyte count greater than 75,000/μl) in response to inflammation or antigenic stimulation is often referred to as a *leukemoid reaction.* Leukemoid reactions usually are characterized by neutrophilia with a significant left shift; however, the term can also be used to describe a severe lymphocytosis, eosinophilia, or monocytosis. In each case the peripheral blood picture can be confused with the corresponding myeloproliferative disease. The neutrophilic leukemoid reaction is characterized by an orderly maturation sequence of neutrophils (e.g., mostly mature neutrophils). Acute myelogenous leukemia is characterized by a predominance of immature neutrophils with a disproportionate number of blasts. Chronic granulocytic leukemia, however, is difficult to differentiate from a leukemoid reaction, because it has the same maturation pattern with mature forms predominating. A diagnosis of granulocytic leukemia is often arrived at by eliminating all possible causes of a leukemoid response. The most common causes of neutrophilic leukemoid reactions are severe localized inflammatory disorders (e.g., pyometra and abscessation), immune-mediated hemoltytic anemia, neoplasia, and *Hepatozoon canis* infection.

An additional characteristic of inflammation and infection is the presence of toxic change in circulating neutrophils. The term *toxic change* is used to describe a constellation of cytoplasmic alternations that may be seen in neutrophils on a peripheral blood film. Cystoplasmic basophilia, vacuolation, and Döhle bodies are the hallmarks of toxic change. Although these changes are usually the result of septicemia or endotoxemia, they can be seen with noninfectious causes of inflammation as well. It is difficult to interpret toxic change noted on blood films prepared from blood samples that have been exposed to EDTA for more than 3 to 4 hours. The morphology of peripheral blood leukocytes will deteriorate over time, and prominent cytoplasmic vacuolation is often present in old samples. This deterioration is the primary reason most reference laboratories request that a fresh unstained blood film be prepared and sent along with the blood sample.

Lymphocytosis as a cause of leukocytosis is much less common in the geriatric dog or cat than in a younger animal. Physiologic lymphocytosis of young dogs and cats is due to excitement or in response to a recent antigenic stimulus (e.g., vaccination). Chronic lymphocytic leukemia should be suspected in any animal with a persistent lymphocytosis (lymphocyte count greater than 20,000/μl). Confirmation of chronic lymphocytic leukemia may be difficult. A bone marrow aspiration biopsy specimen in which the majority of cells present are small lymphocytes is strongly suggestive of leukemia if significant hemodilution of the sample is avoided. A core biopsy is more helpful. In many cases the diagnosis of chronic lymphocytic leukemia is based on eliminating causes of persistent lymphocytosis (e.g., chronic infectious diseases such as canine ehrlichiosis, Rocky Mountain spotted fever, feline leukemia virus infection, and blastomycosis) (Latimer and Meyer, 1989). Response to empirical treatment can be used to differentiate the two causes of lymphocytosis.

Eosinophilia can be a common finding, especially in geographical locations that have a high incidence of external and internal parasitic diseases. Inflammation of tissue that has a high number of resident mast cells (e.g., skin, gastrointestinal tract, urogenital tract, or respiratory tract) can be associated with peripheral eosinophilia; however, in many instances there may be a marked local infiltration of eosinophils in tissue without a concomitant eosinophilia. Eosinophilia is commonly associated with allergies (flea allergic dermatitis and feline asthma), eosinophilic granuloma complex, and disseminated mast cell tumors. It is also seen as a paraneoplastic syndrome resulting from release of cytokines or lymphokines by neoplastic cells (e.g., fibrosarcoma, mammary carcinoma, and lymphosarcoma) (Couto, 1984; Losco, 1986). Idiopathic hypereosinophilic syndrome is seen most often in the cat (Neer, 1991). The cause of this marked eosinophilia is unknown, and treatment is often unsuccessful. Care should be taken when differentiating idiopathic hypereosinophilic syndrome from other causes of marked eosinophilia (e.g., disseminated mast cell tumors). Basophilia is most commonly associated with the causes of eosinophilia.

Monocytosis is a common peripheral blood finding but rarely is responsible for an increase in the total leukocyte count (Latimer and Meyer,

1989). Both acute and chronic inflammation can be associated with a monocytosis. Animals with persistent neutropenia may develop a concomitant monocytosis. It is important not to misinterpret this change as monocytic leukemia; a bone marrow aspiration biopsy will assist in determining the cause of a persistent monocytosis and neutropenia. Monocytosis may occur with chronic stress, hyperadrenocorticism, and excess administration of corticosteroids in the dog.

Leukopenia

Neutropenia is probably the most significant leukopenia seen in the geriatric dog and cat. Lymphopenia and eosinopenia are most often associated with the stress leukogram and do not pose any true threat to the animal's health. Monocytopenia is not recognized as a clinical entity, because the reference range for monocytes is usually reported as fewer than 1500 cells/μl; the same is true for basophils. However, animals that present with neutropenia require aggressive evaluation to determine and correct the underlying cause.

The causes of neutropenia can be divided into two primary categories: (1) decreased production and (2) increased consumption, sequestration, and destruction. Decreased production of neutrophils is associated with bone marrow hypoplasia, as discussed earlier. The most common cause of neutropenia is increased consumption by an acute, overwhelming infectious disease or sequestration in tissue as a result of endotoxic or anaphylactic shock. Neutropenia with a left shift is commonly referred to as a *degenerate left shift* and carries a guarded to poor prognosis. Tissue demand that exceeds the bone marrow's ability to produce adequate numbers of mature cells is seen in severe inflammatory or infectious diseases such as salmonellosis, severe bacterial or aspiration pneumonia, peritonitis, pyothorax, and diffuse suppurative dermatitis. Endotoxemia is associated with increased margination of neutrophils and can result in a severe neutropenia within hours of exposure to endotoxin. Less common causes of neutropenia included immune-mediated leukopenia and hypersplenism. Naturally occurring immune-mediated neutropenia is well recognized in human medicine but has not definitively been diagnosed in the dog or cat. Anecdotal reports of corticosteroid-responsive neutropenia have circulated through the veterinary medical community for several years; in these cases, other causes of neutropenia have been ruled out before the administration of corticosteroids. The lack of a readily available test for antileukocyte antibody is probably responsible for the paucity of published case reports of immune-mediated neutropenia in veterinary medicine. An aspiration bone marrow biopsy that reveals hypercellular marrow with a left shift of the granulocytic series and leukophagia would support the diagnosis of immune-mediated disease.

Platelet Disorders

Platelets are small cytoplasmic fragments that are released from megakaryocytes into the circulation. Platelets are released as long ribbons or pro-platelets that fragment into small individual platelets in the circulation. Megakaryocytes share the common pluripotential marrow stem cell that, under the appropriate growth factor influence (megakaryocyte colony–stimulating factor [Meg-CSF]), induces differentiation of the pluripotential stem cell into a committed stem cell of megakaryocytic lineage. Maturation of the megakaryocyte and release of platelets are primarily influenced by thrombopoietin (Jain, 1986). Reviews of megakaryopoiesis have identified numerous factors (interleukins, colony-stimulating factors, and erythropoietin) that can potentiate megakaryocyte production from stem cells or maturation and platelet release (Hoffman, 1989; Mazur, 1987; Williams, 1991). Although the exact mechanisms and factors involved in thrombopoiesis have not been defined, it is generally accepted that the process has dual regulatory mechanisms: primary marrow response to megakaryocyte mass and progenitor cell numbers and secondary response to circulating platelet mass.

Platelets support endothelial integrity and are responsible for primary hemostasis. Petechiae and small ecchymotic hemorrhages in the skin and mucous membranes are common manifestations of thrombocytopenia. Epistaxis (often bilateral), excessive primary bleeding at a venipuncture site, excessive bleeding during surgical procedures, hemorrhagic diarrhea, and hematuria are all associated with decreased numbers of platelets. Although the most frequent cause of hemorrhage is trauma, thrombocytopenia is the major differential diagnosis in cases of spontaneous bleeding or bleeding that is disproportionate to the injury (Weiser, 1989).

Thrombocytopenia

Thrombocytopenia is caused by four primary mechanisms: decreased production, increased consumption, increased destruction, or sequestration (Table 14–4). Bone marrow evaluation is necessary to differentiate decreased platelet production from sequestration, consumption, and destruction of platelets. The disorders discussed for bone marrow hypoplasia can also be associated with thrombocytopenia. Usually bone marrow hypoplasia results in pancytopenia rather than specific cell line deficiency. Dapsone, a sulfone used for treatment of canine subcorneal pustular dermatosis and dermatitis herpetiformis, is associated with a megakaryocytic aplasia that spares other hematopoietic cell lines (Lees et al, 1979). Canine ehrlichiosis is most often associated with megakaryocytic hyperplasia and increased platelet destruction but can progress to generalized bone marrow suppression and thrombocytopenia as a result of bone marrow hypoplasia. In cats, feline leukemia virus is associated with megakaryocytic hypoplasia (Davenport et al, 1982).

Sequestration of platelets in the liver or spleen and excessive blood loss are often discussed in the literature but are not well documented in naturally occurring cases of thrombocytopenia. Splenomegaly and hepatomegaly result in decreased platelet survival owing to increased removal of platelets by the resident macrophages in these organs (Jain, 1986). Any process that decreases blood flow through an organ with a large capillary network has the potential for sequestering platelets within the vasculature.

The more common causes of significant thrombocytopenia are increased consumption and increased destruction of platelets. The primary cause of increased consumption of platelets is DIC, which is a severe secondary complication of many diseases. Vasculitis, neoplasia, liver disease, overwhelming infections (bacterial, viral, and fungal), toxins, severe hemolysis, and heat stroke are commonly associated with DIC. DIC results from widespread activation of the hemostatic process, which progresses from activation of coagulation with formation of microthrombi to excessive bleeding as a result of thrombocytopenia, coagulation factor deficiency, and increased circulating natural anticoagulants (i.e., fibrin [fibrinogen] degradation products [FDPs]). The thrombocytopenia seen in infectious and neoplastic disease is commonly associated with DIC (Grin-

TABLE 14–4. CAUSES OF PLATELET ABNORMALITIES

THROMBOCYTOPENIA

Decreased Production

Primary bone marrow failure
- Myeloproliferative disease
- Myelofibrosis
- Myelotoxicosis (see "Leukopenia" in Table 14–3)
- Immune-mediated megakaryocytic hypoplasia

Increased Consumption

Microangiopathy
DIC
Vasculitis
Endotoxemia
Neoplasia

Increased Destruction

Immune-mediated thrombocytopenia
- Drug-induced thrombocytopenia
- Live virus vaccine-associated thrombocytopenia

Neoplasia
Microangiopathy

Increased Sequestration

Splenomegaly
Portal hypertension
Splenic torsion
Neoplasia (especially splenic hemangiosarcoma or lymphoma)
Endotoxemia

THROMBOCYTOSIS

Reactive thrombocytosis
- Inflammation/infection
- Neoplasia
- Iron deficiency anemia

Primary bone marrow abnormality
- Malignant thrombocytosis
- Megakaryocytic myelosis

ACQUIRED THROMBOCYTOPATHIAS

Hypofunction
- Uremia
- Liver disease
- Hypergammaglobulinemia (multiple myeloma)
- Drug-induced dysfunction
  - Salicylates
  - Nonsteroidal anti-inflammatory agents

Hyperfunction
- Nephrotic syndrome
- Diabetes mellitus
- Hyperadrenocorticism

DIC, Disseminated intravascular coagulation.

dem et al, 1991). The geriatric dog or cat with subclinical decrease in hepatic function can be predisposed to DIC because of the liver's central role in production of coagulation factors and clearance of activated coagulation factors and FDPs.

Diagnosis of DIC is not straightforward. Thrombocytopenia, prolonged coagulation times, decreased antithrombin III activity, increased FDPs, and red cell fragments appear to be the most consistent abnormalities in dogs with DIC (Feldman, 1981). Increased FDPs and thrombocytopenia are considered by some individuals to be sufficient for a diagnosis of DIC in a dog with a significant bleeding diathesis. Antithrombin III, a serine protease inhibitor that is consumed during the coagulation stage of DIC, has been investigated as a marker for DIC. In addition to assisting in the diagnosis of DIC, antithrombin III is useful in determining prognosis and therapy. A continued decrease in antithrombin III activity in the presence of supportive therapy or specific therapy for the underlying cause of DIC indicates a poor prognosis (Green, 1984). Heparin therapy is used to inhibit further microthrombus formation in some patients with DIC. Because heparin is dependent on antithrombin III for activity, adequate concentrations of antithrombin III are necessary for heparin to be effective.

Destruction of platelets can occur by several mechanisms (immune-mediated, neoplasia, drug-associated, and infectious or inflammatory) and is probably the most common cause of thrombocytopenia. The prevalence of canine thrombocytopenias has been reported by Grindem et al (1991). In this study, the cause of thrombocytopenia was not determined in 304 of 987 cases (31 per cent). Infectious thrombocytopenias (224/987, or 23 per cent) and neoplasia (130/987, or 13 per cent) were the most common diseases identified, whereas immune-mediated thrombocytopenia was found in only 48 of 987 cases (5 per cent) of thrombocytopenia in this study. Not surprisingly, the mean age for neoplasia-associated thrombocytopenia was higher than that for the other categories. In fact, the mean age in all the categories in this study was 5.9 years or older.

This study also found a significant difference in the severity of thrombocytopenia when comparing immune-mediated thrombocytopenia to the other causes. The most severe thrombocytopenias were seen in dogs with immune-mediated thrombocytopenia (platelet count: 36,760 ± 50,288/μl, immune-mediated; 124,539 ± 52,464/μl, neoplasia; and 122,189 ± 53,111/μl, infectious or inflammatory). It is most likely that the severe thrombocytopenia associated with immune-mediated disease is responsible for the clinical impression that immune-mediated thrombocytopenia is the most common cause of spontaneous bleeding in the dog. Spontaneous bleeding owing to thrombocytopenia usually does not occur until the platelet count is less than 50,000/μl, and in fact, dogs with platelet counts as low as 10,000 may not show spontaneous hemorrhage (Jain, 1986).

Many infectious agents (bacterial, viral, fungal, rickettsial, and protozoal) are associated with thrombocytopenia. *E. canis* alone has at least four mechanisms by which thrombocytopenia may occur: bone marrow suppression, immune-mediated removal by the mononuclear-phagocyte system, nonimmunologic platelet aggregation and removal by the mononuclear-phagocyte system, and endothelial damage–induced consumption with or without DIC (Breitschwerdt, 1988). In many cases of infectious thrombocytopenia, DIC is most likely the major mechanism causing the decreased circulating platelets. Septic or endotoxemic vascular damage, with resulting intravascular activation of platelets and the coagulation cascade, and septic shock with decreased tissue perfusion resulting in microvascular stasis set the stage for acute fulminant DIC.

Thrombocytopenia is much less common in cats than in dogs. The incidence of feline thrombocytopenia in one cat population was 1.2 per cent, compared with 5.2 per cent in dogs (Grindem et al, 1991; Jordan et al, 1991). Again, infectious and neoplastic diseases made up a significant proportion of the cases reported (29 per cent each). Leukopenia and nonregenerative anemia were commonly associated with thrombocytopenia in these cats and was likely due to concurrent feline leukemia virus infection and myeloproliferative disorders.

Thrombocytosis

Increased numbers of circulating platelets can be the result of three general mechanisms: physiologic thrombocytosis, reactive thrombocytosis, or essential thrombocytosis, a rare myeloproliferative disorder. Physiologic thrombocytosis refers to mobilization of platelets from storage organs such as the spleen (primary site) and lung, rather than increased production by marrow megakaryocytes. Excitement, with resulting release of epinephrine, and strenuous exercise are commonly associated with transient increases in circulating platelets. Platelet counts in physiologic thrombocytosis rarely exceed 1,000,000/μl (Jain, 1986).

Reactive thrombocytosis is characterized by various degrees of thrombocytosis in which platelet counts can exceed 1,000,000/μl and is the result of increased platelet production (megakaryocytic hyperplasia) (Jain, 1986). Iron deficiency (chronic blood loss), acute infectious or inflammatory diseases, hemolytic anemia, neoplasia, splenectomy, and hyposplenic states (corticosteroid-induced hyposplenism and Cushing's disease) are common causes of reactive thrombocytosis. Although most patients with thrombocytosis do not show any abnormalities in hemostasis, excessive thrombocytosis may result in a bleeding diathesis or thrombosis.

Essential thrombocythemia is a rare myeloproliferative disease that has been reported in both the dog and the cat (Hopper et al, 1989; Hammer et al, 1990). The criteria for a diagnosis of essential thrombocythemia include persistent thrombocytosis (platelet counts greater than 1,000,000/μl), marked megakaryocytic hyperplasia in the bone marrow, absence of increased red cell mass, absence of reactive thrombocytosis, absence of collagen fibrosis in the bone marrow, and absence of circulating blast cells (Hopper et al, 1989). It can be very difficult to rule out all causes of reactive thrombocytosis; however, the circulating platelets in essential thrombocythemia may be morphologically or functionally abnormal, and the megakaryocytes present in the marrow may show dysplastic changes (Tablin et al, 1989). Essential thrombocythemia is often associated with other myeloproliferative disorders (Degen et al, 1989).

Qualitative Platelet Disorders

Qualitative platelet disorders, or thrombocytopathies, are being recognized more often in veterinary medicine because of the increased availability of platelet function tests. Many causes of acquired thrombocytopathies are common disease entities in the geriatric dog or cat. Renal and hepatic diseases are probably the most common disorders associated with altered platelet function. In addition, pancreatitis, hypergammaglobulinemia, myeloproliferative disease, hypothyroidism, and cardiomyopathy have all been shown to alter platelet function to some degree. Drug-induced thrombocytopathies have been well documented in veterinary medicine (Rackear et al, 1988; Weitekamp and Aber, 1983). Acquired thrombocytopathies can be divided into disorders that cause hypofunction of platelets and those that cause hyperfunction.

Decreased platelet function is frequently associated with uremia, liver disease, and dysproteinemia. The thrombocytopathy associated with uremia has several mechanisms and has been best documented in human medicine. Platelet release reaction, aggregation, and platelet factor 3 activity are abnormal in uremic patients. In addition, vascular changes with uremia can reduce endothelial adhesion, possibly because of increased production of prostacyclin, a potent inhibitor of platelet adhesion (Deykin, 1983). The uremic toxins that have been incriminated are primarily metabolites of urea, guanidinosuccinic acid, and phenolic acid.

In cases of liver disease, increased circulating FDPs are thought to reduce platelet function. In addition, severe hepatic disease may result in decreased expression of platelet membrane GPIb, a membrane glycoprotein necessary for normal platelet aggregation and adhesion (Rao and Walsh, 1983). Although decreased platelet function occurs with liver disease, the tendency toward bleeding commonly seen with liver dysfunction is multifactorial. Patients with decreased liver function often have thrombocytopenia, dysfibrinogenemia, decreased production of coagulation factors and antithrombin III, enhanced fibrinolysis, increased circulating activated coagulation factors, and increased FDPs. Many of these changes may actually play a more significant role than decreased platelet function in the bleeding diathesis associated with liver dysfunction.

Although several drugs have been shown to decrease platelet function, the most clinically significant are aspirin and the nonsteroidal anti-inflammatory agents. Aspirin irreversibly inhibits cyclooxygenase, the enzyme necessary for generation of endoperoxides, specifically thromboxane A_2, which is necessary for appropriate platelet aggregation (Handagama, 1986). Because the effect is irreversible, replacement of the affected platelets is required for return of normal platelet function. In the geriatric patient, the use of aspirin should be considered in light of potential subclinical renal or hepatic dysfunction, and other analgesics should be used if possible. The nonsteroidal anti-inflammatory drugs (e.g., indomethacin, ibuprofen, and phenylbutazone) can all inhibit platelet function. Unlike aspirin, however, these drugs do not cause irreversible inhibition, but inhibit platelet function only while they are in circulation. These drugs should also be avoided in the geriatric patient with any indication of decreased renal or hepatic function.

Thrombosis associated with hypercoagulability has been described in dogs with nephrotic syndrome, hyperadrenocorticism, and diabetes mellitus (Feldman and Rasedee, 1986; Green, 1984; Green et al, 1985). Nephrotic syndrome is characterized by severe urinary protein loss and is the end result of severe glomerular disease. Hypoalbuminemia, hypercholesterolemia, proteinuria, and ascites or peripheral edema are the classic findings that constitute a diagnosis of nephrotic syndrome. In addition to albumin, other low-molecular-weight proteins are lost into the urine of patients with nephrotic syndrome. Antithrombin III is decreased in dogs with nephrotic syndrome. The combination of hypoalbuminemia, hypercholesterolemia, and decreased antithrombin III activity results in a significant increase in platelet sensitivity to activation and thrombosis. In addition, the underlying cause of the glomerular lesion may contribute to the hypercoagulable state by altering hemodynamics, endothelial integrity, and/or hemostasis through mechanisms specific to that disorder. Many cases of nephrotic syndrome are associated with chronic inflammation–induced amyloidosis. As discussed previously, inflammation can cause significant alterations in hemostasis, often leading to DIC.

Hypercholesterolemia alone is associated with platelet hyperfunction. It is postulated that hypercholesterolemia results in alterations of platelet membrane components, leading to increased sensitivity to activation (Greco and Green, 1987). Hypercholesterolemia and altered endothelial integrity may contribute to the hypercoagulable state associated with diabetes mellitus and hyperadrenocorticism. In animals with Cushing's disease, the presence of thrombocytosis and increased coagulation factors, antithrombin III, fibrinogen, and plasminogen may further complicate the hemostatic state of the patient (Feldman and Rasedee, 1986).

THE LYMPH NODES

One of the most common clinical abnormalities seen in veterinary practice is lymph node enlargement (Table 14–5). The peripheral lymph nodes are frequently evaluated because of their accessibility; however, radiographic and ultrasonographic evaluation of the thorax or abdomen can reveal masses that represent enlarged visceral lymph nodes. Evaluation of changes in lymph nodes usually involves fine-needle aspiration or core biopsy of the affected tissue. If aspiration cytology is not conclusive, an excisional biopsy is preferable to a core biopsy. Histologic evaluation of lymph node architecture is often crucial for a diagnosis of lymphoma, especial in the case of lymphocytic lymphoma. With metastatic lesions or inflammation caused by fungal agents, a core biopsy may miss the affected area and, hence,

TABLE 14–5. DISORDERS AFFECTING THE LYMPH NODES AND LYMPHATIC VESSELS

LYMPH NODE HYPOPLASIA	**LYMPHANGITIS**
Advanced age	Infectious agents
Feline leukemia virus	Bacterial
Malnutrition	Fungal
Hyperadrenocorticism	Neoplasia (metastatic)
Drugs	Trauma
Corticosteroids	
Anti-neoplastic agents	
Radiation therapy	
LYMPH NODE HYPERPLASIA ± INFLAMMATION	**NEOPLASIA**
Infectious agents	Lymphoma
Bacterial *(Mycobacteria, Streptococcus)*	Hematopoietic neoplasia
Viral (FeLV, FIV)	Metastatic neoplasia
Fungal *(Blastomyces, Cryptococcus)*	Melanoma
Rickettsial *(Ehrlichia, Neorichettsia helminthoeca)*	Squamous cell carcinoma
Parasitic *(Leishmania, Toxoplasma)*	Perirectal adenocarcinoma
Algal *(Prototheca)*	Mammary adenocarcinoma
Immune-mediated diseases	Prostatic adenocarcinoma
Chronic dermatopathies (usually eosinophilic)	Osteosarcoma
Vaccine-associated	Mast cell tumors
Feline lymphadenopathies	
Plexiform vascularization of lymph nodes	
FeLV/FIV-associated	
Eosinophilic granulomas complex	
Hypereosinophilic syndrome	

FeLV, Feline leukemia virus; FIV, feline immunodeficiency virus.

the diagnosis. Markedly enlarged lymph nodes often have a necrotic center resulting either from an inflammatory process causing abscessation or from a neoplastic process that has outgrown its blood supply, causing ischemic necrosis. If possible, the smaller lymph nodes should be evaluated in a patient with generalized or regional lymphadenopathy. If a solitary node is markedly enlarged, the center of the lymph node should be avoided during sampling.

Lymph nodes consist of a capsule, subcapsular sinus, cortex, paracortex, postcapillary venules, medullary cords, and medullary sinuses. The primary function of the lymph node is directing the immune response toward antigens that filter into the lymph node from peripheral tissue. Antigens are processed by the dendritic reticular cells (macrophages that are most likely of bone marrow origin) and are presented to the lymphocytes, which make up most of the lymph node cell population. Fine-needle aspiration cytology of a normal lymph node demonstrates primarily small lymphocytes (greater than 90 per cent); smaller numbers of intermediate lymphocytes and lymphoblasts can be found as well. An occasional plasma cell, neutrophil, mast cell, or eosinophil may be present. If a large amount of blood contamination is evident in the aspirate, peripheral blood leukocytes such as neutrophils and eosinophils may occur in higher numbers. The cell population of a lymph node changes significantly with various causes of lymphadenopathy. Both neoplastic and non-neoplastic disorders can be recognized with aspirate cytology.

Non-neoplastic causes of lymphadenopathy can be divided into two categories: hyperplasia or inflammation. Lymphoid hyperplasia is characterized by increased numbers of intermediate lymphocytes, lymphoblasts, and plasma cells. With marked hyperplasia, Mott cells—plasma cells containing Russell bodies (distinct, empty-appearing vesicles that represent dilated endoplasmic reticuli)—are often present. Lymphoid hyperplasia can be the result of systemic or localized antigenic stimulation. Generalized lymphoid hyperplasia can be seen with widespread dermatologic diseases (eosinophilic inflammation as well as hyperplasia may be evident in such cases) or canine ehrlichiosis or as an idiopathic syndrome in cats that may be associated with feline immunodeficiency virus, feline leukemia virus, or argyrophilic bacteria (Kirkpatrick et al, 1989; Mooney et al, 1987). Localized lymphadenopathy is seen in lymph nodes draining sites of local inflammation, including inflammation associated with neoplasia. Because of the high incidence of dental disease in older dogs, the submandibular lymph nodes and tonsils are often mildly enlarged as a result of lymphoid hyperplasia.

Inflammatory lymphadenopathy, or lymphadenitis, is usually accompanied by some degree of lymphoid hyperplasia and is characterized by an increase in reactive lymphoid cells. The predominant cytologic change in lymphadenitis is increased numbers of neutrophils, eosinophils, or macrophages or of a mixed population of inflammatory cells. Suppurative or neutrophilic lymphadenitis is commonly seen with bacterial infection, whereas a granulomatous or pyogranulomatous lymphadenitis is most often seen with fungal diseases such as blastomycosis, coccidioidomycosis, or sporotrichosis. Mycobacterial infections, however, are associated with granulomatous rather than suppurative inflammation, as is brucellosis. Cryptococcosis is unique in that the host may not produce any inflammatory reaction to the organism. Lymph nodes may become completely effaced with the organism and appear soft and gelatinous. A mixed inflammatory response characterized by increases in neutrophils, macrophages, eosinophils, plasma cells, and mast cells is often seen with dermatopathies. Eosinophils may predominate in cases of flea allergy dermatitis or other causes of cutaneous hypersensitivity and the hypereosinophilic syndrome seen in cats. It is important to remember that mast cells and eosinophils are often increased in these disorders, and such increases should not be considered indicative of metastatic mast cell neoplasia.

Neoplastic diseases can cause either generalized or localized lymphadenopathy. Mast cell tumor, squamous cell carcinoma, melanoma, mammary gland adenocarcinoma, and perianal gland adenocarcinoma have a propensity for spread to regional lymph nodes via the lymphatic vessels. Osteosarcoma may metastasize to or infiltrate regional lymph nodes. The presence of neoplastic cells in a lymph node can elicit an immune response and result in lymphoid hyperplasia. Metastatic neoplasia, particularly squamous cell carcinoma, can also be accompanied by neutrophilic inflammation. In the case of squamous cell carcinoma, the keratin produced by the neoplastic squamous cells elicits a profound neutrophilic inflammatory response.

The primary differential diagnosis for generalized lymphadenopathy in the geriatric dog is lymphoma. Lymphoma is the most common hemolymphatic neoplasm in dogs, and the incidence of lymphoma increases with age. The diagnosis of lymphoma is often made cytologically but may require histopathologic confirmation in cases of lymphocytic or intermediate cell lymphoma. Quality cytologic preparations are necessary for diagnosis, and intact cells must be present for evaluation. Many enlarged lymph nodes, regardless of whether they are neoplastic, have necrotic centers. Aspiration into the necrotic center will result in a nondiagnostic sample consisting of necrotic debris and broken cells. Neoplastic lymphocytes have a tendency to be fragile, and gentle handing of the aspirated material is required to provide intact cells for evaluation. With an adequate sample, diagnosis of lymphoblastic lymphoma can be quite straightforward; cytology will demonstrate a homogenous population of large, deeply basophilic lymphoblasts with prominent nucleoli. However, lymphocytic lymphoma, follicular lymphoma, and lymphoma of mixed cell type can be difficult to distinguish from atypical benign hyperplasia. It is very important to obtain diagnostic samples before anticancer therapy is initiated, because the character of the neoplastic cells can change significantly in response to the anticancer drugs used (Carter and Valli, 1988). Once a diagnosis of lymphoma is made, clinical staging for prognosis includes a CBC count, bone marrow biopsy, and serum biochemistry profile. Several bone marrow samples obtained from different sites may be necessary to rule out bone marrow involvement. Even with a thorough evaluation, only 60 per cent of cases with metastasis to bone marrow will be identified (Carter and Valli, 1988). A core biopsy using a Jamshidi needle increases the chances of finding the neoplasm in the bone marrow.

Several studies of prognostic correlations of clinical findings (clinical stage, hypercalcemia, age, and body weight) have suggested that dogs with liver or spleen involvement have a poor prognosis and increased risk of organ failure as a result of tumor lysis syndrome (i.e., therapy-induced tumor necrosis) (MacEwen et al, 1987). Dogs with high-grade disease (lymphoblastic or immunoblastic) appear to have better survival times as well as better response to anticancer therapy (Greenlee et al, 1990).

Unlike canine lymphoma, feline lymphoma has a bimodal age distribution that reflects the feline leukemia virus–associated lymphomas of young cats (mean age at diagnosis, 3 years) and the non–virus-associated lymphomas of older cats (mean age at diagnosis, 7 years). The alimentary form is more common in geriatric cats (average age at diagnosis, 8 years) (Hardy, 1981). Prognosis in the cat is significantly affected by clinical stage, with complete remission occurring in 90 per cent of cases in stages I and II and in 50 per cent of cases in stages III, IV, and V. Additional negative prognostic indicators in the cat are presence of leukemia, anemia, neutropenia, feline leukemia virus infection, and sepsis. Several idiopathic lymphadenopathies have been reported, but all cases were in cats younger than 2 years of age. Plexiform vascularization of lymph nodes is a benign solitary lymphadenopathy that can affect geriatric cats.

Multiple myeloma is an uncommon neoplasm of lymphoid origin. It is seen most often in the dog, occurring in an estimated 3.6 per cent of primary and secondary bone marrow neoplasms (Matus et al, 1986). Multiple myeloma is characterized by proliferation of malignant plasma cells along with production of a monoclonal gammopathy of IgG or IgA isotype. Clinical findings include lameness associated with pathologic fractures and punctate osteolytic lesions, hemorrhage caused by decreased platelet function, polyuria/polydipsia, and retinal hemorrhage resulting from hyperviscosity. Clinicopathologic findings seen with multiple myeloma include nonregenerative anemia, leukopenia, and thrombocytopenia. The hematologic changes are often associated with plasma cell infiltration of the bone marrow. It is important to remember that other causes of bone marrow plasmacytosis should not be confused with multiple myeloma. Ehrlichiosis is associated with a significant infiltration of the bone marrow by plasma cells and can also be associated with a monoclonal gammopathy. Plasma cell proliferation may also be present in the lymph nodes and spleen of any animal demonstrating chronic antigenic stimulation.

The hemorrhagic diathesis associated with multiple myeloma can have several causes. Hyperviscosity alone will increase bleeding times, as the paraproteins present in the serum are thought to interfere with the coagulation cascade. In addition, paraproteins interfere with platelet adhesion and aggregation (Shepard et al, 1972). Serum biochemical abnormalities often indicate renal dysfunction. Renal disease associated with multiple myeloma may be due to concurrent hypercalcemia or glomerular damage associated with filtration of myeloma proteins.

THE SPLEEN

The spleen is primarily an immunologic and hematopoietic organ. The multiple functions of the spleen include hematopoiesis, antigen filtration and processing, removal of defective (e.g., parasitized, antibody-coated, or oxidized) or senescent RBCs, and blood storage.

The spleen has significantly different anatomic characteristics in dogs and cats. The canine spleen is a sinusal spleen characterized by closed, blunt-ended venous vessels, whereas the feline spleen is a nonsinusal spleen with open-ended venous vessels with a thin-walled discontinuous endothelium. Erythrocytes traversing from the arterial to the venous circulation must migrate between a continuous endothelial lining in the dog, which is probably responsible for the increased efficiency of the canine spleen in removing defective less deformable RBCs and nucleated RBCs (NRBCs) compared with the cat spleen.

Splenomegaly is a common clinical finding in small animal medicine. The clinical signs associated with splenomegaly are quite varied and depend on the primary disease process present. In the geriatric patient, the causes of splenomegaly will fall primarily into two categories: disorders that cause localized splenomegaly and those that cause diffuse splenomegaly (Table 14–6). Aside from splenic torsion and trauma, splenic disease appears to be more common in the geriatric patient than the young patient (Johnson et al, 1989).

Relatively noninvasive diagnostic tests useful for evaluation of the patient with splenomegaly include hematology, fine-needle aspiration cytology, ultrasonography, and radiology. However, in many instances histologic evaluation of surgical biopsy specimens obtained during exploratory laparotomy is necessary for a definitive diagnosis. This is especially true with localized splenic masses. Although cytology is quite reliable for diagnosis of diffuse splenic diseases such as hematopoietic neoplasms and some inflammatory diseases, it is not reliable for diagnosis of most splenic masses (Johnson et al, 1989; O'Keefe and Couto, 1987).

Localized Splenomegaly (Splenic Masses)

When evaluating a geriatric dog or cat with a localized splenic mass, it is important to remember that splenic neoplasia may be overemphasized in the literature. In one review (Neer, 1993), non-neoplastic causes of localized splenomegaly constituted a significant percentage of cases reported (49 per cent in dogs; 63 per cent in cats). Two important points concerning localized splenomegaly were stressed: veterinarians

TABLE 14–6. CAUSES OF SPLENOMEGALY

DIFFUSE SPLENOMEGALY

- Inflammatory
  - Suppurative
    - Bacterial emboli
    - Foreign bodies
    - Splenic torsion
    - Toxoplasmosis
  - Eosinophilic
    - Hypereosinophilic syndrome (cat)
    - Eosinophilic gastroenteritis (dog)
  - Granulomatous
    - Systemic mycoses
    - Mycobacterial infections
    - Brucellosis
  - Pyogranulomatous
    - Systemic mycoses
- Noninflammatory, non-neoplastic
  - Chronic antigenic stimulation
    - Chronic bacterial infections
      - Endocarditis
      - Diskospondylitis
      - Brucellosis
    - Immune-mediated diseases
      - Systemic lupus erythematosus
      - Immune-mediated hemolytic anemia
      - Immune-mediated thrombocytopenia
  - Congestion
    - Tranquilizers and barbiturates
    - Congestive heart failure
    - Splenic torsion
  - Extramedullary hematopoiesis
    - Pyometra
  - Immune-mediated hemolytic anemia
    - Chronic anemia of any cause
    - Immune-mediated thrombocytopenia
  - Amyloidosis
- Neoplastic (infiltrative)
  - Leukemia
  - Mastocytoma
  - Lymphoma
  - Myeloma
  - Malignant histiocytosis (dogs)

LOCALIZED SPLENOMEGALY

- Neoplastic lesions
  - Hemangioma
  - Hemangiosarcoma
  - Fibrosarcoma
  - Leiomyosarcoma
  - Leiomyoma
  - Myelolipoma
  - Lymphoma
- Non-neoplastic lesions
  - Hematomas
  - Abscessation
  - Nodular hyperplasia
  - Infarction
  - Cysts (resolution of hematoma)

tend to overemphasize the importance of splenic neoplasia, and the age of the animal may not help differentiate neoplastic from non-neoplastic disease.

A retrospective study of splenomegaly with emphasis on predictors of neoplasia found that anemia, circulating NRBCs, abnormal red cell morphology, and splenic rupture were more commonly associated with splenic neoplasia than with non-neoplastic diseases (Johnson et al, 1989). All the causes of anemia associated with neoplasia may be associated with the anemia seen with splenic neoplasms. Microangiopathic hemolytic anemia syndrome results from altered microvasculature of the neoplastic spleen, which in turn results from damaged endothelium or intravascular fibrin strands. Red cell fragments and poikilocytes such as acanthocytes are commonly seen with splenic neoplasia. Red cell fragments appear to be more prevalent in splenic neoplasia than in other causes of splenomegaly (23 per cent of neoplastic cases versus 3 per cent of non-neoplastic cases) (Neer, 1993). Increased numbers of circulating NRBCs are common because of the decreased pitting ability of the altered vasculature. Thrombocytopenia is often seen as well as the anemia (Kruth and Carter, 1990). Consumption of platelets in DIC and sequestration of platelets within the congested parenchyma of the spleen are likely causes of the decreased circulating platelet mass.

Analyses of fine-needle aspirates of focal splenic lesions are often misleading. Splenic hemangiosarcomas consist of large, cavernous, endothelium-lined vascular spaces intermixed with areas of hemorrhage and necrosis. Fine-needle aspirates may identify only the necrotic or hemorrhagic areas while completely missing the neoplastic nature of the lesion.

Non-neoplastic causes of localized splenic enlargement can result in anemia of chronic inflammation and extravascular hemolytic anemia as a result of enhanced erythrophagocytosis. Anisocytosis, poikilocytosis, target cells, and increased numbers of Howell-Jolly bodies are commonly seen with splenic disease of non-neoplastic origin (Johnson et al, 1989). Again, fine-needle aspiration cytology is probably not helpful in diagnosis of splenic masses.

Diffuse Splenomegaly

Diffuse enlargement of the spleen is associated with inflammatory, hyperplastic, and neoplastic changes. Inflammatory splenomegaly, or splenitis, is often associated with an infectious agent. The nature of the inflammatory response can help determine the nature of the organism involved. Suppurative or neutrophilic splenitis is seen with bacterial infections as the result of hematogenous dissemination from distant lesions (e.g., endocarditis, penetrating wounds, migrating foreign bodies, or splenic torsion). Eosinophilic inflammation is seen in the hypereosinophilic syndrome of cats, in eosinophilic gastroenteritis in dogs, and in association with mast cell neoplasia. Granulomatous inflammation and pyogranulomatous inflammation are associated with systemic mycoses and some bacterial diseases (*Mycobacterium* spp. and *Brucella* spp.).

The spleen is a lymphoid organ and responds to systemic antigenic stimulation just as lymph nodes do. Immune-mediated disease (e.g., immune-mediated hemolytic anemia and/or thrombocytopenias and systemic lupus erythematosus) is often associated with diffuse splenomegaly. In these cases there are increases in plasma cells, in lymphoblasts or immunocytes, and perhaps in active macrophages. Increased erythrophagia is seen in hemolytic disease. Any disease associated with systemic antigenemia has the potential to cause splenic hyperplasia. Hemoparasites, chronic bacteremia (i.e., endocarditis, diskospondylitis, and brucellosis), viremia, and immune-mediated disease likely result in splenic hyperplasia by chronic systemic antigen stimulation.

Most veterinarians are familiar with the congestive splenomegaly associated with tranquilizers and barbiturates. Splenic smooth muscle relaxation results in pooling of blood within the splenic sinusoids. Splenic congestion can also be seen in patients with right heart failure as a result of increased portal blood pressure. Splenic torsion, a disorder most commonly seen in large, deep-chested breeds of dog, causes significant splenic congestion. Splenic torsion is commonly seen in conjunction with gastric dilatation-volvulus. The stagnation of blood flow within the spleen can result in significant splenic necrosis and provides an opportunity for suppurative splenitis to develop secondary to bacterial proliferation in the affected spleen. Splenic torsion is associated with hemoglobinemia, hemoglobinuria, hyperbilirubinemia, and neutrophilic leukocytosis (Stead et al, 1983).

Infiltration of the splenic parenchyma by hematopoietic, lymphoid, or mast cell neoplasms usually causes diffuse splenomegaly. Myeloproliferative diseases (both acute and chronic), lymphoma, systemic mastocytosis, multiple myeloma, and malignant histiocytosis are causes of diffuse splenomegaly that can often be diagnosed by fine-needle aspirate cytology. One exception is chronic lymphocytic leukemia or lymphoma. The normal splenic cytology sample consists primarily of small to intermediate lymphocytes, with small numbers of plasma cells, neutrophils, and macrophages and occasional hematopoietic cells. The predominance of small lymphocytes with chronic lymphocytic neoplasms cannot be differentiated from the normal cytology of the spleen.

In addition to its function as a lymphoid organ, the spleen retains primordial capability as a hematopoietic organ. In any cause of prolonged hypoxia that stimulates maximal hematopoiesis, the spleen can be recruited in an effort to produce RBCs and alleviate the hypoxia. Extramedullary hematopoiesis in the spleen is especially common in cases of hemolytic anemia, immune-mediated thrombocytopenia, hemangiosarcoma, and myelophthisis (and other causes of primary or secondary bone marrow suppression). Splenic extramedullary hematopoiesis appears to be more common in the dog than in the cat (Neer, 1993). Extramedullary hematopoiesis is one of the primary causes of increased circulating NRBCs.

References and Supplemental Reading

Bellamy JE. Cold-agglutinin hemolytic anemia and *Haemobartonella canis* infection in a dog. J Am Vet Med Assoc 173:397, 1978.

Breitschwerdt EB. Infectious thrombocytopenia in dogs. Compend Contin Educ Pract Vet 10:1177, 1988.

Cain GR, Cain JL, Turrel JM, et al. Immune-mediated hemolytic anemia and thrombocytopenia in a cat after bone marrow transplantation. Vet Pathol 25:161, 1988.

Carter RF, Valli VEO. Advances in the cytologic diagnosis of canine lymphoma. Semin Vet Med Surg (Small Anim) 3:167, 1988.

Christopher MM. Relation of endogenous Heinz bodies to disease and anemia in cats: 120 cases (1978–1987). J Am Vet Med Assoc 194:1089, 1989.

Christopher MM, Perman V, Eaton JW. Contribution of propylene glycol-induced Heinz body formation to anemia in cats. J Am Vet Med Assoc 194:1045, 1989.

Cotter SM. Anemia associated with feline leukemia virus infection. J Am Vet Med Assoc 175:1191, 1979.

Couto CG. Tumor-associated eosinophilia in a dog. J Am Vet Med Assoc 184:837, 1984.

Couto CG. Hematologic abnormalities in small animal cancer patients. Part I. Red blood cell abnormalities. In Veterinary Laboratory Medicine in Practice. Trenton, NJ, Veterinary Learning Systems, 1993, p 258.

Couto CG, Boudrieau RJ, Zanjani ED. Tumor-associated erythrocytosis in a dog with nasal fibrosarcoma. J Vet Intern Med 3:183, 1989.

Cowgill LD. Clinical experience and use of recombinant human erythropoietin in uremic dogs and cats. Proc Am Coll Vet Intern Med Forum 9:147, 1991.

Davenport DJ, Breitschwerdt EB, Carakostas MC. Platelet disorders in the dog and cat. Part I. Physiology and pathogenesis. Compend Contin Educ Pract Vet 4:762, 1982.

Degen MA, Feldman BF, Turrel JM, et al. Thrombocytosis associated with a myeloproliferative disorder in a dog. J Am Vet Med Assoc 194:1457, 1989.

Deykin D. Uremic bleeding. Kidney Int 24:698, 1983.

Ettinger SJ. Textbook of Veterinary Internal Medicine. Philadelphia, WB Saunders, 1989, p 2145.

Feldman BF. Coagulopathies in small animals. J Am Vet Med Assoc 179:559, 1981.

Feldman BF, Rasedee A. Haemostatic abnormalities in canine Cushing's syndrome. Res Vet Sci 41:228, 1986.

Fulton R, Weiser MG, Freshman JL, et al. Electronic and morphologic characterization of erythrocytes of an adult cat with iron deficiency anemia. Vet Pathol 25:521, 1988.

Gaunt SD, Baker DC, Green RA. Clinicopathologic evaluation of *N*-acetylcysteine therapy in acetaminophen toxicosis in the cat. Am J Vet Res 42:1982, 1983.

Greco DS, Green RA. Coagulation abnormalities associated with thrombosis in a dog with nephrotic syndrome. Compend Contin Educ Pract Vet 9:653, 1987.

Green RA. Clinical implications of antithrombin III deficiency in animal diseases. Compend Contin Educ Pract Vet 6:537, 1984.

Green RA, Russo EA, Greene RT, et al. Hypoalbuminemia-related platelet hypersensitivity in two dogs with nephrotic syndrome. J Am Vet Med Assoc 186:485, 1985.

Greenlee PG, Filippa DA, Quimby FW, et al. Lymphomas in dogs. A morphologic, immunologic, and clinical study. Cancer 66:480, 1990.

Grindem CB. Bone marrow biopsy and evaluation. Vet Clin North Am [Small Anim Pract] 19:669, 1989.

Grindem CB, Breitschwerdt EB, Corbett WT, et al. Epidemiologic survey of thrombocytopenia in dogs: A report on 987 cases. Vet Clin Pathol 20:38, 1991.

Grindem CB, Corbett WT, Tomkins MT. Risk factors for *Haemobartonella felis* infection in cats. J Am Vet Med Assoc 196:96, 1990.

Hammer AS, Couto CG, Getzy D, et al. Essential thrombocythemia in a cat. J Vet Intern Med 4:87, 1990.

Handagama P. Salicylate toxicity. In Kirk RW, ed. Current Veterinary Therapy IX. Philadelphia, WB Saunders, 1986, p 524.

Hardy WD. Hematopoietic tumors of cats. J Am Anim Hosp Assoc 17:921, 1981.

Harvey JW. Canine hemolytic anemias. J Am Vet Med Assoc 176:970, 1980.

Harvey JW, French TW, Meyer DJ. Chronic iron deficiency anemia in dogs. J Am Anim Hosp Assoc 18:946, 1982.

Harvey JW, French TW, Senior DF. Hematologic abnormalities associated with chronic acetaminophen administration in a dog. J Am Vet Med Assoc 189:1334, 1986.

Harvey JW, Kornick HP. Phenazopyridine toxicosis in the cat. J Am Vet Med Assoc 169:327, 1976.

Harvey JW, Rackear D. Experimental onion-induced hemolytic anemia in dogs. Vet Pathol 22:387, 1985.

Harvey JW, Sameck JH, Burgard FJ. Benzocaine-induced methemoglobinemia in dogs. J Am Vet Med Assoc 175:1171, 1979.

Hjelle JJ. Acetaminophen-induced toxicosis in dogs and cats. J Am Vet Med Assoc 188:742, 1986.

Hoffman R. Regulation of megakaryocytopoiesis. Blood 74:1196, 1989.

Hohenhaus AE. Canine autoimmune hemolytic anemia: Predisposing and prognostic factors. Proc Am Coll Vet Intern Med Forum 10:146, 1992.

Hopper PE, Mandell CP, Turrel JM, et al. Probable essential thrombocythemia in a dog. J Vet Intern Med 3:79, 1989.

Hoskins JD. Canine haemobartonellosis, canine hepatozoonosis, and feline cytauxzoonosis. Vet Clin North Am [Small Anim Pract] 21:131, 1991.

Jain NC. Schalm's Veterinary Hematology. Philadelphia, Lea & Febiger, 1986.

Johnson KA, Powers BE, Withrow SJ, et al. Splenomegaly in dogs: Predictors of neoplasia and survival after splenectomy. J Vet Intern Med 3:160, 1989.

Jonas LD, Thrall MA, Weiser MG. Nonregenerative form of immune-mediated hemolytic anemia in dogs. J Am Anim Hosp Assoc 23:201, 1987.

Jordan HL, Grindem CB, Breitschwerdt EB. Diseases associated with feline thrombocytopenia: A retrospective review of 41 cases. Vet Clin Pathol 20:22, 1991.

King LG, Giger U, Diserens D, et al. Anemia of chronic renal failure in dogs. J Vet Intern Med 6:264, 1992.

Kirkpatrick CE, Moore FM, Patnaik AK, et al. Argyrophilic intracellular bacteria in some cats with idiopathic peripheral lymphadenopathy. J Comp Pathol 101:341, 1989.

Kruth SA, Carter RF. Laboratory abnormalities in patients with cancer. Vet Clin North Am [Small Anim Pract] 20:897, 1990.

La Rue LH, Feldman BF. Red cell gestalt. Compend Contin Educ Pract Vet 7:519, 1985.

Latimer KS, Meyer DJ. Leukocytes in health and disease. In Ettinger SI, ed. Textbook of Veterinary Internal Medicine. Vol 2. Philadelphia, WB Saunders, 1989, p 2181.

Lees GE, McKeever PJ, Ruth GR. Fatal thrombocytopenic hemorrhagic diathesis associated with dapsone administration to a dog. J Am Vet Med Assoc 175:549, 1979.

Lipschitz DA. Effect of age on hematopoiesis in man. Blood 63:502, 1984.

Losco P. Local and peripheral eosinophilia in a dog with anaplastic mammary carcinoma. Vet Pathol 23:536, 1986.

Lowseth LA, Gillett NA, Gerlach RF, et al. The effects of aging on hematology and serum chemistry values in the beagle dog. Vet Clin Pathol 19:13, 1990.

MacEwen EG, Hayes AA, Matus RE. Evaluation of some prognostic factors for advanced multicentric lymphosarcoma in the dog. 147 cases (1978–1981). J Am Vet Med Assoc 190:564, 1987.

MacWilliams PS. Erythrocytic rickettsia and protozoa of the dog and cat. Vet Clin North Am [Small Anim Pract] 17:1443, 1987.

Madewell BR, Feldman BF. Characterization of anemias associated with neoplasia in small animals. J Am Vet Med Assoc 176:419, 1980.

Maede Y. Methionine toxicosis in cats. Am J Vet Res 48:289, 1987.

Matus RE, Leifer CE, MacEwen EG, et al. Prognostic factors for multiple myeloma in the dog. J Am Vet Med Assoc 188:1288, 1986.

Mauch P. Decline in bone marrow proliferation capacity as a function of age. Blood 60:245, 1982.

Mazur EM. Megakaryocytopoiesis and platelet production: A review. Exp Hematol 15:340, 1987.

Mooney S, Patnaik AK, Hayes AA, et al. Generalized lymphadenopathy resembling lymphoma in cats: Six cases (1972–1976). J Am Vet Med Assoc 190:897, 1987.

Neer TM. Hypereosinophilic syndrome in the cat. Compend Contin Educ Pract Vet 13:549, 1991.

Neer TM. Clinical approach to splenomegaly. Proc Am Coll Vet Intern Med Forum 11:97, 1993.

O'Keefe DA, Couto CG. Fine-needle aspiration of the spleen as an aid in the diagnosis of splenomegaly. J Vet Intern Med 1:102, 1987.

Peterson M. Propylthiouracil-associated hemolytic anemia, thrombocytopenia, and antinuclear antibodies in cats with hyperthyroidism. J Am Vet Med Assoc 184:806, 1984.

Peterson ME, Zanjani ED. Inappropriate erythropoietin production from a renal carcinoma in a dog with polycythemia. J Am Vet Med Assoc 179:995, 1981.

Petrites-Murphy MB, Pierce KR, Lowry SR, et al. Role of parathyroid hormone in the anemia of chronic terminal renal dysfunction in dogs. Am J Vet Res 50:1898, 1989.

Petz LD. Drug-induced immune hemolysis. N Engl J Med 313:510, 1985.

Rackear D, Feldman B, Farver T, et al. The effect of three different dosages of acetylsalicylic acid on canine platelet aggregation. J Am Anim Hosp Assoc 24:23, 1988.

Rao AK, Walsh PN. Acquired qualitative platelet disorders. Clin Haematol 12:201, 1983.

Shepard V, Dodds-Laffin W, Laffin R. Gamma A myeloma in a dog with defective hemostasis. J Am Vet Med Assoc 160:1121, 1972.

Stead AC, Frankland AL, Borthwick R. Splenic torsion in dogs. J Small Anim Pract 24:549, 1983.

Tablin F, Jain NC, Mandell CP, et al. Ultrastructural analysis of platelets and megakaryocytes from a dog with probable essential thrombocythemia. Vet Pathol 26:289, 1989.

Taboada J, Merchant SR. Babesiosis of companion animals and man. Vet Clin North Am [Small Anim Pract] 21:103, 1991.

Wardrop KJ, Kramer JW, Abkowitz JL, et al. Quantitative studies of erythropoiesis in the clinically normal, phlebotomized, and feline leukemia virus-infected cat. Am J Vet Res 47:2274, 1986.

Weiser MG. Erythrocyte volume distribution analysis in healthy dogs, cats, horses, and dairy cows. Am J Vet Res 43:163, 1982.

Weiser MG. Erythrocytes and associated disorders. In Ettinger SJ, ed. Textbook of Veterinary Internal Medicine. Vol 2. Philadelphia, WB Saunders, 1989, p 2145.

Weiser MG, Kociba GJ. Sequential changes in erythrocyte volume distribution and microcytosis associated with iron deficiency in kittens. Vet Pathol 20:1, 1983a.

Weiser MG, Kociba GJ. Erythrocytes macrocytosis in feline leukemia virus associated anemia. Vet Pathol 20:687, 1983b.

Weiser M, O'Grady M. Erythrocyte volume distribution analysis and hematologic changes in dogs with iron deficiency anemia. Vet Pathol 20:230, 1983.

Weiss DJ. Potential role of serum inhibitors of erythropoiesis in the anemia associated with infection, renal disease and malignancy in the dog. Vet Clin Pathol 15:7, 1986a.

Weiss DJ. Canine pure red cell aplasia: Identification of antibody-mediated suppression of erythropoiesis. Vet Clin Pathol 15:10, 1986b.

Weiss DJ. Antibody-mediated suppression of erythropoiesis in dogs with red blood cell aplasia. Am J Vet Res 47:2646, 1986c.

Weiss DJ, Armstrong PJ. Nonregenerative anemias in the dog. Compend Contin Educ Pract Vet 6:452, 1984.

Weiss DJ, McClay CB. Studies on the pathogenesis of the decreased erythrocyte survival associated with anemia of inflammatory disease. Vet Clin Pathol 17:18, 1988.

Weiss DJ, Murtaugh M, White JG. Neutrophil-induced erythrocyte injury involves proteolytic cleavage of membrane proteins as well as oxidative damage. Vet Clin Pathol 20:21, 1991.

Weitekamp MR, Aber RC. Prolonged bleeding times and bleeding diathesis associated with moxalactam administration. J Am Med Assoc 249:69, 1983.

Williams N. Is thrombopoietin interleukin 6? Exp Hematol 19:714, 1991.

Woody BJ, Hoskins JD. Ehrlichial diseases of dogs. Vet Clin North Am [Small Anim Pract] 21:75, 1991.

Wrightman SR, Kier AB, Wagner JE. Feline cytauxzoonosis: Clinical features of a newly described blood parasite disease. Fel Pract 7:23, 1977.

Zoumbos NC, Gascón P, Djeu JY, et al. Circulating activated suppressor T lymphocytes in aplastic anemia. N Engl J Med 312:257, 1985.

Zulty JC, Kociba GJ. Cold agglutinins in cats with haemobartonellosis. J Am Vet Med Assoc 196:907, 1990.

CHAPTER 15

The Endocrine and Metabolic Systems

C. B. CHASTAIN

Endocrine and metabolic diseases in older dogs and cats are common. The most common endocrine and metabolic diseases in dogs of this age group are diabetes mellitus (especially hyperosmolar nonketotic), hyperadrenocorticism, insulinoma, and hyperlipidemia. In older cats, hyperthyroidism, diabetes mellitus, and hypokalemia are the most common endocrine and metabolic diseases. Aging, without concurrent disease, is associated with only a slight gradual decline in the functional reserve of endocrine organs (Quadri and Palazzolo, 1991). Because the functional reserve for endocrine organs is many times greater than the resting level, clinical change is generally not evident except under severe stress. The presenting signs of endocrine and metabolic diseases in older dogs and cats are given in Table 15–1.

DISORDERS OF DOGS

Primary Hyperparathyroidism

Primary hyperparathyroidism is generally caused by neoplasia of the parathyroid glands, in which excessive amounts of parathyroid hormone are secreted; the condition is not responsive to the suppressive effects of hypercalcemia (Berger and Feldman, 1987). Affected parathyroid tissue may be found near or in the thyroid gland, the neck, the pericardial sac, or the cranial mediastinum. Affected dogs are usually older than 8 years old.

Clinical Features. The clinical signs of primary hyperparathyroidism are produced by hypercalcemia, bone resorption, and calcium nephropathy resulting from the excessive secretion of parathyroid hormone. Effects and clinical signs resulting from hypercalcemia, excess parathyroid hormone, and the uremic syndrome resulting from calcium nephropathy are listed in Table 15–2. Affected parathyroid tissue is not palpable. Calcium phosphate or oxalate uroliths may occur in affected dogs (Klausner et al, 1987). Bony facial swelling (hyperostosis), loose teeth, and pliability of the mandible ("rubber jaw") are thought to result from demineralization, multiple infractions, hemorrhage, and replacement of bone by fibrous connective tissue and osteoid.

Laboratory Findings and Diagnosis. Persistent hypercalcemia is the best single diagnostic determinant of hyperparathyroidism (Berger and Feldman, 1987). Rarely, serum calcium levels may be normal or only intermittently elevated. Possible causes of hypercalcemia are listed in Table 15–3. The primary causes of serum calcium levels that exceed 15 mg/dl are malignancies, primary hyperparathyroidism, and hypervitaminosis D. Repeated measurements (at least three) of

TABLE 15–1. PRESENTING SIGNS OF ENDOCRINE AND METABOLIC DISEASES IN OLDER DOGS AND CATS

Weight loss and weakness
- Diabetes mellitus
- Hyperthyroidism
- Pheochromocytoma
- Hypercalcemia of malignancy

Anorexia
- Ketoacidotic diabetes mellitus
- Primary hyperparathyroidism
- Gastrinoma
- Hypercalcemia of malignancy

Increased appetite
- Diabetes mellitus
- Hyperthyroidism
- Insulinoma
- Acromegaly

Obesity
- Hyperadrenocorticism
- Insulinoma
- Hypothyroidism

Mental disurbances
- Hyperthyroidism
- Hypothalamic/pituitary tumors
- Hyperadrenocorticism
- Primary hyperparathyroidism
- Hypothyroidism

Pathologic fractures
- Primary hyperparathyroidism

Polyuria and polydipsia
- Diabetes insipidus
- Diabetes mellitus
- Primary hyperparathyroidism
- Hyperadrenocorticism
- Hyperthyroidism
- Hypercalcemia of malignancy

Tetany, muscle spasms, and muscle cramps
- Hyperadrenocorticism
- Postsurgical hypoparathyroidism
- Hypothyroidism

Alopecia
- Hyperadrenocorticism
- Gonadal tumors
- Hypothyroidism

serum calcium levels are recommended in dogs with clinical signs and history suggestive of primary hyperparathyroidism. Although compensatory changes in calcium regulation (hypercalcitoninism) or concurrent diseases that cause hypoalbuminemia can cause normocalcemia in cases of primary hyperparathyroidism, these instances are rare. Early in the development of primary hyperparathyroidism, hypercalcemia often is accompanied by serum phosphorus levels that are below normal or at the low end of the normal range and by decreased plasma bicarbonate levels.

A radioimmunoassay (RIA) for parathyroid hormone and a determination of concurrent serum ionized calcium level may be considered. A two-site immunoradiometric assay for intact human parathyroid hormone has been validated for the dog (Torrance and Nachreiner, 1989a,b). A mid-molecule parathyroid hormone assay has also been validated for the dog (Mallette and Tuma, 1984). Three random plasma samples should be taken and pooled for parathyroid hormone assessment, because single levels often vary considerably. Plasma samples for parathyroid

TABLE 15–2. CLINICAL SIGNS OF PRIMARY HYPERPARATHYROIDISM AND THEIR CAUSES

Excessive parathyroid hormone
- Pathologic fractures
- Facial hyperostosis
- Loosening and loss of teeth
- Painful mastication and malodorous breath
- Bone pain, lameness, or neck pain

Hypercalcemia
- Anorexia and vomiting
- Constipation
- Muscle weakness
- Bradycardia and arrhythmias
- Depression, coma, or seizures
- Polyuria and polydipsia
- Gastric ulcers

Uremic syndrome
- Depression and vomiting
- Diarrhea
- Oral ulcerations
- Anemia
- Dyspnea (compensation for metabolic acidosis)
- Polyuria and polydipsia
- Bleeding tendency (thrombocytopathy)
- Immunosuppression

TABLE 15–3. POSSIBLE CAUSES OF HYPERCALCEMIA

Primary hyperparathyroidism

Increased release of calcium from bone
- Nonparathyroid malignancies
- Acute immobilization
- Hyperthyroidism
- Septic osteomyelitis
- Hypervitaminosis A

Increased renal tubular reabsorption of calcium
- Thiazide diuretics
- Severe hypoadrenocorticism

Spurious laboratory results (hyperlipidemia)

Congenital renal diseases (decreased glomerular clearance and increased circulating complexed calcium)

Hypervitaminosis D
- Owner error in diet
- Calcitriol rodenticides
- Granulomatous disease (blastomycosis)

hormone assay should be shipped to the laboratory overnight with ice.

Ultrasonography of the neck can aid in detecting parathyroid tumors larger than 1 cm in diameter. Skeletal demineralization, or osteopenia (osteomalacia), can be seen radiographically in dogs with primary hyperparathyroidism; however, mineralization must be severely depleted before it becomes evident on routine radiographs. The earliest detectable changes usually are radiolucency of the laminae durae dentes of the teeth, the vertebral bodies, and the dorsal processes of the vertebrae. Subperiosteal cortical resorption and bone cysts may be visualized radiographically in long bones. Multiple pathologic fractures are rare. Subclinical demineralization may be made evident by a technetium pyrophosphate bone scan. When present, nephroliths and uroliths are seen easily in radiographs, because they are composed of calcium phosphate or oxalate. Renal calculi can also be detected by abdominal ultrasonography. Nephrocalcinosis is less distinct in radiographs but may appear as diffuse mild radiopacity of the kidneys.

Management. Emergency treatment is necessary for severe hypercalcemia. Surgical removal of the parathyroid neoplasm is necessary to treat primary hyperparathyroidism. Before surgery the dog should be evaluated for the extent of functional renal impairment. Thoracic radiographs are also indicated to search for metastasis of parathyroid carcinomas or for cranial mediastinal ectopic parathyroid neoplasms. During surgery parathyroid glands should be examined and their sizes compared. Enlarged glands should be removed; however, if all are enlarged, then three glands should be removed, leaving one cranial parathyroid gland.

Transient but serious hypocalcemia may develop 12 to 96 hours after the operation because the source of excess parathyroid hormone has been removed, with unaccommodated parathyroid tissue remaining, and because of rapid calcium uptake by mineral-starved bone. Due to the risk of postsurgical hypocalcemia, prophylactic postsurgical dihydrotachysterol (Hytakerol) has been recommended (Berger and Feldman, 1987). The recommended dosage is 0.02 mg per kilogram body weight per day for 3 days, then 0.01 mg per kilogram body weight per day for 1 week; the dosage is then reduced by 25 to 50 per cent per week, and the medication is discontinued in 2 months. By adjusting oral doses of calcium gluconate and vitamin D to maintain serum calcium levels between 7.5 and 9.0 mg/dl, the production of parathyroid hormone from the remaining parathyroid tissue will normalize without the risk of acute hypocalcemia. If postoperative serum calcium levels are lower than 7.5 mg/dl and no hypocalcemic signs are noted, oral calcium gluconate should be given in divided doses of 50 to 75 mg/kg/day. The production of parathyroid hormone by the remaining parathyroid tissue should normalize in 1 to 3 weeks. Dihydrotachysterol and oral calcium, in that order, can usually be tapered to discontinuation. Skeletal recovery after successful surgery should be nearly complete in 2 months. If serum calcium levels remain elevated after surgery, additional ectopic tissue in the neck or cranial mediastinum should be sought or the diagnosis of primary hyperparathyroidism reevaluated.

Diabetes Mellitus

Diabetes mellitus results from an absolute or relative deficiency of insulin. The most common cause is not known. Possible causes are genetic, pancreatic injury, beta cell exhaustion from insulin antagonism, target tissue insensitivity, and insulin dyshormonogenesis. The most common known cause is pancreatitis (Alejandro et al, 1988). Three types of diabetes mellitus occur: insulin-dependent, noninsulin-dependent, and diabetes secondary to other conditions (e.g., estrus, hyperadrenocorticism, acromegaly, glucagonomas) or drugs (e.g., progestogen, glucocorticoids) (Jeffers et al, 1991). Diabetes mellitus most frequently occurs in small breeds, especially the dachshund and poodle, but all breeds are affected. The age at onset is usually 8 to 9 years.

Clinical Features. The clinical signs of diabetes mellitus depend on the type of insulin insufficiency, the degree of insulin insufficiency, and the conditions preceding the onset of insulin insufficiency. Clinical forms of diabetes are categorized as nonketotic, ketoacidotic, and nonketotic hyperosmolar. Approximately 25 per cent to 50 per cent of dogs with diabetes are seen for examination in a nonketotic state. Dogs with uncomplicated diabetes mellitus have nocturia, polyuria, and polydipsia with mild dehydration and lose weight even though their appetite is excessive. Most dogs are obese but have experienced recent weight loss. Hepatomegaly may be palpable in 10 to 20 per cent of dogs. Cataracts often occur in unregulated diabetic dogs (Fig. 15–1). Ketoacidosis is present in most dogs that initially present with diabetes mellitus. It represents the uncompensated stage of the body's attempts to buffer the ketoacids formed as an alter-

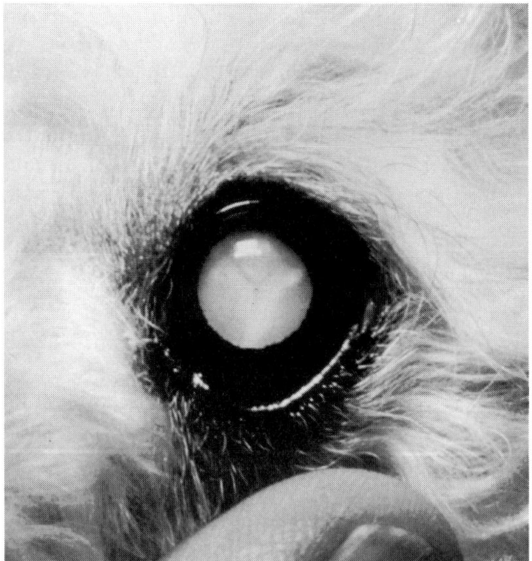

Figure 15–1. Diabetic cataract in a poodle. (From Chastain CB, Ganjam VK. Clinical Endocrinology of Companion Animals. Philadelphia, Lea & Febiger, 1986, p 265.)

perosmolality, in addition to hyperglycemia and glucosuria, are common. Nonketotic hyperosmolar diabetes is characterized by extreme hyperglycemia (glucose levels greater than 500 mg/dl), hyperosmolality, azotemia, and absence of ketonemia or ketonuria. Approximately one fourth to one half of female diabetics have bacterial cystitis at initial presentation.

Management. The initial goals of therapy are to normalize the hyperglycemia, fluid and electrolyte imbalance, and plasma hyperosmolality as carefully as possible. After establishing the diagnosis, dogs should be characterized as having uncomplicated, ketoacidotic, or nonketotic hyperosmolar diabetes. Dogs that are alert, with little or no dehydration and little or no ketonuria, and are also willing and able to eat without vomiting can be treated as having uncomplicated diabetes. Treatment of uncomplicated diabetes mellitus with insulin may begin with subcutaneous administration of an intermediate-acting insulin (NPH

nate energy source during severe or prolonged insulin deficiency (Fig. 15–2).

Nonketotic hyperosmolar syndrome occurs more commonly in older dogs. Cardiac or renal disease impairs the body's ability to retain water and excrete sodium, which leads to nonketotic hyperosmolar coma in affected diabetics. The blood glucose level exceeds 600 mg/dl, serum sodium is often more than 145 mmol/L (mg/dl), and the plasma osmolality exceeds 340 mOsm/L. Each time blood glucose level increases by 100 mg/dl, the plasma osmolality increases by 5.6 mOsm per kilogram body weight. Ketonemia is not present. Dogs with nonketotic hyperosmolar diabetic coma present with, or soon develop, stupor or coma caused by the plasma's hyperosmolality. Central nervous system dysfunction is not likely until the serum osmolality exceeds 340 mOsm/L, usually when blood glucose levels approach 800 mg/dl.

Laboratory Findings and Diagnosis. Overt diabetes mellitus may be diagnosed if repeated fasting blood glucose values exceed 140 mg/dl or if a single fasting or postprandial blood glucose value exceeds 200 mg/dl. Occasionally, fasting blood glucose values may only periodically or transiently exceed 140 mg/dl; this may be caused by a mild to moderate impairment in dogs who have glucose tolerance or a stress-related hyperglycemia. In ketoacidosis, a low blood pH, ketonemia, hypokalemia, hypophosphatemia, and hy-

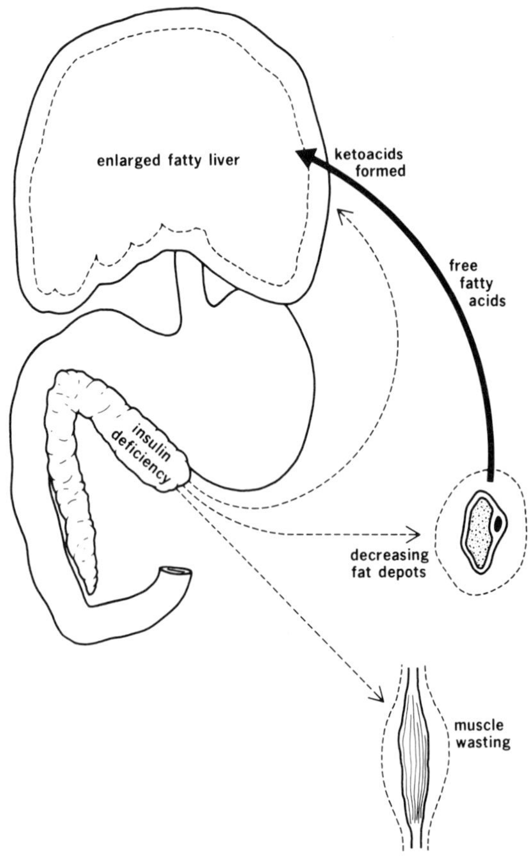

Figure 15–2. The general effects of diabetes mellitus. (From Chastain CB, Ganjam VK. Clinical Endocrinology of Companion Animals. Philadelphia, Lea & Febiger, 1986, p 258.)

or Lente) at 0.5 U/kg 30 minutes before the morning meal. Currently available insulins are listed in Table 15–4. Pork- or beef-origin insulin is most often used in dogs and cats. Pork insulin is identical to dog insulin and similar to human insulin; beef insulin is similar to cat insulin. The response to intermediate insulin should be evaluated 8 to 12 hours after the injection, and the insulin dose should be appropriately modified by 1- to 2-U increments to attain a blood glucose value of 100 to 150 mg/dl in the evening. Morning blood glucose levels should also be measured and should not exceed 200 mg/dl. Crystalline insulin may be given in the evening if evening blood glucose levels exceed 250 mg/dl during the period of morning dosage adjustment. Many cases require a long-acting insulin (Ultralente) or twice-daily intermediate-acting insulin dosing, as insulins have a shorter duration in dogs than previously thought (Goeders et al, 1987). If the insulin dose is 10 U or less, a diluent-to-insulin dilution of 9:1 should be used to facilitate accurate dosing and subcutaneous absorption. Normal saline solution may be used as a diluent if the mixture is used within 24 hours. Otherwise, an insulin diluent formulated for the proper pH and buffer should be used if storage for more than 24 hours is desired.

Exercise and caloric intake should remain as static as possible. It is best to determine caloric requirements based on ideal body weight rather than present body weight. Reduction in excess body fat is beneficial, because obesity reduces insulin receptors and receptor binding of insulin and causes a defect in post–insulin receptor events. Most 10- to 15-kg house dogs are estimated to require 40 to 60 kcal/kg/day. Canned dog food contains approximately 500 to 600 kcal per pound of food. Three to four meals per day may be optimal for diabetics, but this is rarely practical for most dog owners. One fourth of the total daily requirements is generally given in the morning, and three fourths is given 8 to 12 hours after the morning injection of insulin if once-daily insulin injections are being given. The total daily diet should be evenly divided into morning and evening meals if twice-daily insulin injections are required. Increasing the fiber in diets to more than 15 per cent of dry matter and increasing the complex carbohydrates in the diet are possibly beneficial for the control of diabetes mellitus (Nelson and Lewis, 1990). Soluble fiber reduces the postprandial rise in blood glucose and may improve glycemic control in diabetic dogs (Blaxter et al, 1990). Soluble fiber imbibes water, thereby slowing gastric emptying time and reducing the rate of intestinal absorption of glucose. Soluble fiber may be poorly tolerated, causing difficulty in swallowing, poor haircoat, and soft feces. Insoluble fiber may also be beneficial and may be better tolerated, although it can cause constipation. Some commercial high-fiber diets are Prescription Diet (Hills Pet Products) Canine r/d, w/d, and g/d; Science Diet Canine Maintenance Light (Hills Pet Products); and Purina Fit & Trim. To be of value, added fiber must be mixed into the food and not given separately. High-fiber diets should not be given to cachectic diabetic dogs.

TABLE 15–4. TYPES OF INSULINS

Short-acting (up to 8 hours)
Insulin injection USP (regular, crystalline)
Prompt insulin zinc suspension USP (Semilente)
Intermediate-acting (up to 24 hours)
Isophane insulin suspension USP (NPH)
Insulin zinc suspension USP (Lente)
Long-acting (possibly more than 24 hours)
Extended insulin zinc suspension USP (Ultralente)

Frequent monitoring of the initial response to insulin is essential for the successful management of diabetic ketoacidosis. The blood glucose level is generally determined each hour until the blood glucose level is less than 250 mg/dl. This can be done in a little over 1 minute with a few drops of whole blood using glucose oxidase–impregnated strips and a reflectance colorimeter such as Chemstrip bG (Boehringer Mannheim Corporation) and the Accu-Chek II or III monitor (Boehringer Mannheim Corporation) (Joseph et al, 1987). Assessment of serum osmolality also should be included in the initial evaluation of depressed diabetic dogs. The serum of diabetic dogs can become severely hyperosmolar with or without ketoacidosis. If the dog is clinically ill, as shown by such signs as depression, anorexia, weakness, and vomiting, serum hyperosmolality is possible. Tonicity or "effective osmolality" can be calculated in diabetics with the following formula:

$$\text{mOsm/L} = 2\,(\text{Na}) + \text{glucose}/20$$

Normal plasma effective osmolality in the dog is about 280 to 310 mOsm/L; serum osmolality above 340 mOsm/L can be dangerous. Hypotension is particularly likely if hyperosmolality is present, inasmuch as the resulting cellular dehydration of the myocardium weakens myocardial strength of contraction. Proper administration of fluids should improve cardiac output, decrease serum osmolality, reduce hyperglycemia, reduce ketonemia, buffer ketoacids, maintain urinary excretion, and correct electrolyte imbalances. The need for fluid additives, such as potassium phosphate and sodium bicarbonate, is determined by the blood pH and serum potassium concentration. Insulin facilitates the intracellular entry of phosphate as well as potassium. Severe hypophosphatemia (less than 1 mg/dl) can cause hemolytic anemia, seizures, altered mental state, cardiomyopathy, and skeletal muscle weakness (Willard et al, 1987).

Intravenous low-dose administration is the preferred insulin treatment if the dog is severely hypotensive or hypothermic and if adequate supervision is available to prevent malpositioning of catheters and ensure a regular rate of administration. Recommended intravenous low-dose therapy is 0.1 U/kg, followed by a dose of 0.1 U/kg/hour of crystalline insulin diluted in replacement fluids (e.g., lactated Ringer's solution) and administered by slow drip. Low-dose, intramuscular administration of insulin permits more accurate measurement of administered insulin and requires a minimum of equipment and supervision compared with intravenous administration. If the dog is adequately hydrated and has normal cardiovascular function, intramuscular crystalline insulin is effective in 30 minutes and lasts 81 per cent longer than intravenously administered insulin (Nelson et al, 1990). The initial intramuscular dose is 2 U of crystalline insulin, administered in the thigh muscles for small dogs weighing less than 10 kg. Very small dogs (less than 3 kg) should be treated initially with only 1 U of crystalline insulin, followed by 1 U each hour. For dogs weighing more than 10 kg, the initial dose is 0.25 U/kg. Treatment continues each hour thereafter until blood glucose levels are less than 250 mg/dl: for small dogs, 1 U is administered; for dogs weighing more than 10 kg, 0.1 U/kg is administered. Syringes measuring 1 U (Lo-Dose Insulin Syringes; Becton Dickinson and Company) and a fresh dilution of regular insulin in sterile saline solution should be used.

After blood glucose concentration has been reduced to 250 to 150 mg/dl, the administration of intramuscular insulin is discontinued. The mean time required to reduce the blood glucose level to this range is about 4 hours. Fluids are then changed to 5 per cent dextrose solution with potassium phosphate added to prevent dilutional hypokalemia and hypophosphatemia. If the blood glucose level is less than 150 mg/dl, a solution of 5 per cent dextrose with 20 mmol/L of potassium phosphate and potassium chloride (50:50 solution) is administered. Insulin is not given. If the blood glucose level is between 150 and 250 mg/dl, 5 per cent dextrose with potassium phosphate and potassium chloride is given intravenously, and 0.5 U/kg of regular insulin is administered subcutaneously every 6 to 8 hours. Doses are then changed by 1 to 2 U to maintain blood glucose concentrations between 100 and 200 mg/dl at 4 hours after the last injection. When the dog is able to eat without vomiting, fluids and regular administration of insulin can be discontinued. Therapy with an intermediate-acting insulin can then begin in a conventional manner.

Nonketotic hyperosmolar coma should also be treated with regular insulin. Because the coma is due to hyperosmolality, the reduction in hyperglycemia should be gradual to minimize the risk for iatrogenic cerebral edema. Low-dose insulin administration is appropriate and is preferred for the treatment of nonketotic hyperosmolar coma, as well as diabetic ketoacidosis. Once diabetic patients with ketoacidosis or nonketotic hyperosmolar coma are stabilized, willing, and capable of eating without vomiting, they can be treated as uncomplicated diabetic patients.

Possible responses to insulin are illustrated in Figure 15–3. Type A reactions may be caused by the Somogyi effect, an exaggerated response to insulin-induced hypoglycemia, or by a transient effect of intermediate-acting insulin. Transient effects are presumably from excessive insulinase activity (called the *dawn phenomenon*) and are more common than the Somogyi effect. Type B reaction is the desired response. Insulin resistance is arbitrarily defined as the failure to reduce blood glucose to normal levels with the administration of less than 2.2 U/kg per injection (not per day). Insulin resistance may be caused by decreased receptor affinity for insulin, the induction or administration of insulin-antagonistic hormones, insulin-antagonistic endocrinopathies, inactivation of insulin at the site of injection, anti-insulin antibodies, or postreceptor defects in insulin's action (Ihle and Nelson, 1991). Insulin resistance may be corrected by successful management of any concurrent infectious disease, pancreatitis, obesity, pregnancy, estrus, uremia, or insulin-antagonistic endocrinopathy or by discontinuing the administration of insulin-antagonistic drugs.

If the response to long-acting insulin does not produce a type B response, twice-daily intermediate-acting insulin injections are often corrective. If further refinement is necessary or desired, "split-and-mixed" multiple daily injections should be tried. All insulins in the Lente family can be

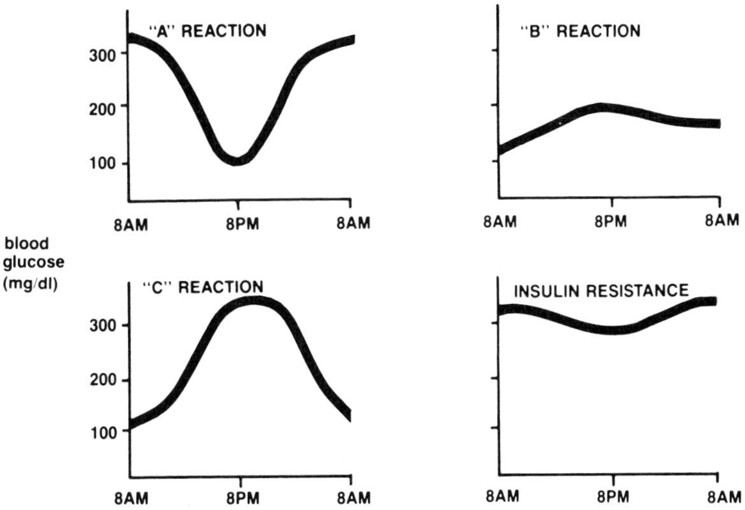

Figure 15–3. Possible responses to a single administration of intermediate or long-acting insulin. (From Chastain CB, Ganjam VK. Clinical Endocrinology of Companion Animals. Philadelphia, Lea & Febiger, 1986, p 286.)

mixed, and regular insulin can be mixed with NPH. However, Lente insulins cannot be mixed with NPH. The best compromise between the insulin's effect and the effort to produce a desired effect is to give a mixture of intermediate-acting insulin and short-acting insulin twice daily, 30 to 60 minutes before the morning and evening meals. A mixture composed of one third short-acting insulin and two thirds intermediate-acting insulin is prepared. Morning and evening meals should each be one half of the calculated daily requirements. Morning and evening dosages are adjusted in 1- to 2-U increments in response to the blood glucose values produced.

The first recheck examination should be scheduled for 2 weeks after the initial discharge. All recommended subsequent rechecks should take place every 3 months, provided the dog is well regulated by the treatment. The owner should keep a log of the parameters (Table 15–5) to be reviewed by the veterinarian at times of apparent poor control and at routine re-examinations. Diabetic dogs should be examined by a veterinarian if abnormalities are detected by monitoring at home for 2 or more consecutive days or whenever ketones are detected in the urine. Diabetics should be physically re-examined, their home monitoring log reviewed, and blood examinations repeated every 3 months.

Glycohemoglobin is the result of a slow, nonenzymatic combination of glucose with certain types of hemoglobin throughout the life of a red blood cell (120 days in the dog). Glycohemoglobin levels parallel the mean blood glucose level over the last 8 to 12 weeks of the cycle. Normal blood glycohemoglobin concentration in dogs is less than 6 per cent. Serum fructosamine is a glycosylation product of serum proteins, particularly albumin. Normal serum fructosamine concentration in dogs is less than 3.5 per cent. Its value reflects the state of glycemic control over the preceding 2 weeks. Recommended components of an outpatient recheck examination are listed in Table 15–6.

TABLE 15–5. HOME ASSESSMENTS OF DIABETES CONTROL

Assess daily:
Attitude
Appetite
Physical activity
Water consumption
Urinary continence
Assess weekly:
Body weight
Assess as necessary:
Urine ketones and glucose

TABLE 15–6. ROUTINE OUTPATIENT ASSESSMENTS OF DIABETES CONTROL

Review of owner's observations and home records
Body weight and routine physical examination
Urinalysis and urine culture (collection by cystocentesis)
Blood and serum examinations:
Hemogram
Blood glucose
Serum urea nitrogen
Cholesterol
Triglycerides
Serum alanine transaminase
Serum alkaline phosphatase
Glycohemoglobin or serum fructosamine

Beta Cell Tumors

Most beta cell tumors in dogs are multihormone producing. Insulin is most frequently produced in enough excess to cause hypoglycemia (Zerbe et al, 1989). Insulinomas are beta cell tumors of the pancreatic islets that predominantly produce an excess of insulin (Fig. 15–4). Even though about 40 per cent of insulinomas appear histologically benign, clinically malignant tumors of the islets outnumber benign tumors by 4:1 (Caywood et al, 1988). The average age of affected dogs is 9 years (range, 3 to 12 years). Breeds larger than 25 kg in body weight—German shepherd dogs, Irish setters, golden retrievers, collies, standard poodles, boxers, and fox terriers—are most often affected (Caywood et al, 1988).

Clinical Features. The presenting signs are either those resulting from a deficient supply of glucose to the brain (neuroglucopenia) or release of catecholamines (adrenergic). The clinical signs of neuroglucopenia include seizures, weakness and incoordination, depression, change in behavior, polyphagia, and syncope (Caywood et al, 1988). Seizures are usually not noticed until blood glucose levels are less than 50 mg/dl. Signs may develop during fasting, exercise, periods of excitement, or eating. Degenerative peripheral polyneuropathy characterized by proprioceptive deficits and depressed reflexes is possible (Braund et al, 1987).

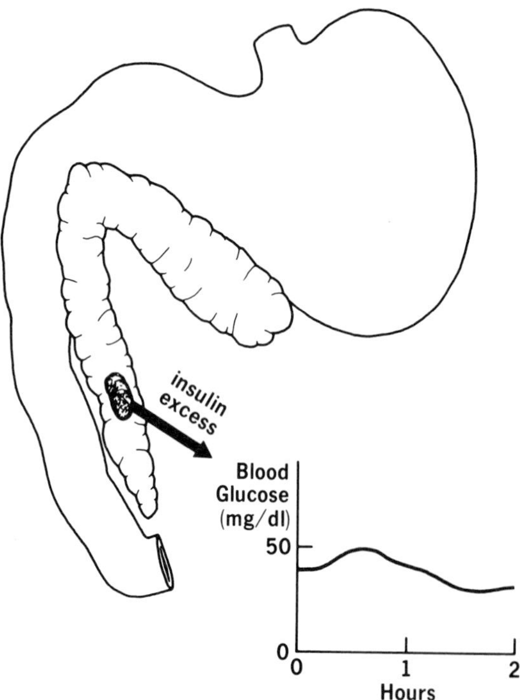

Figure 15–4. The effect of excessive insulin secretion by an insulinoma. (From Chastain CB, Ganjam VK. Clinical Endocrinology of Companion Animals. Philadelphia, Lea & Febiger, 1986, p 304.)

Laboratory Findings and Diagnosis. Postprandial or fasting hypoglycemia (glucose less than 50 mg/dl) is the hallmark of insulinomas in older dogs with muscle weakness, personality changes, and episodic seizures (Caywood et al, 1988). Insulinoma is the most common cause for hypoglycemia in dogs older than 5 years of age. Abnormal routine laboratory findings other than hypoglycemia are uncommon. Liver metastasis from insulinomas usually does not result in elevated serum liver enzyme levels. Mild hypokalemia occurs in about 20 per cent of cases (Leifer et al, 1986). Once fasting hypoglycemia is noted, a fasting immunoreactive insulin (IRI) assay should be done. Shipments of serum to reference laboratories require packing with ice owing to degradation of insulin in unfrozen serum (Reimers et al, 1991). Blood glucose levels should be determined with blood samples drawn at the same time as serum for IRI determination. Normal fasting serum IRI levels in dogs are less than 30 μU/ml (Rogers and Luttgen, 1985). The glucose-to-insulin ratio is generally sufficient for a diagnosis; a ratio of less than 2.5 mg/μU is diagnostic (Rogers and Luttgen, 1985).

Computerized tomography and selective arterial angiography have been successfully used to show pancreatic tumors larger than 2 cm. However, many tumors are smaller than 2 cm, and radiographic proof of the tumor is generally unnecessary for diagnosis or management. Fewer than half are large enough to be detected by ultrasonography (Rogers and Luttgen, 1985).

Management. Excision of insulinomas should be attempted whenever possible (Leifer et al, 1986). Insulinomas in dogs are generally slow-growing malignant tumors. Two thirds appear histologically malignant; 45 per cent of insulinomas have metastases to the liver and regional lymph nodes that are evident at laparotomy. All tumors eventually recur after excision, but excision can eliminate clinical signs in most cases for as long as 3 years. Survival times are shorter without surgery (Rogers and Luttgen, 1985; Leifer et al, 1986). Recommended presurgical, surgical, and postsurgical care is given in Table 15–7. If the insulinoma has been sufficiently excised, blood glucose should rise to normal levels within 2 hours. Postsurgical complications include persistent seizures (Mehlhaff et al, 1985), diabetes

TABLE 15–7. RECOMMENDED SURGICAL CARE FOR ISLET CELL TUMORS

Presurgery
- Feed several small, high-protein meals per day.
- Give no food by mouth for 8 hours before surgery.
- Give 5 to 10 per cent dextrose solution IV at a slow, constant rate for several hours before surgery.
- Monitor serum potassium and blood glucose every 8 hours until time of surgery.

During surgery
- Infuse 10 per cent dextrose solution IV.
- Monitor blood glucose levels every 30 minutes.

Postsurgery
- Measure blood glucose every 8 hours.
- Administer 5 to 10 per cent dextrose solution IV as necessary for hypoglycemia.
- Give no food or water by mouth for 3 days.
- Monitor serum potassium, urea nitrogen, lipase, and amylase at least once a day for 3 days.
- After 3 days, begin feeding small, frequent meals.

IV, Intravenous administration.

mellitus, and trauma-induced pancreatitis. In most cases the hyperglycemia is mild and transient, lasting only 3 to 5 days. If surgical treatment is not possible or unsuccessful, or if hypoglycemic episodes return after surgery, medical therapy is indicated. Initial medical management for hypoglycemia from insulinomas should include feeding small, frequent (three or more) meals high in protein, complex carbohydrates, and fat, plus prednisolone (0.5 mg/kg/day in divided doses). Should dietary management and prednisolone be inadequate, diazoxide (Proglycem) 10 mg/kg/day in divided doses may be tried (Nelson, 1985; Rogers and Luttgen, 1985; Mehlhaff et al, 1985). It is effective in about 70 per cent of cases (Leifer et al, 1986). Common adverse effects are vomiting and anorexia. Chlorothiazide, given in twice-daily doses of 20 to 40 mg/kg, should be used with diazoxide to reduce sodium retention and potentiate hyperglycemic effects.

Hyperadrenocorticism

Spontaneous hyperadrenocorticism may be of pituitary gland or adrenal cortex origin. Pituitary-dependent causes represent about 80 per cent of the total spontaneous cases in dogs. The remaining 10 to 20 per cent of spontaneous cases in dogs are caused by unilateral or bilateral adrenocortical neoplasms. Boston terriers, dachshunds, boxers, miniature poodles, and toy poodles are the breeds most frequently affected with spontaneous hyperadrenocorticism. Brachycephalic breeds have a higher incidence of adrenocorticotropic hormone (ACTH)–producing pituitary tumors than other breeds. Hyperadrenocorticism in dachshunds and poodles is usually caused by bilateral adrenocortical hyperplasia not associated with pituitary tumors. Adrenocortical neoplasms most frequently occur in large breed dogs. Ages affected range from 3 to 15 years; most affected dogs are 7 to 9 years old.

Clinical Features. Most of the clinical signs of hyperadrenocorticism in dogs are caused by excessive levels of cortisol and corticosterone. Possible clinical signs, in order of their reported occurrence, are listed in Table 15–8. Most affected dogs develop a triad of polyuria-polydipsia, pendulous abdomen, and bilateral alopecia (Fig. 15–5). Polyuria-polydipsia is defined as water intake exceeding 100 ml/kg/day and urine production exceeding 50 ml/kg/day. In addition to a pendulous abdomen, affected animals may assume a straight- or stiff-legged stance as a result of muscular weakness. Myotonia or pseudomyotonia in dogs with hyperadrenocorticism results in extensor rigidity of the proximal appendicular muscles. Rigidity usually begins in one hind leg, then progresses to the other hind leg, and finally affects the front legs. The gait is stiff especially after the animal has rested or has been exposed to cold. Sudden development of respiratory distress, right-sided heart failure, or sudden death may be caused by pulmonary thromboembolism (King et al, 1985). Excessive levels of glucocorticoids can produce behavioral changes, psychoses, depression, and mania. Some neurologic clinical abnormalities are more likely the result of an enlarging pituitary tumor or possibly metastasis

TABLE 15–8. POSSIBLE CLINICAL SIGNS OF HYPERADRENOCORTICISM IN DOGS, IN DECREASING ORDER OF OCCURRENCE

Polyuria and polydipsia
Pendulous abdomen
Bilateral alopecia
Hepatomegaly
Polyphagia
Muscular weakness and atrophy
Lethargy
Persistent anestrus or atrophied testes
Hyperpigmentation of the skin
Calcinosis cutis
Heat intolerance
Hypertrophy of the clitoris
Neurologic deficits

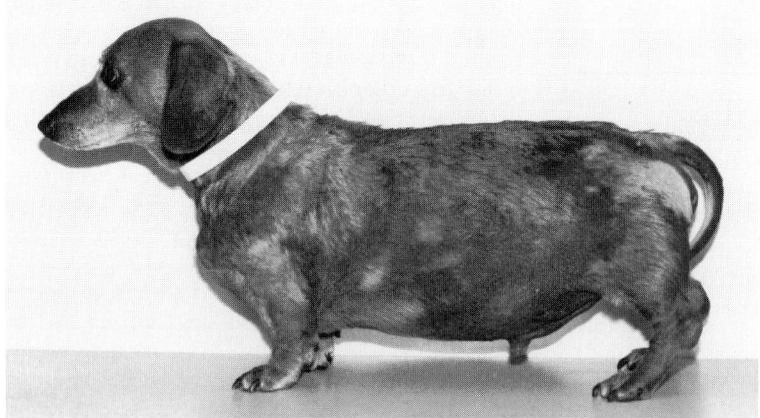

Figure 15–5. Most dogs with hyperadrenocorticism exhibit pendulous abdomen, bilateral alopecia, and polyuria and polydipsia. (From Chastain CB, Ganjam VK. Clinical Endocrinology of Companion Animals. Philadelphia, Lea & Febiger, 1986, p 367.)

from an adrenocortical carcinoma. These signs include seizures, somnolence, aimless wandering, blindness, head pressing, anisocoria, and Horner's syndrome (Nelson et al, 1989). Hypertension is often a manifestation of hyperadrenocorticism.

Laboratory Findings and Diagnosis. The most consistent routine hematologic and serum findings with hyperadrenocorticism are relative and absolute lymphopenia (less than 1000 cells/mm^3) and markedly increased levels of serum alkaline phosphatase (SAP). With the exception of SAP, the increase in serum liver enzymes is usually mild to moderate. Approximately 10 to 20 per cent of dogs with hyperadrenocorticism, especially miniature poodles, develop overt diabetes mellitus caused by insulin antagonism and pancreatic islet exhaustion (Blaxter et al, 1990; Peterson et al, 1986). Well-regulated diabetic dogs have normal plasma cortisol levels and dynamic responses to stimulation and suppression (Zerbe et al, 1988). Arterial blood gases change if thromboembolism occurs; often these changes include a low Po_2 (less than 70 mm Hg) and Pco_2 (less than 30 mm Hg). Urine specific gravity is frequently less than 1.012, unless water is being withheld. The urine should be routinely cultured because the incidence of bacterial infections is about 50 per cent in cases of hyperadrenocorticism.

The ability to suppress plasma cortisol levels to a significant extent with a low dose of dexamethasone usually rules out hyperadrenocorticism. The inability to suppress the plasma cortisol with low-dose administration of dexamethasone (0.01 mg/kg intravenously) may result from hyperadrenocorticism of pituitary or adrenal origin, some drugs, and some nonadrenocortical illnesses. Plasma cortisol samples should be taken at baseline and then 4 and 8 hours later. Normal dogs suppress and maintain plasma cortisol levels to less than 1.5 μg/dl. If the level achieved is less than 50 per cent of the baseline at 4 hours and higher later, pituitary-dependent hyperadrenocorticism is probable (Mack and Feldman, 1990). Exaggerated responses to exogenous stimulation of ACTH are seen in most dogs (more than 80 per cent) with bilateral adrenocortical hyperplasia, more than half of dogs with adrenocortical neoplasms, and in some dogs with nonadrenocortical illnesses. Dogs with adrenocortical carcinomas have exaggerated plasma cortisol values more often and to a greater degree than dogs with adrenocortical adenomas. Dogs should be given 2.2 U/kg intramuscularly of ACTH gel (H.P. Acthar gel) and sampled at baseline and 2 hours later. Normal dogs elevate their plasma cortisol levels up to 20 μg/dl.

A new screening test with a greater potential for diagnostic accuracy is the urine corticoid-to-creatinine (C:Cr) ratio (Jones et al, 1990). Seventy per cent of urine corticoids are free cortisol. However, other steroids may be detected (Rijnberk et al, 1988). The urinary C:Cr ratio is more accurate and more sensitive than the low-dose intravenous dexamethasone suppression test (Rijnberk et al, 1988). Normal values vary among laboratories. Two morning urine samples are preferred. If this test is normal, hyperadrenocorticism is ruled out. If abnormally high, additional tests such as the ACTH stimulation test are needed to confirm the diagnosis and differentiate the cause.

Once the diagnosis of hyperadrenocorticism is determined, a high-dose dexamethasone suppression test (0.1 mg/kg intravenously) should be done to determine the cause and facilitate rendering a prognosis. Suppression is defined as re-

TABLE 15–9. TESTING PROTOCOL FOR HYPERADRENOCORTICISM IN DOGS

Obtain urine for corticoid-to-creatinine ratio.
If urine corticoid-to-creatinine ratio is abnormally high, perform:
- ACTH stimulation test
- Low-dose dexamethasone suppression test
- Abdominal radiography

If the ACTH stimulation test or low-dose dexamethasone suppression test is abnormal and abdominal radiographs are normal, perform abdominal ultrasonography and the high-dose dexamethasone suppression test.
If pituitary-dependent hyperadrenocorticism is suspected, measure endogenous ACTH levels and, if possible, perform a CT scan of pituitary gland.

ACTH, Adrenocorticotropic hormone; CT, computed tomography.

duction from baseline levels by 50 per cent or more. All adrenal tumor–dependent hyperadrenocorticism (ATDH) cases and 10 to 30 per cent of pituitary-dependent cases do not suppress (Emms et al, 1987). Those pituitary-dependent cases that do not suppress are more likely to have macro tumors either larger than 1 cm in diameter or located in the pars intermedia (Nelson et al, 1989). A high-dose dexamethasone suppression test can also be done on an outpatient basis by instructing the owner to give three doses of 0.1 mg/kg of dexamethasone orally at 8-hour intervals before a urine sample for the C:Cr ratio (Rijnberk et al, 1988). Most pituitary-dependent hyperadrenocorticism (PDH) patients suppress their ratio to less than 50 per cent of their mean resting ratio (Rijnberk and Belshaw, 1988). If they don't suppress, an endogenous ACTH test is indicated to differentiate PDH from ATDH with more certainty.

Endogenous ACTH levels fluctuate in bursts throughout the day. Random plasma ACTH samples can be very helpful in differentiating the cause of hyperadrenocorticism in selected cases that cannot be classified otherwise. Plasma ACTH collection and transport require special handling—that is, avoidance of the use of glass tubes, prompt centrifugation, and transport overnight with ice (Hegstad et al, 1990). Normal dogs have endogenous ACTH levels of 10 to 70 pg/ml. High or normal plasma ACTH levels (40 to 500 pg/ml) with concurrently elevated plasma cortisol levels are suggestive of PDH. The magnitude of the endogenous ACTH level above normal often correlates with the size of pituitary tumors producing the excessive ACTH. Low plasma ACTH levels (less than 20 pg/ml) with concurrently elevated plasma cortisol levels are suggestive of ATDH (Tables 15–9 and 15–10).

The most consistent radiographic finding of hyperadrenocorticism is hepatomegaly. Other possible findings include soft tissue mineralization (skin, adrenals, bronchi, branches of the abdominal aorta, kidney, gastric mucosa, and liver capsule), mild osteoporosis, and an enlarged adrenal silhouette (Fig. 15–6). With pulmonary thromboembolism, thoracic radiographs may reveal pleural effusion, blunting of pulmonary arteries, and decreased vascularity of affected lung lobes. The thorax and abdomen should be radiographed to search for adrenal tumors and metastasis. Ultrasonography can also determine the presence of vena cava compression or invasion and is excellent in screening for liver metastasis (Reusch and Feldman, 1991). Tumors as small as 1.2 cm can be detected with ultrasonography (Voorhout, 1990). Routine radiography cannot detect adrenal tumors of 2 cm or less unless they have mineralized (Voorhout, 1990). Magnetic resonance imaging (MRI) or computed tomography (CT) scans are ideal to search for the presence of pituitary tumors (Turrel et al, 1986). MRI is capable of detecting tumors as small as 4 mm in diameter. Cisternography combined with linear tomography has also been useful in detecting pituitary enlargement (Voorhout, 1990).

TABLE 15–10. INTERPRETATION OF LABORATORY TESTS IN PDH AND ATDH

	NORMAL	PDH	ATDH
Urine corticoid-to-creatinine ratio	8–24	High	High
Baseline plasma cortisol (μg/dl)	<1–4	Normal to high	Normal to high
Plasma cortisol after LDDS (μg/dl)	<1.5	>1.5	>1.5
Plasma cortisol after ACTH stimulation (μg/dl)	<20	High	Normal to high
Plasma cortisol after HDDS (μg/dl)	<50 per cent of baseline	<50 per cent of baseline	>50 per cent of baseline
Endogenous plasma ACTH (pg/ml)	10–70	>40	<20

ACTH, Adrenocorticotropic hormone; ATDH, adrenal tumor-dependent hyperadrenocorticism; HDDS, high-dose dexamethasone suppression; LDDS, low-dose dexamethasone suppression; PDH, pituitary-dependent hyperadrenocorticism.

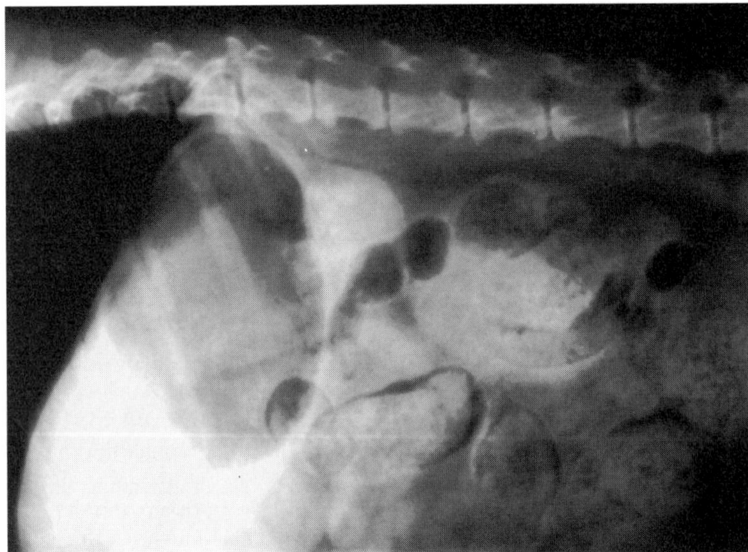

Figure 15–6. A radiograph of enlarged mineralized adrenal tumor in a dog with hyperadrenocorticism.

Management. The treatment of hyperadrenocorticism can be done by pharmacologic control, surgical correction, or a combination. For PDH, the most economical and safest form of treatment is pharmacologic therapy with mitotane (Lysodren). For radiographically demonstrable adrenocortical tumors (enlarged carcinomas), surgical excision should be attempted and, if necessary, pharmacologic control of metastasis used. Adrenocortical hyperplasia is usually treated with mitotane. The recommended dose for adrenal hyperplasia in the dog is 50 mg/kg every day until a satisfactory response is noted. A response should be evident within 10 days of treatment, or a re-evaluation for adrenocortical tumors should be done. An alternative initial treatment consists of giving mitotane for 5 to 14 days with glucocorticoid replacement (Kintzer and Peterson, 1991). An ACTH stimulation test is always necessary before mitotane administration to provide a baseline for evaluation of subsequent effectiveness of treatment. Post-ACTH plasma cortisol levels are below 5 μg/dl after sufficient mitotane treatment. For maintenance, weekly administration of 50 mg/kg is required indefinitely. A dosage of 50 to 150 mg/kg/day can sometimes be effective for inoperable adrenal tumors (Scavelli et al, 1986). The most frequent adverse effects of mitotane are temporary anorexia, weakness, and dizziness for 2 to 12 hours. Pretreatment with low-dose prednisolone may preclude such adverse effects in affected dogs.

If persistent clinical signs of glucocorticoid deficiency (e.g., vomiting, diarrhea, marked depression, or total anorexia) develop, replacement glucocorticoid therapy should be initiated. When necessary, the dose of 0.22 mg/kg/day of prednisone or prednisolone will replace baseline glucocorticoid effects of normal cortisol levels. Addison's disease occurs in about 5 per cent of treated cases and should be suspected if there is poor response to glucocorticoid replacement alone. Then serum sodium and potassium levels should be reassessed.

Re-examination of treated dogs is recommended 6 weeks after dismissal from the hospital and every 3 to 6 months thereafter. About one half of dogs with PDH develop partial resistance to treatment with mitotane because of a compensatory increase in the secretion of ACTH resulting from lowered levels of plasma cortisol. An alternative medical treatment to mitotane is ketoconazole. The dosage required exceeds that required for antifungal effects. It may be used in some dogs to prepare them for surgery or when mitotane cannot be tolerated. Presurgical therapy should begin 4 to 8 weeks before surgery. The dose is 10 to 15 mg/kg bid on an indefinite basis (Feldman et al, 1990). Potential adverse effects include anorexia, vomiting, and lightening of the haircoat. Treatment is ineffective in at least 20 per cent of dogs treated. Mitotane should not be used concurrently with ketoconazole.

Surgical procedures such as adrenalectomy or hypophysectomy are possible means of correcting hyperadrenocorticism. Both procedures require the skill of an experienced surgeon and are expensive compared with drug therapy (Scavelli et al, 1986). Bilateral adrenalectomy should not be performed on a diabetic, because loss of medullary epinephrine allows hypoglycemia to be more severe (Emms et al, 1987). Pituitary macroadenomas and macroadenocarcinomas have been successfully managed with external-beam photon radiotherapy (40 Gy in 10 equal doses over 22 days). Tumor size decreases about 50 per cent every 6 months (Nelson et al, 1989; Dow et al, 1990). Neural and ocular complications are common with radiation exposure to the head.

Treatment of hyperadrenocorticism concurrent with insulin-dependent diabetes mellitus requires insulin therapy until the blood glucose level has been near normal for at least 1 week. Treatment with mitotane is then begun, and the previous insulin dosage is decreased by 50 per cent to reduce the risk of hypoglycemia caused by decreasing concentrations of plasma cortisol yet still inhibit ketogenesis and ketoacidosis. After attaining a satisfactory response to mitotane, the insulin dosage is readjusted to produce more desirable blood glucose levels.

TABLE 15–11. POSSIBLE CLINICAL SIGNS CAUSED BY ADRENAL MEDULLARY PHEOCHROMOCYTOMAS

- Compression of surrounding structures
  - Enlarged caudal superficial abdominal veins
  - Edema of the caudal extremities
  - Weakness of the hind legs
- Secretion of excessive catecholamines
  - Excessive epinephrine secretion
    - Hypotension
    - Noncardiac pulmonary edema
    - Ventricular arrhythmias
  - Predominant excessive norepinephrine secretion
    - Tachycardia and tachyarrhythmias
    - Congestive heart failure
    - Excessive panting
    - Weakness and trembling
    - Epistaxis
    - Seizures
    - Retinal hemorrhage
    - Head pressing
    - Weight loss

Pheochromocytoma

Pheochromocytomas are usually slow-growing, red-brown tumors of the adrenal medulla or sympathetic paraganglia. Pheochromocytomas often occur concurrently with other endocrine neoplasia. The incidence of excess catecholamine-secreting pheochromocytomas in dogs is not known, because the clinical signs of excessive catecholamines are vague, and secretion may be intermittent. Routine screening of peripheral arterial blood pressure and measurements of urinary catecholamine metabolites, the bases for diagnosis of excessive catecholamine secretion by pheochromocytomas, are unfamiliar to most veterinarians. Pheochromocytomas can cause clinical signs by compression or invasion of surrounding structures, especially the caudal vena cava, or by secretion of excessive catecholamines. Clinical signs vary depending on whether an excess of epinephrine or of norepinephrine is predominant. The most common possible clinical signs and their causes are listed in Table 15–11 (Bouayad et al, 1987).

Other clinical signs can include a palpable abdominal mass, ascites, flushing of mucous membranes, fever, constipation, paresthesias, and various neurologic abnormalities caused by hypertension or cerebral hemorrhage. Clinical laboratory findings with pheochromocytomas secreting excessive amounts of catecholamines include hyperglycemia, polycythemia, and hypertriglyceridemia; urinalysis may show proteinuria and hematuria. Measurement of urinary excretion of catecholamines and their metabolites is the standard screening test for these pheochromocytomas.

The diagnosis in dogs can be based on routine abdominal radiography, pneumoperitoneum radiography, angiography, CT scan, or ultrasonography. Abdominal ultrasonography can detect pheochromocytomas larger than 2 cm, and CT scans can detect those larger than 0.5 to 1 cm. Both CT and ultrasonography can detect invasion or compression of the vena cava (Fig. 15–7). Blood pressure response tests to phentolamine, histamine, tyramine, or glucagon are risky and should be reserved for normotensive dogs with equivocal abdominal imaging results. Abdominal radiography may show an enlarged adrenal shadow or adrenal calcification in about one third of cases.

Excision is the only satisfactory treatment for pheochromocytomas. If tachycardia or tachyarrhythmias are present before surgery, the nonselective beta-blocker propranolol hydrochloride may be given in an oral dose of 0.15 to 0.5 mg/kg tid, but only after administration of an oral $alpha_1$- and $alpha_2$-blocker, phenoxybenzamine hydrochloride, has begun. Oral phenoxybenzamine given twice a day at 0.2 to 1.5 mg/kg should begin 10 to 14 days before surgery to stabilize blood pressure. Otherwise, vasoconstriction and severe hypertension may result from unopposed alpha-adrenergic effects. Prazosin (Minipress) has a shorter duration of activity, is a selective

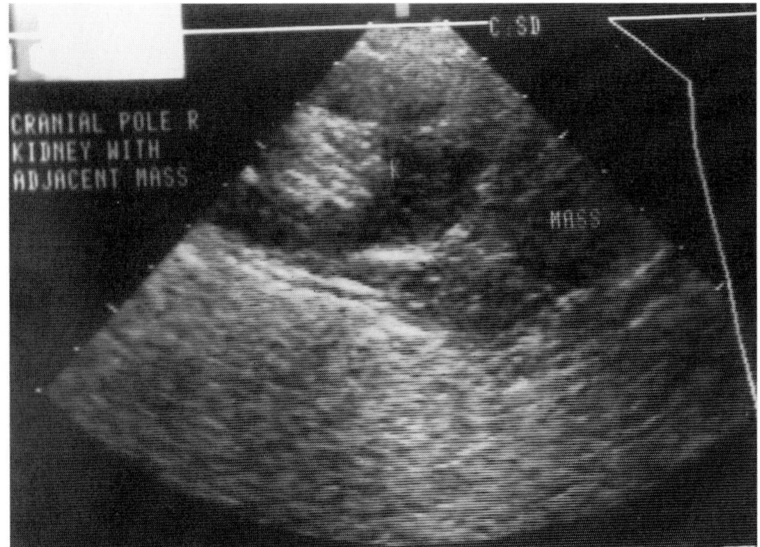

Figure 15–7. An abdominal sonogram showing an enlarged adrenal gland from a pheochromocytoma in a dog.

alpha$_1$-blocker, and may be preferable to phenoxybenzamine.

Preoperative administration of atropine or phenothiazines should be avoided to reduce the risk of tachycardia or sudden hypotension. Equipment for measuring the electrocardiogram and blood pressure should be connected to the dog before induction. Induction should be performed with narcotics or thiobarbiturate combined with glycopyrrolate. Anesthesia should be done with methoxyflurane or enflurane, and nitrous oxide. Phentolamine (Regitine), an alpha blocker for intravenous administration, can be used in a dose of 0.02 to 0.1 mg/kg during surgery to lower blood pressure while manipulating the tumor. Propranolol can be given intravenously in a dose of 0.3 to 1 mg/kg, or lidocaine without epinephrine can be administered intravenously as necessary during the surgery to control tachycardia or tachyarrhythmias. Immediately after the adrenalectomy, the rate of fluid administration should be increased. If blood pressure cannot be maintained, intravenous norepinephrine (Levophed) should be administered carefully. Adrenocortical steroids should not be replaced or supplemented unless both adrenals must be removed.

Hypercalcemia of Malignancy

Hypercalcemia of malignancy (HCM) is more common than primary hyperparathyroidism. Hypercalcemia in adult dogs is defined as equal to or greater than 12 mg/dl. HCM is the most common paraneoplastic disorder of the dog. In comparison with primary hyperparathyroidism, HCM is usually characterized by a more rapid onset of weight loss, lack of overt bone demineralization, and hypercalcemia of greater magnitude. Multicentric and thymic (cranial mediastinal) forms of lymphosarcoma are most commonly associated with hypercalcemia. About 10 per cent of dogs with multicentric lymphosarcoma and half of dogs with thymic forms develop hypercalcemia. More than 80 per cent of dogs with hypercalcemia from lymphosarcoma have a cranial mediastinal mass; most have bone marrow involvement. Breeds considered at a greater-than-expected risk for lymphosarcoma include the boxer, basset hound, St. Bernard, Scottish terrier, and various hunting breeds.

The term *pseudohyperparathyroidism* has been used to describe any hypercalcemia resulting from malignancy not caused by metastasis to bone. About 50 to 80 per cent of malignancies that cause hypercalcemia in people are associated with parathyroid hormone-related peptide (PTH-rP) (Rosol and Capen, 1988). PTH-rP has also been demonstrated in apocrine gland adenocarcinomas (AGACs) of the anal sac in dogs (Rosol et al, 1990). The degree of hypercalcemia caused by an AGAC is linearly related to the PTH-rP produced. Other malignancies that often cause HCM are multiple myeloma and a variety of carcinomas.

The second most common cause of hypercalcemia in dogs is AGACs of the anal sacs. More than 90 per cent of dogs affected with AGAC of the anal sacs are female dogs with an average age of 10 years. It is the most common malignant perineal tumor in older female dogs. German shepherd dogs may have a higher than expected incidence of AGACs of the anal sacs. About 80 per cent of the AGACs are unilateral, and despite the relative lack of anaplastic appearances, more than 90 per cent have metastasized to the iliac or sublumbar lymph nodes by the time of diagnosis. This tumor usually, but not invariably, causes hypercalcemia. It is often occult and is not discovered until a digital examination of the anus and rectum is done. About 60 per cent of affected dogs have a perineal mass or dyschezia (Ross et al, 1991).

Clinical Features. Many of the clinical signs of HCM are attributable to hypercalcemia and are identical to those seen in animals with primary hyperparathyroidism (Table 15–12). Clinical signs are often not evident until the serum calcium concentration exceeds 14 mg/dl. Additional clinical signs may be produced by the nonparathyroid tumor itself, including such signs as enlarged lymph nodes, perianal tumors, mammary tumors, cough from lung metastasis, and others. The osteomalacia seen in subjects with primary hyperparathyroidism is not evident radiographically in subjects with humorally mediated HCM. Signs of AGACs of the anal sacs include tenesmus, constipation, ribbon stools, perineal swelling, polyuria/polydipsia, pelvic limb edema, and cough. AGAC of the anal sacs metastasizes early. Most cases, but not all, have hypercalcemia and hypophosphatemia until renal failure occurs.

Laboratory Findings and Diagnosis. The clinical diagnosis of HCM is based on correction of elevated serum calcium levels after the removal, destruction, or suppression of the nonparathyroid neoplasm suspected to be producing hypercalcemia-promoting substances. A minimal data base, necessary to arrive at a tentative diagnosis of HCM, requires a thorough and accurate history. Physical examination should include palpation of the skeleton, all superficial lymph nodes, anal sacs, and deep abdominal structures and an ophthalmologic examination. Other causes of hypercalcemia include hypervitaminosis D, primary hypoadrenocorticism, end-stage renal failure, granulomatous diseases (i.e., blastomycosis), and primary or metastatic bone neoplasia. Elevated serum alkaline phosphatase levels occur more often, and to a greater magnitude, in animals with HCM than in dogs with primary hyperparathyroidism. Calcium nephropathy is present in most cases of HCM. Urinalysis usually shows isosthenuria or hyposthenuria, and calcium phosphate or oxalate crystals may be found. Mineralization of soft tissue outside the kidneys is rare in dogs with HCM.

Malignancies causing hypercalcemia are occult in nearly half the cases. Recommended laboratory data useful in detecting occult nonparathyroid malignancies and differentiating HCM from primary hyperparathyroidism include a hemogram, serum chemistry panel, urinalysis, thoracic and abdominal radiographs, bone marrow biopsy, and an aspirate biopsy of the lymph nodes. A low serum phosphorus level with hypercalcemia is suggestive of excessive parathyroid hormone (PTH) or PTH-rP production. Radiologic examination of the bones for subperiosteal resorption should include the dental arcade and the metacarpals and phalanges. Radiographs of the thorax and abdomen are also recommended to search for nonparathyroid malignancies or skeletal demineralization typical of primary hyperparathyroidism. Thyroid or bone radioisotope scans may be useful in selected cases. AGACs of the anal sacs metastasize in more than 50 per cent of cases; this is usually recognized by enlargement of the iliac lymph nodes (Ross et al, 1991).

Management. Ideally, the nonparathyroid tumor responsible for HCM should be excised or totally destroyed by radiation or immunotherapy. Within 2 days of excision, the hypercalcemia should be resolved. Hypercalcemic crisis resulting from serum calcium levels in excess of 14 mg/dl occurs more often with HCM than with primary hyperparathyroidism. Clinical signs of hypercalcemic crisis can include constipation, muscle tremors, and mental depression. Serum calcium levels that exceed 18 mg/dl can result in renal failure and shock, rapidly leading to death. It is advisable to attempt to reduce serum calcium levels with an intravenous solution of sterile isotonic saline solution with added potassium chloride (10 mmol/L) and furosemide (1 mg/kg) every 2 hours. In addition to the dilutional effects of an intravenous saline solution, sodium loading with saline solution and treatment with furosem-

TABLE 15–12. POSSIBLE CLINICAL SIGNS OF HYPERCALCEMIA OF MALIGNANCY

Polyuria and polydipsia
Vomiting
Constipation
Weight loss
Anemia
Weakness and depression

ide inhibit calcium's reabsorption in the renal tubules. Thiazide diuretics can aggravate hypercalcemia and should be avoided.

Other means of reducing hypercalcemia can be considered after conservative attempts with intravenous administration of saline solution, furosemide, and glucocorticoids have failed. Etidronate disodium (Didronel IV), a diphosphonate that inhibits osteoclastic activity, should be tried if conservative therapy has been unsuccessful. The dosage is 7.5 mg/kg diluted in at least 250 ml of saline solution and given intravenously over a minimum of 2 hours each day for 3 consecutive days. Other treatments for refractory hypercalcemia include calcitonin and gallium nitrate. Calcitonin (Calcimar) 4 U/kg intravenously or subcutaneously is effective, but it has a short duration and is expensive. Gallium nitrate (Ganite) inhibits bone resorption but is nephrotoxic to the tubules.

There is no known successful medical treatment for AGAC of the anal sacs; excision is recommended. AGACs of the anal sacs should not be confused with the more common perianal gland adenomas in older male dogs. One half of excised AGACs of the anal sacs recur. Mean survival after excision is 1 year (Ross et al, 1991).

DISORDERS OF CATS

Hyperthyroidism

Hyperthyroidism in cats is usually caused by a solitary adenoma or multinodular adenomatous hyperplasia. Thyroid carcinomas (mixed compact and follicular carcinomas and, occasionally, follicular and papillary carcinomas) are rare in cats, making up only 2 per cent of all hyperthyroid cases (Turrel et al, 1988). Hyperthyroidism is the most commonly diagnosed endocrinopathy in the cat (Peterson, 1984). Older cats (6 to 20 years old) are most often affected.

Clinical Features. Clinical signs are caused by an increased metabolic rate and increased sensitivity to catecholamines. Most thyroid tumors (90 per cent) are palpable. The most frequently recognized clinical sign is weight loss despite a good appetite. Other common signs are listed in Table 15–13. Less common clinical signs include anorexia, apathy, mild fever, polypnea and dyspnea, irritability when handled, muscle weakness and tremors, congestive heart failure, unkempt haircoat, hair loss, and increased nail growth (Fig. 15–8). In about 10 per cent of affected cats, severe depression, anorexia, and weakness occur.

TABLE 15–13. COMMON CLINICAL SIGNS OF HYPERTHYROIDISM IN CATS, IN DECREASING ORDER OF OCCURRENCE

Weight loss
Polyphagia
Hyperactivity
Tachycardia
Polyuria and polydipsia
Vomiting
Cardiac murmur
Diarrhea and increased fecal volume

This "apathetic hyperthyroidism" is usually associated with cardiac arrhythmias or congestive heart failure (Meric, 1989). Cardiac complications can be life threatening. More than 80 per cent of thyrotoxic cats have cardiomegaly, and 10 to 15 per cent have congestive heart failure (Jacobs et al, 1986). Some have pulmonary edema and pleural effusion, and two thirds have sinus tachycardia (heart rates exceeding 240 beats/min) and tachyarrhythmias. One third have increased QRS voltages in lead II exceeding 0.9 mV. Many have second-degree atrioventricular blocks and left anterior fascicular blocks. Echocardiograms usually reveal hypertrophy of the left ventricular caudal wall, enlarged left atrial diameter, and hypertrophy of the interventricular septum (Bond et al, 1988). Hypertension occurs in 87 per cent of cats with hyperthyroidism (Kobayashi et al, 1990). However, hypertensive vascular accidents are not common.

Hypertrophic cardiomyopathy will resolve after therapy. The left ventricular caudal wall and the interventricular septal wall thicknesses decrease after therapy if they were hypertrophic as

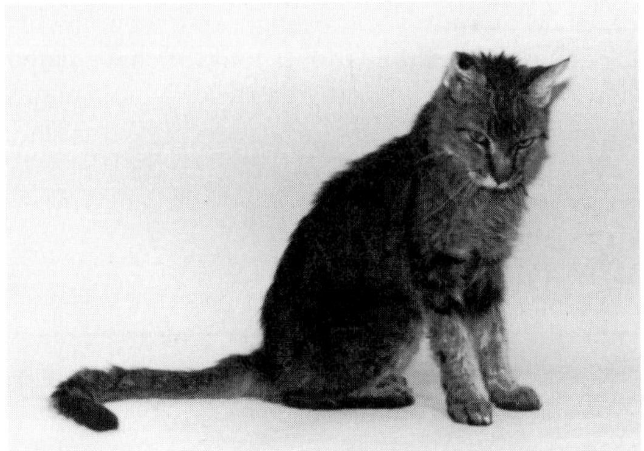

Figure 15–8. A hyperthyroid cat presented for weight loss despite a good appetite.

a result of hyperthyroidism (Bond et al, 1988). If the cardiomyopathy is congestive, it is not reversible. Changes in the electrocardiogram revert to normal in at least 80 per cent of cats whose serum thyroxine (T_4) and triiodothyronine (T_3) levels are successfully lowered. No other form of hypertrophic cardiomyopathy can be so effectively corrected. All cases of feline cardiomyopathy should be screened by measuring serum T_4 and T_3 levels to rule out or substantiate hyperthyroidism as a cause (Meric, 1989).

Laboratory Findings and Diagnosis. Laboratory findings associated with feline hyperthyroidism include a stress leukogram, mild to moderate erythrocytosis, macrocytosis, increased serum inorganic phosphorus, increased fecal fat, hyperbilirubinemia, and elevated serum hepatic enzymes. Hypercalcemia may occur if a carcinoma is present (Turrel et al, 1988). Increased serum enzymes of hepatic origin occur in more than one half of affected cats. These serum enzymes include alkaline phosphatase, lactic dehydrogenase, aspartate transaminase, and alanine transaminase. All older cats demonstrating weight loss and elevated levels of serum liver enzymes should be screened for hyperthyroidism by measurement of serum T_4 levels. The definitive diagnosis of feline hyperthyroidism is usually based on elevated serum T_4 levels (i.e., greater than 4 μg/dl) (Broome et al, 1988; Meric, 1989). Cats with early or mild hyperthyroidism combined with a severe nonthyroidal illness may have baseline serum T_4 levels in the high normal range (Peterson et al, 1990). In such cases, the serum T_4 level should be rechecked in 1 to 2 weeks. If both T_4 measurements are normal but hyperthyroidism is suspected, a T_3 suppression test or a thyrotropin-releasing (TRH) hormone stimulation test should be performed.

A T_3 suppression test is done by giving 25 μg of T_3 (Cytomel) orally tid until seven doses are administered. Two to 4 hours after the last dose of T_3, serum T_4 and T_3 samples should be taken. Cats with hyperthyroidism have an unsuppressed serum T_4 of greater than 1.5 μg/dl and less than 50 per cent drop from baseline T_4 levels. The serum T_3 level should be normal to elevated to verify that the last T_3 dose was administered and absorbed (Peterson et al, 1990). TRH stimulation test can be performed by administering 0.1 mg/kg of TRH (Thypinone) intravenously. Normal cats double their baseline serum T_4 level by 4 hours after the injection, whereas hyperthyroid cats show no significant change after TRH stimulation. Hypersalivation and vomiting are common adverse effects. Thyroid scans (1 mCi sodium pertechnetate given intravenously) can detect aberrant "hot" thyroid nodules or metastasis (Fig. 15–9). An image of a nodule that is darker than the salivary glands is diagnostic of hyperthyroidism. Scans also indicate whether involvement is unilateral or bilateral. Scans of carcinomas often reveal multiple nodular lesions in the neck, thoracic inlet, and cranial mediastinum (Turrel et al, 1988). When unilateral hyperthyroid neoplasia exists, the contralateral lobe should not be evident on a thyroid scan. If serum T_4 or T_3 levels are persistently high, any thyroid tissue visible on thyroid scans should be excised if surgery is planned. Recent treatment with methimazole (Tapazole) increases the uptake of pertechnetate or ^{131}I in otherwise normal atrophied

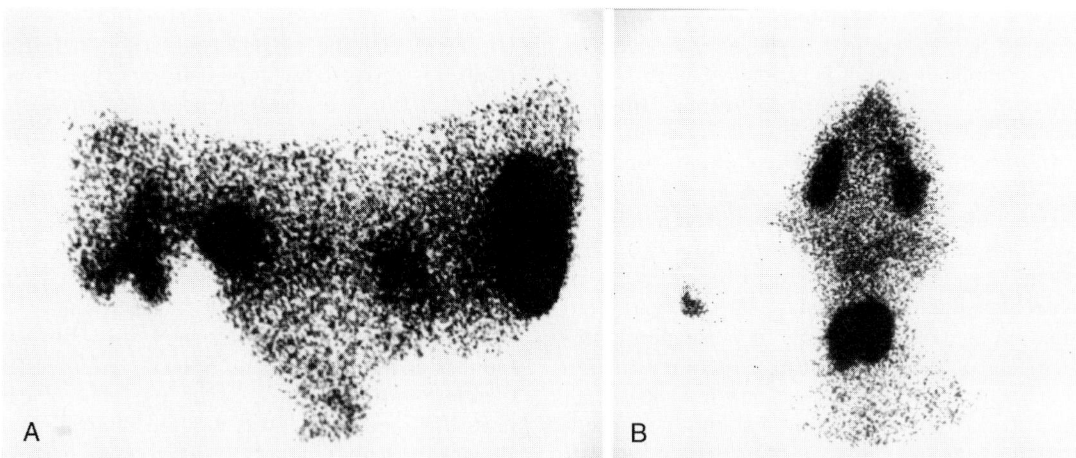

Figure 15–9. *A*, A lateral view of a thyroid scan using pertechnetate in a cat with bilateral multinodular adenomatous hyperplasia. *B*, A ventrodorsal view of a thyroid scan using pertechnetate in a cat with bilateral multinodular adenomatous hyperplasia.

thyroid lobes (Broome et al, 1988) and therefore should not be used before thyroid scans or radioiodine therapy.

Management. Treatment of hyperthyroidism can be accomplished with antithyroid drugs, radioactive iodine, and surgery. If surgery is planned, the hypermetabolism and hypersensitivity to catecholamines should first be medically controlled. Methimazole is preferred to suppress glandular hypersecretion, because it has a higher bioavailability and a longer duration of effect than propylthiouracil in cats (Trepanier and Peterson, 1991). Treatment with methimazole is begun with a dose of 5 mg every 8 hours and continued for 2 weeks before the thyroidectomy. Because methimazole primarily blocks organification in the thyroid, stored hormone continues to be released and must be allowed to dissipate before surgery. Serum T_4 levels begin to drop within 24 to 48 hours of treatment, but serum T_4 levels of less than 4 μg/dl should be confirmed before surgery is done. If there is little decline in serum T_4 levels after 2 weeks of treatment, methimazole can be increased to a dose of 20 to 30 mg/day.

Because of the risks of the surgical procedure and the poor risk inherent in doing surgery on debilitated aged cats, thyroidectomies should be done by an experienced surgeon. Presurgical thyroid scans are recommended, because bilateral involvement may not be grossly evident based on intraoperative appearance (Meric, 1989). If an external parathyroid is evident, a modified extracapsular technique has been recommended over intracapsular (subcapsular) thyroidectomy (Welches et al, 1989). The subcapsular method is best to preserve the parathyroid gland, but postsurgical relapse of hyperthyroidism is a greater risk (Flanders et al, 1987). Staged bilateral thyroidectomy has the fewest postoperative complications but is expensive and requires two periods of anesthesia. Overall, surgery-related mortality rates are 5 to 10 per cent.

In one study using three techniques for bilateral thyroidectomy in cats, there was about a 25 per cent incidence of hypocalcemia within 3 days (Welches et al, 1989). After the surgery, serum calcium levels should be monitored for signs of hypocalcemia for at least 3 days. Parathyroid function may be temporarily or permanently impaired by postsurgical trauma. Treatment for hypocalcemia is usually unnecessary in at least half the cases. However, treatment should be considered if serum calcium levels have fallen below 7 mg/dl. Severe hypocalcemia should be treated with an intravenous dose of calcium gluconate, 1 to 3 ml of 10 per cent, followed by 6 to 8 ml in 100 ml of saline solution bid. In addition, dihydrotachysterol 0.03 mg/kg/day is given for 3 days, followed by a dosage of 0.01 to 0.02 mg/kg/day (Meric, 1989). Persistent hypocalcemia may be controlled with an oral dose of dihydrotachysterol 0.02 mg/kg/day and calcium gluconate 750 mg/kg/day. Most patients can be weaned off, as accessory parathyroid tissue occurs in at least 64 per cent of cats. Also, serum calcium can normalize through a PTH-independent mechanism (Flanders et al, 1991).

After a unilateral thyroidectomy, serum T_4 levels should be monitored. Because the remaining thyroid gland will have been suppressed, serum T_4 levels will be low and may remain so for 2 to 3 months, but replacement therapy with thyroid hormone should not be administered unless marked lethargy occurs or low serum T_4 levels persist for more than 3 months. If a bilateral thyroidectomy is done, a dose of 0.05 to 0.1 mg of sodium levothyroxine should be given daily. When the cat has recovered from the thyroidectomy, the replacement dosage of thyroxine can be gradually reduced to allow any remaining normal ectopic thyroid tissue to hypertrophy and possibly eliminate the need for replacement of thyroid hormone. Other possible postsurgical problems include Horner's syndrome or laryngeal paralysis. The recurrence rate within 3 years after thyroidectomy may be 5 to 10 per cent (Meric, 1989; Swalec and Birchard, 1990).

Therapy with radioactive iodine ^{131}I can be safer than a thyroidectomy in many cats. Anesthetics are not necessary, and no hypoparathyroidism results. Therapy with ^{131}I is also a valuable salvage procedure when subtotal thyroidectomy is not curative. The disadvantages of ^{131}I therapy are the need for 3 to 5 weeks of isolation, difficulty in accurately titrating the dose so that the hyperthyroidism is corrected without causing hypothyroidism, and the need for specialists to administer the treatment and monitor the post-treatment isolation. An intravenous dose of 4 to 5 mCi of ^{131}I is administered to deliver approximately 20,000 rads to the "hot" nodules (Meric and Rubin, 1990). Improvement should be noticeable within 1 to 2 weeks. More than half of cats so treated have normal serum T_4 levels in 4 days; 74 per cent have normal levels in 8 days. Retreatment is advisable if serum T_4 levels are elevated 6 months after therapy. Seven per cent of cats have low serum T_4 levels without clinical signs. Recent treatment with antithyroid drugs may decrease the response to ^{131}I (Meric et al, 1986). Antithyroid drug therapy should be discontinued at least 4 weeks before ^{131}I treatment (Meric, 1989). About 8 per cent of cats may relapse after fixed-dose therapy with ^{131}I. Most relapses occur within 9 months of the initial treatment. Serum T_4 levels should be re-evaluated 6 months and 12 months after treatment for hyperthyroidism in cats. Carcinomas are treated with 3 to 10 times the usual dose of ^{131}I (20 to 30 mCi). Or instead, cobalt 60 may be used at 48 Gy in 12 fractions of four each, three times per week (Turrel et al, 1988).

If a thyroidectomy or therapy with radioactive iodine is not possible or is undesirable, indefinite therapy using methimazole may be tried as a last resort. The maintenance dose for methimazole is 2.5 to 20 mg/day. Adverse effects (anorexia, vomiting, lethargy, self-induced excoriation of face and neck, bleeding, and icterus) occur in 10 to 20 per cent of treated cats in the first month. Ten to 20 per cent have eosinophilia, lymphocytosis, and a slight leukopenia. Three to 4 per cent have agranulocytosis and thrombocytopenia. One in five are antinuclear antibody (ANA) positive (one half after 6 months of treatment), but no lupus syndrome occurs. Ten to 15 mg/day should be given initially and the serum T_4 and hemogram routinely monitored every 3 to 6 months. Hyperthyroid levels return in 2 days after cessation. Methimazole's effects last longer than the duration in the plasma because it is concentrated in the thyroid (Peterson et al, 1988).

Diabetes Mellitus

As in dogs, the most common cause of diabetes mellitus in cats is unknown. However, the incidence of islet cell amyloidosis is higher in diabetic cats than in nondiabetic cats. An insulin-related protein, possibly from proinsulin or preproinsulin, is involved in the formation of feline islet amyloid (O'Brien et al, 1985). Selective islet cell amyloidosis may contribute to the loss of ability to secrete insulin in normal amounts (O'Brien et al, 1986). Megestrol acetate or other progestogens can precipitate diabetes mellitus in predisposed cats. Three fourths of diabetic cats are older than 7 years of age.

Clinical Features. The clinical signs of diabetes in cats are similar to those in dogs. However, cats do not develop clinically significant diabetic cataracts. Diabetic cats are more likely than dogs to develop a peripheral polyneuropathy, which is characterized by a plantigrade stance, depressed patella reflexes, apparent paraesthesias, and weakness.

Laboratory Findings and Diagnosis. Persistent fasting hyperglycemia (greater than 140 mg/dl) is the hallmark of diabetes mellitus. The renal threshold for glucose in cats (about 290 mg/dl) is much higher than in dogs (about 180 mg/dl).

Management. The management of diabetes is similar for both cats and dogs, except that 20 to 50 per cent of diabetic cats have noninsulin-dependent diabetes mellitus and do not require insulin. These cats do not have ketonuria or anorexia and the degree of hyperglycemia is mild. They may be maintained with avoidance of stress and hypoglycemic drugs. High-fiber diets are possibly beneficial in overweight diabetic cats. Prescription Diet Feline (Hills Pet Products) w/d or r/d and Science Diet Feline Maintenance Light (Hills Pet Products) are high-fiber, low-caloric-density diets for cats. Soft, moist foods are not recommended, because they contain corn syrup and propylene glycol, which will rapidly increase the blood glucose level. Obesity should be corrected and then prevented from recurring. Older diabetic cats usually require 60 to 70 kcal per kilogram of ideal body weight (Nelson, 1988). However, high-fiber diets should not be used if the cat is cachectic.

If high-fiber diets and calorie control alone are not effective in normalizing blood glucose levels within 1 week, hypoglycemic drugs should be tried. Glipizide (Glucotrol) has been reported to be effective in selected cases, particularly if the serum insulin level is greater than 20 μU/ml during an intravenous glucose tolerance test. The recommended dosage of glipizide is 5 mg two to three times per day with food. Possible adverse effects are vomiting, hypoglycemia, blood dyscrasias, or hepatopathy. Response to glipizide therapy should be evaluated for 1 month. If, during the trial course of therapy, clinical signs become worse, ketoacidosis occurs, the blood glucose level exceeds 300 mg/dl, or the owners are dissatisfied, glipizide therapy should be discontinued.

Insulin therapy is necessary if ketonuria, anorexia, or a failed response to diet and hypoglycemic drugs has occurred. Maintenance insulin therapy usually requires twice-daily subcutaneous injections of intermediate- or long-acting insulin (Wallace et al, 1990). At least one fourth of poorly regulated diabetic cats do not absorb long-acting insulin well enough to control their diabetes; intermediate-acting insulins are more reliable. A 1:9 dilution of 100 U/ml insulin with the proper insulin diluent to make 10 U/ml is recommended to facilitate accurate measurement and reliable subcutaneous absorption. It is best to use 0.5-ml syringes with 27-gauge needles. The use of morning urine glucose samples for regulation of diabetes is not helpful in detecting over- or underdosage of insulin (McMillan and Feldman, 1986).

Hypokalemia

Low serum potassium levels (3.6 mmol/L or less) may occur with increased, normal, or subnormal total body potassium concentration. About 98 per cent of the body's exchangeable potassium (approximately 150 mmol/L) is intracellular. Hypokalemia is due primarily to either potassium loss or to redistribution (intracellular shift), although anorexia can aggravate hypokalemia by preventing the intake necessary to compensate for potassium losses. Shifts to the inside of cells are due to acute metabolic alkalosis, insulin, anabolic steroids, or stimulation of adrenergic receptors (Table 15–14). Acute alkalosis may be caused by overtreatment with bicarbonate or overventilation during anesthesia (Chew et al, 1991). Specific causes of potassium loss are vomiting, diarrhea, or urinary losses. Urinary losses occur from diuretic therapy with potassium-wasting drugs, diuresis with potassium-deficient fluid therapy, mineralocorticoid excess, and renal tubular acidosis (Eger et al, 1983). Chronic acidosis, such as occurs with chronic renal failure, or the oral administration of acidifiers can cause potassium depletion (Dow et al, 1989).

Clinical Features. Severe depletion of potassium can cause muscular weakness, stiff gait, apparent muscle pain, ileus, arrhythmias, and primary polyuria. Weakness is often of acute onset and associated with apparent pain. Persistent ventroflexion of the neck is a characteristic finding in cats. Hypermetria and a wide-based stance are also common.

TABLE 15–14. CAUSES OF HYPOKALEMIA

Poor dietary intake
Anorexia
Inability to eat
Excessive use of potassium-free fluid therapy
Increased fluid loss
Gastrointestinal: vomiting, diarrhea
Renal: diuretics, renal tubular acidosis, chronic renal failure, administration of urinary acidifiers, hyperaldosteronism
Intracellular fluid shift
Insulin therapy
Anabolic steroid administration
Mineralocorticoid administration

Laboratory Findings and Diagnosis. Serum potassium concentrations of less than 3.6 mmol/L are diagnostic for hypokalemia. Serum potassium levels of less than 3.0 mmol/L indicate severe hypokalemia. The serum bicarbonate level is often elevated. Serum creatine kinase activity can be elevated with severe hypokalemia because of resulting rhabdomyolysis. Pseudohypokalemia can be caused by extreme serum elevations of glucose, proteins, lipids, or urea nitrogen. The history should be evaluated for recent vomiting, diarrhea, use of potassium-wasting diuretics, and insulin or anabolic steroid therapy. Metabolic alkalosis with hypokalemia is usually due to vomiting of gastric acid or administration of diuretics. Fractional excretion of potassium can be determined as follows:

$$\text{Urine K/Serum K} \times \text{Serum Cr/Urine Cr} \times 100.$$

Low fractional excretion suggests nonrenal potassium losses. Fractional excretion of potassium in excess of 4 per cent suggests an inappropriate renal loss. Chronic hypokalemia can cause tubular nephropathy and impair the urine-concentrating ability of the kidneys.

Management. Long-term successful management of hypokalemia is dependent on finding and correcting the cause. It is impractical to measure total body potassium for clinical purposes. Repeated measurement of serum potassium concentration during therapy, with appropriate adjustments of fluid rates, is the only means of safely administering potassium. Immediate therapy is necessary for severe and acute hypokalemia. Oral potassium should be given whenever possible. An estimated beginning oral dose of potassium gluconate (Tumil-K) is 1 mmol/kg bid. The dosage should be adjusted based on serum potassium concentrations. Potassium can be given subcutaneously if diluted in isotonic fluids such as lactated Ringer's solution (up to 30 mmol potassium chloride per liter of lactated Ringer's solution). Potassium given intravenously should never exceed the rate of 0.5 mmol/kg/hour. An estimated daily potassium requirement for moderate to severe hypokalemia is 4 to 8 mmol/kg. Chloride (as in physiologic saline or potassium chloride) is necessary if metabolic alkalosis is present with hypokalemia. Dextrose infusions should be avoided, as they stimulate insulin release and an intracellular shift of potassium. Intravenous solutions of more than 40 mmol per liter may cause phlebitis. Dopamine (Intropin) (0.5 μg/kg/min) may be used in some instances to shift intracellular potassium extracellularly.

References and Supplemental Reading

Alejandro R, Feldman EC, Shienvold FL, et al. Advances in canine diabetes mellitus research: Etiopathology and results of islet transplantation. J Am Vet Med Assoc 193:1050, 1988.

Berger B, Feldman EC. Primary hyperparathyroidism in dogs: 21 cases (1976–1986). J Am Vet Med Assoc 191:350, 1987.

Blaxter AC, Cripps PJ, Gruffydd-Jones TJ. Dietary fiber and postprandial hyperglycaemia in normal and diabetic dogs. J Small Anim Pract 31:229, 1990.

Bond BR, Fox PR, Peterson ME, et al. Echocardiographic findings in 103 cats with hyperthyroidism. J Am Vet Med Assoc 192:1546, 1988.

Bouayad H, Feeney DA, Caywood DD, et al. Pheochromocytoma in dogs: 13 cases (1980–1985). J Am Vet Med Assoc 191:1610, 1987.

Braund KG, Steiss JE, Amling KA, et al. Insulinoma and subclinical peripheral neuropathy in two dogs. J Vet Intern Med 1:86, 1987.

Broome MR, Feldman EC, Turrel JM. Serial determination of thyroxine concentrations in hyperthyroid cats. J Am Vet Med Assoc 192:49, 1988.

Caywood DD, Klausner JS, O'Leary TP, et al. Pancreatic insulin-secreting neoplasms: Clinical, diagnostic, and prognostic features in 73 dogs. J Am Anim Hosp Assoc 24:577, 1988.

Chew DJ, Leonard M, Muir WW. Effect of sodium bicarbonate infusion on serum osmolality, electrolyte concentrations, and blood gas tensions in cats. Am J Vet Res 52:12, 1991.

Dow SW, Fettman MJ, Curtis CR, et al. Hypokalemia in cats: 186 cases (1984–1987). J Am Vet Med Assoc 194:1604, 1989.

Dow SW, LeCouteur RA, Rosychuk RAW, et al. Response of dogs with functional pituitary macroadenomas and macrocarcinomas to radiation. J Small Anim Pract 31:287, 1990.

Eger CE, Robinson WF, Huxtable CRR. Primary hyperaldosteronism (Conn's syndrome) in a cat; a case report and review of comparative aspects. J Small Anim Pract 24:293, 1983.

Emms SG, Johnston DE, Eigenmann JE, et al. Adrenalectomy in the management of canine hyperadrenocorticism. J Am Anim Hosp Assoc 23:557, 1987.

Feldman EC, Bruyette DS, Nelson RW, et al. Plasma cortisol response to ketoconazole administration in dogs with hyperadrenocorticism. J Am Vet Med Assoc 197:71, 1990.

Flanders JA, Harvey HJ, Erb HN. Feline thyroidectomy: A comparison of postoperative hypocalcemia associated with three different surgical techniques. Vet Surg 16:362, 1987.

Flanders JA, Neth S, Erb HN, et al. Functional analysis of ectopic parathyroid activity in cats. Am J Vet Res 52:1336, 1991.

Goeders LA, Esposito LA, Peterson ME. Absorption kinetics of regular and isophane (NPH) insulin in the normal dog. Domest Anim Endocrinol 4:43, 1987.

Hegstad RL, Johnston SD, Pasternak DM. Effects of sample handling on adrenocorticotropin concentration measured in canine plasma, using a commercially available radioimmunoassay kit. Am J Vet Res 51:1941, 1990.

Ihle SL, Nelson RW. Insulin resistance and diabetes mellitus. Compend Contin Educ Pract Vet 13:197, 1991.

Jacobs GJ, Hutson C, Dougherty J, et al. Congestive heart failure associated with hyperthyroidism in cats. J Am Vet Med Assoc 188:52, 1986.

Jeffers JG, Shanley KJ, Schick RO. Diabetes mellitus induced in a dog after administration of corticosteroids and methylprednisolone pulse therapy. J Am Vet Med Assoc 199:77, 1991.

Jones CA, Refsal KR, Lippert AC, et al. Changes in adrenal cortisol secretion as reflected in the urinary cortisol/creatinine ratio in dogs. Domest Anim Endocrinol 7:559, 1990.

Joseph RJ, Allyson K, Graves TK, et al. Evaluation of two reagent strips and three reflectance meters for rapid determination of blood glucose concentrations. J Vet Intern Med 1:170, 1987.

King RR, Mauderly JL, Hahn FF, et al. Pulmonary function studies in a dog with pulmonary thromboembolism associated with Cushing's disease. J Am Anim Hosp Assoc 21:555, 1985.

Kintzer PP, Peterson ME. Mitotane (o,p'-DDD) treatment of 200 dogs with pituitary-dependent hyperadrenocorticism. J Vet Intern Med 5:182, 1991.

Klausner JS, O'Leary TP, Osborne CA. Calcium urolithiasis in two dogs with parathyroid adenomas. J Am Vet Med Assoc 191:1423, 1987.

Kobayashi DL, Peterson ME, Graves TK, et al. Hypertension in cats with chronic renal failure or hyperthyroidism. J Vet Intern Med 4:58, 1990.

Leifer CE, Peterson ME, Matus RE. Insulin-secreting tumor: Diagnosis and medical and surgical management in 55 dogs. J Am Vet Med Assoc 188:60, 1986.

Mack RE, Feldman EC. Comparison of two low-dose dexamethasone suppression protocols as screening and discrimination tests in dogs with hyperadrenocorticism. J Am Vet Med Assoc 197:1603, 1990.

Mallette LE, Tuma SN. A new radioimmunoassay for the midregion of canine parathyroid hormone. Miner Electrolyte Metab 10:43, 1984.

McMillan FD, Feldman EC. Rebound hyperglycemia following overdosing of insulin in cats with diabetes mellitus. J Am Vet Med Assoc 188:1426, 1986.

Mehlhaff CJ, Peterson ME, Patnaik AK, et al. Insulin-producing islet cell neoplasms: Surgical considerations and general management in 35 dogs. J Am Anim Hosp Assoc 21:607, 1985.

Meric SM. Diagnosis and management of feline hyperthyroidism. Compend Contin Educ Pract Vet 11:1053, 1989.

Meric SM, Hawkins EC, Washabau RJ, et al. Serum thyroxine concentrations after radioactive iodine therapy with hyperthyroidism. J Am Vet Med Assoc 188:1038, 1986.

Meric SM, Rubin SI. Serum thyroxine concentrations following fixed-dose radioactive iodine treatment in hyperthyroid cats: 62 cases (1986–1989). J Am Vet Med Assoc 197:621, 1990.

Nelson RW. Medical management of canine hyperinsulinism. J Am Vet Med Assoc 187:78, 1985.

Nelson RW. Dietary therapy for diabetes mellitus. Compend Contin Educ Pract Vet 10:1387, 1988.

Nelson RW, Brown SA, Jones RJ, et al. Absorption kinetics of regular insulin in dogs with alloxan-induced diabetes mellitus. Am J Vet Res 51:1671, 1990.

Nelson RW, Ihle SL, Feldman EC. Pituitary macroadenomas and macroadenocarcinomas in dogs treated with mitotane for pituitary-dependent hyperadrenocorticism: 13 cases (1981–1986). J Am Vet Med Assoc 194:1612, 1989.

Nelson RW, Lewis LD. Nutritional management of diabetes mellitus. Semin Vet Med Surg 5:178, 1990.

O'Brien TD, Hayden DW, Johnson KH, et al. High dose intravenous glucose tolerance test and serum insulin and glucagon levels in diabetic and non-diabetic cats: Relationships to insular amyloidosis. Vet Pathol 22:250, 1985.

O'Brien TD, Hayden DW, Johnson KH, et al. Immunohistochemical morphometry of pancreatic endocrine cells in diabetic, normoglycaemic glucose-intolerant and normal cats. J Comp Pathol 96:357, 1986.

Peterson ME. Feline hyperthyroidism. Vet Clin North Am (Small Anim Pract) 14:809, 1984.

Peterson ME, Graves TK, Gamble DA. Triiodothyronine (T3) suppression test: An aid in the diagnosis of mild hyperthyroidism in cats. J Vet Intern Med 4:233, 1990.

Peterson ME, Kintzer PP, Hurvitz AI. Methimazole treatment of 262 cats with hyperthyroidism. J Vet Intern Med 2:150, 1988.

Peterson ME, Winkler B, Kintzer PP, et al. Effect of spontaneous hyperadrenocorticism on endogenous production and utilization of glucose in the dog. Domest Anim Endocrinol 3:117, 1986.

Quadri SK, Palazzolo DL. How aging affects the canine endocrine system. Vet Med 86:692, 1991.

Reimers TJ, Lamb SV, Bartlett SA, et al. Effects of hemolysis and storage on quantification of hormones in blood samples from dogs, cattle, and horses. Am J Vet Res 52:1075, 1991.

Reusch CE, Feldman EC. Canine hyperadrenocorticism due to adrenocortical neoplasia: pretreatment evaluation of 41 dogs. J Vet Intern Med 5:3, 1991.

Rijnberk A, Belshaw BE. Advances in the diagnosis and treatment of canine hyperadrenocorticism. Vet Ann 28:146, 1988.

Rijnberk A, van Wees A, Mol JA. Assessment of two tests for the diagnosis of canine hyperadrenocorticism. Vet Rec 122:178, 1988.

Rogers KS, Luttgen PJ. Hyperinsulinism. Compend Contin Educ Pract Vet 7:829, 1985.

Rosol TJ, Capen CC. Pathogenesis of humoral hypercalcemia of malignancy. Domest Anim Endocrinol 5:1, 1988.

Rosol TJ, Capen CC, Danks JA, et al. Identification of parathyroid hormone-related protein in canine apocrine adenocarcinoma of the anal sac. Vet Pathol 27:89, 1990.

Ross JT, Scavelli TD, Matthiesen DT, et al. Adenocarcinoma of the apocrine glands of the anal sac in dogs: A review of 32 cases. J Am Anim Hosp Assoc 27:349, 1991.

Scavelli TD, Peterson ME, Matthiesen DT. Results of surgical treatment for hyperadrenocorticism caused by adrenocortical neoplasia in the dog: 25 cases (1980–1984). J Am Vet Med Assoc 189:1360, 1986.

Swalec KM, Birchard SJ. Recurrence of hyperthyroidism after thyroidectomy in cats. J Am Anim Hosp Assoc 26:433, 1990.

Torrance AG, Nachreiner R. Human-parathormone assay for use in dogs: Validation, sample handling studies, and parathyroid function testing. Am J Vet Res 50:1123, 1989a.

Torrance AG, Nachreiner R. Intact parathyroid hormone assay and total calcium concentration in the diagnosis of disorders of calcium metabolism in dogs. J Vet Intern Med 3:86, 1989b.

Trepanier LA, Peterson ME. Pharmacokinetics of methimazole in normal cats and cats with hyperthyroidism. Res Vet Sci 50:69, 1991.

Turrel JM, Feldman EC, Nelson RW, et al. Thyroid carcinoma causing hyperthyroidism in cats: 14 cases (1981–1986). J Am Vet Med Assoc 193:359, 1988.

Turrel JM, Fike JR, LeCouteur RA, et al. Computed tomographic characteristics of primary brain tumors in 50 dogs. J Am Vet Med Assoc 188:851, 1986.

Voorhout G. X-ray-computed tomography, nephrotomography, and ultrasonography of the adrenal glands of healthy dogs. Am J Vet Res 51:625, 1990.

Wallace MS, Peterson ME, Nichols CE. Absorption kinetics of regular, isophane, and protamine zinc insulin in normal cats. Domest Anim Endocrinol 7:509, 1990.

Welches CD, Scavelli TD, Matthiesen DT, et al. Occurrence of problems after three techniques of bilateral thyroidectomy in cats. Vet Surg 18:392, 1989.

Willard MD, Zerbe CA, Schall WD, et al. Severe hypophosphatemia associated with diabetes mellitus in six dogs and one cat. J Am Vet Med Assoc 190:1007, 1987.

Zerbe CA, Boosinger TR, Grabau JH, et al. Pancreatic polypeptide and insulin-secreting tumor in a dog with duodenal ulcers and hypertrophic gastritis. J Vet Intern Med 3:178, 1989.

Zerbe CA, Refsal KR, Schall WD, et al. Adrenal function in 15 dogs with insulin-dependent diabetes mellitus. J Am Vet Med Assoc 193:454, 1988.

CHAPTER 16

The Urinary System

DONALD R. KRAWIEC, CARL A. OSBORNE, JODY P. LULICH, and HOWARD B. GELBERG

Because older dogs and cats are generally not as active as younger dogs, owners are more likely to interpret inactivity as an inevitable consequence of the aging process. As a result, if dogs and cats have disease processes that result primarily in inactivity, owners are less likely to seek veterinary attention when this problem is noticed. Likewise, it may be difficult for veterinarians to determine whether nonspecific problems in geriatric dogs and cats should be further evaluated. It is uncommon not to find abnormalities on evaluation of a serum chemistry profile of a geriatric dog or cat. Determining which abnormality is actually affecting the animal's health and well-being and, therefore, should undergo further evaluation, requires judgment in the absence of certainty. This is a major concern because of the fragile nature of geriatric dogs and cats and their inability to handle stressful situations. Hospitalizing a geriatric animal or performing diagnostic procedures to pursue an inconsequential problem can adversely affect the animal. Because of the frequency of major medical problems related to the urinary system, the veterinarian must be aware of the more common urologic disorders affecting geriatric dogs and cats.

UROLOGIC DISORDERS OF THE DOG

Renal failure is the second leading cause of nonaccidental death in dogs. The average age at onset is 6.95 years (Lewis et al, 1987). Other urologic disorders that are primarily seen in middle-age or geriatric dogs include urinary incontinence, prostate disease, and urinary bladder tumors. Diagnosis of urologic disorders can be a challenge, because the signs of disease are often insidious, nonspecific, and atypical in older dogs. For instance, the first sign of renal failure in older dogs may be nocturia or urinary incontinence rather than polyuria. Polyuria occurs at any age in dogs with renal failure, but in older dogs, increased urine output may stress the urethral sphincter, which may also be altered. Likewise, the urinary bladder may have reduced urine-holding capacity. Therefore, polyuria-induced urinary incontinence and nocturia may be the first abnormalities noticed by the owners.

Chronic Renal Failure

Kidneys of geriatric dogs and humans are smaller in weight and size than those of younger individuals; this is reflected in decreased glomerular numbers, decreased tubular size and weight, and increased mesangium and fibrosis (Cowgill and Spangler, 1981; Samiy, 1983). These changes in morphology are associated with decreased renal blood flow; glomerular filtration; urinary concentration ability; and ability to maintain sodium, water and acid–base homeostasis (Table 16–1). Concentrations of renin, aldosterone, and activated vitamin D may also be decreased (Samiy, 1983).

TABLE 16–1. STRUCTURAL AND FUNCTIONAL CHANGES OBSERVED IN AGING HUMAN KIDNEYS

FUNCTIONAL CHANGES	STRUCTURAL CHANGES
1. Progressive reduction in renal blood flow and glomerular filtration. a. Renal fraction of cardiac output declines with age. b. Structural changes in renal vasculature may be associated with increased vascular resistance. c. Glomerular capillary surface area declines. d. Despite a decline in glomerular filtration rate, serum creatinine concentration may remain normal, because reduced muscle mass results in reduced production of creatinine. e. This reduction may contribute to reduced ability to excrete excessive water. 2. Impaired tubular reabsorption and secretion. a. Impaired urine concentrating capacity (and impaired thirst) may be associated, in part, with a change in renal blood flow from cortical to medullary portions of the kidney. b. Ability to conserve (and excrete) sodium is impaired. c. Ability to excrete potassium is impaired. d. Ability to excrete hydrogen ions after an acid load is impaired. 3. Impaired hormone production. a. Production of 1,25-vitamin D (calcitriol) is impaired. b. Renin/aldosterone production is decreased. 4. Blunted compensatory increases of function in response to nephron damage.	1. Progressive reduction in renal weight and volume. 2. Reduced numbers of normal glomeruli. 3. Increased degree of glomerular sclerosis. 4. Reduction in tubular number, volume, and length. 5. Progressive increase in renal interstitial tissue.

Adapted from Lonergan ET. Aging and the kidney: Adjusting treatment to physiologic change. Geriatrics 43:27, 1988; and Kater LW, Haensly WE. Kidney in the aging cat. Neutral lipid and adenyl cylase histochemistry. Am J Vet Res 38:897, 1977.

Decrease in renal function over time is likely due to a number of causes. One proposed mechanism of decreased renal function associated with aging is the consumption of high-protein diets. One identifiable clinical sign of renal aging in rats is proteinuria. Proteinuria is associated with significant renal structural abnormalities (Samiy, 1983). High-protein meals cause varying degrees of glomerular hyperfiltration, which can damage the glomerular vascular endothelium and result in protein leakage into the glomerular mesangium and proteinuria (Brenner et al, 1982). Hyperfiltration-mediated movement of proteins into the mesangium has been linked to inflammation and sclerosis. Progressive sclerosis of the glomerulus will eventually result in the destruction of its attached tubule. One study has shown that healthy individuals who eat meat as a part of their diet have significantly higher proteinuria and blood pressures than do vegetarians (Wiseman et al, 1987).

It is unlikely that the slow deterioration of renal function over time, whether due to dietary protein or to other causes, by itself results in renal failure. Fortunately, the kidneys have a great reserve of functional nephrons. However, geriatric dogs are less able to tolerate other types of renal diseases because of reduced renal reserve. Therefore, it is important to try to identify and eliminate potentially reversible causes of renal disease in older dogs. For example, poor renal perfusion owing to heart failure can result in ischemic renal disease and renal failure if not identified early and treated. Hypercalcemia, diabetes mellitus, urinary tract infections, and urinary obstructions are other potentially reversible diseases that may have a serious impact on the kidneys if not managed. These disorders pose an even greater threat to geriatric dogs with reduced renal reserve. Veterinarians should also be very careful when considering the use of nephrotoxic drugs in geriatric dogs. Geriatric kidneys are less able to tolerate potential side effects and may be unable to handle routinely recommended dosages.

Standard recommendations for the conservative treatment of renal failure can usually be followed when treating geriatric dogs (Polzin and Osborne, 1986). Recommendations aimed at decreasing the progressive nature of chronic renal failure include decreasing dietary protein intake, controlling hypertension, and maintaining normal serum phosphorus levels. Commercial diets recommended for dogs and cats with renal failure should be designed to reduce protein, salt, and phosphorus intake (e.g., Prescription Diet Canine k/d or u/d, Hill's Pet Products, Topeka, KS). Because renal failure is a dynamic process associated with varying degrees of dysfunction, it is not possible to select a single desirable level of dietary protein intake for all dogs. The general therapeutic goal is to feed enough protein so that the dog maintains nitrogen balance without metabolizing endogenous proteins for energy. In general, it is recommended that dogs with serum creatinine less than 4.5 mg/dl be maintained on 2.0 to 2.2 g/kg/day of high biologic quality dietary protein. Dogs with serum creatinine levels greater than 4.5 mg/dl should be fed approximately 1.3 g/kg/day of protein (Polzin and Osborne, 1986). Dogs fed protein-restricted diets should have adequate amounts of dietary fat and carbohydrate to fulfill 100 per cent of their daily caloric needs. This will facilitate utilization of dietary protein for anabolism and not as a source of energy. Because the quantity of protein required varies among older dogs, individual animals should be carefully monitored for excesses and deficiencies of dietary protein. If dogs continue to manifest signs of uremia attributable to excess dietary protein, further adjustments of dietary protein should be considered. On the other hand, loss of muscle mass associated with decreased protein intake should be corrected by increasing dietary protein.

Hypertension is generally first treated by restricting dietary salt intake. However, controlled studies designed to determine the optimal amount of reduction of sodium chloride needed to benefit hypertensive dogs with renal failure have not been performed. Currently available commercial diets formulated for dogs with renal failure contain sodium levels of between 0.21 and 0.26 per cent of dry matter (e.g., Prescription Diet Canine k/d or u/d, Hill's Pet Products). Homemade diets that provide a dog with 35 mg sodium/kg/day would closely approximate commercial renal failure diets (Polzin and Osborne, 1983). Other medications that have been advocated for treatment of hypertension in dogs with renal failure include diuretics, sympatholytic agents, and vasodilators (Cowgill and Kallet, 1983).

Hyperphosphatemia is initially managed by feeding low-phosphorus diets. Because most of the phosphorus in diets is found in the protein portion, reduction of dietary protein results in a corresponding reduction in dietary phosphorus. Aluminum hydroxide– and aluminum carbonate–containing antacids (administered at a dosage of 30 to 90 mg/kg/day) have been recommended as oral phosphate-binding agents (Polzin and Osborne, 1986). These drugs are considered if proper hydration and dietary protein restriction are ineffective in correcting hyperphosphatemia. Serum phosphorus levels should be maintained below 6 mg/dl, and fractional excretion of urinary phosphorus should be maintained below 30 per cent (Finco, 1983; Finco and Barsanti, 1983). Additional recommendations for treatment of dogs with renal failure are summarized in Table 16–2.

Urinary Incontinence

The average age of dogs presented with acquired urinary incontinence is between 5.3 and 8.3 years (DiBartola and Adams, 1983; Osborne et al, 1980; Rosin and Barsanti, 1981). The most common causes of urinary incontinence in dogs are urethral incompetence, urinary tract infection, and polyuria/polydipsia (Krawiec, 1989). Urethral incompetence (commonly referred to as *hormone-responsive incontinence*) often occurs in spayed female dogs and infrequently in intact female and neutered and intact male dogs. Urinary tract infection usually causes urge incontinence and is more common in females than males. Polyuria can be produced by a number of pathologic abnormalities and by certain medications (Hardy, 1982; Hardy and Osborne, 1980). Eliminating or ameliorating the increased urine output may eradicate or substantially decrease incontinence. Behavioral problems or debilitating diseases may also cause incontinence. Older dogs may become more dependent on their owners and may urinate when they get excited while greeting their owners. These dogs may have to

TABLE 16–2. THERAPEUTIC RECOMMENDATIONS FOR PATIENTS WITH COMPENSATED CHRONIC RENAL FAILURE

Recommendations for slowing the progression of failure
Reduce dietary protein
Control hypertension
Treat hyperphosphatemia
Recommendations for making the animal feel better
Reduce dietary protein
Furnish unlimited access to water
Avoid stress
Treat acidosis
Furnish vitamin B and C dietary supplements
Treat clinical hypocalcemia with vitamin D and calcium

be retrained to empty their urinary bladders more frequently or become less excited in stressful situations. Debilitated animals may have to be trained to void on newspapers or may require help to go outside to urinate (Krawiec, 1988).

Determination of the causes of urinary incontinence requires careful evaluation of information obtained from the history, physical examination, and laboratory tests. The history should include detailed information about the nature of the incontinence. Urethral incompetence is most often seen while the dog is relaxing or asleep. The physical examination should include a neurologic examination; abdominal palpation to evaluate the bladder for distention, tenderness, and irregularities; inspection and palpation of the external genitalia; and digital rectal examination. The physical examination should also include evaluation of the urine stream and of the dog's behavior while urinating. To assess urethral tone, dogs should be interrupted while urinating to assess their ability to stop urinating midstream. Residual urine volume should be measured after voiding is completed to determine whether the dog can completely empty the urinary bladder. Residual urine volumes should not be greater than 0.2 to 0.4 ml/kg (Moreau, 1982). A urinalysis should be performed routinely to detect urinary tract infection. Other tests that may be included are a complete blood cell count, serum chemistry profile, abdominal radiography, and abdominal ultrasonography.

Therapy should be directed at the specific cause of the urinary incontinence. If a specific cause cannot be identified, nonspecific treatment of the incontinence should be considered. Medications are available that can increase or decrease bladder contraction or urethral contraction (Krawiec, 1989). For these medications to be used appropriately, it is imperative to localize the problem to the urinary bladder or urethra and to determine whether the problem is one of excessive contraction or relaxation.

Urinary Bladder Tumors

Urinary bladder tumors are the most common neoplasm of the urinary tract in older dogs, with the average age at diagnosis being 9.1 to 9.4 years (Burnie and Weaver, 1983; Osborne et al, 1968). Bladder neoplasia may occur more frequently in female dogs than in males (Hayes, 1976). Scottish terriers, Shetland sheepdogs, beagles, collies, cocker spaniels, springer spaniels, dachshunds, boxers, Labrador retrievers, West Highland white terriers, and cairn terriers are the most common breeds affected by bladder tumors (Hayes, 1976; Osborne et al, 1968). Transitional cell carcinomas, the most common urinary bladder tumor of older dogs, may occur as a papillary projection into the bladder lumen and/or infiltrate into the wall. Squamous cell carcinomas and adenocarcinomas may also occur and probably develop as a result of metaplasia of transitional cells.

A urinary bladder tumor should be suspected in any older dog with persistent hematuria, pollakiuria, dysuria, and/or incontinence that is not responsive to antimicrobials or other routine therapy. Bladder masses can be identified by contrast cystography, bladder ultrasonography, and/or cystoscopy. Definitive diagnosis is based on light microscopic evaluation of a bladder biopsy specimen, which may be obtained via cystoscopy, laparoscopy, cystotomy, or catheter biopsy. Cytologic evaluation of urine sediment or needle aspiration biopsies of the bladder mass may provide definitive evidence of neoplasia (Crow and Klausner, 1983). Bladder tumors should be staged according to the TMN system. Patients with poorly differentiated tumors with distant metastasis have the worst prognosis, whereas those with superficial, solitary, well-differentiated tumors have the best prognosis (Crow and Klausner, 1983).

Successful treatment of urinary bladder tumors is primarily dependent on early diagnosis. Unfortunately, however, most bladder tumors are identified at an advanced stage, and therapy for such patients is often aimed at relieving urinary discomfort, maintaining urinary continence, and preventing hydronephrosis and hydroureter. Curative treatment is rarely attainable. Surgically accessible tumors should be removed along with a wide zone of healthy tissue. Widespread tumors or tumors involving the neck region may be debulked. Total cystectomy with urinary diversion may be attempted but has been unrewarding. Nonsurgical therapy includes radiation and chemotherapy. At the University of Illinois Veterinary Teaching Hospital, we are currently using a combination of intravesicular and parenteral cisplatin and/or doxorubicin along with intravesicular hyperthermia. Symptomatic therapy includes treatment of secondary urinary tract infection and urolithiasis and chemical cauterization of the bladder to minimize bleeding. Methenamine mandelate (10 mg/kg PO every 6 hours or intravesicular instillation of a dilute formalin solution) may be used to cauterize the bladder mucosa (Crow and Klausner, 1983; Macy, 1986). Piroxicam, a nonsteroidal anti-inflammatory drug, has also been shown to minimize discomfort.

TABLE 16–3. AGE AT DIAGNOSIS OF CATS WITH CHRONIC RENAL DISEASE SEEN AT THE UNIVERSITY OF ILLINOIS VETERINARY TEACHING HOSPITAL (JULY 1981 TO DECEMBER 1986)

AGE (yr)	TOTAL NO. OF CATS SEEN DURING THE PERIOD (%)	NO. OF AFFECTED CATS (%)	PERCENTAGE OF AFFECTED CATS IN TOTAL POPULATION
0–1	1934 (38)	6 (4.8)	0.31
1–2	628 (12)	1 (0.8)	0.16
2–4	830 (16)	7 (5.6)	0.84
4–7	644 (13)	6 (4.8)	0.93
7–10	408 (8)	14 (11.2)	3.43
10–15	488 (10)	42 (33.6)	8.61
>15	166 (3)	49 (39.2)	29.52
Total	5098	125	2.45

UROLOGIC DISORDERS OF THE CAT

Chronic Renal Disease and Chronic Renal Failure

Demographics. Records of 131 cats with chronic renal disease seen at the University of Illinois Veterinary Teaching Hospital between July 1981 and December 1986 were evaluated for breed, age at onset of renal disease, sex, owner's primary complaint, clinical and necropsy diagnosis, and concurrent disease. Chronic renal disease and renal failure in cats are often thought to be an inevitable consequence of aging. The average age at the time of diagnosis of 125 cats with chronic renal disease was 12.8 years (median, 14 years) in our hospital population (Table 16–3). The average of cats with chronic renal failure was 13.4 years (median, 15 years). Gender was identified in 119 of the 131 cats. Neutered males represented the largest group with renal disease (48 cats, or 40.3 per cent). Forty-three cats (36.1 per cent) were spayed females, 16 (13.5 per cent) were intact males, and 12 (10.1 per cent) were intact females. Most cats with renal disease were domestic mixed breed cats (102 cats, or 81.6 per cent), followed by Siamese (14.4 per cent) and Persians (4 per cent). A prototype of feline renal failure is presented in Table 16–4.

Owners' Complaints. The most common clinical sign identified by owners of cats with chronic renal failure was anorexia, followed by polyuria/polydipsia (Table 16–5). Other signs observed, in decreasing order of frequency, were lethargy and depression, vomiting, weight loss, oral cavity abnormalities, neurologic abnormalities (e.g., vestibular disease, ataxia, rear limb paresis, disorientation), diarrhea, and blindness.

Diagnosis. Of 131 cats with chronic renal disease, 100 cats were diagnosed clinically as having a chronic renal disorder. Fifty-four (41.5 per cent) cats evaluated either died or were euthanized; their kidneys were available for light microscopic examination. The most common morphologic lesion identified was membranous glomerulonephropathy, which was identified as the only histopathologic abnormality in 10 cats and as the primary lesion in an additional five cats. Membranoproliferative glomerulonephropathy was identified in three cats. Quantitative

TABLE 16–4. FELINE RENAL FAILURE PROTOTYPE

1. 10 years of age and older
2. Siamese, Abyssinian, Burmese, Maine Coon, or Russian Blue breed
3. Male or female
4. Clinical signs (nonlocalizing)
   a. Anorexia
   b. Weight loss
   c. Vomiting
   d. Dehydration
   e. Polyuria, polydipsia
5. Kidney size: variable (small, normal, large)
6. Laboratory findings
   a. Serum chemistry profile
      1. Constant
         a. Azotemia
         b. Hyperphosphatemia
         c. Acidemia
      2. Variable
         a. Calcium
         b. Potassium
         c. Sodium
         d. Chloride
         e. Albumin
   b. Urinalysis
      1. Impaired urine concentration
      2. Proteinuria (nonglomerular)
      3. Infectious inflammation
   c. Hemogram indicative of nonregenerative anemia

TABLE 16–5. PRESENTING COMPLAINT AND CONCURRENT DISEASE IN CATS WITH CHRONIC RENAL DISEASE SEEN AT THE UNIVERSITY OF ILLINOIS VETERINARY TEACHING HOSPITAL (JULY 1981 TO DECEMBER 1986)

	NUMBER OF CATS (%)*
Presenting complaint	
Anorexia	46 (29.9)
Polyuria/polydipsia	31 (20.1)
Lethargy and depression	17 (11.0)
Vomiting	15 (9.9)
Weight loss	11 (7.1)
Oral cavity problems	8 (5.2)
Neurologic problems	8 (5.2)
Diarrhea	5 (3.2)
Respiratory abnormalities	5 (3.2)
Lower urinary tract problem	4 (2.6)
Blind	4 (2.6)
Concurrent disease	
Neoplasia	27 (30.3)
Hyperthyroidism	16 (18.0)
Liver disease	11 (12.4)
Cardiac disease	11 (12.4)
Lower urinary tract disease	8 (9.0)
Retinal detachment	6 (6.7)
Diabetes mellitus	4 (4.5)
Hypertension	3 (3.4)
Pneumonia	3 (3.4)

*More than one presenting complaint and/or concurrent disease may be present in a given individual.

urine protein determinations were not performed in any of these cases. There was no significant difference between the serum albumin levels of cats with severe glomerular lesions (mean serum albumin, 2.95 g/dl) and those of cats without glomerular lesions (mean serum albumin, 3.0 g/dl). The mean urine protein level of cats with severe membranous lesions was 136 mg/dl, whereas the average urine protein level of cats without glomerular lesions was 65 mg/dl. The average urine specific gravities of the two groups were the same (1.018). Chronic tubulointerstitial nephritis was the only lesion identified in eight cats and the primary lesion identified in an additional cat. Twenty-two cats had a combination of glomerular and tubulointerstitial changes. Renal neoplasia was identified in three cats, and hydronephrosis and renal hypoxia were each identified in a single cat.

Concurrent Diseases. The most common disorder associated with chronic renal disease was neoplasia (see Table 16–5). The most common neoplasms identified were thyroid adenoma and adenocarcinoma (seven cats), followed by squamous cell carcinoma (five cats). Other types of neoplasms present were lymphosarcoma, hepatocellular carcinoma, abdominal mesothelioma, mast cell tumor, nasal adenocarcinoma, biliary carcinoma, bronchiogenic carcinoma, salivary gland carcinoma, intestinal adenocarcinoma, and pancreatic acinar cell adenoma. The most common clinical entity that affected cats with chronic renal disease was hyperthyroidism (16 cats). Neoplasia, hyperthyroidism, and chronic renal failure are all diseases that primarily affect older cats. This illustrates the need to evaluate older cats thoroughly for occult disease, even if a primary abnormality has been identified.

Liver disease was present in 11 cats with chronic renal disease: 3 cats had hepatic neoplasm, 1 cat had hepatic lipidosis, and the remaining cats had nonspecific hepatocellular degeneration/vacuolization or undefined liver disease. Lower urinary tract disease was identified in eight cats: two cats had idiopathic lower urinary tract disease, and the remainder had bacterial cystitis. Idiopathic retinal detachment was identified in six cats: three cats with retinal detachment had hypertension, and the other three cats were not evaluated for hypertension. We recommend that any cat with unexplained retinal detachment be evaluated for renal failure and hypertension.

Diabetes mellitus was present in four cats with renal disease. Two of the four cats were identified as having glomerular disease on the basis of light microscopic examination of renal tissue. The other two cats' kidneys were not evaluated by light microscopy, and the cats were identified as having a clinical glomerular problem.

Cardiac disease was identified in 11 cats, with hypertrophic cardiomyopathy diagnosed in 6 of the 11. There is a high association between hypertrophic cardiomyopathy and hyperthyroidism, but only one of these six cats was diagnosed with hyperthyroidism.

Chronic Nephritis

Cats often develop a slow deterioration of renal function that leads to renal failure, end-stage kidney disease, and death. Regardless of the initiating cause, this deterioration is usually characterized histologically by fibrosis and mononuclear cell infiltration (chronic tubulointerstitial nephritis). Because of the long-standing nature of the disease and its nondistinctive lesions, the cause of chronic nephritis is not identified.

Chronic nephritis is usually not identified until renal failure (azotemia and inappropriate urine-concentrating capacity [urine specific gravity between 1.008 and 1.034]) has occurred. Chronic renal failure also includes a nonregenerative normochromic, normocytic anemia, bilateral reduction in renal size, illness for months to years, and evidence of renal osteodystrophy. Therapy for chronic nephritis is aimed at slowing the progression of the disease and ameliorating the signs of uremia. Typically, treatment involves reducing salt intake to control hypertension, restricting dietary protein and phosphorus, providing unlimited access to water, avoiding stress, providing dietary supplementation with water-soluble vitamins, treating acidosis, using recombinant erythropoietin or anabolic agents to promote red blood cell production, and controlling hypocalcemia (Osborne and Polzin, 1983).

Glomerulonephropathy

Glomerulonephropathy in cats is an immune-mediated inflammatory disorder (August and Leib, 1984; DiBartola and Chew, 1986). Two forms of glomerulonephropathy may occur: antiglomerular basement membrane nephritis and immune complex nephritis. Antiglomerular basement membrane nephritis occurs after development of antibodies directed against the glomerular basement membrane; this antigen–antibody interaction results in complement activation and inflammation. This glomerulopathy has not yet been described in cats. However, immune complex nephritis does occur in cats and is associated with immune complex deposition in the glomerular capillary network. Numerous chronic inflammatory disorders (e.g., feline leukemia virus infection, feline infectious peritonitis, systemic lupus erythematosus, and endocarditis) have been implicated as a cause of immune complex nephritis. However, immune complex nephritis in cats also occurs as an idiopathic disorder (i.e., the inciting antigenic stimulus is not identifiable). Cats with glomerulonephropathy may subsequently develop renal failure and/or nephrotic syndrome. Specific therapy for glomerulonephropathy should be aimed at identifying and treating the primary inflammatory disorder causing chronic antigenic stimulation. Unfortunately, however, this is often not possible. One of the newest therapies for glomerulonephropathy-induced edema is enalapril, an angiotensin converting enzyme (ACE) inhibitor that acts as a diuretic by decreasing aldosterone levels. Enalapril also decreases angiotensin concentration and thus acts as a vasodilator as well. Enalapril has the added advantage of decreasing intraglomerular pressures and the hypertension-induced glomerular damage seen in many cases of glomerulonephropathy (Heeg et al, 1987). The dosage of enalapril for cats with hypertension or glomerulonephropathy-induced edema is 0.25 mg/kg every 12 hours. Enalapril should not be used in combination with other diuretics, as profound life-threatening hypotension may occur.

Renal Amyloidosis

Renal amyloidosis primarily affects older cats of both sexes and numerous breeds, with a hereditary tendency in Abyssinian cats (Chew et al, 1982). In cats, amyloid deposition occurs primarily in the medullary interstitium, although it can also be found in renal cortical areas and glomeruli. Renal amyloidosis in cats typically is characterized by renal failure and uremia. Proteinuria may or may not be severe depending on the degree of glomerular involvement. Amyloidosis is not an inflammatory disease but is associated with various inflammatory diseases, neoplasms, endocrine disorders, and hypervitaminosis A (Chew and DiBartola, 1983). In most instances, however, an underlying abnormality cannot be identified or eliminated. A definitive diagnosis of amyloidosis can be made only by evaluation of renal tissue obtained by renal biopsy or at necropsy. Therapy should be aimed at identifying and removing underlying inflammatory disease and treating the cat symptomatically for renal failure. No specific therapy to prevent deposition or facilitate the removal of amyloid in cats is known.

Perirenal Cysts (Pseudocysts)

Perirenal cyst is an uncommonly recognized disorder characterized by progressive abdominal enlargement owing to accumulation of fluid in a cyst-like structure surrounding one or both kidneys (Lulich et al, in press). Perirenal cysts have primarily been seen in male or neutered male cats but have also been observed in females. This condition can be differentiated from hydronephrosis, polycystic kidneys, and neoplasia by ultrasonography or intravenous urography, which usually reveals a normal-size kidney encased in a fluid-filled sac. The cause of perirenal cysts in cats is unknown. Affected cats may or may not be azotemic but generally are brought to the veterinarian because of progressive abdominal distention. Therapy is aimed at surgically removing the cyst and correcting any identifiable causes (Lulich et al, in press).

DIAGNOSIS AND MANAGEMENT OF CHRONIC RENAL FAILURE IN OLDER DOGS AND CATS

Diagnosis

Renal disease can be unilateral or bilateral; it can also be self-limiting and benign or progressive and lead to renal failure. Chronic renal failure is usually irreversible and progressive and in many instances eventually leads to end-stage renal failure and death. A number of causes of chronic renal failure have been described (Table 16–6) (Krawiec and Gelberg, 1990). The diagnostic work-up for older dogs and cats suspected of having chronic renal disease includes a history, physical examination, and appropriate laboratory diagnostic tests (Ross, 1986). A problem-specific data base for feline renal failure is outlined in Table 16–7. Signs commonly associated with chronic renal failure are summarized in Table 16–8. The most common clinical signs are anorexia, polyuria/polydipsia, lethargy, depression, vomiting, and weight loss (Cowgill, 1983; DiBartola et al, 1987; Krawiec and Gelberg, 1990).

Laboratory Abnormalities

Laboratory abnormalities consistent with polyuric chronic renal failure are listed in Table 16–9 and include a normochromic, normocytic nonregenerative anemia; elevations in levels of serum urea nitrogen, creatinine, and phosphorus; decreased serum calcium concentration; and impaired urine concentration. In addition, glomerular abnormalities are associated with hypoalbuminemia, hypoproteinemia, hypercholesterolemia, and proteinuria (Cowgill, 1983; Osborne et al, 1983). The anemia of chronic renal failure is likely due to a number of abnormalities, including decreased erythropoietin, decreased red blood cell precursors owing to uremia-induced bone marrow toxicity, decreased red blood cell survival, blood loss owing to platelet abnormalities or excessive blood sampling, chronic inflammation, and malnutrition. Loss of urine-concentrating ability is often the first functional abnormality identified in older dogs and cats with renal failure. This abnormality occurs when there is a loss of approximately 66 per cent of the total functional capacity of both kidneys and may manifest itself as polyuria and polydipsia (Cowgill, 1983; Osborne et al, 1983). Many nonrenal pathologic and physiologic disorders are associated with impaired urine-concentrating capacity (Table 16–10) (Hardy, 1982).

TABLE 16–6. SOME TREATABLE CAUSES OF AZOTEMIA WITH PRIMARY RENAL FAILURE

- I. Specific treatment available
  - A. Prerenal causes
    - Decreased renal perfusion
      - Dehydration
      - Cardiovascular dysfunction
      - Severe hypoalbuminemia
      - Hypoadrenocorticism
    - Increased urea metabolism
      - Gastrointestinal hemorrhage
      - Extensive tissue necrosis
      - High-protein diet
      - Catabolic drugs
        - Glucocorticoids
        - Antineoplastic agents
        - Tetracyclines (antianabolic?)
        - Excessive thyroid supplementation
  - B. Postrenal causes
    - Rent in excretory pathway
    - Urinary tract obstruction
      - Uroliths
      - Operable neoplasms
      - Herniated urinary bladder
      - Blood clots
      - Spay granuloma
      - Others
  - C. Primary renal causes
    - Acute tubular necrosis
      - Ischemia
        - Prolonged hypovolemia
        - Nonsteroidal anti-inflammatory toxicity
        - Thromboembolic disorders
      - Nephrotoxins, including
        - Aminoglycoside antimicrobials
        - Ethylene glycol
        - Heme pigments
        - Amphotericin B
        - Cisplatin
    - Hypercalcemic nephropathy
    - Bacterial and fungal urinary tract infection
    - Some glomerulonephropathies
    - Immune disorders
    - Adverse drug reactions
    - Heat stroke
- II. No specific treatment available
  - A. Inherited and congenital disease
  - B. Polycystic disease; perirenal pseudocysts
  - C. Amyloidosis
  - D. Feline infectious peritonitis
  - E. Neoplasia
  - F. Periarteritis nodosa
  - G. Idiopathic

TABLE 16–7. PROBLEM-SPECIFIC DATA BASE FOR RENAL FAILURE

I. Minimum Data Base
  A. Medical history checklist
    1. Age?
    2. Breed?
    3. Duration of illness?
    4. Previous illness or injury?
    5. Past history of renal disease? Recent evaluation indicating adequate renal function?
    6. Exposure to possible nephrotoxins?
    7. Recent trauma, surgery, or anesthesia?
    8. Diet: Type? Frequency of feeding? Supplements? Recent diet changes? Preferences?
    9. Water consumption: Increased, decreased, unknown, or no change? If change noted, when?
    10. Micturition?
      Frequency? Quantity? Color? Odor? Changes?
      Urinary incontinence?
      Micturition in abnormal locations?
    11. Detection of signs not directly referable to the urinary tract
      Anorexia?
      Vomiting?
      Diarrhea?
      Weight loss?
      Constipation?
      Others?
    12. Are clinical signs increasing in severity, decreasing in severity, or remaining the same?
    13. Medication history: Medications given? When given? Dosage? Response? Tolerance?
  B. Physical examination checklist
    1. Temperature, pulse, and respiratory rate?
    2. Hydration status (skin pliability, xerostoma, etc.)?
    3. Body weight?
    4. Mouth: Mucosal ulcers? Discoloration of tongue? Pallor of mucous membranes? Loose or missing teeth? Enlargement of maxillary tissues?
    5. Cardiovascular system: Pulse rate and character? Mucous membrane color? Capillary refill time? Heart sounds? Venous distention? Arterial blood pressure (if available)?
    6. Kidneys: both palpable? Bilaterally symmetric? Position? Size? Shape? Consistency? Contour? Pain?
    7. Urinary bladder: Size (before and after micturition)? Shape? Consistency? Position? Pain? Wall thickness? Intraluminal masses (Consistency? Attached? Grating sensation?)?
    8. Urethra (if possible?): Position? Size? Shape? Consistency? Intraluminal masses (Consistency? Attached? Grating sensation?)?
    9. Penis/prepuce/vulva: Shape? Consistency? Discharge? Pain?
    10. Ophthalmoscopic examination of fundus for evidence of hypertension: Retinal detachment? Hemorrhage? Others?
  C. Laboratory data checklist
    1. Urinalysis, including urine sediment
    2. Kidney function tests (serum creatinine and urea nitrogen)
    3. Hematocrit, total plasma protein concentration (complete blood cell count?)

II. Further Diagnostic Considerations
  A. Serum biochemical profile (Na, Cl, K, P, TCO_2, Ca, albumin, others) to identify associated complications and extrarenal causes of azotemia (i.e., hypoadrenocorticism, hyponatremia, others)
  B. Urine culture, especially if microburia, dysuria, or hematuria is detected
  C. Survey abdominal radiography to verify kidney number, size, shape, and position
  D. Urine protein-to-creatinine ratio to quantify protein loss in animals with proteinuria
  E. Intravenous urography
  F. Renal ultrasonography
  G. Renal biopsy

Azotemia, the elevation of serum urea and creatinine concentrations, occurs when approximately 75 per cent of the total functional capability of both kidneys is lost. Azotemia can be caused by disorders other than renal failure and therefore can be interpreted only after analyzing other historical, physical, and laboratory abnormalities. Prerenal azotemia can be caused by dehydration, shock, ischemia, or a high-protein meal, and postrenal azotemia can be caused by urethral or bilateral ureteral obstruction or rupture of the lower urinary tract. Prerenal azotemia is usually identified in dogs and cats with azotemia and concentrated urine, whereas postrenal azotemia is usually identified by finding physical or radiographic evidence of urethral or ureteral

TABLE 16–8. SIGNS OF CHRONIC RENAL FAILURE

- Neurvous system abnormalities
  - Lethargy
  - Weakness
  - Seizures
  - Coma
  - Peripheral neuropathy
  - Blindness
- Gastrointestinal system signs
  - Stomatitis
  - Vomiting
  - Diarrhea
  - Anorexia
  - Weight loss
- Hematologic system abnormalities
  - Anemia
  - Bleeding tendency
- Skeletal system signs
  - Extraosseous calcification
  - Osteodystrophy
- Endocrine system signs
  - Insulin resistance
  - Impotence
  - Infertility
  - Renal secondary hyperparathyroidism
  - Hypertension
  - Impaired growth
- Dermatologic system signs
  - Pruritus
  - Dehydration
  - Edema
- Urinary system signs
  - Polyuria
  - Oliguria
  - Anuria
  - Nocturia
- Serum chemistry abnormalities
  - Azotemia
  - Hyperphosphatemia
  - Hyper- or hypocalcemia
- Potential life-threatening alterations
  - Severe dehydration
  - Severe acidosis
  - Severe hypo- or hyperkalemia
  - Severe hypocalcemia

obstruction or evidence of urine in the abdominal cavity.

Renal Function Tests

Fractional electrolyte excretion (FE) data may provide qualitative information concerning renal function. FE is defined as the ratio of the renal clearance of an electrolyte to the renal clearance of creatinine. Kidneys maintain electrolyte homeostasis by increasing or decreasing the fractional excretion of many metabolites filtered by glomeruli according to need. In renal failure, there are fewer functional nephrons doing the same amount of work. Therefore, as renal function decreases, FE will proportionately increase to maintain homeostasis. Fractional excretion of sodium, potassium, and phosphorus is increased in dogs and cats with renal failure, because each surviving nephron must excrete a larger percentage of filtered electrolyte to maintain homeostasis. Ultimately, as the failure progresses, maximum FE will be attained, and total body

TABLE 16–9. LABORATORY DATA THAT MAY BE ABNORMAL IN CHRONIC RENAL DISEASE

- Urinalysis
  - Significant proteinuria
  - Urine casts
  - Bacteriuria
  - Pyuria
  - Hematuria
- Complete blood cell count
  - Anemia
  - Inflammatory leukon*
- Serum chemistry profile
  - Increased urea nitrogen
  - Increased creatinine
  - Increased phosphorus
  - Increased or decreased potassium
  - Increased or decreased sodium
  - Increased cholesterol
- Other abnormalities
  - Decreased glomerular filtration rate
  - Hypertension
  - Decreased or increased renal size
  - Retinal hemorrhage or detachment
  - Acidosis
  - Platelet function deficiency
  - Tendency toward thrombosis†

*May be seen in pyelonephritis.
†May be seen in glomerulonephritis.

TABLE 16–10. CAUSES OF POLYURIA

- Water diuresis (urine specific gravity, 1.001–1.007)
  - Excessive ingestion of water
  - Central diabetes insipidus
  - Renal diabetes insipidus
  - Pyometra
- Solute diuresis (urine specific gravity: cat, 1.008–1.034; dog, 1.008–1.029)
  - Diabetes mellitus
  - Hyperthyroidism
  - Post relief of urethral obstruction
- May produce either a solute or a water diuresis (urine specific gravity: cat, 1.001–1.034; dog, 1.008–1.029)
  - Liver failure
  - Hypercalcemia
  - Chronic renal failure
  - Drugs
  - Hypokalemia
  - Hyperadrenocorticism
  - Hypoadrenocorticism

electrolyte levels will start to increase, resulting in elevations in serum electrolyte concentrations. Elevations of FE occur before other signs of renal failure, making this an excellent method for defining early nonazctemic polyuric renal failure (Fig. 16–1).

Quantitative evaluation of renal function is determined by calculating glomerular filtration rate (GFR) (Cowgill, 1983; Osborne et al, 1983; Ross, 1986). GFR is defined as the milliliters of plasma that are cleared of a substance per minute per kilogram body weight. Laboratory tests measure function by determining the plasma clearance of substances that are removed or cleared by the kidney. The three most common tests used to determine GFR are exogenous creatinine clearance, endogenous creatinine clearance, and inulin clearance. The inulin clearance test is the most accurate evaluation of renal function available, but the easiest test to perform in a clinical setting is the endogenous creatinine clearance (CrCl) test. This test is not as accurate as exogenous creatinine or inulin clearance, because noncreatinine chromogens will falsely evaluate serum creatinine concentration. These chromogens are not excreted in urine and therefore will falsely reduce GFR values. The accuracy of CrCl can be enhanced by removing noncreatinine chromogens from the sample before determining serum creatinine levels. However, this is rarely done by commercial laboratories using autoanalyzers. Noncreatinine chromogen serum levels do not progressively increase as GFR declines, and therefore, their effect becomes negligible as serum creatinine levels increase.

Endogenous creatinine clearance is often measured over a 24-hour period. All urine produced over this time is collected, the urine volume is measured, and the urine creatinine concentration is ascertained from an aliquot of the well-mixed total urine volume. The urinary bladder may be "washed" with a small volume of sterile water or normal saline solution at the beginning and at the end of the study. The washes are removed from the urinary bladder to ensure that all urine in the bladder is removed. The first wash is discarded, but the wash at the end of the study is added to the total urine collected. The combination of wash and urine is mixed well, and an aliquot of this mixture is used to calculate the urine creatinine concentration and urine volume. Cats usually void in a litterbox, and nonabsorbable litter can be substituted for commercial litter. Voided urine can then be eluted from the nonabsorbable litter, allowing 24-hour urine volume to be measured. The urine used for total urine volume and urine creatinine concentration in the CrCl formula consists of the urine produced + volume of fluid used to flush the bladder + volume of fluid used to elute the urine from the nonabsorbable litter. Blood is drawn 12 hours after the start of the CrCl test, and the serum creatinine concentration is determined. The formula for calculating endogenous creatinine clearance is shown in Figure 16–1.

Electrolyte Evaluations

Serum phosphorus and calcium concentrations commonly become abnormal in dogs and cats with chronic renal failure (Cowgill, 1983; Osborne et al, 1983; Ross, 1986). Serum phosphorus levels usually begin increasing at the same time azotemia occurs. Because fractional excretion of phosphorus by the kidneys reaches a maximum when approximately 75 per cent of renal function is impaired, serum levels of phosphorus increase. However, phosphorus and calcium remain soluble in plasma only when concentrations are within physiologic limits. Elevation of either beyond this limit results in precipitation of both in tissue. When serum phosphorus concentration increases, serum calcium concentration tends to decrease. Serum calcium concentrations also fall because of impaired production of 1,25-vitamin D (calcitriol) by the kidneys. Low serum calcium and vitamin D levels result in the compensatory

$$\text{FE} = \frac{\text{Urine electrolyte} \times \text{Serum creatinine}}{\text{Serum electrolyte} \times \text{Urine creatinine}} \times 100$$

$$\text{CrCl} = \frac{\text{Urine creatinine} \times \text{Urine volume}}{\text{Serum creatinine} \times \text{Urine collection time (min)} \times \text{Body weight (kg)}}$$

$$\text{Urine protein (mg/kg/day)} = \frac{\text{Urine protein (mg/dl)/Urine creatinine (mg/dl)} - 0.006}{0.033}$$

Figure 16–1. Formulas for the determination of fractional excretion of electrolytes (FE), creatinine clearance (CrCl), and 24-hour urine protein excretion (urine protein). The formula for urine protein excretion was derived from data obtained in experiments using dogs.

secretion of increased quantities of parathyroid hormone (PTH). PTH enhances calcium reabsorption from the distal renal tubules and increases calcium reabsorption from bone, resulting in a return of serum calcium levels to normal. However, increased serum calcium concentration in the presence of increased phosphorus causes further precipitation of calcium and phosphorus in tissue. Therefore, calcium levels are again decreased, resulting in further release of PTH and further bone demineralization. These events are collectively called *renal secondary hyperparathyroidism.*

Persistent renal secondary hyperparathyroidism causes osteodystrophy as a result of (1) the effect of PTH on bone demineralization and (2) extraosseous mineralization owing to enhancement of calcium and phosphorus precipitation in tissue. Mineralization of the kidneys results in inflammation and dysfunction, accelerating the progression of renal failure. In addition, hyperparathormonemia induces other changes that contribute to uremia. It has been associated with decreased reabsorption of bicarbonate and worsening of acidosis, decreased tubular reabsorption and excess excretion of amino acids, decreased tubular reabsorption of sodium, neuromuscular disturbances, pruritus, pancytopenia, sexual dysfunction, anemia, hemorrhagic diathesis, and increased susceptibility to infection.

Sodium and potassium are also affected by renal failure. Total body sodium is often elevated in renal failure, even though serum levels are often normal. Because renal failure may predispose dogs and cats to the development of hypertension, the quantity of sodium in the diet is often reduced. Serum potassium levels usually will not rise as long as the dog or cat is polyuric.

Radiography

Survey abdominal radiography will facilitate evaluation of the shape, size, and contour of the kidneys. Acute renal failure, some forms of amyloidosis, polycystic kidneys, hydronephrosis, and neoplasms are often associated with normal-size or enlarged kidneys. Chronic tubulointerstitial nephritis, pyelonephritis, and glomerulonephritis are usually associated with small, irregularly shaped kidneys. Intravenous urography can be performed to enhance visualization of the kidneys in dogs and cats with poor abdominal contrast. It can also be used as an aid in the diagnosis of polycystic kidneys, hydronephrosis, and perirenal pseudocysts and may be helpful in identifying renal pelvic dilation associated with pyelonephritis.

Ultrasonography

Ultrasonography may allow visualization of renal changes that cannot be detected by survey radiography or intravenous urography (Walter et al, 1987). Ultrasonography is especially helpful in evaluation of the architectural changes associated with renal neoplasia, cystic disease, perirenal pseudocysts, and nephrolithiasis. Renal ultrasound may also facilitate differentiation of chronic inflammatory disorders (e.g., tubulointerstitial nephritis, glomerulonephritis) from acute renal disorders.

Kidney Biopsy

Most diagnostic tests previously described will only provide information concerning renal function and gross morphology. A renal biopsy is required if a precise morphologic diagnosis is desired. However, in general, evaluation of renal biopsy specimens is not of prognostic or therapeutic value in dogs and cats with chronic renal failure. The histologic appearance of tubulointerstitial nephritis is the same regardless of the initiating cause, and polycystic kidneys, pseudocystic disease, and hydronephrosis usually can be identified without evaluation of biopsy specimens. Renal biopsies are required to definitively diagnose amyloidosis and renal neoplasia (DiBartola et al, 1987), and if necessary, they may also be performed to help differentiate acute and chronic renal failure. Renal biopsies can be obtained during abdominal surgery, with the aid of ultrasound, or with a blind percutaneous technique. Specific techniques for obtaining renal biopsy specimens are discussed in detail elsewhere (Cowgill, 1983; Finco et al, 1983).

Management

The seven principles guiding treatment of renal failure, the therapeutic options for the management of renal failure, and a therapy-specific data base for monitoring renal failure are outlined in Tables 16–11, 16–12, and 16–13.

Therapy for Uremic Crisis in Polyuric Renal Failure

Uremic crisis is a serious manifestation of renal failure. Dogs and cats with uremic crisis can no longer adequately compensate for abnormalities caused by renal dysfunction and will likely continue to deteriorate and die if not treated quickly and correctly. Uremic crisis may occur with chronic renal failure if kidney disease has pro-

TABLE 16–11. SEVEN PRINCIPLES GUIDING TREATMENT OF RENAL FAILURE

1. No therapy will eliminate renal lesions; renal lesions must heal spontaneously. The polysystemic metabolic and biochemical disorders caused by generalized renal lesions, however, may be modified or eliminated by appropriate therapy.
2. Detect and eliminate reversible nonrenal disorders that may have precipitated or aggravated a uremic crisis.
3. Evaluate the potential reversibility of renal disease and renal dysfunction with the knowledge that adequate renal function is not synonymous with total renal function.
4. Formulate specific therapy to eliminate or control underlying causes with the objective of preventing further renal destruction.
5. Formulate supportive and symptomatic therapy that minimizes alterations in fluid, electrolyte, acid–base, endocrine, and nutrient balance and, therefore, sustain life until the processes of regeneration, repair, and compensatory adaptation allow the kidneys to regain adequate function to re-establish homeostasis. Formulate supportive and symptomatic therapy according to whether the patient has oliguric or nonoliguric primary renal failure.
6. Administer drugs to animals with renal failure only after consideration of their routes and rates of metabolism and elimination and their potential to induce adverse reactions in the uremic environment.
7. Avoid overtreatment.

gressed to end-stage renal failure or if a prerenal or postrenal abnormality is superimposed on primary chronic renal failure. Differentiating end-stage renal failure from potentially treatable renal abnormalities is of major importance, as end-stage renal failure can be effectively treated only with dialysis or kidney transplantation. Some of the abnormalities (e.g., dehydration, congestive heart failure, diabetes mellitus, infectious diseases) that may have caused the renal decompensation are treatable. If the inciting cause of the decompensation can be eliminated, the signs of uremia will often subside.

Because dogs and cats in uremic crisis are dehydrated, estimation and replacement of the fluid deficits are usually the first therapeutic steps. Replacement of fluid deficits will increase renal blood flow and may halt any ongoing renal ischemic damage caused by dehydration. Polyionic, isotonic fluids should be used for replacement. The potassium concentration of the replacement fluids should be adjusted based on whether the dog or cat is hypokalemic, normokalemic, or hyperkalemic. Fluid deficits should be replaced over a 4- to 5-hour period, but if the dog or cat is in shock, fluid may be administered at a faster rate. After rehydration, fluid diuresis may be instituted. By facilitating urinary excretion of prerenal toxins with enhanced urine flow, induced diuresis may hasten the onset of recovery. Intensive diuresis is usually reserved for dogs and cats with severe uremia (Table 16–14) (Finco and Low, 1980). Although intensive diuresis can be time consuming, it will facilitate return of the dog or cat to a compensated state of homeostasis.

Intensive diuresis is performed in two stages. The first stage involves administering an intravenous fluid load. Polyionic replacement fluids should be used for this purpose. In the second stage, a diuretic is administered to remove the fluid. Before starting this therapy, it is important to accurately determine the animal's body weight. Monitoring the animal's body weight is crucial, because rapid increases or decreases in body weight usually reflect excesses or deficiencies in hydration. Fluid volumes equaling 3 to 5 per cent of the animal's body weight should be administered over 1 hour; a diuretic is then administered. A number of diuretics can be used; the most common are 20 per cent dextrose solution, furosemide, and mannitol.

Twenty per cent dextrose is administered at a dose of 25 to 65 ml/kg. Initially, 2 ml/min is administered over the first 10 to 15 minutes; the rest is administered at a rate of 1 ml/min. The advantages of using dextrose are that it will provide energy and can easily be found in urine. Polyuric dogs and cats should develop glucosuria within minutes of beginning 20 per cent dextrose administration. If glucosuria cannot be identified, the dog or cat may be oliguric, and therefore, further dextrose administration should be discontinued. The disadvantage of using 20 per cent dextrose solution is that it is time consuming to administer and should be administered in a central vein. The animal should be producing 3 ml/hour per kilogram body weight by the time half of the dextrose is administered. If the animal is not producing urine at this rate, the dextrose should be discontinued, and the animal should be reassessed for oliguria.

Mannitol solution at a dose of 0.5 g per kilogram body weight given intravenously over 5 minutes or furosemide at a dose of 2 to 4 mg per kilogram body weight can be substituted for dextrose. The main advantage of using these two diuretics is their ease of administration. The combination of fluid load followed by diuretic may be repeated two to three times a day. While performing intensive diuresis, fluid input and urine output should be monitored carefully. Under most circumstances, quantitative monitoring of urine output requires the use of an indwelling

TABLE 16–12. THERAPEUTIC OPTIONS FOR THE MANAGEMENT OF RENAL FAILURE IN DOGS AND CATS

TREATABLE ABNORMALITY	CLINICAL CORRELATES	THERAPEUTIC OPTIONS*
Negative fluid balance	Dehydration Vomiting/diarrhea Polyuria/nocturia Adipsia Hypernatremia Hyperproteinemia	Unlimited access to water If vomiting or unwilling to drink, consider parenteral fluid administration
Undernutrition	Weight loss due to tissue loss Hypoalbuminemia Proteinuria Leukopenia	Provide balanced diet to minimize deficits and excesses in fluid, acid–base, electrolyte, calorie, and endocrine balance and to minimize production of metabolic wastes Minimize anorexia
Metabolic acidosis	Reduced serum concentrations of total CO_2 or HCO_3 Decreased blood pH	Dietary protein reduction Prescription Diet k/d, others Homemade diets Avoid diets producing acidic urine Sodium bicarbonate (10 mg/kg q 8–12 hr)† Potassium citrate (40–60 mg/kg q 12 hr)† (*caution:* may enhance intestinal absorption of aluminum, resulting in toxicity)
Hyperphosphatemia	Elevated serum phosphorus concentration Extraosseous mineralization Increased serum parathyroid hormone concentration Increased urinary fractional excretion of phosphorus Renal osteodystrophy	Correct dehydration Dietary protein reduction Prescription Diet k/d, others Homemade diets Intestinal phosphate-binding agents Aluminum hydroxide (30–90 mg/kg/day)† (*caution:* use with citrate salts may enhance intestinal absorption of aluminum resulting in toxicity) Calcium carbonate (100 mg/kg/day)† Others
Hypoproliferative anemia	Typically normocytic, normochromic anemia Pale mucous membranes Anorexia Weakness Depression	Minimize blood sampling Erythropoietin replacement Consider if hematocrit below 20 per cent Epogen (50–100 U/kg three times/wk); increase dose interval when hematocrit > 35 per cent Androgen therapy (?) Decanandrolin (1–1.5 mg/kg/wk); double dose if no response in 3 months
Systemic hypertension	Increased arterial blood pressure Retinal lesions (hemorrhage, detachment, others)	Gradual dietary sodium reduction Enalapril (0.25 mg/kg q 12–24 hr)† Diltiazem (7.5 mg q 8–12 hr)† Propranolol (0.3 to 1.0 mg/kg q 8–12 hr)† Others Combinations
Hypokalemic	Muscle weakness Ventral neck flexion in cats Decreased serum potassium concentration	Oral potassium supplementation Potassium gluconate (2–4 mEq q 8–12 hr)† Potassium citrate (40–60 mg/kg q 12 hr) Parenteral potassium supplementation
Hypernatremia	Elevated serum sodium concentration Dehydration Depression	Correct dehydration Proper use of sodium-containing medications

TABLE 16–12. THERAPEUTIC OPTIONS FOR THE MANAGEMENT OF RENAL FAILURE IN DOGS AND CATS *Continued*

TREATABLE ABNORMALITY	CLINICAL CORRELATES	THERAPEUTIC OPTIONS*
Hyperkalemia	Oliguria/anuria Weakness Muscle trembling Electrocardiographic abnormalities Spiked T waves Reduced P waves Bradycardia Prolonged PR interval	Correct dehydration with polyionic fluids containing reduced quantities of potassium Promote polyuria Avoid potassium supplementation
Hypocalcemia	Decreased serum calcium concentration Muscle twitching	Verify absolute hypocalcemia First correct hyperphosphatemia Oral calcium supplementation† Vitamin D therapy Calcitriol (1.5–3.5 ng/kg/day)†
Hypercalcemia	Increased serum calcium concentration Polydipsia/polyuria Weakness Anorexia	Correct dehydration Correct hyperphosphatemia Others
Urinary tract infection	Microburia Pyuria, hematuria, proteinuria Positive urine culture	Appropriate antimicrobial therapy Avoid nephrotoxic drugs (i.e., aminoglycosides, amphotericin B) Adjust dosage according to route of elimination and degree of renal dysfunction
Progression of renal failure	Progresive decrease in creatinine clearance Progressive increase of serum creatinine concentration Progressive increase in the magnitude of proteinuria	Eliminate underlying causes of renal failure Correct reversible components of renal failure Prerenal azotemia Postrenal azotemia Minimize iatrogenic renal damage Avoid nephrotoxic drugs Avoid unnecessary urinary catheterization Avoid unnecessary urinary system surgery Avoid unnecessary contrast radiographic procedures Dietary modification Provide only necessary quantities of high biologic value protein Minimize phosphorus Gradual calorie reduction Gradual sodium reduction Avoid saturated lipids Others Avoid diets producing acidic urine Minimize hypokalemia Control hypertension

*Management options should be instituted sequentially, and only if necessary.
†Values represent starting dose and should be adjusted on the basis of laboratory and clinical response.

TABLE 16–13. THERAPY-SPECIFIC DATA BASE FOR MONITORING RENAL FAILURE

I. Minimum Follow-up Data
  A. History checklist
    1. Diet: Type? Compliance? Frequency of feeding? Willingness to eat? Quantity consumed? Supplements?
    2. Water consumption: Increased? Decreased? No change? Unknown?
    3. Micturition: Frequency? Quantity? Color? Odor?
    4. Amelioration of polysystemic signs
      a. Anorexia?
      b. Vomiting?
      c. Diarrhea?
      d. Weight loss?
      e. Constipation?
      f. Others?
    5. Medication history: Medications given? When given? Dosage? Compliance? Response?
  B. Physical examination checklist
    1. Temperature, pulse, and respiratory rate?
    2. Amelioration of clinical signs
      a. Dehydration?
      b. Gastrointestinal signs: Mucosal ulcers? Discoloration of tongue?
      c. Cardiovascular signs
        (1) Pale mucous membrane color?
        (2) Abnormal pulse rate and character?
        (3) Delayed capillary refill time?
        (4) Venous distention?
        (5) Elevated arterial blood pressure?
      d. Abnormal kidney size, shape, consistency, contour, pain?
  C. Laboratory data checklist
    1. Urinalysis
    2. Kidney function tests (serum creatinine and urea nitrogen)
    3. Hematocrit, total plasma protein concentration (CBC?)

II. Problem-Specific Considerations
  A. Urinary tract infection: Quantitative urine culture
  B. Protein-losing glomerulonephropathy
    1. Urine protein-to-creatinine ratio
    2. Serum albumin concentration
  C. Obstructive uropathy: Ultrasonography or contrast radiography (intravenous urography, cystography, etc.) to verify continued patency of urinary tract
  D. Divalent ion disorders
    1. Serum concentrations of phosphorus, calcium, parathyroid hormone (?), and 1,25-vitamin D (?)
    2. Evaluate for signs of osteodystrophy
      a. Loose or missing teeth?
      b. Enlargement of maxillary tissue?
      c. "Rubber jaw"?
  E. Acidosis: Serum concentrations of total CO_2, HCO_3, and hydrogen ion (pH)
  F. Anemia
    1. Hematocrit
    2. Total plasma protein concentration
  G. Hypertension
    1. Arterial blood pressure
    2. Ophthalmoscopic examination for retinopathies: Detachment? Hemorrhage? Others?
  H. Potassium disorders
    1. Serum concentration of potassium
    2. Evaluate for signs of hypokalemia
      a. Muscle weakness
      b. Renal concentration
    3. Evaluate for signs of hyperkalemia
      a. Auscultate heart rate and rhythm
      b. Electrocardiogram

urinary catheter; urine production should match fluid administration. Body weight should also be monitored. Increasing body weight may indicate fluid retention, whereas decreasing body weight may indicate dehydration. If an animal is producing less urine than fluids being administered and is gaining weight, fluids can be reduced and the dosage of diuretic increased. On the other hand, if urine output is greater than fluid input and the animal is losing weight, fluids can be increased and the dosage of diuretic decreased.

After 12 to 24 hours of therapy, the animal's serum urea nitrogen, creatinine, sodium, potassium, and phosphorus concentrations should be re-evaluated. The magnitude of the animal's azotemia should progressively decrease as a result of use of this protocol. If the concentrations of serum urea nitrogen and creatinine are unchanged after 1 or 2 days of intensive diuresis, the animal is likely in end-stage renal failure. In

TABLE 16–14. OUTLINE OF INTENSIVE DIURESIS THERAPY FOR PATIENTS PRESENTING IN UREMIC CRISIS

1. Rehydrate with a balanced electrolyte solution in 4 to 6 hours.
2. Weigh animal after rehydration.
3. Place an indwelling catheter in the urinary bladder to monitor urine output.
4. Evaluate acid–base status.
5. Intravenously administer a fluid load equal to 3 to 5 per cent of the animal's body weight.
6. Administer a diuretic.
7. Administer two or three cycles of fluid load followed by diuretic every 24 hours.
8. Fluid input and urine output should be approximately equal.
9. Re-evaluate serum chemistry data every 24 hours while diuresing
10. Potassium levels should be maintained greater than 3 mEq/L.
11. When serum urea nitrogen and creatinine are stable, stop diuretic, slowly reduce fluids, and start feeding.

animals that respond to intensive diuresis, a point will be eventually reached at which diuresis will no longer reduce the magnitude of azotemia. The concentrations of serum urea nitrogen and creatinine at which this stabilization will occur depends on the magnitude of renal dysfunction. When the azotemia has stabilized, diuresis can be discontinued and the animal given maintenance quantities of fluid. Remember that maintenance fluid requirements for polyuric animals are higher than for normal animals. Until the animal is able to drink water, fluid input should match urine output. Body weight should continue to be monitored, and rates of fluid administration should be adjusted according to daily weight gains or losses. Maximal reduction of azotemia will usually occur within 2 to 4 days. By this time or shortly thereafter, the animal should be feeling better. As the patient's condition improves, subcutaneous fluids can be substituted for intravenous fluids, and oral fluids, medications, and food can be given. Parenteral fluids can be withdrawn when the animal can maintain hydration. Conservative therapy for renal failure should then be initiated. If the animal is not improving after 2 to 4 days of diuresis, either it is in end-stage renal failure or there is an additional nonrenal abnormality contributing to the disease syndrome.

In many instances intensive diuresis is an unnecessarily aggressive form of therapy for uremia. If the uremia is not severe, diuresis induced with intravenously administered fluid alone given in an amount of 1.5 to 3 times the maintenance dose per day may be adequate. In other instances, diuresis induced by administering fluids subcutaneously may be sufficient to achieve the desired results. Care should be taken to ensure that the dog or cat can tolerate the amount of fluids administered. For dogs and cats with concomitant heart failure, fluids should be given at a slower rate, and the animal should be monitored more closely for fluid overload. In general, replacement fluids are used for diuresis. These fluids contain relatively little potassium, and therefore, diuresis can rapidly deplete serum potassium levels. For this reason, serum potassium concentration should be monitored and maintained above 3 mEq/L. Potassium chloride can be added to intravenously administered fluids, but the rate of potassium administration should not exceed 0.5 mEq/kg/hour.

The acid–base status of dogs and cats in uremic crisis should also be evaluated. Blood gas determinations should be performed, if possible. If blood gas determinations are not possible, urine pH can provide indirect evidence of acid–base status. Urine pH should be maintained between 6 and 7. Often rehydration alone will significantly correct metabolic acidosis. Therefore, except in cases of severe acidosis, the clinician should rehydrate the animal and then determine whether bicarbonate therapy is necessary. Bicarbonate replacement can be calculated from the following formula:

Bicarbonate replacement (mEq) = body weight (kg) $\times$ 0.3 $\times$ (25 $-$ patient's plasma HCO_3 concentration).

This formula can be used if plasma bicarbonate concentration data are available. If plasma bicarbonate levels are not available, bicarbonate replacement can be determined by estimating the severity of acidosis. Mild acidosis can be treated with 1.5 mEq of bicarbonate per kilogram body weight; moderate acidosis, with 3.0 mEq bicarbonate per kilogram body weight; and severe acidosis, with 4.5 mEq bicarbonate per kilogram body weight. Regardless of how bicarbonate supplementation is determined, half of the calculated dosage should be given as a bolus over 5 minutes, with the rest placed in the patient's fluids and administered over 6 hours. After bicarbonate therapy, the animal's acid–base status should be re-evaluated before additional bicarbonate therapy is administered.

Conservative Treatment of Chronic Renal Failure

Chronic renal failure in dogs and cats is often an idiopathic, irreversible, and progressive disorder. The irreversible nature of the disorder makes it impossible to abate the damage that has already occurred. In most instances, specific therapy for the disorder cannot be given because of difficulty in identifying a treatable cause. However, conservative therapy aimed at ameliorating the consequences of renal dysfunction is possible. Conservative therapy for chronic renal failure, therefore, is aimed at slowing the progression of failure and minimizing the polysystemic, metabolic, biochemical, endocrine, and nutritional abnormalities seen in uremia (see Table 16–2) (DiBartola and Chew, 1986). Conservative therapy is conservative (1) for the veterinarian, as it is easy to implement and monitor for effectiveness; (2) for the owner, because it requires very little time or extra effort to accomplish; and (3) for the dog or cat, because it is not stressful and affects their everyday life very little. However, appropriate caution must be taken when prescribing medications for patients in renal failure (Tables 16–15 and 16–16).

Recommendations for treatment of mild to moderate chronic renal failure that is specifically aimed at delaying the progression of chronic renal failure include reduction of dietary protein and control of hypertension, hyperphosphatemia, and acidosis. The diets of dogs and cats in renal failure should contain reduced quantities of high-quality protein. Commercial and homemade renal failure diets for cats should provide approximately 20 per cent protein calories and approximately 3.3 to 3.5 g of protein/kg/day. The diet should also provide 70 to 80 kcal/kg/day. Energy requirements should be calculated with only non-protein components (supplied as carbohydrate and fat) of the diet. Cats have unique vitamin and mineral requirements, and before a homemade diet is instituted, the current literature should be consulted to be sure the recommendations will provide an adequately balanced diet for the cat.

The precise timing for initiation of protein restriction in renal failure remains a matter of personal opinion. Some believe that every dog and cat should eat less protein regardless of their level of renal function, and that restriction should be instituted at the first sign of renal disease. Others believe that protein restriction should not be started until the dog or cat develops signs of uremia. A moderate approach would be to institute protein restriction when urine-concentrating capacity becomes impaired or when fractional urinary excretion of phosphorus is elevated. The clinician should strive to keep serum urea nitrogen levels below 30 mg/dl. If the underlying disease is progressive, azotemia and hyperphosphatemia will eventually occur, despite dietary modification. Dietary protein should not be restricted to the degree that protein malnutrition will likely occur. A checklist of factors that may minimize uremic anorexia is presented in Table 16–17.

Hypertension is a complicating factor of renal failure in dogs and cats with renal failure. Hypertension will damage glomerular vascular endothelium, resulting in leakage of albumin and other serum protein into the glomerular space. Protein outside the vascular system is irritating to the glomerulus, induces inflammation, and eventually causes the destruction of the glomerulus and connecting tubule. Therefore, it is important to identify and treat dogs and cats with renal failure–associated hypertension. Hypertension associated with chronic renal failure is usually first treated by moderately reducing dietary sodium intake. The failing kidney requires time to adjust to reduced sodium intake. Based on this logic, low-sodium food is usually introduced slowly into the diet of dogs and cats with renal failure. This can be accomplished by adding salt to the diet and then withdrawing the added salt over 2 to 4 weeks. Adaptation can also be performed by mixing the low-sodium food with regular maintenance food, which usually has high salt levels. The regular food is then withdrawn over 2 to 4

TABLE 16–15. SOME COMMON DRUGS THAT SHOULD GENERALLY BE AVOIDED IN PATIENTS WITH RENAL FAILURE

1. Prophylactic antimicrobial agents (unless there is need for urinary tract catheterization)
2. Catabolic drugs
   a. Glucocorticoids
   b. Antineoplastic agents
   c. Tetracycline (?)
3. Nonsteroidal anti-inflammatory agents (especially if fluid volume is depleted)
4. Urine acidifiers
   a. Ammonium chloride
   b. Methionine
   c. Others
5. Urinary antiseptic agents
   a. Methenamine mandelate
   b. Nalidixic acid
6. Magnesium and phosphorus-containing antacids
7. Nephrotoxic drugs
   a. Aminoglycoside antimicrobials
   b. Amphotericin B
   c. Cisplatin

TABLE 16–16. RISK FACTORS THAT MAY PREDISPOSE GERIATRIC PATIENTS TO ADVERSE DRUG EVENTS

1. Decline in function of various organs and systems associated with aging.
2. Increased likelihood of multiple diseases affecting more than one organ or body system.
3. Altered absorption, distribution, biotransformation, and excretion of drugs
   a. Reduced renal clearance
   b. Potential for reduced hepatic biotransformation and clearance
   c. Decreased binding of some drugs to protein
   d. Altered distribution of drugs associated with
      (1) Reduced total body water
         (a) Reduced thirst
         (b) Impaired urine concentration
      (2) Reduced muscle mass and increased body fat
4. Greater likelihood of exposure to
   a. Multiple drugs
   b. Nephrotoxic drugs

Modified from Aucoin DP. Drug therapy in the geriatric animal. Vet Clin North Am 19:41, 1989.

TABLE 16–17. CHECKLIST OF FACTORS THAT MAY MINIMIZE UREMIC ANOREXIA

1. Correct underlying abnormalities: minimize deficits and excesses in
   a. Fluid balance
   b. Serum concentrations of nitrogenous wastes
   c. Serum electrolyte concentrations
      (1) Potassium
      (2) Sodium
      (3) Calcium
      (4) Phosphorus
   d. Serum hydrogen ion concentration
   e. Serum concentrations of hormones
      (1) Parathyroid hormone
      (2) Erythropoietin
      (3) Vitamin D
      (4) Angiotensin
      (5) Renin
   f. Others
2. Enhance palatability of diet
   a. When changing diet
      (1) Switch food gradually
      (2) Maintain texture and flavor similar to usual diet
   b. Try flavoring agents
      1. Clam juice
      2. Tuna juice
      3. Chicken broth
      4. Water
      5. Liquid elemental diets (Feline Renal Care [Pet-Ag], Impact {Sandoz Nutrition] with taurine added, or Ensure [Ross Laboratories] with taurine added)
      6. Garlic
      7. Brewer's yeast
      8. Carnitine (?)
   c. Warm food to body temperature
3. Modify feeding patterns
   a. Emphasize frequent small meals
   b. Offer rewards
      (1) Favorite foods
      (2) Maintenance foods
   c. Hand feed
   d. Avoid adverse associations with eating
      (1) Medications
      (2) Injections
      (3) Others
   e. Prevent food aversion: Do not offer diets designed for long-term management of renal failure during periods of nausea and vomiting
4. Minimize vomiting
   a. Correct underlying abnormalities (see factor 1, above)
   b. Pharmacologic antiemetics
      1. Metoclopramide (0.25–0.5 mg/kg q 12 hr)
      2. Cimetidine (2.5–5 mg/kg q 12 hr)
5. Implement pharmacologic appetite stimulation
   a. Diazepam (0.2–0.3 mg/kg q 12 hr)
   b. Oxazepam (0.2–0.4 mg/kg q 24 hr)
   c. Cyproheptadine (2–4 mg/kg q 24 hr)
   d. Propofol
   e. B vitamins
   f. Anabolic agents
6. Enteral feeding
   a. Hand feeding
   b. Nasogastric tube feeding

weeks. Some drugs that have been recommended for treatment of hypertension in dogs and cats include diuretics, vasodilators, calcium channel blockers, and ACE inhibitors.

Another therapeutic modality recommended for slowing the progression of renal failure is to reduce serum phosphorus concentrations to the normal range. Most of the phosphorus in diets is found in the protein component. Hyperphosphatemia, therefore, is controlled by restricting dietary protein. Phosphorus should be restricted in any dog or cat in renal failure that has elevated serum phosphorus levels and/or elevated fractional urinary excretion of phosphorus. Phosphorus may be restricted if the fractional urinary phosphorus excretion exceeds 30 per cent (Wiseman et al, 1987). Serum phosphorus levels should be kept in the normal range (3.0 to 6.0 mg/dl). Phosphate-binding antacids have been advocated to reduce serum phosphorus levels, but unfortunately, they are generally not palatable to cats and may induce anorexia and constipation. Therefore, oral phosphate-binding agents should be used only after efforts have been made to reduce hyperphosphatemia by maintaining adequate hydration and by modifying the diet.

Other recommendations are aimed at ameliorating the signs of uremia (see Table 16–14). These recommendations include restriction of dietary protein, providing an unlimited supply of water, avoidance of stress, supplementation of water-soluble vitamins, treatment of acidosis with sodium bicarbonate or potassium citrate, using recombinant erythropoietin to promote red blood cell formation, and control of hypocalcemia. Nonrenal disease conditions superimposed on chronic renal failure can have devastating consequences. Therefore, dogs and cats in renal failure should not be allowed to roam unsupervised out of the owner's house, and environmental stresses, including visits to the veterinarian and hospitalization, should be minimized. Dogs and cats in renal failure cannot conserve water-soluble vitamins, and therefore, vitamins B and C should be supplemented in their diets. The precise requirements of these vitamins have not been determined for cats in renal failure, although requirements for normal cats are approximately six to eight times greater than the normal requirement for dogs.

Oral sodium bicarbonate or potassium citrate may be used to treat severe acidosis. In general, bicarbonate supplementation should not be instituted until plasma bicarbonate levels are below approximately 18 mEq/L or urine pH drops below 6. Alkalosis should not be induced. The empirically established dosage for bicarbonate supplementation is 8 to 10 mg/kg q 12 hours. Bicarbonate usually is supplied as sodium bicarbonate and therefore should be used with caution in hypertensive dogs and cats. The recommended starting dosage of potassium citrate is 40 to 60 mg/kg every 8 to 12 hours. Dosage of sodium bicarbonate and potassium citrate should be titrated by evaluating blood bicarbonate or serum TCO_2 concentrations.

Anabolic agents have been advocated to treat the nonregenerative anemia that accompanies chronic renal failure, but there is no evidence that such agents are effective. We do not recommend the use of anabolic agents. Recombinant human erythropoietin is effective in correcting this anemia, but because dogs and cats develop antierythropoietin antibodies, leading to severe anemias despite administration of recombinant human erythropoietin, we generally do not consider use of this drug until the packed cell volume falls below 20 per cent.

Hypocalcemia is treated by restricting dietary phosphorus and reducing serum phosphorus concentration. Severe clinical hypocalcemia may be treated with calcium and administration of 1,25-vitamin D (calcitriol) (see Table 16–12). Clinical hypocalcemia is often a late sign of uremia and therefore is usually associated with a grave patient prognosis. Dosages of calcium and vitamin D supplements should be standardized for each dog or cat. Caution must be used so as not to induce hypercalcemia. The 1,25-vitamin D (calcitriol) should not be given until the serum phosphorus concentration is reduced to 6 mg/dl or less. Correction of hypocalcemia without reducing the magnitude of hyperphosphatemia may result in mineralization of tissue with calcium phosphate.

References and Supplemental Reading

August JR, Leib MS. Primary renal diseases of the cat. Vet Clin North Am 14:1247, 1984.

Brenner BM, Meyer TW, Hostetter TH. Dietary protein intake and the progressive nature of kidney disease: The role of hemodynamically mediated glomerular injury in the pathogenesis of progressive glomerular sclerosis in aging, renal ablation and intrinsic renal disease. N Engl J Med 307:652, 1982.

Burnie AG, Weaver AD. Urinary bladder neoplasia in the dog: A review of seventy cases. J Small Anim Pract 24:129, 1983.

Chew DJ, DiBartola SP. Feline renal amyloidosis. In Kirk RW, ed. Current Veterinary Therapy VIII. Philadelphia, WB Saunders, 1983, p 976.

Chew DJ, DiBartola SP, Boyce JT, et al. Renal amyloidosis in related Abyssinian cats. J Am Vet Med Assoc 181:139, 1982.

Cowgill LD. Diseases of the kidney. In Ettinger SJ, ed. Textbook of Veterinary Internal Medicine. Vol 2, 2nd ed. Philadelphia, WB Saunders, 1983, p 1793.

Cowgill LD, Kallet AJ. Recognition and management of hypertension in the dog. In Kirk RW, ed. Current Veterinary Therapy VIII. Philadelphia, WB Saunders, 1983, p 1025.

Cowgill LD, Spangler WL. Renal insufficiency in geriatric dogs. Vet Clin North Am 11:727, 1981.

Crow SE, Klausner JS. Management of transitional cell carcinomas of the urinary bladder. In Kirk RW, ed. Current Veterinary Therapy VIII. Philadelphia, WB Saunders, 1983, p 1119.

DiBartola SP, Adams WM. Urinary incontinence associated with malposition of the urinary bladder. In Kirk RW, ed. Current Veterinary Therapy VIII. Philadelphia, WB Saunders, 1983, p 1089.

DiBartola SP, Chew DJ. Glomerular disease in the dog and cat. In Kirk RW, ed. Current Veterinary Therapy IX. Philadelphia, WB Saunders, 1986, p 1132.

DiBartola SP, Rutgers HC, Zack PM, et al. Clinicopathologic findings associated with chronic renal disease in cats: 74 cases (1973–1984). J Am Vet Med Assoc 190:1196, 1987.

Finco DR. The role of phosphorus restriction in the management of chronic renal failure in the dog and cat. In Seventh Annual Kal Kan Symposium for the Treatment of Small Animal Diseases. Vernon, CA, Kal Kan Foods, 1983, p. 131.

Finco DR, Barsanti JA. Treatment of mineral imbalances of chronic renal failure. In Kirk RW, ed. Current Veterinary Therapy VIII. Philadelphia, WB Saunders, 1983, p 1019.

Finco DR, Barsanti JA, Crowell WA. The urinary system. In Pratt PW, ed. Feline Medicine. Santa Barbara, CA, American Veterinary Publications, 1983, p 363.

Finco DR, Low DG. Intensive diuresis in polyuric renal failure. In Kirk RW, ed. Current Veterinary Therapy VII. Philadelphia, WB Saunders, 1980, p 1091.

Hardy RM. Disorders of water metabolism. Vet Clin North Am 12:353, 1982.

Hardy RM, Osborne CA. Water deprivation and vasopressin concentration tests in the differentiation of polyuric syndromes. In Kirk RW, ed. Current Veterinary Therapy VII. Philadelphia, WB Saunders, 1980, p 1080.

Hayes HM. Canine bladder cancer: Epidemiologic features. Am J Epidemiol 104:673, 1976.

Heeg JE, De Jong PE, Van Der Hem GK, et al. Reduction of proteinuria by angiotensin converting enzyme inhibition. Kidney Int 32:78, 1987.

Krawiec DR. Urinary incontinence in dogs and cats. Mod Vet Pract 69:17, 1988.

Krawiec DR. Diagnosis and treatment of acquired canine urinary incontinence. Comp Anim Pract 1:12, 1989.

Krawiec DR, Gelberg HB. Chronic renal disease in the cat. In Kirk RW, ed. Current Veterinary Therapy X. Philadelphia, WB Saunders, 1990, p 1170.

Lewis LD, Morris ML Jr, Hand MS. Small Animal Nutrition III. Topeka, KS, Mark Morris Associates, 1987.

Lulich JP, Osborne CA, Polzin DJ. Cystic disease of the kidney. In Osborne CA, Finco DR, eds. Canine and Feline Nephrology and Urology. Philadelphia, Lea & Febiger, in press.

Macy DW. Chemotherapeutic agents available for cancer treatment. In Kirk RW, ed. Current Veterinary Therapy IX. Philadelphia, WB Saunders, 1986, p 467.

Moreau PM. Neurogenic disorders of micturition in the dog and cat. Compend Contin Educ Pract Vet 4:12, 1982.

Osborne CA, Finco DR, Low DG. Pathophysiology of renal disease, renal failure and uremia. In Ettinger SJ, ed. Textbook of Veterinary Internal Medicine. Vol 2. 2nd ed. Philadelphia, WB Saunders, 1983, p 1733.

Osborne CA, Low DG, Perman V, et al. Neoplasms of the canine and feline urinary bladder: Incidence, etiologic factors, occurrence and pathologic features. Am J Vet Res 29:2041, 1968.

Osborne CA, Oliver JE, Polzin DE. Non-neurogenic urinary incontinence. In Kirk RW, ed. Current Veterinary Therapy VII. Philadelphia, WB Saunders, 1980, p 1128.

Osborne CA, Polzin DJ. Conservative medical management of feline chronic polyuric renal failure. In Kirk RW, ed. Current Veterinary Therapy VIII. Philadelphia, WB Saunders, 1983, p 1008.

Polzin DJ, Osborne CA. Conservative medical management of canine chronic polyuric renal failure. In Kirk RW, ed. Current Veterinary Therapy VIII. Philadelphia, WB Saunders, 1983, p 997.

Polzin DJ, Osborne CA. Update—conservative medical management of chronic renal failure. In Kirk RW, ed. Current Veterinary Therapy IX. Philadelphia, WB Saunders, 1986, p 1167.

Rosin AE, Barsanti JA. Diagnosis of urinary incontinence in dogs: Role of the urethral pressure profile. J Am Vet Med Assoc 178:814, 1981.

Ross LA. Assessment of renal function in the dog and cat. In Kirk RW, ed. Current Veterinary Therapy IX. Philadelphia, WB Saunders, 1986, p 1103.

Samiy AH. Renal disease in the elderly. Med Clin North Am 67:463, 1983.

Walter PA, Feeney DA, Johnston GR, et al. Ultrasonographic evaluation of renal parenchymal diseases in dogs: 32 cases (1981–1986). J Am Vet Med Assoc 191:999, 1987.

Wiseman MJ, Hunt R, Goodwin A, et al. Dietary composition and renal function in healthy subjects. Nephron 46:37, 1987.

CHAPTER 17

The Skeletal System

JACEK J. DE HAAN and BRIAN S. BEALE

Veterinarians and owners make continuous progress in the quality of medical care they provide to canine and feline pets. Great improvement in preventive medicine—vaccinations, heartworm prevention, dental care, and routine physical examinations and checkups—has resulted in increased life expectancy of these dogs and cats, but along with this longevity has come an increasing number of geriatric patients with age-related problems. The concurrent increased life expectancy in pets and in humans has brought about more sensitivity to the diseases that come with advanced age and, especially, to improving the quality of life for the aged.

Providing veterinary care to older pets is extremely important, because as the family's attachment to the pet grows over the years, so does the number of clinical problems that require increasing veterinary attention. Musculoskeletal diseases are very common in geriatric patients seen by veterinarians, and about 20 per cent of all aged dogs present with orthopedic problems (Reichenbach, 1989).

PHYSICAL EXAMINATION

Physical examination is the most important diagnostic tool available to all veterinarians dealing with musculoskeletal disorders. It is cost effective, it does not require sophisticated equipment, and it can lead to a diagnosis or a list of differential diagnoses and a diagnostic plan within a relatively short period of time. A correctly performed physical examination allows accurate diagnosing of many disorders and can make orthopedic surgery very rewarding.

For the physical examination to be successful, a systematic approach and a good understanding of all musculoskeletal diseases are essential. Orthopedic examination should start with the signalment, which should include the age, breed, and sex of the patient (Brinker et al, 1990; Newton, 1985; Whittick and Simpson, 1990). Many orthopedic disorders are seen only at a certain age, and the frequency of many of them is strongly affected by the breed of the animal.

Next, the patient's chief complaint should be determined. At this stage it is extremely important to distinguish between objective observations and subjective interpretations of the owner. In many cases, when asked about the chief complaint, the owner will answer, for example, that the dog has hip dysplasia. The owner's interpretation of the pet's clinical signs is not necessarily correct. In such a case, a correctly formulated complaint should be something like "lameness in both rear legs." This lameness can be caused not only by hip dysplasia, but also by a neurologic disorder, back pain, or a bilateral knee problem. An incorrect definition of the complaint will frequently lead to misdiagnosis.

The next step is to obtain the patient's history, which should include questions pertinent to the musculoskeletal system and primary complaint, as well as questions concerning the pet's environment, other past and present illnesses, surgeries, and treatments. It is essential to identify the manner of onset (acute or slow and progressive) and the duration of the clinical signs seen by the owner. In the case of lameness, the veterinarian must ask if the same extremity has always been involved, if the degree of lameness has changed over time, if rest or exercise changes clinical presentation, and if the symptoms change during the day. Owners' responses should be critically evaluated, because many slowly progressive disorders go unnoticed for a prolonged period of time and then are suddenly noticed at an advanced stage of the disease and assumed to be of acute origin. Most owners spend long hours with their pets. They walk and play with them and observe their daily activity. Many of them are able to notice even relatively small changes in the gait, behavior, and daily routine of their pets, so they can provide valuable information that can be helpful in arriving at the final diagnosis. It is sometimes difficult to distinguish between the owner's interpretation and the clinical signs themselves, but well-directed questions will usually help solve this problem. Questions about the daily routine of the pet should reveal, among other things, the animal's normal physical activity and whether the animal stays mostly outside or inside. Another consideration is whether there are other animals in the house. Also, the intended use of the animal may be important in advising the best treatment and giving long-term prognosis. For instance, recommendations for the treatment of degenerative joint disease in a 12-year-old poodle will be different from those for the treatment of the same disease in a young hunting dog. Before treating an animal, it is also necessary to know all previous treatments prescribed by other veterinarians or administered by the owner on the recommendation of breeders, friends, or others.

Before focusing on the physical examination of the musculoskeletal system, examination of all other body systems must be performed. Examination of the musculoskeletal system should start with observation of the animal standing and then at different gait speeds. The animal should be observed at rest for unequal weight bearing and abnormal conformation of the bones, joints, and muscles. Observation of walk and trot should allow the diagnosis of a lameness and the determination of the affected legs. Hypermetria, shortened stride, and any other gait abnormality should be noticed as well. In some cases of very subtle disorder, it may be necessary to exercise the animal to elicit lameness or pain. Walking the animal in tight circles or up and down stairs may be helpful in some cases.

Some neurologic disorders may result in signs suggestive of an orthopedic problem. While watching the gait of the animal, it is necessary to distinguish between ataxia resulting from neurologic disorders and musculoskeletal lameness. Conscious proprioception should be tested in the front and rear legs in all examined animals. If there is any suspicion of a neurologic disorder, a full neurologic examination should be performed.

A "hands-on" orthopedic examination should start with the animal standing. The animal's limbs should be assessed for any asymmetry in size, shape, heat, and sensitivity. The rear legs are examined with the veterinarian behind the animal, and the front legs are examined with the veterinarian in front of the animal. Attention should be placed on the neck and back, followed by a thorough examination of all four limbs. The examination should start proximally and slowly progress in the distal direction. All joints should be assessed for changes in size and shape, as well as in temperature and sensitivity to touch. Joint effusion and periarticular changes resulting in increased joint size should be noticed at that time.

Manipulation of all joints should be performed with the animal in lateral recumbency. The examined limb should be uppermost. When manipulating joints it is important to isolate a single joint to prevent misdiagnosis owing to pain elicited from an adjacent joint. Joint manipulation should include assessment of the normal range of motion, response to hyperextension or hyperflexion of the joint, and stability of the ligaments supporting the joint. During manipulation, crepitus, abnormal noises, and other pathologic responses should be noted. Examination of the stifle joint should include evaluation for cranial cruciate ligament rupture and for patellar luxation. The hip joint must be evaluated for laxity of the joint capsule. This evaluation can be performed by attempting to induce Bardens' and Ortolani's signs. If there are doubts about what is normal for the patient, then comparison with the opposite leg can be attempted.

Because of pain, some animals will resist physical examination and make it virtually impossible. In such cases sedation or sometimes even general anesthesia may be required to make complete manipulation of all joints possible. It is important to realize that by sedating or anesthetizing an animal, the veterinarian may lose some valuable information on reactions of the patient to manipulation of the joints.

Physical examination can be facilitated by use

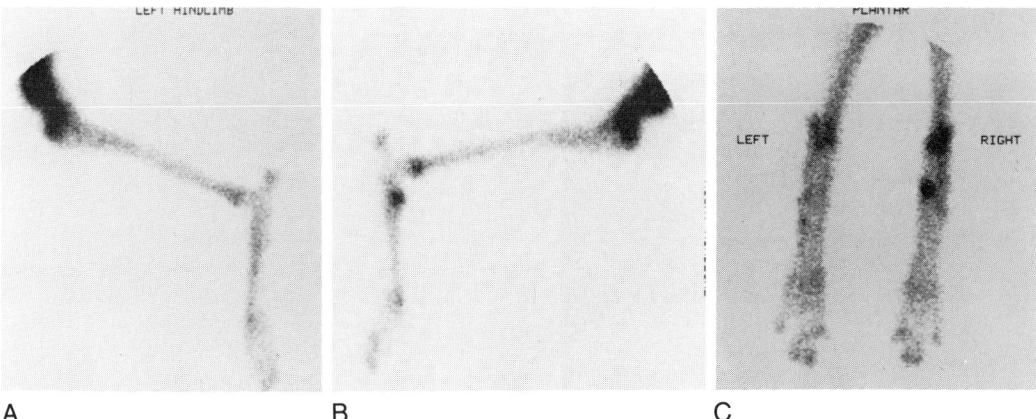

Figure 17–1. Lateral bone scans of the left (*A*) and right (*B*) hindlimbs and a craniocaudal bone scan of both hindlimbs (*C*). Focally increased uptake is identified in the right distal tibia and the medial aspect of the right distal tarsus. The left hindlimb is normal.

of a measuring tape and goniometer. Both instruments are very inexpensive, easy to use, and allow more objective measurement and recording of the examination findings. A goniometer can be used to measure normal standing angles and range of motion of all joints. A measuring tape is useful in objective assessment of muscle mass. Leg circumference can be measured at specific locations during the first examination and later at follow-up examinations to more objectively assess progression of the disease. Where available, the additional use of force plate analysis is helpful.

Other diagnostic procedures commonly performed in orthopedic patients include radiographs and joint taps. In addition, if systemic disease is suspected, a complete blood cell count, biochemistry profile, and urinalysis are indicated. Other diagnostic procedures available at some large referral centers include bone scintigraphy (Fig. 17–1), computerized tomography, magnetic resonance imaging, and arthroscopy.

DISORDERS OF DOGS

Degenerative Joint Disease

Geriatric dogs may have many orthopedic diseases affecting their quality of life. The most common is degenerative joint disease, a noninflammatory disorder of the joints that results in deterioration of the hyaline articular cartilage and other articular components. Other terms commonly used to describe degenerative joint disease are *arthrosis* and *osteoarthrosis*. HOWEVER, the term *osteoarthritis* is misleading and should not be used, because it implies the presence of an inflammatory condition.

Routine radiographic examination of older dogs often reveals evidence of degenerative joint disease. In many cases multiple joints are involved, with the hip joint being the most commonly affected. In older dogs the degenerative joint disease is usually an incidental observation, unrelated to the main clinical problem (Olsewski et al, 1983). Degenerative joint disease may be primary or secondary in origin (Alexander, 1980). Primary degenerative joint disease is a result of the aging process and the normal wear and tear of the articular cartilage, without any extra-articular inciting cause. The diagnosis of primary degenerative joint disease is made when no cause for the disorder can be found. Secondary degenerative joint disease, which is much more common, can be caused by a developmental disease, such as hip dysplasia (Fig. 17–2), osteochondritis dissecans (Fig. 17–3), or a fragmented coronoid process in the elbow (Fig. 17–4). Secondary degenerative joint disease may also be the result of an acquired, traumatic injury such as cranial cruciate ligament rupture (Fig. 17–5), an intra-articular fracture (Fig. 17–6), or an injury to one of the growth plates that results in growth deformity and abnormal use of the joints (Vaughan, 1990; Alexander, 1984). Because of the nonspecific joint changes in some dogs, it is sometimes very difficult or even impossible to distinguish between primary and secondary degenerative joint disease (Fig. 17–7).

Primary Degenerative Joint Disease

Aging results in degenerative changes in articular cartilage. The aging process changes the biochemical, histologic, and mechanical properties of the cartilage (Miles and Eichelberger, 1964;

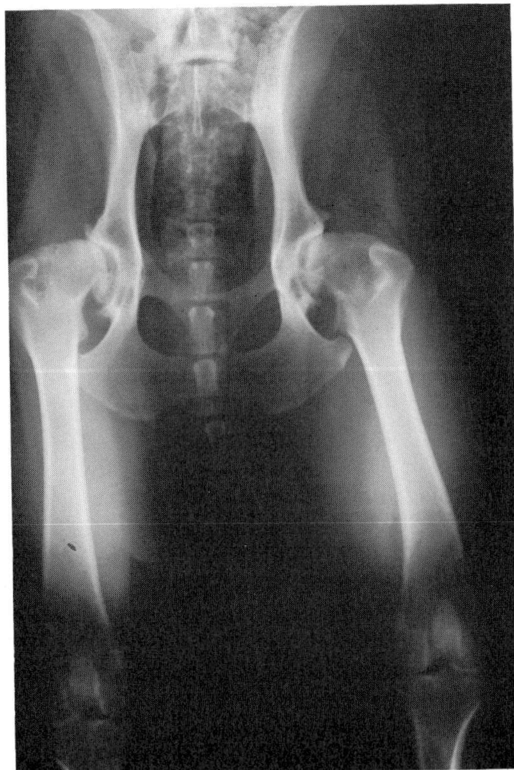

Figure 17–2. Ventrodorsal radiograph of the pelvis of a dog with severe hip dysplasia.

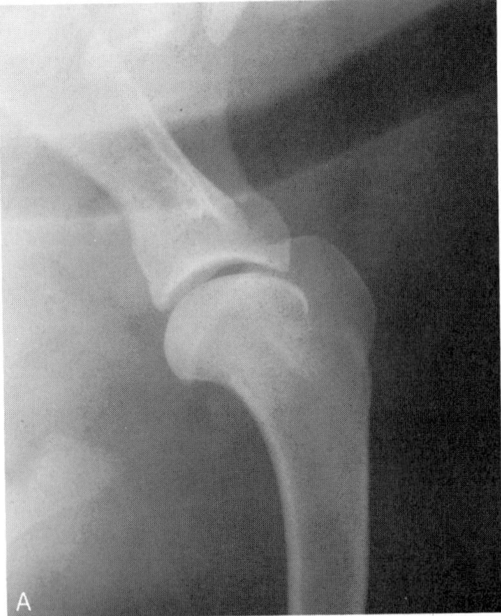

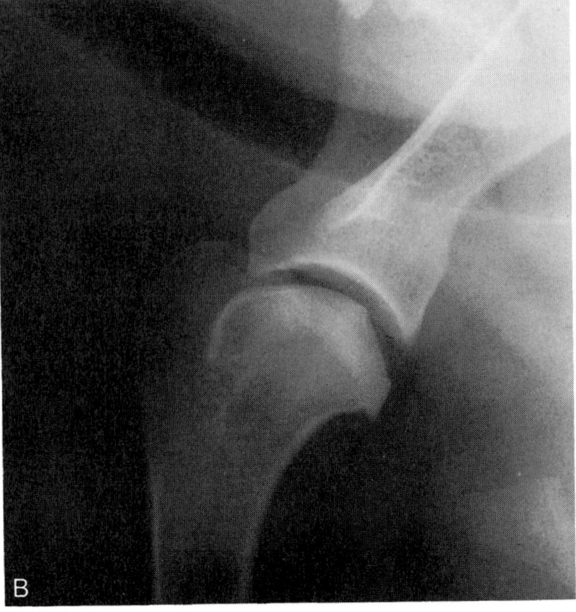

Figure 17–3. Lateral radiographs of the left (*A*) and right (*B*) shoulder of a dog. Osteochondritis dissecans and degenerative joint disease are visible in the right shoulder. The left shoulder is normal.

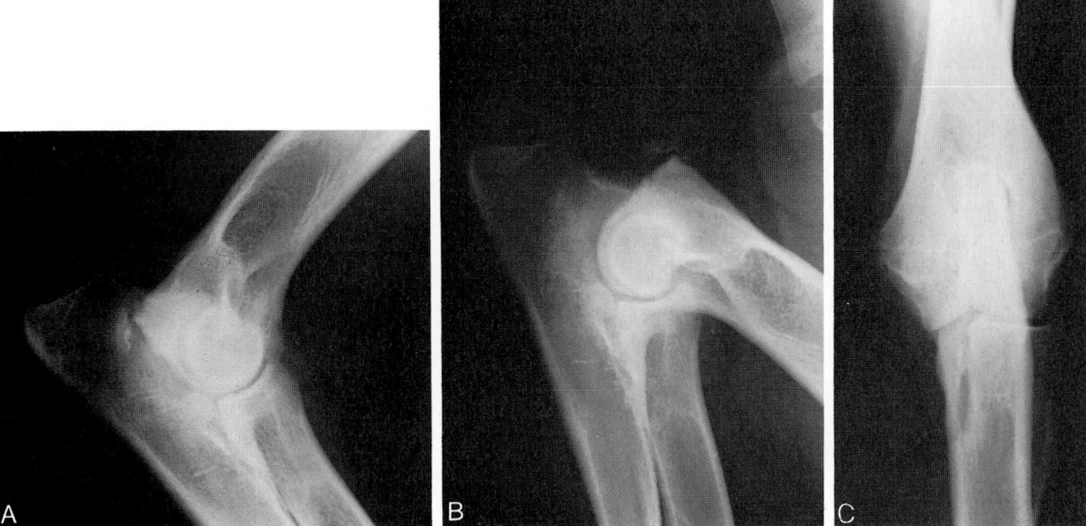

Figure 17–4. Lateral (*A*), lateral flexed (*B*), and craniocaudal (*C*) radiographs of the elbow of a dog. Degenerative joint disease consistent with the diagnosis of a fragmented medial coronoid process is present.

Clark, 1991a). During the normal aging of canine articular cartilage, the amount of proteoglycans decreases. In addition, proteoglycans become smaller, their glycosaminoglycan ratio changes, and they acquire higher keratan sulfate and lower chondroitin sulfate content (Inerot et al, 1978). As proteoglycan size and content decrease, articular cartilage loses its viscoelastic properties and becomes more susceptible to damage.

A large survey of canine stifle joints in 150 cadavers revealed that 20 per cent of the dogs had degenerative joint disease of at least one of the stifles, and 60 per cent of the affected stifles had primary degenerative joint disease (Tirgari and Vaughan, 1975). The average age of the 150 dogs was 9.6 years, and the aging process was probably involved in the cause of the primary degenerative joint disease. During the same survey, the authors also encountered 12 dogs with primary shoulder degenerative joint disease (Tirgari and Vaughan, 1973). In all cases the abnormality was bilateral. Because the average age of the dogs was 11 years and there was no known underlying disease, the changes were most likely age related. This survey demonstrates the high frequency of primary degenerative joint disease in geriatric dogs.

Dogs with primary degenerative joint disease present with a history of chronic progressive lameness. Most of the patients have a stiff, short

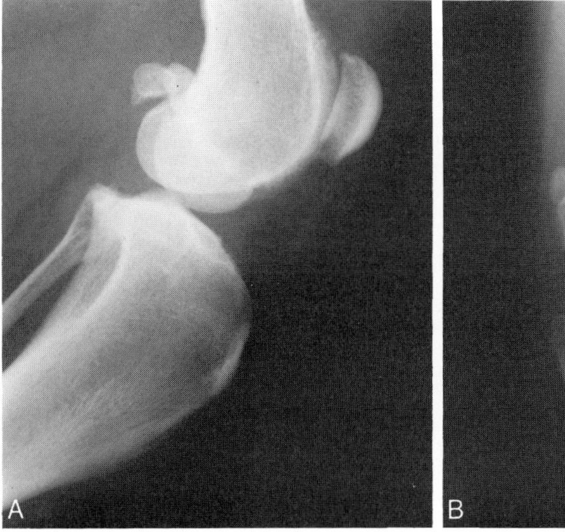

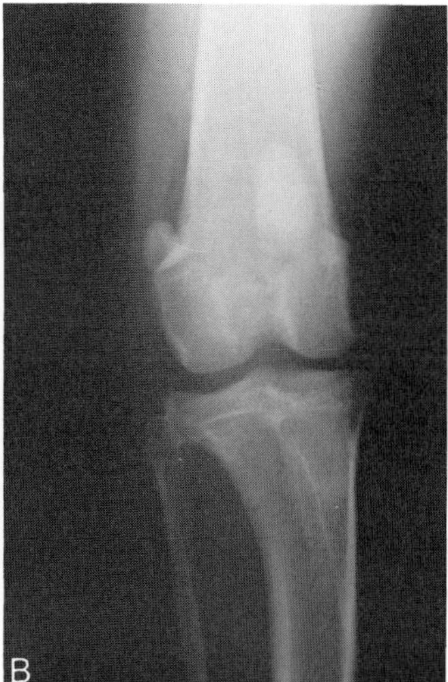

Figure 17–5. Lateral (*A*) and craniocaudal (*B*) radiographs of the left stifle of a dog. Degenerative joint disease and a moderate amount of joint effusion are visible.

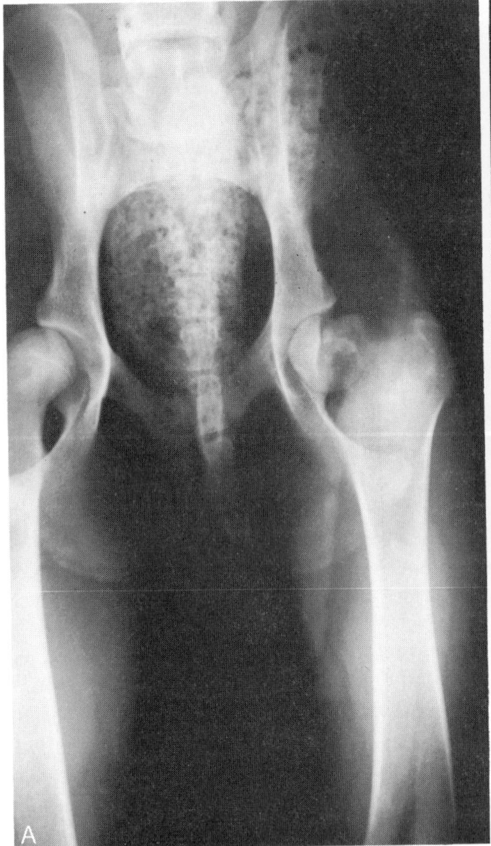

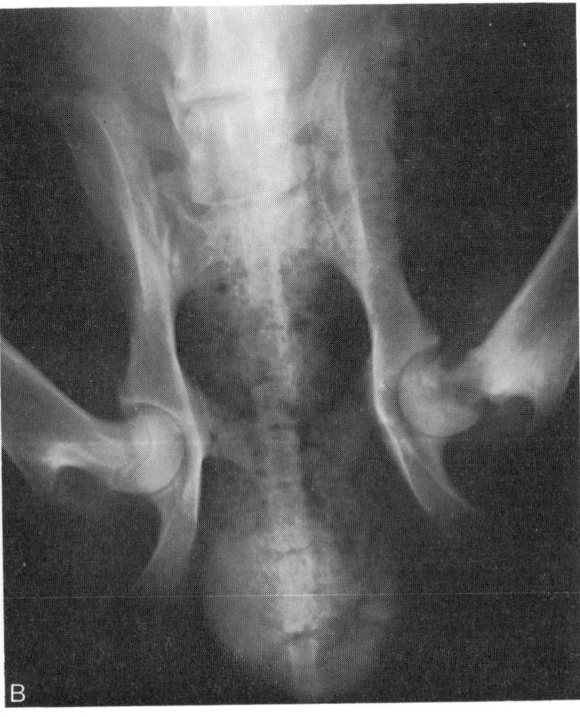

Figure 17–6. Extended (*A*) and flexed (*B*) ventrodorsal radiographs of both hips of a young dog. An old femoral capital epiphyseal fracture with resorption of bone of the left femoral neck is present.

Figure 17–7. Lateral radiograph of the tarsus of a dog demonstrating soft tissue swelling and severe degenerative joint disease.

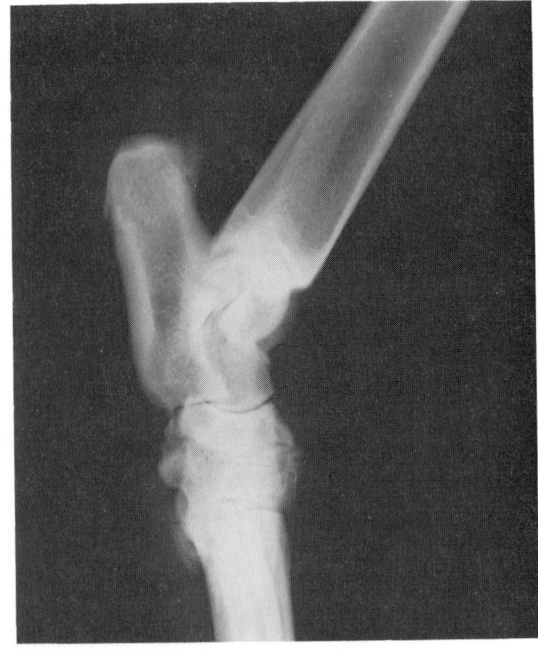

gait, especially in the morning. Usually they can warm out of the lameness during the day. Many dogs exhibit decreased function; for instance, they are reluctant to climb stairs or to jump into the car. The lameness can be aggravated after long exercise, and owners may notice acute worsening of signs after increased activity (Alexander, 1984; Vaughan, 1990). Bilateral disease involving the hip or stifle may be misinterpreted by the owner or the veterinarian as a back problem. Physical examination of the affected joint will reveal decreased range of motion, enlargement of the joint owing to thickening of the joint capsule and periarticular osteophytes, pain and crepitation on flexion and extension, and some degree of joint effusion. Usually there will also be muscle atrophy in the affected extremity (Alexander, 1984; Vaughan, 1990).

Radiographic examination is indicated to confirm the diagnosis and to rule out neoplasia, septic or immune-mediated arthritis, and other less common diseases. The most frequent radiographic changes seen with degenerative joint disease include periarticular osteophytes, subchondral bone sclerosis, joint effusion, and thickening of the periarticular soft tissues. Some animals show arthritic changes on survey radiographs without any clinical signs of disease (Farrow, 1984). Occasionally the diagnosis is questionable, and in such cases arthrocentesis, cell count, and cytologic examination and culture of the synovial fluid should be performed. Synovial fluid changes seen with degenerative joint disease usually include a mild increase in leukocyte count, with the predominant cell being mononuclear.

The goal of treating dogs with degenerative joint disease is to relieve the pain, provide them with good quality of life, and return them to functional status. The owner must understand that there is no cure for degenerative joint disease and that in most cases treatment is continued for the life of the pet. The treatment usually consists of one or more of the following: weight reduction, exercise modification, and medication (Clark, 1991b). If the response to the conservative management is insufficient, surgery can be considered (Table 17–1).

The most important first step is maintaining a lean body weight; weight reduction for overweight dogs is essential. Every pound of excess weight increases both the stress on the joints and the wear and tear of the cartilage, worsening the clinical signs and accelerating the progression of the disease. Obesity alone tends to limit the physical activity of the patients, eventually resulting in muscle atrophy and less support provided by the muscles to the joints. The weight reduction program is often very difficult to implement owing to owner noncompliance. Also, some breed standards inadvertently favor heavily built (overweight) dogs. It is not enough to tell the owner that the dog needs to lose weight; the veterinarian must present a well-designed weight reduction program. These programs should include an optimal body weight goal and a timetable to achieve it, weekly rechecks of the body weight, diet modification, and instructions concerning the total caloric intake. To achieve weight reduction, dogs should be fed 60 per cent of the calories required to maintain the desired body weight (Lewis et al, 1987).

TABLE 17–1. TREATMENT OF PRIMARY DEGENERATIVE JOINT DISEASE

Conservative Management
Weight reduction
Exercise modification
Medical treatment
Nonsteroidal anti-inflammatory drugs
Glucocorticosteroids
Polysulfated glycosaminoglycans
Surgical Management
Arthrodesis
Excision arthroplasty
Total joint replacement

The second important step in patient management is exercise modification. Dogs with degenerative joint disease must keep their physical activity below the level that results in aggravation of clinical signs. Owners should eliminate activities that result in increased pain or stiff gait the following day. All unusual peak activity, such as long Sunday morning walks, should be discontinued. During the course of the day, dogs with degenerative joint disease need several short periods of light to moderate activity. Non–weight-bearing forms of exercise, such as swimming, are particularly useful to preserve muscle tone while sparing joint surfaces. The exercise program must be adjusted, based on its results, to each individual dog. Many dogs with degenerative joint disease improve sufficiently with weight reduction and exercise modification so that they do not require any additional measures.

Medical treatment of degenerative joint disease consists usually of nonsteroidal anti-inflammatory drugs. The first choice for treatment of dogs is aspirin (acetylsalicylic acid) at a dose of up to 25 mg/kg orally, three times daily. Side effects of aspirin include gastrointestinal ulceration and impaired platelet function. The owner should be warned about the possible complications and should return if the dog exhibits any sign of vomiting, gastrointestinal blood loss, or other bleeding problems. To decrease gastrointestinal side effects, buffered forms of aspirin may be used. Another commonly used nonsteroidal anti-inflammatory drug is phenylbutazone in a recommended dosage of 1 mg/kg three times daily. The potential side effects include gastrointestinal ulceration, bone marrow suppression, and nephrotoxicity.

A large number of other nonsteroidal anti-inflammatory drugs approved for use in humans are currently on the market, and although it is tempting to use them in dogs, so far there is no evidence that they are more effective than aspirin in relieving clinical signs of degenerative joint disease in animals. These drugs are not approved by the Food and Drug Administration for use in dogs, so veterinarians should be extremely cautious administering or prescribing them to their patients.

Another group of drugs commonly used for treatment of degenerative joint disease is the glucocorticosteroids, very potent anti-inflammatory drugs. Their administration results in reduction of clinical signs and improved function of the patient. However, the short-term improvement is overshadowed by the side effects, especially with chronic use. These include polydipsia; polyuria; increased appetite, which can lead to weight gain; loss of proteoglycans; and destruction of the joint cartilage; in addition, catabolic side effects can lead to a decrease in muscle mass and weakening of the tendons and ligaments. Many dogs treated long term with glucocorticosteroids suffer cranial cruciate ligament rupture or hyperextension injuries of the carpus or tarsus. Because of these effects, glucocorticosteroids should be used only short term and only orally to relieve acute aggravation of the clinical signs. They are a last-resort treatment, and if administered, they should be given on alternate days and at the smallest effective dose. Prednisone can be started at a dosage of 0.5 to 1 mg/kg once a day, but the dosage should be decreased as soon as desired clinical response is achieved. Before administration of glucocorticosteroids, the veterinarian should rule out any possibility of infection (e.g., septic arthritis, discospondylitis) or traumatic injury (e.g., cranial cruciate ligament rupture), which would make the use of glucocorticosteroids contraindicated. Glucocorticosteroids should never replace weight reduction and exercise modification but should be used only in combination with them. Intra-articular administration of glucocorticosteroids has detrimental effects on the joint cartilage and is contraindicated in dogs.

Polysulfated glycosaminoglycans (Adequan, Luitpold Pharmaceuticals, Inc., Shirley, NY) is a new drug for the treatment of degenerative joint disease in aged patients. Polysulfated glycosaminoglycans have a chondroprotective effect in a medial meniscectomy and cranial cruciate ligament transection model of canine osteoarthrosis (Altman et al, 1989a,b; Hannan et al, 1987). Joint cartilage from dogs treated with polysulfated glycosaminoglycans shows less swelling, lower activity of cartilage-degrading enzymes, and more normal appearance on histopathologic examination. In one study, intramuscular administration of polysulfated glycosaminoglycans in growing puppies, 6 weeks to 8 months of age and susceptible to hip dysplasia, resulted in significant reduction of subluxation of the hip joint and decreased pathologic changes (Lust et al, 1992). There are anecdotal reports of successful clinical use of polysulfated glycosaminoglycans in dogs with degenerative joint disease, but there are no controlled studies supporting their use for treatment of naturally occurring degenerative joint disease in dogs. In clinical cases we use polysulfated glycosaminoglycans at a dose of 4 mg/kg intramuscularly twice a week for a total of six to eight treatments. If the dog initially improves but the clinical signs return, this treatment regimen can be repeated. Before the drug is prescribed, the owner must be informed that polysulfated glycosaminoglycans are not approved by the Food and Drug Administration for use in dogs but have been approved for intramuscular and intra-articular use in horses. After intramuscular injection, polysulfated glycosaminoglycans inhibit coagulation and platelet aggregation for up to 24 hours, and therefore, they should not be given to dogs with bleeding disorders or concomitantly with any drugs that would cause prolonged bleeding time (Beale et al, 1990). In clinical use, we have not encountered any complications with intramuscular administration of polysulfated glycosaminoglycans at a dose of 4 mg/kg. It should be noted, however, that not all dogs improve after treatment.

If conservative management of a geriatric dog fails to relieve clinical signs of degenerative joint disease, surgical treatment should be considered. If possible, surgery should be performed before significant muscle atrophy occurs, as this could limit function after surgical treatment. There are three types of procedures for treatment of end-stage degenerative joint disease in dogs: arthrodesis, excision arthroplasty, and total replacement of the joint with an implant. If the dog is in good general health and is a good candidate for surgery, age alone is not a contraindication for surgical treatment, and excellent results can be achieved even in aged patients.

Arthrodesis is surgical fusion of a joint. Successful arthrodesis of the carpus, tarsus (Fig. 17–8), elbow, stifle, and shoulder joint can be performed (Moore and Withrow, 1981). A good result can be achieved with arthrodesis of any of the above joints; however, carpal arthrodesis provides the best functional result (Fig. 17–9).

Excision arthroplasty of the hip joint (femoral head and neck ostectomy) is commonly performed for treatment of painful diseases of the hip joint (Fig. 17–10). In dogs weighing up to 20 kg, this procedure, if performed correctly, is very successful and can result in almost normal function. Many different modifications of this procedure for large dogs have been described. Soft tissue interposition between the proximal femur and the pelvis can be performed, but the results seem to be inconsistent, and this is a controversial procedure (Lewis, 1992; Prostredny et al, 1991). Excision arthroplasty of the shoulder joint and radial head have been described, but they are not performed very commonly, and functional results are less predictable.

Total hip replacement is currently routinely performed at many referral institutions, and results are excellent (Olmstead et al, 1983; Parker et al, 1984; DeYoung et al, 1992). Total hip replacement eliminates pain and returns function of the hip joint to near normal. The complication rate is currently less than 10 per cent and is decreasing as the surgical technique improves. The development of a modular total hip system has improved application of implants as a result of a more customized fit (Fig. 17–11). In the future, replacements of other joints in clinical patients are likely.

Secondary Degenerative Joint Disease

During their lives many dogs sustain some type of developmental or acquired joint disease that in time results in progressive degenerative joint disease. Secondary degenerative joint disease is very common in geriatric dogs. A survey of cadaver material has shown that 20 per cent of examined dogs had stifle degenerative joint disease and that some type of primary mechanical derangement was present in 20 of the 54 affected joints (Tirgari and Vaughan, 1975).

The most common developmental causes of degenerative joint disease are hip dysplasia, pa-

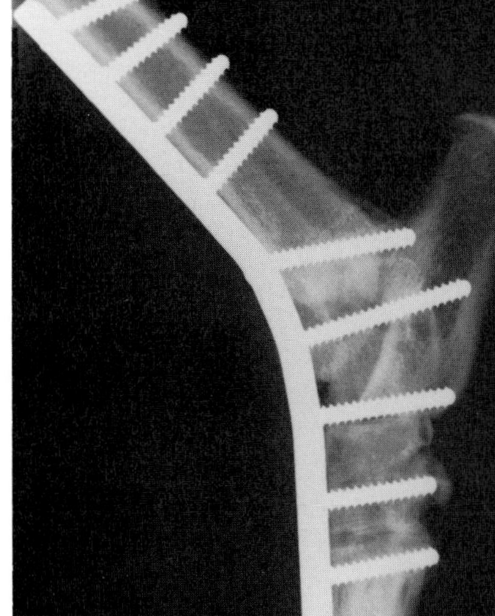

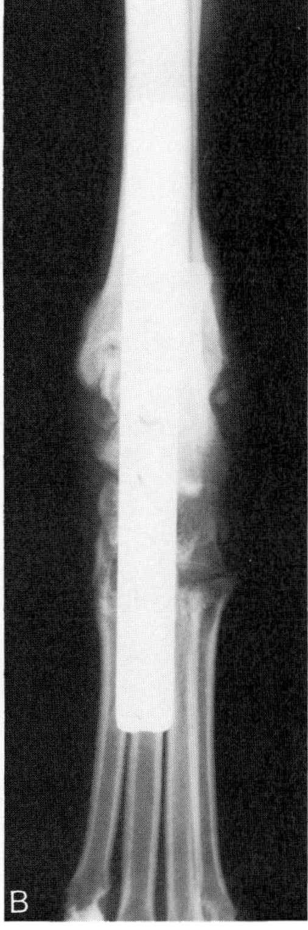

Figure 17–8. Lateral (*A*) and craniocaudal (*B*) radiographs of the right tarsus of a dog showing pantarsal arthrodesis of the joint. The tarsus was stabilized using a plate.

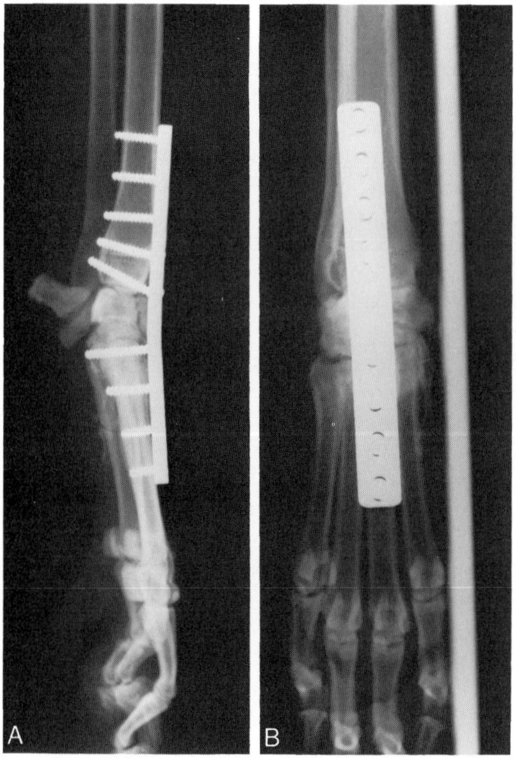

Figure 17–9. Lateral (*A*) and craniocaudal (*B*) radiographs of the right carpus of a dog demonstrating pancarpal arthrodesis performed using a bone plate.

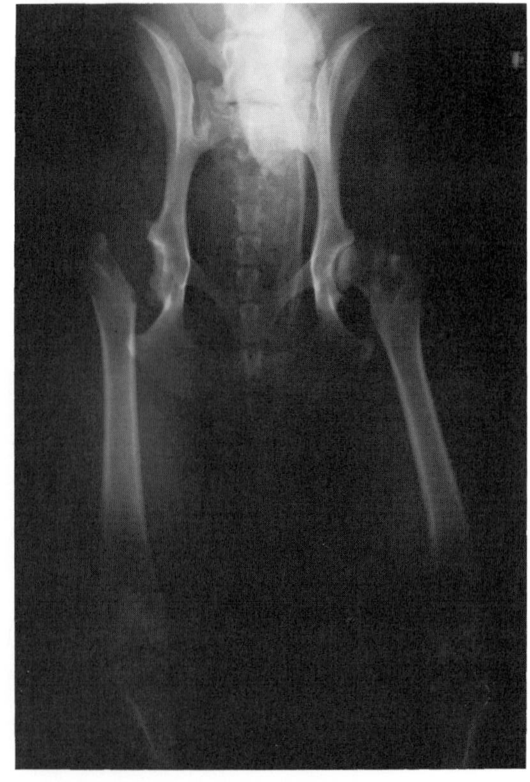

Figure 17–10. Ventrodorsal radiograph of the pelvis of a dog. A femoral head and neck ostectomy was performed on the right side. The left hip has changes consistent with hip dysplasia.

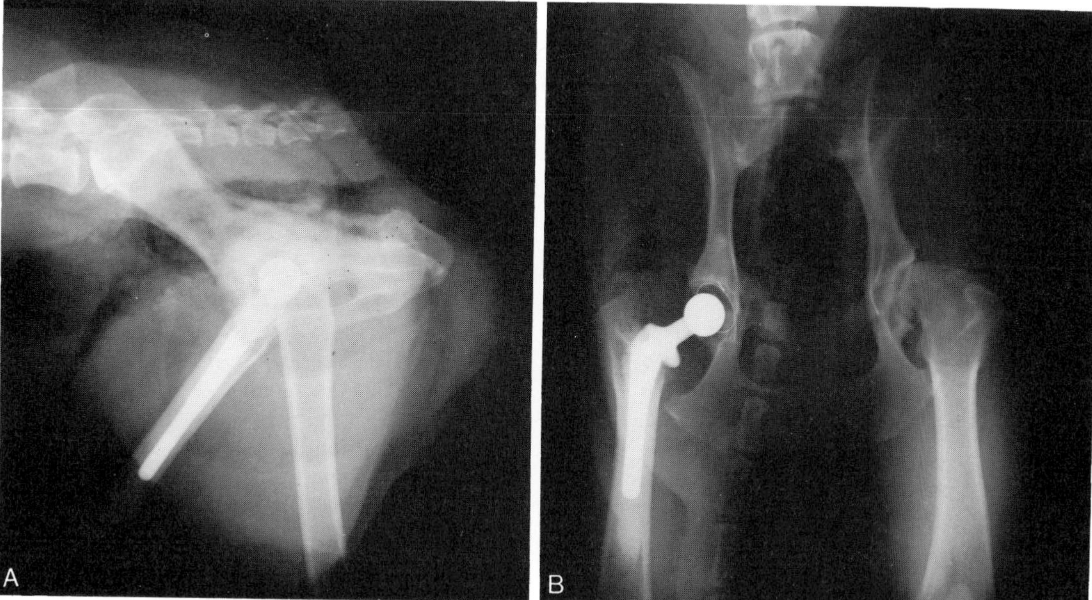

Figure 17–11. Lateral (*A*) and ventrodorsal (*B*) radiographs of the pelvis of a dog. A total hip replacement was performed on the right hip. Hip dysplasia is evident on the left side.

tellar luxation in the stifle, a fragmented coronoid process and nonunited anconeal process in the elbow, and osteochondrosis of one of the joints. The traumatic causes of degenerative joint disease include joint dislocation, ligamentous instability, growth deformity secondary to premature growth plate closure, intra-articular fracture, and malunion resulting in abnormal stress on the joint. Generally speaking, the diagnosis and treatment of dogs with secondary degenerative joint disease is similar to those for primary degenerative joint disease. However, in addition to the treatment recommended previously for primary degenerative joint disease, it is important to find and, if possible, surgically correct the underlying disease.

Senile Osteoporosis

Osteoporosis is a reduction in quantity, or atrophy, of the bone. Senile osteoporosis is caused by advanced age of the individual. Atrophy of the bone can also be secondary to a metabolic disease or disuse (Fig. 17–12). Senile osteoporosis is an important clinical problem in human orthopedic surgery. It affects large numbers of postmenopausal women and, to a lesser degree, older men. It results in a high incidence of pathologic fractures in elderly humans. Some of these are caused by minor trauma that would not be sufficient to fracture normal healthy bone. A lack of estrogen in postmenopausal women is one of the most important causative factors in people.

In geriatric dogs there is a gradual decrease of the bone mass, but the clinical significance of senile osteoporosis in older dogs is limited. Osteoporosis in dogs is not severe enough to cause the problems commonly seen in geriatric humans (Weigel and Alexander, 1981). The majority of the fractures seen in small animals are secondary to automobile accidents and are seen mostly in young animals. In one survey, 80 per cent of fractures occurred in animals 3 years old or younger (Phillips, 1979).

The primary importance of senile osteoporosis in dogs is its influence on fracture healing (Weigel and Alexander, 1981). In older animals callus formation is slower, and fractures need more time to heal. For that reason, the likelihood of delayed union, nonunion, muscle atrophy, and disuse osteoporosis is increased. To prevent this, the use of rigid internal fixation, which allows early return of function, and an autogenous cancellous bone graft to stimulate bone healing is recommended in older dogs.

Metabolic Osteoporosis

In addition to orthopedic problems, older dogs also have an increased frequency of metabolic

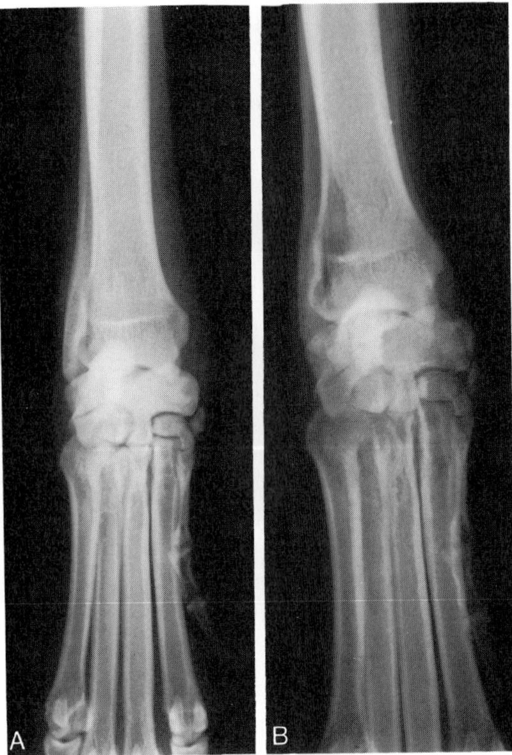

Figure 17–12. Craniocaudal radiographs of the right carpus of a dog. The first radiograph (*A*) demonstrates normal bone density; the second (*B*), taken 2 months later, shows disuse osteoporosis. The dog did not use the right front limb during the 2 months between radiographs.

disorders, which usually result first in systemic signs but eventually can also affect the musculoskeletal system. Endocrine diseases can especially alter the metabolism of the bone, resulting in osteoporosis, pathologic fractures, and weakening of the ligaments. Disorders of the parathyroid and adrenal glands are the most common metabolic diseases affecting the musculoskeletal system (Buckley, 1984).

Primary hyperparathyroidism, an excessive production of parathyroid hormone caused by neoplasia or hyperplasia of the parathyroid gland, is seen in older dogs. The clinical signs are usually related to the hypercalcemia and not to the musculoskeletal system. High levels of parathyroid hormone in blood result in increased bone resorption, but usually this is not clinically detectable.

Renal failure can lead to secondary hyperparathyroidism. Increased concentration of parathyroid hormone stimulates bone resorption, which can lead to enlarged, soft maxillary bones (rubber jaw) and loss of the lamina dura around the teeth. Most dogs with renal failure are presented because of signs related to such failure, but some may demonstrate bony abnormalities. Secondary hyperparathyroidism can also be the result of low-calcium, high-phosphorus diets and malabsorption (Buckley, 1984).

Hyperadrenocorticism (Cushing's syndrome) is common in older dogs and can be caused by increased production of endogenous glucocorticosteroids or by excessive iatrogenic administration of glucocorticosteroids. Catabolic effects of glucocorticosteroids can affect the musculoskeletal system and result in osteoporosis, muscle atrophy, and weakening of the ligaments supporting the joint. Most cushingoid dogs are also overweight, aggravating clinical signs.

Other endocrine disorders that can induce osteoporosis are hyperthyroidism and diabetes mellitus (Buckley, 1984). Treatment of orthopedic problems related to systemic metabolic diseases should be directed toward the primary cause; the musculoskeletal disease is treated only symptomatically.

Neoplasia

The incidence of tumors involving the musculoskeletal system is relatively low in older dogs. The most common are malignant primary bone tumors, listed here in order of decreasing frequency: osteosarcoma, chondrosarcoma, fibrosarcoma, and hemangiosarcoma.

Osteosarcoma. Osteosarcoma is the most common primary bone tumor in the dog. Osteosarcoma occurs usually in middle age to older dogs belonging to giant and large breeds. The preferred locations are the proximal humerus and the distal radius, but the distal femur and proximal tibia are also commonly affected (Fig. 17–13). The most common clinical signs are lameness, pain, and local swelling of the extremity. As the disease progresses, the dog may sustain pathologic fractures and develop systemic signs secondary to metastatic disease, usually in the thorax.

The diagnosis of osteosarcoma is based on the history, physical examination, and radiographic findings, and it should be confirmed with a biopsy and histopathologic examination. Radiographic signs of osteosarcoma include cortical destruction and periosteal new bone formation. Aggressive tumors usually have a poorly demarcated zone between normal and abnormal bone and between the tumor itself and the surrounding soft tissues. Osteosarcomas usually do not cross the joints. Pathologic fractures can be seen occasionally.

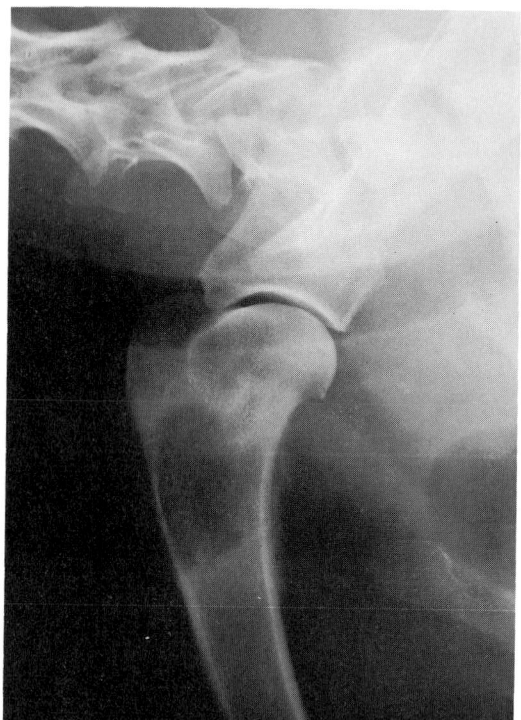

Figure 17–13. Radiograph of the right proximal humerus of a dog reveals an osteolytic and proliferative lesion involving the metaphysis. The radiographic changes are indicative of osteosarcoma.

Thoracic radiographs are necessary to evaluate the chest for the presence of visible pulmonary metastasis. Bone scintigraphy can be helpful in determining the size of the tumor and makes complete resection of the tumor easier (Lamb et al, 1990; Parchman et al, 1989). A combination of bone scintigraphy and radiography helps in evaluating the skeleton for metastatic or multicentric neoplasia, which is of great importance for the diagnosis, treatment, and long-term prognosis of the patient (Parchman et al, 1989; Hahn et al, 1990). Bone scintigraphy is of no value in differentiating among different types of primary bone tumors (Berg et al, 1990).

Traditionally, treatment of appendicular osteosarcoma has consisted of limb amputation with subsequent administration of chemotherapy, usually cisplatin. Mean survival time after amputation alone is 190 days (median, 168 days). If combined with two cisplatin treatments, the mean survival time can be extended to 315 days (median, 290 days) (Thompson and Fugent, 1992). Amputation combined with six cisplatin treatments can extend the survival time to a median of 413 days (Kraegel et al, 1991). Despite chemotherapy, most dogs die because of intrapulmonary or bone metastatic disease. Chemotherapy appears to be ineffective for the treatment of clinically evident metastatic osteosarcoma in the dog (Ogilvie, 1993).

There have been a number of reports of limb-sparing procedures for the treatment of appendicular osteosarcoma (LaRue et al, 1989; Berg et al, 1992). Generally, limb-sparing surgery consists of segmental tumor resection and application of a frozen cortical allograft and a bone plate for limb reconstruction. Surgery is usually combined with other treatment modalities such as chemotherapy (i.e., cisplatin) and irradiation. Reported mean and median survival times after limb reconstruction and cisplatin treatment either alone or combined with irradiation are 12 and 8 months, respectively (LaRue et al, 1989). Partial ulnectomy and some form of adjuvant therapy (immunotherapy, radiation therapy, or chemotherapy) were also described as a therapy for osteosarcomas of the ulna (Straw et al, 1991). In addition to cases of appendicular osteosarcomas, cases of axial skeletal osteosarcomas were reported in the mandible, maxilla, spine, cranium, ribs, nasal cavity, paranasal sinuses, and pelvis. The median survival time for surgically treated dogs was 154 days (Heyman et al, 1992).

Chondrosarcomas. Chondrosarcomas are the second most common bone tumors. They occur mostly in large breed dogs and usually affect flat bones (Fig. 17–14). There is no age predisposition, and clinical signs depend on the location of the tumor. Chondrosarcomas metastasize via a hematogenous route to the lungs, but at a later stage of the disease than do osteosarcomas. Treatment consists of surgical excision.

Fibrosarcomas. Primary fibrosarcomas of the appendicular skeleton are rare and occur predominantly in older, large breed dogs (Wesselhoeft Ablin et al, 1991). It is difficult to differentiate between primary fibrosarcomas of the bone and soft tissue fibrosarcomas secondarily invading the bone. Fibrosarcomas of the appendicular skeleton are treated by amputation of the involved limb or by limb-sparing surgery, along with chemotherapy with cisplatin. Primary appendicular bone fibrosarcomas are generally not very sensitive to chemotherapy, but because of their low frequency, the effect of treatment and the occurrence of local regrowth and distant metastasis are not well documented (Wesselhoeft Ablin et al, 1991).

Hemangiosarcomas. Primary hemangiosarcomas of the bone are rare and are seen most commonly in medium and large breed dogs. Clinical signs include lameness, localized swell-

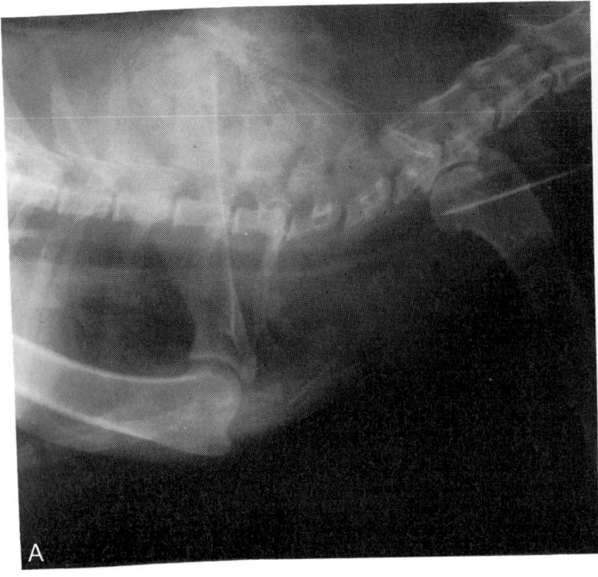

Figure 17–14. Lateral (*A*) and craniocaudal (*B*) radiographs of the left scapula of a dog revealing a highly proliferative and destructive lesion consistent with the diagnosis of chondrosarcoma.

ing, and pain. Primary hemangiosarcomas start in the medullary cavity and lead to lysis of the cortical bone and sometimes pathologic fractures (Goldschmidt and Thrall, 1985). Metastasis to the lung, spleen, liver, and right atrium is common.

Other Malignant Tumors. Other malignant tumors that can originate in the bone are liposarcomas, plasma cell myelomas, lymphosarcomas, and giant cell tumors (Goldschmidt and Thrall, 1985). Bone can also be affected by primary benign tumors and by local and distant metastasis of soft tissue tumors.

Bone Infarction

Bone infarction is localized areas of aseptic necrosis of the medullary bone and other components of the medullary cavity secondary to interruption of the blood supply to the bone (Ansari, 1991). Bone infarction is seen most commonly in older dogs; mean and median ages are about 10 years (Dubielzig et al, 1981). Most of the affected dogs belong to small breeds (median weight, 10 kg) (Dubielzig et al, 1981). The cause of bone infarction in the dog is unknown. Most dogs have no specific history or physical examination findings that can be attributed to infarction. A complete blood cell count and biochemistry profile, including alkaline phosphatase and calcium levels, are usually within normal limits.

Bone infarction is usually an incidental finding on survey radiographs of the skeleton. Radiographic changes consistent with bone infarction include radiodense areas located within the medullary cavity of the bone (Fig. 17–15). The margins of the lesions are well demarcated.

Bone infarcts can be associated with malignant bone tumors, most commonly osteosarcomas (Dubielzig et al, 1981; Riser et al, 1972). The causative relationship between bone infarction and malignant bone tumors in the dog is not established. Extrapolation of human information would suggest that bone infarction is the primary problem and that infarcted areas can undergo malignant transformation (Ansari, 1991). If bone infarction is diagnosed in a dog without any evidence of neoplasia, then the dog should be followed very closely to detect potential development of secondary neoplasia and to start early treatment. In almost all cases, the clinical signs

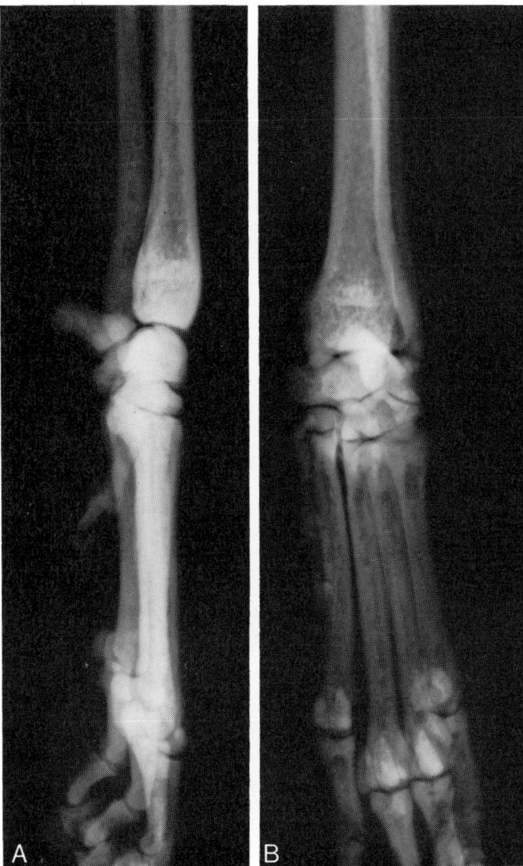

Figure 17–15. Lateral (*A*) and craniocaudal (*B*) radiographs of the distal front limb of a dog demonstrating enostosis compatible with the diagnosis of multiple bone infarction.

on presentation are related to the malignant bone tumor and are not attributed to the bone infarction. Prognosis for affected dogs depends on the prognosis of the primary bone tumor and is usually poor.

Hypertrophic Osteopathy

Hypertrophic osteopathy is an uncommon condition seen most often in geriatric patients (Susaneck and Macy, 1982). Hypertrophic osteopathy results in periosteal new bone formation affecting first the distal bones (metacarpals and metatarsals) of all four extremities (Susaneck and Macy, 1982). As the disease progresses, the periosteal reaction spreads in the proximal direction. The joints are not involved.

Patients with hypertrophic osteopathy present because of pain, lameness, and swelling of all four limbs. Radiographic changes include bilaterally symmetric periosteal new bone formation and soft tissue swelling, which starts along the shafts of the metatarsal and metacarpal bones. As the disease progresses, the periosteal new bone formation spreads proximally to the humerus and femur (Susaneck and Macy, 1982). The exact mechanism causing hypertrophic osteopathy is not known, but almost all affected dogs have thoracic disease, usually metastatic, or, less commonly, primary lung tumor (Fig. 17–16). Other possible causes of hypertrophic osteopathy include lung abscess, inflammatory lung disease, heartworm disease, bacterial endocarditis, *Spirocerca lupi* infection, and abdominal tumors (Hesselink and van den Tweel, 1990; Brodey, 1971). Increased periosteal bone formation is believed to occur as a result of enhanced blood flow to the distal limbs secondary to peripheral vasodilation caused by the primary disease. It is not known whether this effect is mediated through changes in the autonomic nervous system, release of humoral factors, or direct effects on the circulatory system. Treatment of hypertrophic osteopathy is directed toward the primary cause of the syndrome and usually consists of resection of the thoracic mass. In patients with lung tumors, a lobectomy or pulmonectomy can be performed. If the surgery is successful, signs of hypertrophic osteopathy will regress. In one report, regression occurred for 2 weeks to 7 months after surgery but was limited by recurrence of metastatic lung nodules (Brodey, 1971). The prognosis for the dog depends on the type of primary disease, and because most patients have metastatic lung tumors, prognosis is usually guarded.

DISORDERS OF CATS

Orthopedic disorders in cats are being seen with increasing frequency, most likely because older cats are being kept as family pets. Although many orthopedic disorders of the cat mimic those of the dog, some are unique to the cat. Treatment of orthopedic diseases of the cat may differ from that for the dog. Skeletal disorders affecting older cats include degenerative joint disease, polyarthritis, neoplasia, hypertrophic osteopathy, and hypervitaminosis A.

Degenerative Joint Disease

Because of less severe clinical signs and a lower number of developmental diseases, degenerative joint disease is seen less frequently in older cats than in older dogs. Clinical signs,

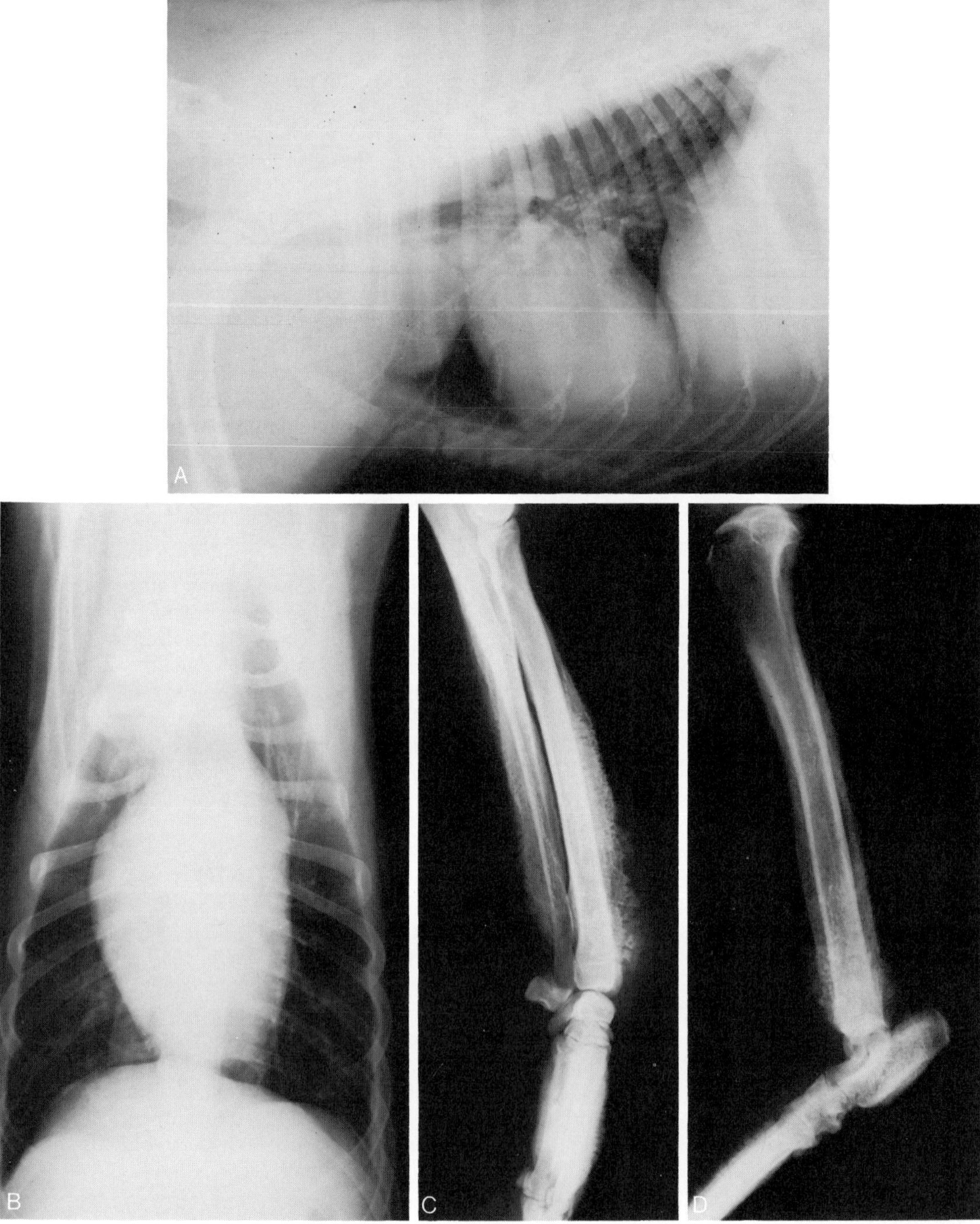

Figure 17–16. Lateral (*A*) and ventrodorsal (*B*) thoracic radiographs of a dog showing a dense soft tissue mass in the right cranial lung lobe. Radiographs of the distal front limb (*C*) and distal hindlimb (*D*) demonstrate periosteal proliferation involving the diaphyses of all long bones consistent with a hypertrophic osteopathy.

radiographic appearance, and synovial fluid cytology mimic those seen in the dog. Both primary and secondary degenerative joint disease occur. Primary degenerative joint disease can occur in any joint and is thought to be due to normal wear and tear associated with aging. Secondary degenerative joint disease is usually caused by a developmental disease resulting in abnormal forces acting on a joint (hip dysplasia, patellar luxation), traumatic instability of a joint (e.g., ruptured cranial cruciate ligament, collateral ligament instability, or hyperextension injury), or anatomic damage to articular surfaces (e.g., osteochondrosis, articular fractures).

Hip dysplasia is typically thought to affect primarily young, large breed dogs. Interestingly, cats may also be afflicted (Fig. 17–17) (Kolde, 1974; Holt, 1978; Hayes et al, 1979). Purebred cats, especially Persian cats, are predisposed (Hayes et al, 1979). Hip dysplasia in the cat may be seen as a separate entity or in association with medial patellar luxation (Giger et al, 1992). Clinical signs include lameness, pain and crepitus on hip extension, muscle atrophy, and sometimes a "bunny-hop" gait. The onset of clinical signs may be insidious, not appearing until later in life; some cats may not have any clinical signs. If treatment is indicated, conservative treatment may be tried initially using an appropriate dosage of nonsteroidal anti-inflammatory drug or a chondroprotective drug such as polysulfated glycosaminoglycans. Persistent lameness that does not respond to medical therapy can be successfully treated by surgical excision of the femoral head and neck.

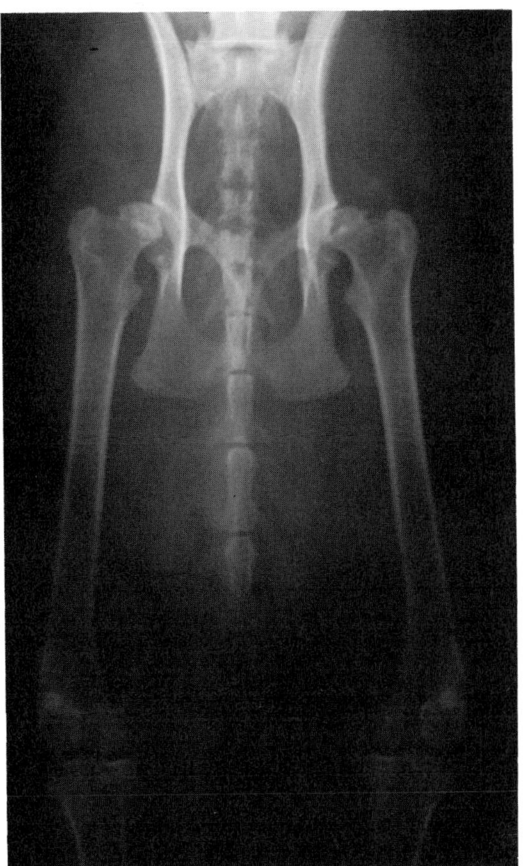

Figure 17–17. Ventrodorsal radiograph of the pelvis of a cat. Bilateral degenerative joint disease and subluxation of the hip joints consistent with hip dysplasia are present.

Patellar luxation is usually seen in young cats, but occasionally geriatric cats will be presented for lameness associated with degenerative joint disease secondary to patellar luxation. Medial luxation is most common (Johnson, 1986; Giger et al, 1992). Patellar luxation is graded from 1 to 4, with higher numbers representing greater severity. Surgical correction is recommended for grades 2 to 4. Repair techniques include imbrication of the lateral fascia, release incisions on the medial side, trochlear wedge recession, and tibial crest transposition.

Cranial cruciate ligament rupture and a deranged stifle joint are two commonly seen traumatic injuries to the stifle. A deranged stifle joint is characterized by severe instability associated with cranial and/or caudal cruciate ligament rupture, collateral ligament rupture, and meniscal tear. Conservative treatment of isolated cranial cruciate ligament rupture is often successful in resolving lameness (Scavelli and Schrader, 1987). Surgical stabilization of the joint should be performed if lameness persists after conservative management (Alexander et al, 1977). Surgical stabilization speeds recovery and probably lessens the chance of secondary degenerative joint disease. A deranged stifle joint always requires surgical repair. Damaged meniscal tissue must be excised by partial or total meniscectomy. Stabilization of the joint can be achieved by several techniques: reconstruction of the torn ligaments (Phillips, 1982), transarticular pinning (Welches and Scavelli, 1990), or transarticular external skeletal fixation (Aron, 1988).

Occasionally, the fibrocartilaginous menisci within the stifle undergo mineralization (Whiting and Pool, 1985). Clinical signs are not always present but can include lameness and swelling of the joint. The cause of this condition is unknown; however, meniscal calcification has been observed in cats without pre-existing stifle instability, as well as in cats with cranial cruciate ligament instability. If lameness is associated with these conditions, meniscectomy is recommended.

Polyarthritis

Polyarthritis, an inflammatory joint disease involving two or more joints, is occasionally seen in geriatric cats (Fig. 17–18). Polyarthritis is characterized by inflammatory changes in the synovial membrane and fluid. Nonerosive forms of polyarthritis are most common, but erosive forms do occur. Erosive polyarthritis in the cat often results from bacterial sepsis, bacterial L-forms infection, and chronic progressive polyarthritis. Clinical signs of any form of polyarthritis include multiple limb lameness, swelling of multiple joints (with the carpal and tarsal joints most commonly affected), and sometimes systemic illness. Infectious, immune-mediated, and idiopathic causes occur.

Early radiographic changes associated with polyarthritis are subtle and may include thickening of the synovial membrane, distention of the joint capsule, and slight widening of the joint space attributable to effusion. These joint findings are nonspecific and may occur as early changes in erosive or nonerosive polyarthritis. Radiographic abnormalities are more severe in the later stages; included is mild periosteal proliferation of the bones adjacent to the affected joint space that progresses to destruction of the articular cartilage. Evidence of secondary osteomyelitis may also be noted. Pathologic fractures and/or fibrous or bony ankylosis are present in severe disease and make the prognosis for recovery guarded. Treatment depends on the cause of the polyarthritis. Depending on the cause of the disease, antimicrobial agents, glucocorticosteroids, and cytotoxic immunosuppressive drugs are used.

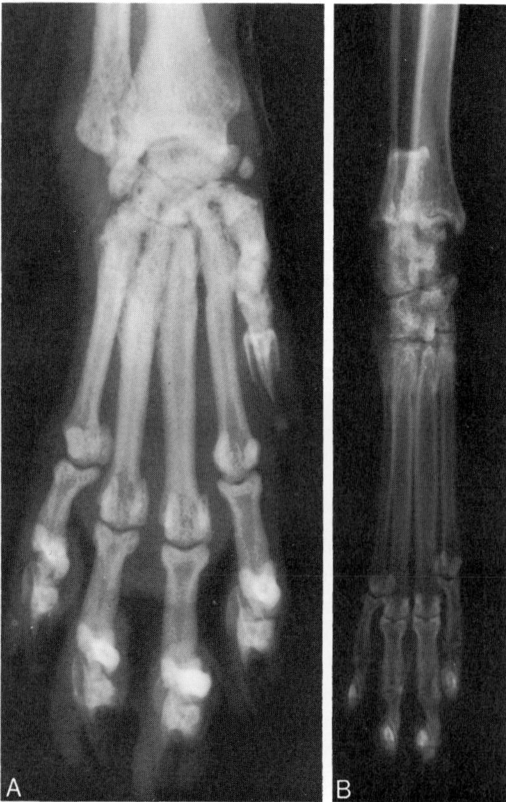

Figure 17–18. Craniocaudal radiographs of the carpus (*A*) and tarsus (*B*) of a cat. Marked destructive changes with some bony proliferation involving the tarsus and carpus are present. The lesions are consistent with immune-mediated polyarthritis in the cat.

Infectious arthritis may occur by a hematogenous route or by direct inoculation of the joint. Geriatric cats may become more susceptible to infectious arthritis if they are immunocompromised secondary to neoplastic processes or feline immunodeficiency virus or feline leukemia virus infections. Causative agents include *Mycoplasma*, bacteria, fungi (e.g., *Histoplasma, Cryptococcus*), and viruses (Schrader and Sherding, 1989). Treatment should be determined based on cytology and histopathology of the synovial membrane, microbiologic identification of the offending organism, and antimicrobial sensitivity testing results.

Chronic progressive polyarthritis is an immune-mediated arthritis that has two forms: periosteal proliferative and deforming, rheumatoid-like. Although both forms can occur in all ages of cats, the proliferative form has been most frequently associated with young adult cats, and the deforming form has been seen more commonly in older cats. Chronic progressive polyarthritis is reported to occur exclusively in male cats and has been linked to concurrent infection with feline syncytium-forming virus and feline leukemia virus (Pedersen et al, 1980). The pathogenesis is probably immune mediated (Schrader and Sherding, 1989).

Clinical signs of the periosteal form include fever, malaise, weight loss, lameness, generalized stiffness, lymphadenopathy, and joint swelling, which is usually most severe in the carpus and tarsus (Schrader and Sherding, 1989). Periarticular periosteal swelling generally appears several weeks after onset of clinical signs. Clinical signs of the deforming form are more insidious and include onset of a chronic, progressive lameness and stiffness that are not associated with an acute febrile stage (Schrader and Sherding, 1989).

Diagnosis is made by identification of characteristic radiographic and synovial fluid analysis findings. Radiographic changes of the periosteal form include periarticular swelling and periosteal bone proliferation of the tarsi, carpi, metatarsi, and metacarpi. Changes seen with the deforming form include periarticular swelling, erosion of subchondral bone, collapse of joint spaces (tarsi and carpi), and subluxation. Synovial fluid analysis of both forms is consistent with a purulent, nonseptic inflammatory process with a nucleated cell count of 4000 to 70,000 per mm^3 and a predominance of nondegenerate neutrophils (Pedersen et al, 1980). Lymphocytic-plasmocytic synovitis is evident on histopathologic examination of synovial biopsy specimens.

Treatment with immunosuppressive drugs is recommended. The prognosis is guarded for both forms, but cats afflicted with the periosteal form tend to respond better to treatment. Prednisone is tried initially at a dosage of 2 to 4 mg/kg/day. Long-term, alternate-day prednisone may be required. The best long-term results can be achieved with combination chemotherapy using prednisone (10 mg orally every other day), azathioprine (7.5 mg orally every other day), and cyclophosphamide (7.5 mg orally daily for 4 consecutive days of each week) (Pedersen et al, 1980).

Idiopathic polyarthritis is usually associated with lameness, stiffness, and swelling of the carpi and tarsi. The cause is unknown, but an immune-mediated mechanism is likely. Typically, the only radiographic change seen is joint capsular distention. Synovial fluid analysis is consistent with nonseptic purulent inflammation with a predominance of 4000 to 30,000 nondegenerate neutrophils per mm^3. Treatment with a short course of prednisone (2 mg/kg orally every day, tapering over a period of 3 weeks) is usually curative, but this condition can recur. Underlying causes, such as drug-induced polyarthritis (e.g., by antimicrobial agents such as a trimethoprim-sulfonamide combination and cephalosporins), enteropathic polyarthritis, polyarthritis associated with chronic disease, and systemic lupus erythematosus, should be ruled out before starting treatment.

Neoplasia

Many types of primary neoplasia can occur in bones of older cats; the most common are osteosarcoma and chondrosarcoma. Metastatic neoplasia in the bone is frequently seen with local invasion from adjacent soft tissue tumors (fibrosarcoma and squamous cell carcinoma) or distant metastasis of carcinoma cells from other sites in the body. Mammary adenocarcinoma is frequently associated with distant bone metastasis. Biopsy and a histopathologic diagnosis are mandatory before appropriate treatment and prognosis can be provided. The behavior of most bone tumors in the cat tends to mimic that seen in the dog, with the exception of osteosarcoma of the appendicular skeleton.

Osteosarcoma. Osteosarcoma is the most common skeletal neoplasia in both the dog and cat (Fig. 17–19). It is most common in middle-age and geriatric cats. The most common site is the metaphysis of long bones. The biologic behavior of osteosarcoma involving the appendicular skeleton in the cat is different from that seen in the dog. Osteosarcoma in dogs is associated with early metastasis and short survival. Osteosarcoma in cats, however, is associated with distant metastasis in less than 10 per cent of cases (Turrel and Pool, 1982). In addition, cats generally have a good long-term prognosis after amputation of the affected limb, even without adjunctive chemotherapy. In one study, more than 50 per cent of cats were alive more than 5 years after amputation of the affected limb (Bitetto et al, 1987). Osteosarcoma involving the axial skeleton has a poor prognosis and is associated with short survival times (Bitetto et al, 1987).

Chondrosarcoma. Chondrosarcoma is most common in middle-age and geriatric cats. The scapula is affected most often, although the tumor is also seen in the skull, pelvis, and long bones (Schrader and Sherding, 1989). Amputation or wide surgical excision is the treatment of choice. Radiotherapy or chemotherapy may be useful as an adjunct to surgery. At the present time, the prognosis is less favorable than with osteosarcoma (Schrader and Sherding, 1989).

Fibrosarcomas. Fibrosarcomas in geriatric cats are usually solitary and most commonly affect bones of the skull and appendicular skeleton (Schrader and Sherding, 1989). Solitary fibrosarcomas behave differently from the multicentric form associated with feline sarcoma virus infection seen in younger cats. Radiographic changes include the appearance of a soft tissue mass that may be associated with distortion and lysis of adjacent bony structures. Pathologic fractures are common (Schrader and Sherding, 1989). These tumors are locally aggressive and are slow to metastasize. Wide surgical excision is the treatment of choice. If tumor-free margins cannot be achieved, adjunctive therapy should be considered.

Squamous Cell Carcinoma. Squamous cell

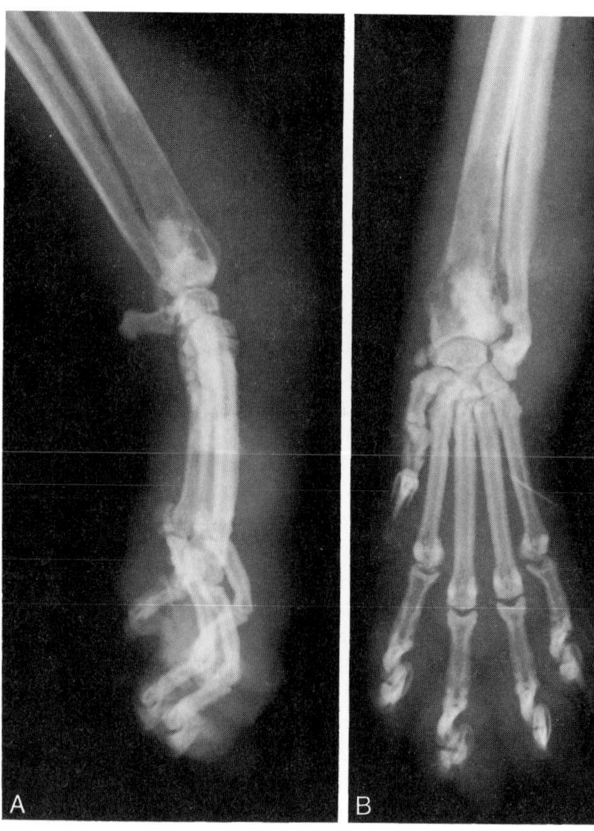

Figure 17–19. Lateral (*A*) and craniocaudal (*B*) radiographs of the distal left front limb of a 7-year-old spayed female cat. A destructive lesion involving the distal diaphysis and metaphysis of the radius indicative of osteosarcoma is present.

carcinoma is the most common oral tumor in geriatric cats; however, this tumor may affect almost any location, including long bones, digits, skull, and nose (Harvey, 1985). Radiographic changes include the appearance of a soft tissue mass that may be associated with distortion and lysis of adjacent bone. These tumors are locally aggressive, and distant metastasis occurs late in the disease process. Wide surgical excision is the treatment of choice. If wide margins (including the deep margin) cannot be achieved, adjunctive radiotherapy and/or chemotherapy should be considered.

Hypertrophic Osteopathy

Hypertrophic osteopathy has been reported less frequently in the cat than in the dog, but the clinical signs are similar to those seen in the dog: pain, lameness, and swelling of the distal aspects of all four limbs (Carr, 1971; Richards, 1977; Roberg, 1977; Nafe et al, 1981; Gram et al, 1990). As in the dog, the specific cause is unknown; however, the condition is most frequently associated with an intrathoracic mass. Diagnosis is made by identifying an intrathoracic or intra-abdominal mass and periosteal new bone formation involving the bones of the distal extremities. Treatment involves removal of the predisposing mass within the thoracic or abdominal cavity. Prognosis is usually poor owing to the malignant nature of the primary disease.

Hypervitaminosis A

Excessive consumption of foods or supplements high in vitamin A can lead to hypervitaminosis A. This metabolic disorder is most frequently associated with diets having a high liver content (Lucke et al, 1968; Clark et al, 1970; Goldman, 1992). Special care should be taken to avoid long-term feeding of such diets when trying to stimulate appetite in anorexic cats. Clinical signs associated with hypervitaminosis A include lameness, cervical spinal pain, stiffness, and reluctance to move. The clinical signs are attributable to periarticular exostoses, most commonly affecting the cervical and thoracic vertebrae, sternebrae, and forelimbs. Diagnosis is made by identifying excessive oral intake of a food high in vitamin A and the characteristic exostoses on radiographic examination. Treatment of affected cats should include introduction of a balanced commercial diet and symptomatic pain relief. At this time there is no available treatment to eliminate the exostoses already formed.

References and Supplemental Reading

Alexander JW. Pathogenesis and biochemical aspects of degenerative joint disease. Compend Contin Educ Pract Vet 2:961, 1980.

Alexander JW. Aging and the joints. Compend Contin Educ Pract Vet 6:1074, 1984.

Alexander JW, Shumway JD, Lau RE, et al. Anterior cruciate ligament repair. Feline Pract 7:38, 1977.

Altman RD, Dean DD, Muniz OE, Howell DS. Prophylactic treatment of canine osteoarthritis with glycosaminoglycan polysulfuric acid ester. Arthritis Rheum 32:759, 1989a.

Altman RD, Dean DD, Muniz OE, Howell DS. Therapeutic treatment of canine osteoarthritis with glycosaminoglycan polysulfuric acid ester. Arthritis Rheum 32:1300, 1989b.

Ansari MM. Bone infarcts associated with malignant sarcomas. Compend Contin Educ Pract Vet 13:367, 1991.

Aron DN. Traumatic dislocation of the stifle joint: Treatment of 12 dogs and one cat. J Am Anim Hosp Assoc 24:333, 1988.

Beale BS, Goring RL, Clemmons RM, Altman D. The effect of semi-synthetic polysulfated glycosaminoglycan on the hemostatic mechanism in the dog. Vet Surg 19:57, 1990.

Berg J, Lamb CR, O'Callaghan MW. Bone scintigraphy in the initial evaluation of dogs with primary bone tumors. J Am Vet Med Assoc 196:917, 1990.

Berg J, Weinstein MJ, Schelling SH, Rand WM. Treatment of dogs with osteosarcoma by administration of cisplatin after amputation or limb-sparing surgery: 22 cases (1987–1990). J Am Vet Med Assoc 200:2005, 1992.

Bitetto WV, Patnaik AK, Schrader SC, et al. Osteosarcoma in cats: 22 cases (1974–1984). J Am Vet Med Assoc 190:91, 1987.

Brinker WO, Piermattei DL, Flo GL. Handbook of Small Animal Orthopedics and Fracture Treatment. 2nd ed. Philadelphia, WB Saunders, 1990, p 267.

Brodey RS. Hypertrophic osteoarthropathy in the dog: A clinicopathologic survey of 60 cases. J Am Vet Med Assoc 159:1242, 1971.

Buckley JC. Pathophysiologic considerations of osteopenia. Compend Contin Educ Pract Vet 6:552, 1984.

Carr SH. Secondary hypertrophic pulmonary osteoarthropathy in a cat. Feline Pract 1:25, 1971.

Clark DM. Current concepts in the treatment of degenerative joint disease. Compend Contin Educ Pract Vet 13:1439, 1991b.

Clark DM. The biochemistry of degenerative joint disease and its treatment. Compend Contin Educ Pract Vet 13:275, 1991a.

Clark L, Seawright AA, Hrdlicka J. Exostosis in hypervitaminotic A cats with optimal calcium-phosphorus intakes. J Small Anim Pract 11:553, 1970.

DeYoung DJ, DeYoung BA, Aberman HA, et al. Implantation of an uncemented total hip prosthesis. Technique and initial results of 100 arthroplasties. Vet Surg 21:168, 1992.

Dubielzig RR, Biery DN, Brodey RS. Bone sarcomas associated with multifocal medullary bone infarction in dogs. J Am Vet Med Assoc 179:64, 1981.

Farrow CS. The radiology of aging: Its clinical applications. Compend Contin Educ Pract Vet 6:1114, 1984.

Giger U, Green PA, Smith GK. Hip dysplasia and patellar luxation in cats. In Proceedings of the North Am Vet Conf, Orlando, FL, 1992, p 321.

Goldman AL. Hypervitaminosis A in a cat. J Am Vet Med Assoc 200:1970, 1992.

Goldschmidt MH, Thrall DE. Malignant bone tumors in the dog. In Newton CD, Nunamaker DM, eds. Textbook of Small Animal Orthopaedics. Philadelphia, JB Lippincott, 1985, p 887.

Gram WD, Wheaton LG, Snyder PW, et al. Feline hypertrophic osteopathy associated with pulmonary carcinoma. J Am Anim Hosp Assoc 26:425, 1990.

Hahn KA, Hurd C, Cantwell HD. Single-phase methylene diphosphate bone scintigraphy in the diagnostic evaluation of dogs with osteosarcoma. J Am Vet Med Assoc 196:1483, 1990.

Hannan N, Ghosh P, Bellenger C, Taylor T. Systemic administration of glycosaminoglycan polysulphate (Arteparon) provides partial protection of articular cartilage from damage produced by meniscectomy in the canine. J Orthop Res 5:47, 1987.

Harvey HJ. Oral tumors. Vet Clin North Am 15:493, 1985.

Hayes HM, Wilson GP, Burt JK. Feline hip dysplasia. J Am Anim Hosp Assoc 15:447, 1979.

Hesselink JW, van den Tweel JG. Hypertrophic osteopathy in a dog with a chronic lung abscess. J Am Vet Med Assoc 196:760, 1990.

Heyman SJ, Diefenderfer DL, Goldschmidt MH, Newton CD. Canine axial skeletal osteosarcoma. A retrospective study of 116 cases (1986 to 1989). Vet Surg 21:304, 1992.

Holt PE. Hip dysplasia in a cat. J Small Anim Pract 19:273, 1978.

Inerot S, Heinegard D, Audell L, Olsson S. Articular-cartilage proteoglycans in aging and osteoarthritis. Biochem J 169:143, 1978.

Johnson ME. Feline patellar luxation. A retrospective case study. J Am Anim Hosp Assoc 22:835, 1986.

Kolde DL. Pectineus tenectomy for treatment of hip dysplasia in a domestic cat: A case report. J Am Anim Hosp Assoc 10:564, 1974.

Kraegel SA, Madewell BR, Simonson E, Gregory CR. Osteogenic sarcoma and cisplatin chemotherapy in dogs: 16 cases (1986–1989). J Am Vet Med Assoc 199:1057, 1991.

Lamb CR, Berg J, Bengtson AE. Preoperative measurement of canine primary bone tumors using radiography and bone scintigraphy. J Am Vet Med Assoc 196:1474, 1990.

LaRue SM, Withrow SJ, Powers BE, et al. Limb-sparing treatment for osteosarcoma in dogs. J Am Vet Med Assoc 195:1734, 1989.

Lewis DD. Femoral head and neck excision and the controversy concerning adjunctive soft tissue interposition. Compend Contin Educ Pract Vet 14:1463, 1992.

Lewis LD, Morris ML, Hand MS. Small Animal Clinical Nutrition III. Topeka, Kansas, Mark Morris Associates, 1987, p. 6–2.

Lucke VM, Baskerville A, Bardgett PL, et al. Deforming cervical spondylosis in the cat associated with hypervitaminosis A. Vet Rec 82:141, 1968.

Lust G, Williams AJ, Burton-Wurster N, et al. Effects of intramuscular administration of glycosaminoglycan polysulfates on signs of incipient hip dysplasia in growing pups. Am J Vet Res 53:1836, 1992.

Miles JS, Eichelberger L. Biochemical studies of human cartilage during the aging process. J Am Geriatr Soc 12:1, 1964.

Moore RW, Withrow SJ. Arthrodesis. Compend Contin Educ Pract Vet 3:319, 1981.

Nafe LA, Herron AJ, Burk RL. Hypertrophic osteopathy in a

cat associated with renal papillary adenoma. J Am Anim Hosp Assoc 17:659, 1981.

Newton CD. Examination of the orthopaedic patient. In Newton CD, Nunamaker DM, eds. Textbook of Small Animal Orthopaedics. Philadelphia, JB Lippincott, 1985, p 125.

Ogilvie GK, Straw RC, Jameson VJ, et al. Evaluation of single-agent chemotherapy for treatment of clinically evident osteosarcoma metastases in dogs: 45 cases (1987–1991). J Am Vet Med Assoc 202:304, 1993.

Olmstead ML, Hohn RB, Turner TM. A five-year study of 221 total hip replacements in the dog. J Am Vet Med Assoc 183:191, 1983.

Olsewski JM, Lust G, Rendano VT, Summers BA. Degenerative joint disease: Multiple joint involvement in young and mature dogs. Am J Vet Res 44:1300, 1983.

Parchman MB, Flanders JA, Erb HN, et al. Nuclear medical bone imaging and targeted radiography for evaluation of skeletal neoplasms in 23 dogs. Vet Surg 18:454, 1989.

Parker RB, Bloomberg MS, Bitetto W, Rodkey WG: Canine total hip arthroplasty: A clinical review of 20 cases. J Am Anim Hosp Assoc 20:97, 1984.

Pedersen NC, Pool RR, O'Brien T. Feline chronic progressive polyarthritis. Am J Vet Res 41:522, 1980.

Phillips IR. A survey of bone fractures in the dog and cat. J Small Anim Pract 20:661, 1979.

Phillips IR. Dislocation of the stifle joint in the cat. J Small Anim Pract 23:217, 1982.

Prostredny JM, Toombs JP, VanSickle DC. Effect of two muscle sling techniques on early morbidity after femoral head and neck excision in dogs. Vet Surg 20:298, 1991.

Reichenbach T. Aging in canine pets. Calif Vet July/August: 11, 1989.

Richards CD. Hypertrophic osteoarthropathy in a cat. Feline Pract 7:41, 1977.

Riser WH, Brodey RS, Biery DN. Bone infarctions associated with malignant bone tumors in dogs. J Am Vet Med Assoc 160:411, 1972.

Roberg J. Hypertrophic pulmonary osteoarthropathy. Feline Pract 7:18, 1977.

Scavelli TD, Schrader SC. Nonsurgical management of rupture of the cranial cruciate ligament in 18 cats. J Am Anim Hosp Assoc 23:337, 1987.

Schrader SC, Sherding RG. Disorders of the skeletal system. In Sherding RG, ed. The Cat: Diseases and Clinical Management. New York, Churchill Livingstone, 1989, p 1247.

Straw RC, Withrow SJ, Powers BE. Primary osteosarcoma of the ulna in 12 dogs. J Am Anim Hosp Assoc 27:323, 1991.

Susaneck SJ, Macy DW. Hypertrophic osteopathy. Compend Contin Educ Pract Vet 4:689, 1982.

Thompson JP, Fugent MJ. Evaluation of survival times after limb amputation, with and without subsequent administration of cisplatin, for treatment of appendicular osteosarcoma in dogs: 30 cases (1979–1990). J Am Vet Med Assoc 200:531, 1992.

Tirgari M, Vaughan LC. Clinico-pathological aspects of osteoarthritis of the shoulder in dogs. J Small Anim Pract 14:353, 1973.

Tirgari M, Vaughan LC. Arthritis of the canine stifle joint. Vet Rec 96:394, 1975.

Turrel JM, Pool RR. Primary bone tumors in the cat: A retrospective study of 15 cats and a literature review. Vet Radiol 23:152, 1982.

Vaughan LC. The geriatric cat and dog. Orthopedic problems in old dogs. Vet Rec 126:379, 1990.

Weigel J, Alexander JW. Aging and the musculoskeletal system. Vet Clin North Am [Small Anim Pract] 11:749, 1981.

Welches CD, Scavelli TD. Transarticular pinning to repair luxation of the stifle joint in dogs and cats: A retrospective study of 10 cases. J Am Anim Hosp Assoc 26:207, 1990.

Wesselhoeft Ablin LA, Berg J, Schelling SH. Fibrosarcoma of the canine appendicular skeleton. J Am Anim Hosp Assoc 27:303, 1991.

Whiting PG, Pool RR. Intrameniscal calcification and ossification in the stifle joints of three domestic cats. J Am Anim Hosp Assoc 21:579, 1985.

Whittick WG, Simpson S. Examination of the orthopedic patient. In Whittick WG, ed. Canine Orthopedics. 2nd ed. Philadelphia, Lea & Febiger, 1990, p 61.

CHAPTER 18

Neuromuscular Disorders

G. DIANE SHELTON

Neuromuscular disorders affect components of the motor unit. The motor unit consists of (1) a single motoneuron whose cell body resides within the central nervous system in either the nuclei of cranial nerves or the ventral horns of the spinal cord, (2) the axon of each motoneuron within its respective cranial or peripheral nerve, (3) the neuromuscular junction, and (4) the myofibers innervated by that nerve. Specific abnormalities affecting components of the motor unit can occur as acquired conditions in the geriatric dog and cat.

EVALUATION FOR NEUROMUSCULAR DISORDERS

History and Physical Examination

An accurate history, including all previous medical problems and therapies, should be obtained. Thorough systemic and neurologic examinations should be performed. Weakness, a motor sign, is common to all motor unit abnormalities. Muscle strength may be evaluated by observing the animal's gait as it walks and, if necessary, after it has exercised more strenuously. Because the clinical expression of weakness may vary considerably in severity and distribution, other tests, such as wheelbarrowing, hopping, or hemiwalking, may be necessary to specifically define a paresis. The presence of ataxia or analgesia indicates sensory deficits. Other clinical signs, including dysphagia (pharyngeal dysfunction), regurgitation (esophageal dysfunction), and dysphonia and dyspnea (laryngeal dysfunction) indicate involvement of selected motor units serving visceral functions. Muscle tone and spinal reflexes should be assessed, and the presence of muscle atrophy or swelling should be noted. After the examination, it should be possible to tentatively localize the disorder to a specific part of the motor unit.

Routine and Special Laboratory Evaluations

A complete blood cell count, serum chemistry profile (including electrolytes and creatine kinase [CK]), and urinalysis should be performed on all patients to evaluate possible underlying metabolic abnormalities.

Serum CK levels are elevated in muscle disorders associated with myonecrosis or increased cell membrane permeability. Although serum CK is a sensitive indicator of the presence and severity of myonecrosis, modest elevations can occur after intramuscular injections or with neuropathies (Cardinet, 1989). The presence of persistently elevated serum CK levels is *not necessarily diagnostic of myositis*. Other noninflammatory muscle disorders producing significant myonecrosis may result in marked elevations in serum CK levels. Histologic and histochemical examination of a muscle biopsy specimen is an absolute requirement to obtain a diagnosis in these cases.

Evaluation of plasma lactate levels before and after exercise should be done in all dogs with exercise intolerance and muscle weakness. Lactic acid is the end product of glycolysis when further oxidative metabolism is impaired. (For a review of lactic acidemia, see Robinson [1989].) Elevations in plasma lactate levels may be physiologic, as in hypoxic/ischemic injury, or pathologic, as when associated with disorders of oxidative metabolism. In several cases studied by this author, lactic acidemia associated with muscle weakness, atrophy, exercise intolerance, and lipid storage myopathy was documented as an acquired disorder in older dogs (Shelton, 1993).

Adrenal gland and thyroid gland status should be evaluated in cases of chronic muscle weakness and atrophy, particularly if other clinical signs are present suggesting an endocrine abnormality. Myopathy associated with hypothyroidism and myopathy and myotonia associated with hyperadrenocorticism have been described (Braund et al, 1980, 1981; Duncan et al, 1977; Greene et al, 1979; Hoskins et al, 1980). Although a direct association has not yet been proven, hypothyroidism may result in peripheral neuropathies that may respond at least partially to thyroid supplementation (Bichsel et al, 1988).

Serum antinuclear antibody (ANA) titers may be useful in the evaluation of inflammatory myopathies. Immune-mediated diseases have been postulated as an underlying cause of these disorders, and a positive ANA titer would support an immune abnormality (Shelton, 1991)

Serum *Toxoplasma gondii* and *Neospora caninum* titers may also be useful in evaluation of inflammatory myopathies. Infections in older dogs may result in clinical signs of multifocal central nervous system involvement along with polymyositis (Dubey, 1992). Cysts may be observed within the myofibers in a muscle biopsy sample. Other infectious agents, including *Ehrlichia canis* (Buoro et al, 1990) and *Borrelia burgdorferi* may result in an inflammatory myopathy, and testing should be performed for these agents, particularly in endemic areas.

"Myasthenia-like" syndromes and delayed neuropathies have been associated with organophosphate toxicity, and evaluation of plasma cholinesterase levels may be indicated if there has been previous exposure (Shelton, 1989a; Wheeler, 1991).

A radioimmunoassay for the detection of serum acetylcholine receptor antibodies (Shelton, 1992a) and an immunocytochemical assay for the detection of serum antibodies against masticatory muscle type 2M fibers (Shelton and Cardinet, 1989) are currently available as aids in the diagnosis of acquired myasthenia gravis and masticatory muscle myositis. A positive acetylcholine receptor antibody titer is diagnostic of acquired myasthenia gravis. Although a positive serum assay is highly suggestive of masticatory muscle myositis, a muscle biopsy should also be performed.

Analysis of cerebrospinal fluid is critical in the evaluation of lower motor neuron disorders in which nerve root involvement is suspected. Evaluation of protein concentration and cell counts is important in the diagnosis of these disorders.

Electrodiagnostic Evaluation

Electrophysiologic evaluation is an important adjunct to the diagnosis of neuromuscular disorders and is usually performed with the animal under anesthesia. Electromyography involves the detection and characterization of electrical activity (potentials) recorded from the patient's muscles. A systematic study of individual muscles permits an accurate determination of the distribution of affected muscles. Evaluation of motor and sensory nerve conduction velocities provides information about the integrity of nerve fibers in peripheral nerves. Evaluation of the amplitude of the evoked potential after repetitive nerve stimulation may provide information about the integrity of neuromuscular transmission. Single-fiber electromyography may be a more sensitive indicator of disorders of neuromuscular transmission, but it is technically difficult and must be performed by individuals highly trained in the procedure (Hopkins, 1992).

Examination of Muscle and Nerve Biopsy Specimens

The muscle biopsy allows direct examination of portions of most motor unit components, as well as supportive, connective, and vascular tissue. If fresh frozen sections are used, histologic and cytologic details are preserved, and many biochemical and immunochemical reactions within cells and tissues can be localized. Frozen sections may also be used in specific biochemical assays for enzymes and substrates (Cardinet, 1989).

Sensory and/or motor fascicles of certain

nerves can also be sampled (Braund, 1991). Although the basic pathologic reactions of axonal degeneration and demyelination can be defined, the histologic changes in many biopsy specimens are not pathognomonic of a particular disease, and several conditions can produce similar structural alterations.

Electromyographic evaluation aids in identifying affected muscles and/or nerves for biopsy. An involved muscle should be sampled. End-stage muscle should be avoided, as essential diagnostic features may no longer be present. If electromyographic procedures cannot be performed, then routinely evaluated muscles, such as the vastus lateralis, triceps brachii, cranial tibial, or extensor carpi radialis, should be sampled in generalized disorders and specific muscles (i.e., temporalis or masseter) in focal disorders.

The muscle biopsy should be taken with the dog or cat under general anesthesia, usually after electrophysiologic evaluation. Using sterile technique, an open biopsy procedure should be used in which a small incision is made in the skin overlying the muscle to be sampled, the subcutaneous tissues are separated, and the fascia overlying the muscle is incised and retracted. A cylinder of muscle approximately 0.5 × 0.5 × 1 cm should be taken along the longitudinal length of the muscle fibers. After collection, the sample should be wrapped in a saline-dampened gauze sponge (not dripping wet, merely moistened), placed in a watertight container, and kept cold until delivery to the laboratory for processing. For optimal results the sample should be shipped on cold packs in a well-insulated Styrofoam container and received by the laboratory within 24 hours for freezing and processing. It is important to consult with the pathologist *before* collecting a biopsy specimen, because once a muscle is placed in formalin or handled incorrectly, it is of limited diagnostic value. For muscle and peripheral nerve specimens it is advisable to use a laboratory specialized in handling these tissues.

Techniques used for the collection of peripheral nerve biopsies have been described (Braund, 1991), with fascicular biopsies of the common peroneal, ulnar, tibial, and caudal cutaneous antebrachial nerve the most commonly performed procedures.

SPECIFIC NEUROMUSCULAR DISORDERS

Neuropathies

Polyneuropathies are disorders affecting many peripheral nerves. They may affect lower motor neurons, sensory neurons, or both. Although polyneuropathies in general are relatively common in clinical practice, the specific cause of a polyneuropathy, as in humans, is most often not discovered. Mononeuropathies may also occur but will not be discussed.

Pathophysiology. Polyneuropathies are the result of degeneration or destruction of the neuronal cell body in the ventral horn of the spinal cord gray matter, primary demyelination, or axonal degeneration (with secondary demyelination).

Diagnosis. The diagnosis of a polyneuropathy is dependent on clinical signs of a lower motor neuron disorder (i.e., decreased muscle tone, hyporeflexia, and, in chronic cases, muscle atrophy), electromyography and nerve conduction studies, and histopathologic and histochemical evaluation of properly performed muscle and peripheral nerve biopsy specimens (Figs. 18–1 and 18–2). Additional laboratory testing, including analysis of cerebrospinal fluid, is warranted in these cases. A complete metabolic screening is important for potentially treatable causes of neuropathies, including hypoglycemia secondary to an insulinoma (Shahar et al, 1985), hypothyroidism (Bichsel et al, 1988), and hyperglycemia secondary to diabetes mellitus (Johnson et al, 1983, Katherman et al, 1983; Kramek et al, 1984).

Causes. Most cases of peripheral neuropathies in small animals are idiopathic in nature. The most common polyneuropathy of the dog is coonhound paralysis (CHP), although the true incidence is not known. Currently it is thought that a protein constituent of raccoon saliva may induce a delayed hypersensitivity against myelin, but this has not yet been proven. Although the development of polyradiculoneuritis after exposure to a raccoon is unequivocal in CHP, dogs without contact with raccoons have been found with a clinicopathologic entity similar to CHP. Other probable causes of peripheral neuropathy in small animals include presumed immune-mediated, metabolic, including diabetes mellitus, hypothyroidism, hypoadrenocorticism, and hyperinsulinism secondary to an insulinoma; toxic; paraneoplastic; and degenerative disorders that are rare and breed specific.

Treatment. If the underlying cause of the disorder can be identified (e.g., diabetes mellitus or insulinoma), treatment of the cause may result in some improvement of clinical signs. Most dogs with CHP recover spontaneously, and only careful nursing (soft bedding and frequent turning) is required. In the presumed immune-mediated neuropathies, corticosteroid therapy has been only marginally successful. Because the majority

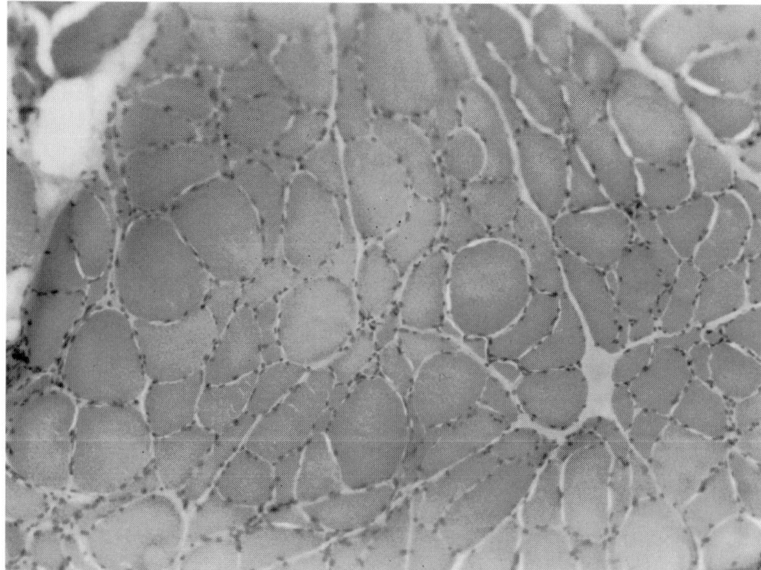

Figure 18–1. Frozen section of a limb muscle biopsy showing variation in myofiber size, with atrophic fibers having an angular shape. The angular atrophied fibers were of both fiber types (H & E stain; ×100).

of peripheral neuropathies have an unknown underlying etiology, therapeutic recommendations cannot be given.

Disorders of Neuromuscular Transmission

Disorders of neuromuscular transmission may be the result of presynaptic (hypocalcemia, botulism, tick paralysis), synaptic cleft (cholinesterase inhibitors), or postsynaptic (myasthenia gravis) defects (Shelton, 1989a; Wheeler, 1991). The most common disorder of neuromuscular transmission in small animals is acquired myasthenia gravis (MG). Acquired (immune-mediated) MG is a result of antibody-mediated destruction of postsynaptic acetylcholine receptors. Although this disorder is common in the dog, it appears to be rare in the cat.

History and Clinical Signs. Acquired MG affects numerous breeds of dogs. There is a bimodal age-related incidence, with peaks at 1 to 3 years of age and at 9 to 13 years of age (Shelton et al, 1992a). Signs of muscular weakness may be focal (with selective involvement of the esopha-

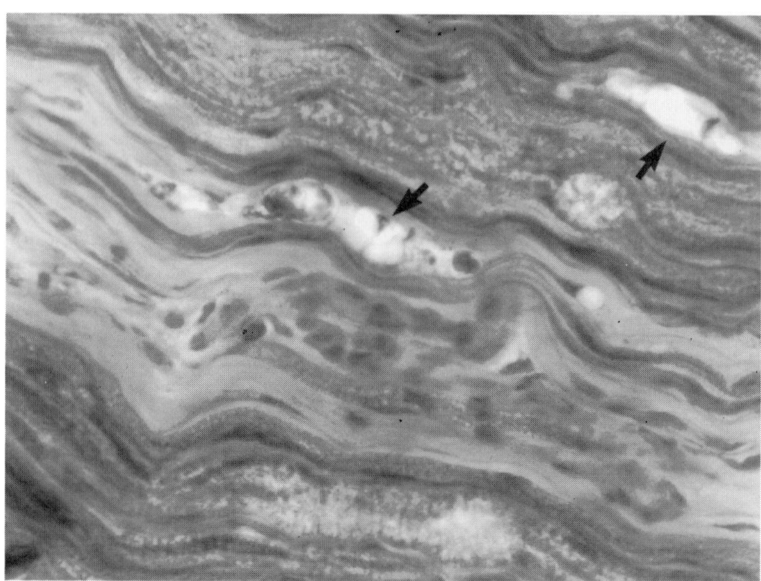

Figure 18–2. Frozen section of a peripheral nerve biopsy showing myelin degeneration. The arrows indicate myelin ovoids (modified trichrome stain; ×400).

geal, pharyngeal, and facial muscles) or diffuse (with signs of generalized muscle weakness). From one study it was estimated that one fourth of the canine patients presented with idiopathic megaesophagus had focal myasthenia gravis (Shelton et al, 1990). Signs of generalized muscle weakness may vary considerably, ranging from exercise intolerance, which improves with rest, to acute tetraplegia with hyporeflexia. Dogs with focal or generalized signs and megaesophagus often present with pneumonia secondary to aspiration. In the older age group, thoracic radiographs may reveal the presence of a cranial mediastinal mass.

Diagnostic Tests. Intravenous administration of edrophonium chloride (Tensilon) (0.1 mg/kg) should result in transient improvement in muscle strength, although some dogs that are severely affected may not show a positive response. Some improvement in muscle strength may be observed in dogs with other neuromuscular disorders, although the improvement is usually not dramatic. False-positive and false-negative results may occur with the Tensilon test (Oh and Cho, 1990).

A decline in the amplitude of successive potentials (i.e., a decrementing response) using repetitive nerve stimulation that reverses with edrophonium chloride is highly suggestive of myasthenia gravis. False-negative results can occur with this testing procedure, and false-positive results may occur if the stimulus frequency used is too high. Single-fiber electromyography may provide a more sensitive technique for evaluating neuromuscular synaptic function (Hopkins, 1992).

Quantitation of the serum acetylcholine receptor antibody titer using antigen-specific immunoprecipitation radioimmunoassay is both sensitive and specific and documents an immune response against acetylcholine receptors. False-positive results do not occur, but false-negative values may be found in rare "seronegative" cases (Shelton, 1989b).

Treatment. Anticholinesterase drugs are the mainstay of treatment for acquired MG and result in improved neuromuscular transmission (Shelton, 1992a). Pyridostigmine bromide (Mestinon) (1.0 to 3.0 mg/kg PO, bid) is the anticholinesterase of choice over neostigmine (Prostigmin), as fewer cholinergic side effects have been described (Physician Desk Reference, 1993). Pyridostigmine is available in tablet, elixir, and injectable forms. The elixir form is preferred for dogs with megaesophagus, as delivery to the stomach may be more reliable than with the tablet form. The elixir should be diluted 1:1 in water, as it may be irritating if given undiluted. For cases in which regurgitation is severe and treatment cannot be given orally, injectable pyridostigmine (1/30th of the oral dose) should be used. A gastric feeding tube should be placed in severe cases in which nothing can be taken orally. Such a tube will facilitate maintenance of nutrition and drug therapy. Addition of corticosteroids is recommended for cases that do not respond optimally to anticholinesterase drugs alone.

Insecticides containing long-acting anticholinesterases reversibly or irreversibly bind acetylcholinesterase, permitting continuous cholinergic stimulation. Acetylcholine accumulates at central, muscarinic, and nicotinic cholinergic synapses, with resulting clinical signs that include excessive salivation, diarrhea, ataxia, incoordination, muscle tremors, convulsions, and respiratory paralysis. Specific treatment, including atropine (0.1 to 0.2 mg/kg SC, prn) to chemically compete with acetylcholine binding to acetylcholine receptors and oximes (pralidoxime chloride, 20 mg/kg IM, tid) to release the inhibited acetylcholinesterase, along with supportive therapy as required, is usually adequate for routine clinical cases. Diphenhydramine has been shown to block the effects of nicotinic receptor overstimulation in cases of fenthion intoxication in dogs (Clemmons et al, 1984). An important source of organophosphate insecticide poisoning in the cat occurs with the use of chlorpyrifos-based products for the control of ectoparasites (Fikes, 1990).

MYOPATHIES

Myopathies are broadly classified as inflammatory and noninflammatory (Shelton, 1991) (Table 18–1). Although representative disorders from both categories occur in geriatric dogs and cats, the noninflammatory myopathies, particularly the endocrine and metabolic myopathies, are most common in this age group.

Inflammatory Myopathies

Masticatory Muscle Myositis

Masticatory muscle myositis (MMM) is an inflammatory muscle disorder limited to the muscles of mastication in dogs (Shelton and Cardinet, 1989). The muscles of mastication in the dog are composed predominantly of type 2M fibers, which differ from the type 2A fibers in limb muscles. Type 2M fibers are selectively affected and

TABLE 18–1. INFLAMMATORY AND NONINFLAMMATORY MYOPATHIES

Inflammatory Myopathies	Noninflammatory Myopathies
Infectious	Metabolic
Toxoplasma gondii	Lipid storage
Neospora caninum	Electrolyte abnormalities
Hepatozoon canis	Endocrine
Leptospirosis	Glucocorticoid excess
Microfilariasis	Cushing's syndrome
Postviral infection (?)	Hypothyroidism
Presumed immune-mediated	
Masticatory muscle myositis	
Polymyositis	
Dermatomyositis	
Extraocular myositis	
Paraneoplastic	
Thymoma	
Other neoplasms	
Drug-induced	
D-Penicillamine	
Trimethoprim-sulfadiazine	

destroyed in this disorder. Previously this condition was known as *eosinophilic* and/or *atrophic myositis*, but in reality, circulating or tissue eosinophils are not commonly found in this disorder. The acute phase, evidenced by muscle swelling, and the atrophic phase, evidenced by muscle atrophy, are probably separate stages of the same disease process.

History and Clinical Signs. Onset of clinical signs may be acute or chronic. Cases with an acute onset usually present with bilateral swelling of the temporalis and masseter muscles and, in some cases, exophthalmia owing to swelling of the pterygoid muscles. The animal may be febrile with conjunctivitis and enlarged lymph nodes and tonsils. Trismus is frequently present, and the dog exhibits pain when the jaws are manipulated and opening is attempted. A hallmark of this disorder is the inability to open the jaws even under anesthesia. With the chronic disorder, muscle atrophy may be marked, leaving the patient with a "skull-like" appearance.

Diagnosis. Measurement of serum CK levels should be performed, although elevations may be modest owing to the limited amount of muscle mass involved. Electromyographic examination helps define the distribution of involvement in acute cases, but in severely atrophied muscles with significant replacement of muscle by connective tissue, abnormal potentials may not be detected.

A muscle biopsy is essential to the diagnosis, and changes consistent with an inflammatory myopathy are usually observed (Fig. 18–3). Detection of immunoglobulin G (IgG) within type 2M fibers is observed using immunocytochemical methods (Shelton and Cardinet, 1989). Serologic testing confirms the presence of circulating antibodies against masticatory muscle type 2M fibers (Shelton and Cardinet, 1989).

Treatment. Immunosuppressive doses of corticosteroids usually result in clinical improvement and a return of jaw mobility. Long-term maintenance on alternate-day corticosteroid treatment is usually required.

Polymyositis

Although not as common as MMM, polymyositis (PM) is a generalized inflammatory myopa-

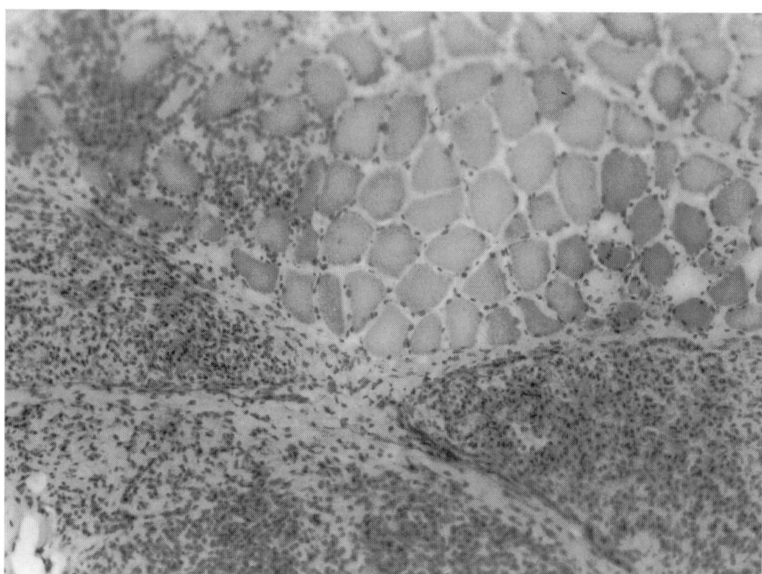

Figure 18–3. Frozen section of a limb muscle biopsy from a dog with polymyositis showing mononuclear cell infiltration (H & E stain; ×100).

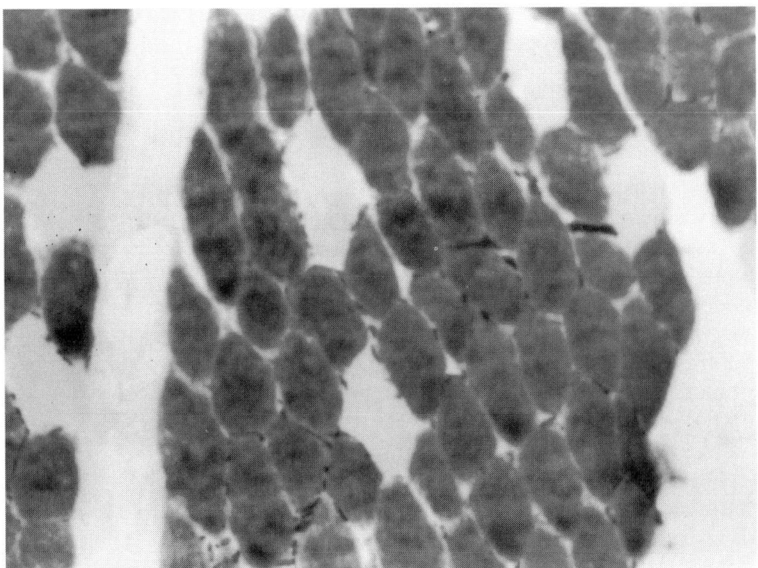

Figure 18–4. Frozen section of a limb muscle biopsy from a dog with confirmed hypothyroidism. There is a marked shift in myofiber types to a type 1 predominance (adenosine triphosphatase stain; pH 4.3; ×100).

thy. Underlying causes include infectious agents (*T. gondii, N. caninum, E. canis*) and ill-defined immune-mediated mechanisms. PM may also occur as a paraneoplastic disorder and is described in association with thymoma in dogs and cats (Aronsohn et al, 1984; Carpenter and Holzworth, 1982; Klebanow, 1992). I have recently processed muscle biopsy specimens from two dogs with confirmed disseminated mast cell tumor and severe polymyositis. Elevations in serum CK are usually marked, and muscle biopsy results should be diagnostic.

Noninflammatory Myopathies

Endocrine Myopathies

Myopathies have been described in association with several endocrine disorders and are a common cause of weakness in the geriatric dog. In some cases, the myopathy may be subclinical (Braund et al, 1980).

Hypothyroid Myopathy. Myopathies have been reported to occur in dogs in association with hypothyroidism. Clinical signs such as muscle weakness, stiffness, and muscle atrophy support a neuromuscular disorder. Although not fully documented, megaesophagus may also occur in hypothyroid dogs, with resolution of the esophageal dilatation occurring after thyroid replacement therapy. Laryngeal paralysis has also been reported in association with hypothyroidism (Harvey et al, 1983), although the majority of these cases probably are related to a peripheral neuropathy.

DIAGNOSIS. The clinical diagnosis of hypothyroidism is discussed in Chapter 15. The diagnosis of muscle involvement is dependent on electrophysiologic evaluation followed by muscle and nerve biopsies. Nonspecific findings such as fibrillation potentials and positive sharp waves may be found in hypothyroid dogs, with bizarre high-frequency discharges occurring in some dogs. The bizarre high-frequency discharges, in my experience, have been found in cases with muscle hypertrophy and stiffness and a shift in percentage of fiber types to type 1 fibers (Fig. 18–4). In dogs in which weakness and muscle atrophy are prominent, selective type 2 fiber atrophy may be the only abnormal finding. In some cases, changes consistent with neuropathy (angular atrophy of both type 1 and type 2 fibers) may be observed. The presence of nemaline rods in type 1 fibers or abnormal glycogen inclusions may be observed in some dogs.

TREATMENT. Thyroid supplementation should be initiated. Adequate studies have not been performed to evaluate whether clinical signs and pathologic abnormalities within muscle and nerve biopsy samples resolve after treatment.

Hyperthyroid Myopathy. Clinical signs of neuromuscular dysfunction have been described in hyperthyroid cats, and in one study, weakness attributable to muscle dysfunction was relatively common (Joseph and Peterson, 1992). Clinical presentation of muscle weakness included ventroflexion of the neck, muscle tremors, gait disturbances (e.g., ataxia, incoordination, inability to jump), muscle atrophy, and collapse. Serum CK levels were high in some cats. Myotatic reflexes were normal to exaggerated. Diminished reflexes were rarely observed, and areflexia was not recognized. Electromyographic studies were incomplete in these cats, and no histopathologic examinations of muscle biopsy specimens have been reported in the literature. Further studies are necessary to document the pathologic basis of clinical weakness in hyperthyroid cats.

Myasthenia gravis has not been documented to be associated with hyperthyroidism in cats, although two cats on methimazole treatment with associated muscle weakness tested positive for acetylcholine receptor antibodies (Shelton, unpublished observation). The mechanism may be similar to the drug-induced myasthenia gravis reported in humans associated with D-penicillamine treatment (Bever et al, 1982).

Treatment. Re-establishment of a euthyroid state can be achieved by the use of antithyroid drugs, radioactive iodine, or surgical thyroidectomy. With correction of hyperthyroidism most neuromuscular signs have been reported to resolve (Joseph and Peterson, 1992).

Glucocorticoid Excess. Muscle weakness and myopathy have been associated with naturally occurring hyperadrenocorticism in dogs and with iatrogenic hyperadrenocorticism in cats and dogs (LeCouteur et al, 1989). Dogs appear to be particularly sensitive to the effects of exogenous corticosteroids, and significant atrophy, particularly of the masticatory muscles, and muscle weakness may develop. Clinical signs consistent with a neuromuscular disorder include a stiff, stilted gait, muscle weakness, and atrophy. In some severely affected dogs with Cushing's syndrome, pelvic limb rigidity and inability to walk have been noted (Fig. 18–5).

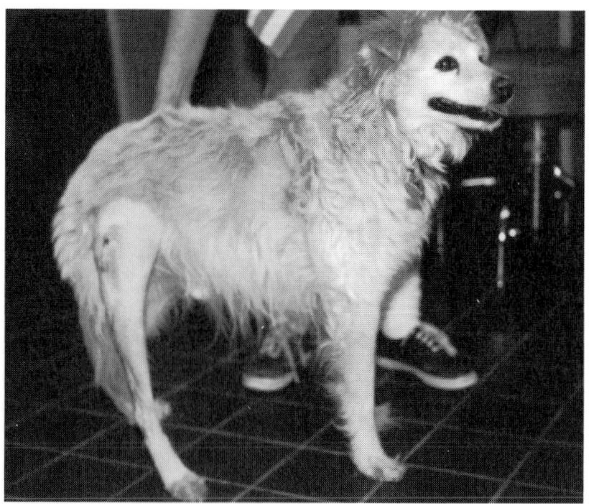

Figure 18–5. Pelvic limb rigidity in a dog with Cushing's syndrome and myotonia. (Courtesy of Don Levesque, DVM, Veterinary Neurological Center, Phoenix, AZ.)

Diagnosis. Usually animals with Cushing's syndrome show other clinical signs consistent with glucocorticoid excess, including polydipsia, polyuria, alopecia, and a pendulous abdomen, although this is not absolute. A discussion on the laboratory diagnosis of Cushing's syndrome and iatrogenic Cushing's syndrome may be found in Chapter 15. Electrophysiologic studies followed by a muscle biopsy are required for pathologic confirmation of the neuromuscular disorder. Bizarre high-frequency discharges may be seen in electromyographic studies in dogs.

Cushing's Myopathy. Examination of muscle biopsy specimens may show variable changes ranging from selective type 2 fiber atrophy (Fig. 18–6) in dogs with severe muscle weakness to

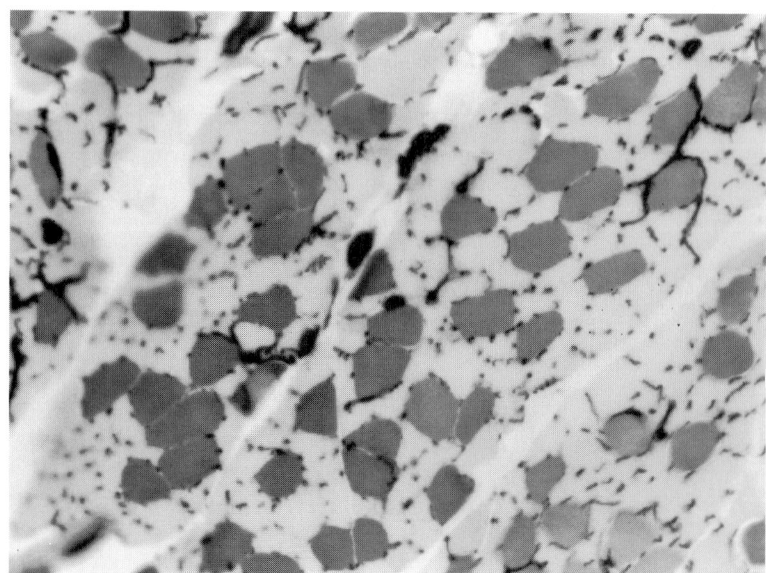

Figure 18–6. Type 2 myofiber atrophy in a muscle biopsy from a dog with Cushing's syndrome, muscle atrophy, and weakness (adenosine triphosphatase stain; pH 4.3; ×100).

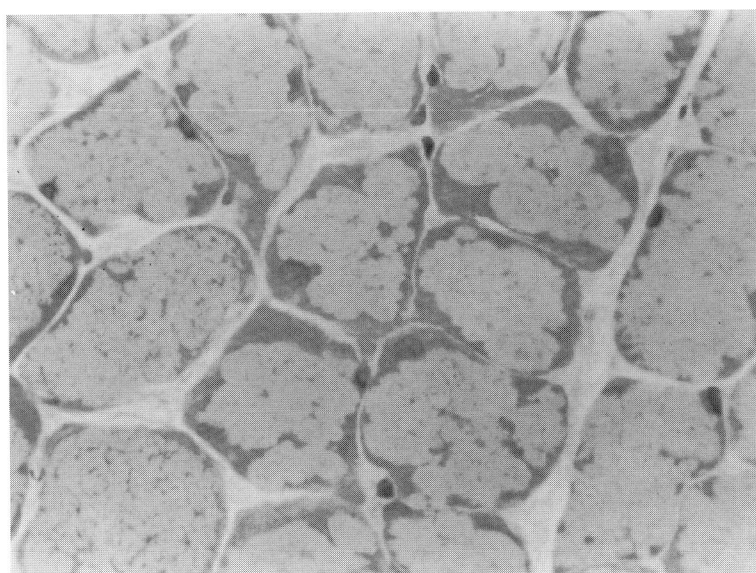

Figure 18–7. Muscle biopsy section from a dog with Cushing's syndrome and myotonia showing myofibers having a cross between lobulated and ragged red–like cytoarchitectural changes (H & E stain; ×400).

"ragged red"–like fibers and lipid storage in dogs with pelvic limb rigidity and so-called Cushing's "myotonia" (Fig. 18–7). Peripheral neuropathies have also been reported to occur along with neuropathies in glucocorticoid excess, although this has not been my experience.

TREATMENT. A discussion of therapy for Cushing's syndrome and iatrogenic Cushing's syndrome may be found in Chapter 15. Clinical signs have been reported to improve after therapy for hyperadrenocorticism, but most dogs have a poor prognosis for complete resolution of a myopathy despite control of elevated cortisol levels. Return of muscle strength should occur in cases of iatrogenic Cushing's syndrome.

Hypoadrenocorticism. Muscle weakness occurs frequently in association with hypoadrenocorticism (Addison's disease) in dogs and cats (Greco and Peterson, 1989; Schrader, 1986). Resolution of clinical signs usually occurs after diagnosis and treatment of the disorder. Dysphagia and megaesophagus may occur in association with muscle weakness, and these signs should also resolve. Although clinical signs of weakness are probably related to alterations in electrolyte levels, one report documents the occurrence of a reversible megaesophagus associated with deficient glucocorticoid secretion without a mineralocorticoid deficiency (Bartges and Nielson, 1992).

Metabolic Myopathies

Electrolyte Disorders. Electrolyte disorders are an important cause of muscular weakness in dogs and cats. Cats appear to be particularly sensitive to electrolyte imbalances. Electrolyte evaluation should be part of a general screen in any animal showing muscle weakness.

HYPOKALEMIC MYOPATHY. Hypokalemic myopathy has been well documented in the cat (Dow et al, 1987). It is important to differentiate this disorder from polymyositis in this species, as the clinical presentation may be identical. As in polymyositis, ventroflexion of the neck (Fig. 18–8) and generalized muscle weakness with a moderately to markedly elevated CK may be found. Serum potassium concentrations are normal in cases of polymyositis and less than 3.5 mEq/L in

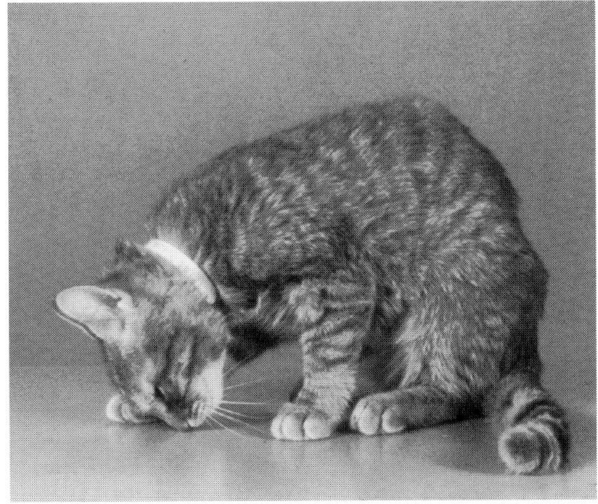

Figure 18–8. Ventroflexion of the neck in a cat with hypokalemic myopathy and generalized muscle weakness. (Courtesy of Mike Podell, DVM, The Ohio State University, Columbus, OH.)

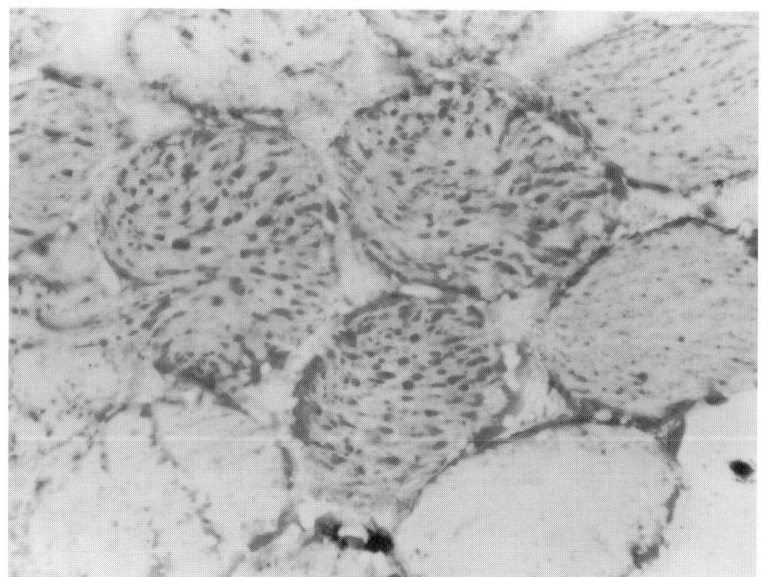

Figure 18–9. Increased neutral lipid within a fresh frozen muscle biopsy section from a dog with muscle pain, atrophy, and weakness associated with low muscle carnitine levels (Oil-red-O stain; ×400).

cases of hypokalemic myopathy. Muscle biopsy samples from cats with hypokalemic myopathy are usually normal. In one series of cases, improvement in muscle strength in hypokalemic cats was noted after changing the diet to one with a higher potassium content or after dietary supplementation with potassium (Dow et al, 1987).

HYPERKALEMIA. Secondary hyperkalemia and muscle weakness may occur in association with numerous clinical conditions, including metabolic acidosis, hypoadrenocorticism, renal failure, or hyperaldosteronism. Iatrogenic causes include intravenous potassium administration and the use of potassium-retaining diuretics. Initial clinical signs are usually referable to cardiovascular abnormalities.

OTHER ELECTROLYTE ABNORMALITIES. Electrolyte abnormalities, including hypernatremia, hypo- or hypercalcemia, hypo- or hypermagnesemia, and hypo- or hyperphosphatemia, may result in signs of neuromuscular dysfunction, although specific myopathies associated with these disorders have not been reported. Clinical signs should resolve with normalization of serum electrolyte levels. Muscle biopsy specimens from cases involving electrolyte abnormalities in dogs and cats have not been abnormal.

Lipid Storage Disorders. Myopathies associated with storage of neutral lipid within myofibers have been recognized in older dogs (Shelton, 1993). In humans, most lipid storage myopathies recognized to date are associated with a derangement of carnitine metabolism, either primary or secondary (Engel, 1986). Others occur with mitochondrial abnormalities that do not involve carnitine, and in still others, the basis of the lipid storage remains unknown.

In dogs the most common presenting clinical signs include muscle pain (acute and chronic), weakness, and muscle atrophy. Less frequently reported clinical presentations include stiffness, lameness, cramping, exercise intolerance, and tremors. A presumptive diagnosis of a lipid storage myopathy is based on histopathologic observation of increased intramyofiber lipid within a fresh frozen muscle biopsy section, using a stain for neutral lipid (Fig. 18–9). Resting plasma lactate levels are usually elevated. Organic acid abnormalities as assessed by gas chromatography mass spectrometry of urine are usually present and include lactic and pyruvic aciduria. Elevations in plasma and urine alanine may be present, and abnormalities in plasma, urine, and muscle carnitine levels may be found (Shelton, 1993).

TREATMENT. L-carnitine (50 mg/kg bid) has been used in a number of dogs with lipid storage myopathy, with varying results. Dogs with the most severe metabolic abnormalities did the poorest, while other dogs returned to normal. Other treatments used in human medicine include a low-fat, high-carbohydrate diet and cofactor treatment with riboflavin and coenzyme Q. The benefits of these additional treatments are not fully established.

References and Supplemental Reading

Aronsohn MG, Schunk KL, Carpenter JL, et al. Clinical and pathologic features of thymoma in 15 dogs. J Am Vet Med Assoc 184:1355, 1984.

Bartges JW, Nielson DL. Reversible megaesophagus associated with atypical primary hypoadrenocorticism in a dog. J Am Vet Med Assoc 201:889, 1992.

Bever CT, Chang HW, Penn AS, et al. Penicillamine-induced myasthenia gravis: Effects of penicillamine on the acetylcholine receptor. Neurology 32:1077, 1982.

Bichsel P, Jacobs G, Oliver JE. Neurologic manifestations associated with hypothyroidism in four dogs. J Am Vet Med Assoc 192:1745, 1988.

Braund KG. Nerve and muscle biopsy techniques. Progress in Veterinary Neurology 2:35, 1991.

Braund KG, Dillon AR, Mikeal RL, et al. Subclinical myopathy associated with hyperadrenocorticism in the dog. Vet Pathol 17:134, 1980.

Braund KG, Dillon AR, August JR, et al. Hypothyroid myopathy in two dogs. Vet Pathol 18:589, 1981.

Buoro IBJ, Kanui TI, Atwell RB, et al. Polymyositis associated with *Ehrlichia canis* infection in two dogs. J Small Anim Pract 31:624, 1990.

Cardinet GH III. Skeletal muscle function. In Kaneko JJ, ed. Clinical Biochemistry of Domestic Animals. San Diego, Academic Press, 1989, p 462.

Carpenter JL, Holzworth J. Thymoma in 11 cats. J Am Vet Med Assoc 181:248, 1982.

Clemmons RM, Meyer DJ, Sundlof SF, et al. Correction of organophosphate-induced neuromuscular blockade by diphenhydramine. Am J Vet Res 45:2167, 1984.

Dow SW, LeCouteur RA, Fettman MJ, et al. Potassium depletion in cats: Hypokalemic polymyopathy. J Am Vet Med Assoc 191:1563, 1987.

Dubey JP. *Neospora caninum* infections. In Kirk RW, Bonagura JD, eds. Current Veterinary Therapy XI. Philadelphia, WB Saunders, 1992, p 263.

Duncan ID, Griffiths IR, Nash AS. Myotonia in canine Cushing's disease. Vet Rec 100:30, 1977.

Engel AG. Carnitine deficiency syndromes and lipid storage myopathies. In Engel AG, Banker BQ, eds. Myology. New York, McGraw-Hill, 1986, p 1663.

Fikes JD. Organophosphorus and carbamate insecticides. Vet Clin North Am [Small Anim Pract] 20:353, 1990.

Greco DS, Peterson ME. Feline hypoadrenocorticism. In Kirk RW, ed. Current Veterinary Therapy X. Philadelphia, WB Saunders, 1989, p 1042.

Greene CE, Lorenz MD, Munnell JF, et al. Myopathy associated with hyperadrenocorticism in the dog. J Am Vet Med Assoc 174:1310, 1979.

Harvey HJ, Irby NL, Watrous BJ. Laryngeal paralysis in hypothyroid dogs. In Kirk RW, ed. Current Veterinary Therapy VIII. Philadelphia, WB Saunders, 1983, p 694.

Hopkins AL. Single fiber electromyography in the dog. Proc Am Coll Vet Intern Med Forum, 10:768, 1992.

Hoskins JD, Nafe LA, Cho DY. Myopathy associated with hyperadrenocorticism in a dog: A case report. Vet Med Small Anim Clin 77:760, 1980.

Johnson CA, Kittleson MD, Indrieri RJ. Peripheral neuropathy and hypotension in a diabetic dog. J Am Vet Med Assoc 183:1007, 1983.

Joseph RJ, Peterson ME. Review and comparison of neuromuscular and central nervous system manifestations of hyperthyroidism in cats and humans. Progress in Veterinary Neurology 3:114, 1992.

Katherman AE, Braund KG. Polyneuropathy associated with diabetes mellitus in a dog. J Am Vet Med Assoc 182:522, 1983.

Klebanow ER. Thymoma and acquired myasthenia gravis in the dog: A case report and review of 13 additional cases. J Am Anim Hosp Assoc 28:63, 1992.

Kramek BA, Moise NS, Cooper B, et al. Neuropathy associated with diabetes mellitus in the cat. J Am Vet Med Assoc 184:42, 1984.

LeCouteur RA, Dow SW, Sisson AF. Metabolic and endocrine myopathies of dogs and cats. Semin Vet Med Surg 4:146, 1989.

Oh SJ, Cho HK. Edrophonium responsiveness not necessarily diagnostic of myasthenia gravis. Muscle Nerve 13:187, 1990.

Physicians Desk Reference. Montvale, NJ, Medical Economics Data, 1993.

Robinson BH. Lactic acidemia. In Scriver CR, Beaudet AL, Sly WS, Valle D, eds. The Metabolic Basis of Inherited Disease. New York, McGraw-Hill, 1989, p 869.

Schrader LA. Hypoadrenocorticism. In Kirk RW, ed. Current Veterinary Therapy IX. Philadelphia, WB Saunders, 1986, p 972.

Shahar R, Rousseaux C, Steiss J. Peripheral polyneuropathy in a dog with functional islet B-cell tumor and widespread metastasis. J Am Vet Med Assoc 187:175, 1985.

Shelton GD. Disorders of neuromuscular transmission. Semin Vet Med Surg [Small Anim] 4:126, 1989a.

Shelton GD. Canine seronegative acquired myasthenia gravis. Proc Am Coll Vet Intern Med Forum 7:999, 1989b.

Shelton GD. Differential diagnosis of muscle diseases in companion animals. Progress in Veterinary Neurology 2:27, 1991.

Shelton GD. Canine myasthenia gravis. In Kirk RW, Bonagura JD, eds. Current Veterinary Therapy XI. Philadelphia, WB Saunders, 1992a, p 1039.

Shelton GD. Megaesophagus secondary to acquired myasthenia gravis. In Kirk RW, Bonagura JD, eds. Current Veterinary Therapy XI. Philadelphia, WB Saunders, 1992b, p 580.

Shelton GD. Canine lipid storage myopathies. Proc Am Coll Vet Intern Med Forum 11:707, 1993.

Shelton GD, Cardinet GH III. Canine masticatory muscle disorders. In Kirk RW, ed. Current Veterinary Therapy X. Philadelphia, WB Saunders, 1989, p 816.

Shelton GD, Willard MD, Cardinet GH III, et al. Acquired myasthenia gravis. Selective involvement of esophageal, pharyngeal and facial muscles. J Vet Intern Med 4:281, 1990.

Wheeler SJ. Disorders of the neuromuscular junction. Progress in Veterinary Neurology 2:129, 1991.

CHAPTER 19

The Nervous System

T. MARK NEER

Relatively few neurologic conditions occur in dogs and cats that are identified specifically with old age. Some neurologic diseases occur that, because of their pathogenesis, would have no predilection based on age (e.g., trauma, inflammatory/infectious diseases, and/or toxicities). This discussion is organized according to neuroanatomic areas affected and the neurologic signs produced from lesions in these areas. These neuroanatomic areas and signs include the following:

- forebrain disease: change in attitude, seizures, circling, blindness, compulsive walking
- cerebellar disease: ataxia, dysmetria, intention tremor
- spinal cord disease: paraparesis, tetraparesis
- vestibular disease: ataxia, head tilt, nystagmus
- brain stem disease: paresis of limbs associated with cranial nerve deficits
- lumbosacral disease: urinary bladder, tail, and anal sphincter dysfunction
- peripheral nerve disease: deficits associated with lower motor neuron disease
- tremors
- deafness

Diseases and/or disorders that affect the myoneural junction or muscular system are discussed in Chapter 18.

HISTORICAL, PHYSICAL, AND NEUROLOGIC EXAMINATIONS

History. A thorough history should be obtained before complete physical and neurologic examinations are performed on old dogs and cats. The history may be the key component for developing a differential diagnosis list and/or for placing the animal's problem into a specific disease category (e.g., neoplastic, infectious, vascular). Many times the history will direct the initial diagnostic plan and therapeutic approach or even help establish a diagnosis of a clinical syndrome (e.g., geriatric vestibular disease). In addition, prognosis may be strongly based on the historical information. The areas of primary interest to include in the history are as follows:

1. Reason for presentation (i.e., why is the owner concerned about the pet?)
2. Summary of past medical/surgical problems
3. Description of the problem as seen by the owner; this includes the following:
   a. Onset of action: a very abrupt or subtle beginning?
   b. Progression of the problem since onset: is the problem static, improving, or worsening?
   c. Was or is there any asymmetry in the problem? This may be helpful in localizing spinal cord lesions that may have begun as an asymmetric problem but had developed into a symmetric problem by the time the animal was presented to the veterinarian.
   d. Has there been a change in the pattern of a long-standing problem (e.g., has the seizure frequency/severity of an idiopathic epileptic animal suddenly changed?)?
4. Is the animal presently on any medication?

Table 19–1 lists the categories of neurologic disease and their typical history with regard to onset/progression and type of neurologic deficits.

Physical Examination. The importance of a thorough physical examination in old dogs and cats with a neurologic problem cannot be overemphasized. Older animals are more likely to have a disease of another body system masquerading as a primary neurologic problem. The physical examination may define the body system that is associated with the primary neurologic problem or the source of metastatic CNS neoplasia. For example, the presence of fever, anterior uveitis, and chorioretinitis may lead to a diagnosis of an infectious disease. Older dogs and cats are also more likely to have diseases of other body systems coexisting with a primary neurologic problem that may affect the animal's overall prognosis.

Neurologic Examination. A complete discussion of the different aspects of the neurologic examination will not be done here, as this information can be found in several veterinary neurology textbooks. Instead, this discussion will focus on those aspects of the neurologic examination that differ or should be assessed differently because the dog or cat is older. These comments are at times subjective and are based solely on experience and not necessarily on scientifically controlled studies. This information is intended to be used as a guideline and to heighten the clinician's powers of observation. The main point is that there are significant differences between young and older dogs and cats with regard to the neurologic examination.

As dogs and cats mature to old age, the senses of sight and hearing become decreased by several processes, and as a result, reactions to response tests may be altered. Obviously, reflexes or reactions directly involving hearing and vision are affected, but in addition to these, the animal may be hypersensitive to external stimuli (i.e., sensitive to noise if blind and sensitive to touch if deaf). It is important to initially work slowly with a geriatric patient that has diminished senses and to handle the patient for a few minutes before beginning the neurologic examination. Animals that are blind may appear to be slightly hypermetric in their gait and during postural testing. In addition, they may have brisk myotatic tendon reflexes as a result of increased sensitivity to touch. Therefore, even if both gait and postural test reactions are normal, the clinician should not overinterpret "hyperreflexia" of the myotatic tendon reflexes.

Iris atrophy is a common aging change in older dogs and cats, especially those older than 8 years of age (Fig. 19–1). It is a common cause of incomplete pupillary light reflexes and therefore should always be ruled out before optic or oculomotor nerve deficits are considered as the cause of pupillary light reflex abnormalities. Clues that iris atrophy may exist include (1) irregular pupil margins, (2) strands of iris that span across portions of the pupil, and (3) the presence of large holes in the iris stroma or iris dilator muscle that resemble multiple pupillary openings (Smedes, 1992). In some breeds of dogs, especially cocker spaniels, the palpebral reflex may be less complete when compared with that in younger dogs of the same breed. This appears to be a result of motor weakness to eyelid closure and not sensory loss, because sensation to the head and face is normal. These animals usually have had no history of a previous episode of facial nerve paralysis, either idiopathic or secondary to

TABLE 19–1. NEUROLOGIC DISEASES IN THE OLDER DOG AND CAT AND TYPICAL PRESENTING HISTORIES

CATEGORY	ONSET AND PROGRESSION	NEUROLOGIC DEFICITS
Idiopathic syndromes	Usually acute and nonprogressive	Vary with syndrome
Trauma	Acute, nonprogressive	Symmetric or asymmetric
Vascular	Acute, nonprogressive	Symmetric or asymmetric; common to have lateralization if spinal cord affected
Toxic	Acute, usually progressive	Usually symmetric
Infectious/inflammatory	Acute, progressive	Multifocal deficits
	Subtle, progressive	Symmetric
Metabolic	Acute, progressive	Usually symmetric
	Chronic, progressive	
	Episodic (seizures, weakness)	
Degenerative	Subtle, chronic, progressive	Usually symmetric
Neoplasia	Subtle, chronic, progressive	Symmetric or asymmetric
	Acute, progressive (seizures)	

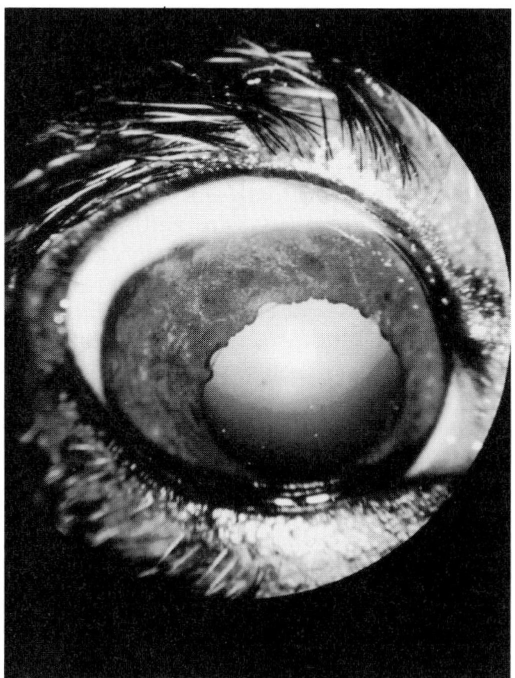

Figure 19–1. Iris atrophy in an 11-year-old mixed breed dog with a dilated pupil.

otitis media. It is uncertain whether this finding represents a partial palsy or is just an age-related change.

The older dog and cat may not be as responsive and alert to external stimuli as the younger animal. When assessing functions such as object following, menace reflex, and response to auditory stimuli, the veterinarian should not always overinterpret a depressed response as indicating neurologic deficits. A depressed response could represent nothing more than a change in the animal's general interest in these external stimuli. The older dog with degenerative disease of the coxofemoral joints may have what appears to be slow tarsal replacement (proprioceptive testing). This response may result from the reluctance of the dog to flex the hip because of pain. Therefore, mild slowing of tarsal replacement should not be assumed to have a neurologic cause. Certainly, however, prolonged "knuckling over" of the foot would not be caused by orthopedic disease.

NEUROLOGIC DISORDERS IN THE DOG

Forebrain Disease

Disorders that are likely to cause forebrain signs (e.g., changes in attitude, seizures, circling, blindness, or compulsive walking) in the geriatric patient include neoplasia, inflammatory disease, vascular disease, senile degeneration, and metabolic disorders. Diseases that show no association with age but may also cause these signs include toxins, infections, and trauma.

Neoplasia

Brain tumors are classified as either primary (arising from tissue inherent to the brain and its coverings) or secondary (reaching the brain by local extension or hematogenous metastasis). The most common primary tumors of dogs are neuroepithelial (gliomas), meningeal (meningiomas), and lymphoid (reticulosis, lymphosarcoma) in origin. Brain tumors are recognized most frequently in dogs older than 6 years of age. Glial cell neoplasms and pituitary gland tumors occur most commonly in brachycephalic breeds, whereas meningiomas are recognized most often in dolichocephalic breeds (Kornegay, 1986). The brain is also another common site for metastasis of systemic neoplasms. Metastatic brain tumors usually include nasal adenocarcinomas and their direct extension, as well as distant metastasis from melanoma, hemangiosarcoma, mammary gland adenocarcinoma, pancreatic adenocarcinoma, undifferentiated carcinomas, and adenocarcinoma of multiple origins.

Clinical Findings. Regardless of whether the tumor is primary or metastatic, the signs that develop are the result of primary or secondary tumor effects (Table 19–2). As a general rule, the clinical signs associated with primary brain tumors are slowly progressive (over several weeks to months), in contrast to metastatic brain neoplasms, which have signs that are rapid in onset and a clinical course that is generally shorter, with death occurring in days or weeks after initial diagnosis (Fenner, 1990). This difference may be due to the high prevalence of infarction and/or hemorrhage associated with metastatic CNS neo-

TABLE 19–2. EFFECTS OF BRAIN TUMORS

Primary effects
Infiltration of nervous tissue
Compression of adjacent anatomic structures
Secondary effects
Hydrocephalus
Disruption of cerebral circulation
Local necrosis
Hemorrhage
Disturbance of CSF flow dynamics
Elevated intracranial pressure
Cerebral edema
Brain herniation

plasia, although spontaneous hemorrhage may occur with primary CNS tumors. The factors determining clinical signs and progression are tumor location, size, type, and tendency to result in hemorrhage. For example, a tumor in the midbrain will generally impair movement of cerebrospinal fluid (CSF) more rapidly than will a cerebellar tumor; a small lesion in the midbrain will cause severe signs early in the course of the disease, whereas a lesion of similar size in the cerebrum may cause very subtle changes that go unnoticed for months.

Many dogs with brain tumors have long histories of "vague" signs that are often overlooked until signs of brain dysfunction are well developed. These signs include subtle behavior alterations that may progress slowly over many months. Whether these vague signs are due to headaches will remain speculative, as this is a "verbalized" phenomenon in humans and is impossible to recognize in dogs or cats. However, dogs and cats may exhibit abnormal behavior that is consistent with the presence of a headache, such as avoiding physical contact with humans or hiding during the day (LeCouteur, 1990).

The objective clinical signs of brain neoplasms include seizures, altered behavior, circling, head pressing, compulsive walking, altered consciousness, and locomotor disturbances. Cerebral tumors typically cause behavior changes, seizures, visual deficits, and circling. Brain stem tumors cause depression, head tilt, cranial nerve deficits, weakness, and ataxia. Cerebellar tumors will cause ataxia, head tilt, circling, and tremor. Seizure is the most common clinical sign of a brain neoplasm, especially in the rostral cerebrum (Holliday et al, 1987). Choroid plexus papillomas have also been associated with such non-neurologic signs as vomiting and bradycardia (Hammer et al, 1990; Zaki and Nafe, 1980). In addition, acute onset of blindness may be the only clinical sign of intracranial neoplasia. Chiasmatic neoplasia, even in the absence of other neurologic signs, should be an important consideration in older dogs with acute, unexplained vision loss.

Diagnosis. If the neurologic examination indicates a focal brain lesion (i.e., cranial nerve deficits, motor weakness, postural test reaction deficits, and/or circling), then the likelihood is high that primary brain disease exists as a result of a focal mass (i.e., neoplasia, granuloma, or hemorrhage). If only seizures and/or behavioral/mentation changes are present, metabolic diseases (e.g., hypoglycemia, hepatic disease) should also be included in the differential diagnosis along with primary brain disease. The minimum laboratory evaluation of a dog with signs of a brain lesion should include a hemogram, serum chemistry panel, and urinalysis. If the neurologic examination strongly supports the presence of a focal lesion, these tests are unlikely to be abnormal. These screening tests are most beneficial in older dogs that have only seizures or mentation changes as the primary signs and in which the probability of metabolic disease is more likely. The major objective of these tests is to eliminate extracranial causes of cerebral dysfunction. Further evaluation for extracranial disorders may include fasting and 2-hour postprandial bile acid determinations; determination of blood ammonia levels and serum insulin-to-glucose ratios; endocrine tests (thyroid-stimulating hormone [TSH] stimulation, test, adrenocorticotropic hormone [ACTH] stimulation test); and determination of a blood lead level if the history and/or hemogram so indicate.

If results of the minimum laboratory evaluation are normal and/or the neurologic examination indicates that the problem is most likely intracranial, then further diagnostic tests are indicated. Abdominal and thoracic radiographs may be helpful in defining a primary neoplasia elsewhere. For example, one study found that dogs with brain metastasis from hemangiosarcoma (HSA) also had a high incidence of pulmonary metastasis (Waters et al, 1989). Further tests may include plain film skull radiographs, CSF analysis, and/or special imaging techniques such as computerized tomography (CT) or magnetic resonance imaging (MRI). Plain film skull radiographs in dogs are of limited value in the diagnosis of a primary brain tumor; however, they may be helpful in the detection of neoplasms of the skull or nasal cavity that have affected the brain by local extension (Smith et al, 1989). Skull radiographs may reveal erosion or hyperostosis of the calvarium in association with a primary brain tumor (e.g., meningioma) or may document areas of mineralization within a neoplasm (LeCouteur, 1989). CSF analysis is often helpful in evaluating patients suspected of having an intracranial neoplasm; fluid collected from the cerebellomedullary cistern will usually be altered by an intracranial neoplasm, especially if the tumor communicates with the ventricles or subarachnoid space. Although CSF changes are often nonspecific, when combined with the history and neurologic examination, such changes may provide an accurate diagnosis (Nafe, 1990). CSF analysis may reveal a definitive diagnosis if neoplastic cells are visualized, but this is unusual unless the neoplasm is lymphosarcoma. Unless neoplastic cells are present, CSF analysis will provide only indirect evidence that a tumor exists. In general, increased CSF protein content and normal to increased CSF white blood cell counts are considered the typical changes seen with brain neoplasms (Bailey and Higgins, 1986). The presence of increased numbers of neutrophils in CSF does not exclude the diagnosis of a neoplasm. Increased neutrophils may occur secondary to inflammation and/or necrosis of the surrounding nervous tissue (Bailey and Higgins, 1986; Carrillo et al, 1986). Meningiomas are more commonly associated with a neutrophilic CSF pleocytosis; however, pleocytosis can be seen with other tumors as well (Bailey and Higgins, 1986; Carrillo et al, 1986; Foster et al, 1988). Choroid plexus papillomas may cause dramatic increases in CSF protein concentration (Zaki and Nafe, 1980). Primary intracranial neoplasia is generally associated with a CSF white blood cell (WBC) count of fewer than 50 cells/μL with variable elevations of CSF protein. In contrast, metastatic or invasive neoplasia is associated with higher WBC counts and protein levels (Nafe, 1990).

Special Imaging Techniques. Because most intracranial neoplasms are not visible with plain film radiographs, the development of CT and MRI have revolutionized the diagnosis and treatment of intracranial neoplasms (Fig. 19–2). These techniques allow for precise localization of tumors, facilitate brain biopsy, determine the feasibility of surgical removal of a neoplasm, allow for a high degree of certainty about tumor type and for localization before radiation therapy, improve the owner's ability to make decisions regarding care, and enable the veterinarian to more accurately advise owners regarding therapy and prognosis.

The CT features of most intracranial tumors in dogs are similar to those of comparable tumors in humans (Ambrose et al, 1975; Kornegay, 1990a). One large series of cases (50 dogs) found that meningiomas could be distinguished from tumors within the brain parenchyma, because they usually were broad-based, peripherally located masses that enhanced homogeneously with contrast material (Turrel et al, 1986). Among the parenchymal tumors, astrocytomas are not easily distinguished from oligodendrogliomas, because both tumors have similar ring-like and nonuniform enhancement, and poorly defined tumor margins. Choroid plexus tumors are seen as well-defined, hyperdense masses that have marked uniform contrast enhancement. Pituitary tumors are distinguished readily by their location, minimal peritumoral edema, uniform contrast enhancement, and well-defined margins. In addition to defining primary brain tumors, CT may be helpful in identifying nasal tumors that have extended into the rostral cerebrum (Moore et al, 1991). These dogs may have no clinical signs of nasal disease.

MRI is optimal for demonstrating the amount

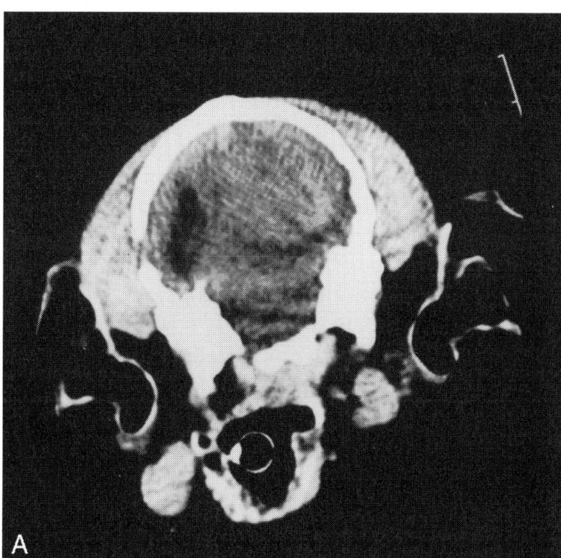

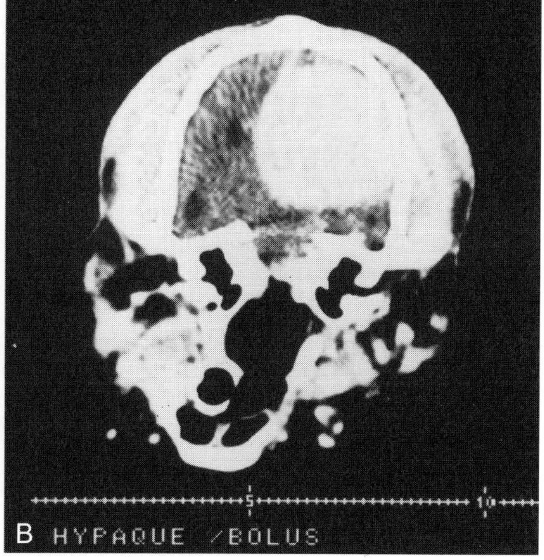

Figure 19–2. Transverse computed tomographic (CT) images from a 15-year-old miniature poodle with a 2-month history of grand mal seizures, right cortical blindness, and right postural test reaction deficits. *A*, A homogeneous mass is present in the left occipital cortex. *B*, Iodine-enhanced image revealing a large, regularly shaped mass. In both views the left lateral ventricle has been compressed and obliterated by the mass. Histopathologic analysis confirmed the mass to be a meningioma.

of nasal or cerebral involvement and also shows more detail of the anatomic features of these masses than CT (Sackman et al, 1989). Also, images obtained by means of MRI are superior to those obtained by CT for certain brain regions (e.g., brain stem) (Panciera et al, 1987). Even though CT and MRI have added significantly to the ability to localize tumors and despite the fact that certain tumors do have characteristic CT and MRI changes, biopsy and histopathology still remain the definitive methods for diagnosis of brain tumor type. Ideally an intracranial lesion should undergo biopsy before therapy of any type. However, biopsy is not always attempted because of the risks involved (e.g., attempting to biopsy a brain stem neoplasm may involve significant morbidity) (LeCouteur and Turrel, 1986). The advantages of a histopathologic diagnosis are that (1) a more accurate patient prognosis and determination of potential response to therapy can be given to the owner based on the biologic behavior of the neoplasm and (2) some inflammatory and non-neoplastic masses may also be seen with CT and MRI, and these may be confused with neoplasia, only to be differentiated by histopathology (Plummer et al, 1991).

Treatment. Control of secondary tumor effects, such as increased intracranial pressure or cerebral edema, and tumor eradication (or reduction) are the main goals of therapy for an intracranial neoplasm (LeCouteur and Turrel, 1986). Palliative therapy for dogs with brain tumors consists of the administration of glucocorticoids for reducing edema and, in some cases, retarding tumor growth (Kornegay, 1986). Some animals with brain tumors demonstrate dramatic improvement in clinical signs for weeks to months with sustained glucocorticoid therapy. Should seizure therapy be needed, phenobarbital is the drug best suited for control of generalized seizures (LeCouteur and Child, 1989).

Eradication or reduction of a neoplasm is the primary consideration for the long-term survival of a dog with a brain tumor. Four methods of therapy for a brain tumor are available for use in dogs: surgery, irradiation, chemotherapy, and immunotherapy (biologic response modification) (LeCouteur, 1990).

Surgery. Neurosurgical intervention is an essential consideration in the management of intracranial neoplasms. This may involve complete excision, partial removal (also called *cytoreduction* or *debulking*), or biopsy (LeCouteur, 1989). The location, size, and extent of a neoplasm, along with its invasiveness, may limit the possibility of complete surgical removal. Meningiomas, particularly those located over the cerebral convexities or in the frontal lobes of the cerebrum, can be completely (or almost completely) removed by surgery (LeCouteur, 1989). In contrast, significant morbidity and mortality are associated with surgical removal of neoplasms located in the caudal fossae and brain stem.

Limited information is available concerning surgical management of secondary brain tumors. Calvarial tumors such as osteosarcomas, chondrosarcomas, and multilobular osteochondromas have been removed successfully. The prognosis for tumor-free survival after removal of a calvarial osteosarcoma may be better than that after removal of osteosarcomas of long bones (LeCouteur, 1990). In addition, those patients that underwent surgery plus cobalt 60 radiation therapy had longer survival times than those that underwent surgery alone.

Irradiation. Irradiation may be used for the treatment of primary brain tumors either alone or in conjunction with other treatments such as total reduction or cytoreduction. Metastatic neoplasms may also be managed with radiation therapy in certain instances (LeCouteur, 1990). The objective of radiation therapy is to destroy the neoplasm while minimizing damage to any normal tissue within the irradiated area (LeCouteur, 1990). External beam megavoltage irradiation (cobalt 60) is currently used for treatment of brain tumors in dogs. Careful treatment planning by experienced personnel is essential to the success of radiation therapy. Brain tumors may also respond to megavoltage irradiation (Heidner et al, 1991; LeCouteur et al, 1987). One report described four dogs that were administered radiation with a cobalt 60 teletherapy unit (Turrel et al, 1984). Complete tumor regression, as determined from CT scans, improvement in clinical signs, and reduction in medication, were documented in all dogs. The median survival time for irradiated dogs was 322 days, compared with 56 days in eight dogs given symptomatic treatment.

Functional pituitary macroadenomas and macrocarcinomas are sensitive to radiation therapy. In six treated dogs, survival times ranged from 157 to 1298 days, with a median of 743 days (Dow et al, 1990). These dogs still required adrenal suppressive therapy, as pituitary hypersecretion of ACTH persisted for at least 1 year after completion of radiation therapy. In a retrospective study, 25 of 86 dogs with brain tumors that received megavoltage radiation treatment had a median survival time of 4.9 months (Heidner et al, 1991). Boron neutron capture therapy (Moore et al, 1989) and brachytherapy or interstitial radiation therapy (Heidner et al, 1991) may have a role in the treatment of brain tumors in the future.

Chemotherapy and Immunotherapy. Several factors affect the use of chemotherapeutic agents for the treatment of brain tumors. The blood–brain barrier may prevent exposure of all or some of the tumor to a chemotherapeutic agent that is injected parenterally. The tumor cell heterogeneity may be such that only certain cells within a tumor are sensitive to a given agent, or the tumor may be sensitive only at dosages that are toxic to normal brain tissue or other organs (LeCouteur, 1990). The mainstay of palliative therapy for brain tumors is glucocorticoids. The primary effect of these drugs is relief of peritumoral edema and inflammation, although some reduction in tumor size or a slowed rate of tumor growth is possible. Dexamethasone is preferred in acute and severe cases, whereas prednisone or prednisolone may be used for maintenance. Methylprednisolone has been helpful in the treatment of spinal cord edema and may also be beneficial in the treatment of acute peritumoral brain edema (Hoerlein et al, 1985).

Glucocorticoids play an important role in specific antineoplastic therapy for lymphosarcoma, leukemia, and hemolymphatic tumors that affect the CNS. Glucocorticoids readily penetrate the blood–brain barrier and have direct antitumor activity in these types of neoplasia. Dosages and specific protocols vary depending on the type of neoplasia and the veterinarian's preference (Rosenthal, 1989). Table 19–3 lists the suggested chemotherapy protocol for CNS lymphosarcoma. In dogs receiving intrathecal therapy, cytosine arabinoside, the agent of choice, was administered at a dosage of 20 mg/m^2 of body surface as a bolus injection after an equal volume of CSF was withdrawn. The total dose was diluted in 2 to 4 ml of lactated Ringer's solution and was injected twice weekly for six treatments. In dogs with the potential for tentorial herniation, radiation therapy should be considered before intrathecal therapy is instituted, because the rapid reduction in tumor mass produced by radiation will decrease CSF pressure, allowing intrathecal chemotherapy to be used more safely.

TABLE 19–3. CHEMOTHERAPY PROTOCOL FOR CNS LYMPHOSARCOMA

DRUG	DOSAGE
Induction of remission	
Cyclophosphamide	50 mg/m^2 PO 4 days/wk for 8 wk
Vincristine	0.5 mg/m^2 IV once a week for 8 wk
Cytosine arabinoside	100 mg/m^2/day, IV continuous infusion for 4 days
Prednisone	40 mg/m^2 PO once a day for 1 wk, then 20 mg/m^2 every other day for 8 wk
Maintenance therapy	
Chlorambucil	2 mg/m^2 PO every other day
Prednisone	20 mg/m^2 PO every other day

From Couto CG, Cullen J, Pedroia V, et al. Central nervous system lymphosarcoma in the dog. J Am Vet Med Assoc 184:809, 1984.

The nitrosoureas (carmustine, lomustine, and semustine) are alkylating agents that cross the blood–brain barrier in sufficient amounts to be at least partially effective against some brain tumors. Their primary use is in the treatment of tumors of glial cell origin. The use of carmustine for the treatment of primary brain tumors has been described (Cook, 1990; Dimski and Cook, 1990). The recommended dosage for carmustine is 50 mg/m^2 given intravenously every 4 to 6 weeks. The primary side effect seen in dogs has been acute transient bone marrow suppression, with neutrophil and thrombocyte nadirs occurring 7 to 10 days after treatment. Interstitial pneumonia and fibrosing alveolitis have been reported to occur in human patients receiving long-term carmustine therapy (Aronin et al, 1980; Weiss and Issell, 1982). This complication has not occurred in dogs (Cook, 1990).

Immunotherapy involves modifying a dog's immune response so that the tumor is eliminated immunologically. This mode of therapy is currently in its infancy but holds much promise (Ingram et al, 1990). Treatment involves the use of interleukin-2–stimulated autologous lymphocytes to attack tumor cells.

Prognosis. Information is limited concerning median survival times for dogs that have received only palliative therapy for brain tumors (i.e., therapy to control secondary effects of a tumor without an attempt to eradicate the tumor); expected median survival times are 60 to 80 days after CT diagnosis of a primary brain tumor (Turrel et al, 1984). Brain tumors of any histologic type or location always carry a poor prognosis. Most dogs with brain tumors eventually die or are euthanized as a direct result of their tumor. Radiation therapy appears to be the most successful treatment and has certainly been shown to be an effective mode of therapy to increase survival times while also allowing good quality of life. If surgery is performed, postoperative radiation therapy appears to be beneficial in improving survival duration.

Inflammatory Disease Causing Forebrain Signs

Granulomatous Meningoencephalitis. Granulomatous meningoencephalitis (GME) is an idiopathic disease of the CNS seen primarily in adult female dogs, most often in purebred small breed dogs (80 per cent small breeds, with poodles comprising 30 per cent of cases). Disseminated, focal, and ocular forms of GME exist, but the disseminated and focal forms are most common. In disseminated GME, the distribution is primarily in the white matter of the cerebrum, caudal brain stem, cerebellum, and cervical spinal cord. The neurologic signs will be dependent on the type of GME and its distribution and, if the focal form is present, the location of the inflammatory focus. With disseminated GME, the clinician is more likely to see multifocal forebrain signs, whereas with focal GME, seizures may be the primary sign if the inflammatory focus is in the cerebrum.

Dogs with disseminated GME, particularly those with forebrain and midbrain involvement, seem to suffer a more acute and fulminating clinical course, whereas those with focal disease tend to have subtle signs at the beginning and a more prolonged clinical course. Although glucocorticoids may improve the neurologic status initially, most researchers agree that GME is a progressive disease. The most helpful diagnostic test is CSF analysis (Bailey and Higgins, 1986; Cuddon and Smith-Maxie, 1984; Sorjonen, 1990; Thomas and Eger, 1989). Abnormalities include elevated protein content and increased white blood cell count (primarily mononuclear cells, both lymphocytes and macrophages). Whether glucocorticoid use before collection of CSF is a significant factor in causing the CSF to become normal, thereby masking the diagnosis, is debated. Cytologic findings in the CSF of patients with GME can give a strong indication for GME but do not permit absolute differentiation of GME from canine distemper and other chronic encephalitides (Gearhart et al, 1986; Sarfaty et al, 1986). In addition, CT may play an important role in defining focal mass lesions of GME (Plummer et al, 1991; Sisson et al, 1989; Speciale et al, 1992).

Treatment. Symptomatic treatment with glucocorticosteroids has proved successful in temporarily alleviating clinical signs and/or slowing disease progression (Thomas and Eger, 1989). Prednisone has been the most frequently used glucocorticoid; dosages ranging from 2 to 4 mg/kg/day appear to be adequate. The author has also found dexamethasone and methylprednisolone to be useful. Cessation of glucocorticoid therapy is invariably associated with rapid and dramatic clinical deterioration, and therefore, glucocorticosteroids should not be discontinued. Radiation therapy may prove to be very beneficial for the treatment of focal GME.

Necrotizing Meningoencephalitis of Pug Dogs. A unique, nonsuppurative meningoencephalitis associated with extensive cerebral necrosis has been described in pug dogs as old as 7 years of age (Cordy and Holliday, 1989). Dogs with acute disease are presented with a sudden onset of seizure activity and neurologic deficits referable to involvement of the cerebrum, brain stem, and meninges. Dogs may have difficulty walking, be weak or uncoordinated, circle, have a head tilt, head press, exhibit blindness with normal pupillary light reflexes, or show signs of cervical rigidity and pain. These neurologic signs progress rapidly, and within 5 to 7 days the dogs develop uncontrollable seizures, become recumbent, and drift into a comatose state. Dogs with slowly progressive disease are presented because of generalized or partial motor seizures but are usually neurologically normal after the seizures. Diagnosis should be suspected on the basis of the signalment and characteristic clinical and laboratory features. CSF analysis is characterized by an increased nucleated cell count, with the predominant cell type being the small lymphocyte. Definitive diagnosis requires necropsy or brain biopsy. There is no specific treatment for this disease, although treatment with phenobarbital may decrease the severity and frequency of the seizures for a short time.

Vascular Disease Causing Forebrain Signs

Primary cerebrovascular disease is rare in the dog. When present, cerebrovascular disease usually develops secondary to other conditions such as renal disease, septic or neoplastic emboli, coagulopathies, endocarditis, infection with parasites such as *Dirofilaria immitis*, cardiomyopathy, and hypothyroidism. In addition to these diseases, cerebral thrombosis and hemorrhage have been associated with L-asparaginase administration (Swanson et al, 1986). Vascular disorders have an acute onset with a nonprogressive course. The area of brain involvement dictates the signs that will be seen. Seizure activity is the most common cortical sign seen in animals with primary vascular disease (Stoffregen et al, 1985; Swayne et al, 1988). A tentative diagnosis of vascular disease is largely based on the history of acute onset of lateralizing CNS deficits. CSF analysis may be normal or reveal increased protein content, xanthochromia, and/or dull brown coloration. CT and MRI or angiography may be helpful in further defining a lesion and its location. A definitive diagnosis may require necropsy. Treatment is directed at treating the specific underlying disease (e.g., antimicrobial agents for endocarditis or thyroid supplementation for hypothyroidism), but if an underlying disorder cannot be documented, then supportive care and glucocorticosteroids constitute the primary treatments. Many animals make a dramatic improvement over the first 3 to 10 days after the onset of signs, although some never return to normal functional status (Meric, 1992).

Metabolic Disorders Causing Forebrain Signs

Metabolic disorders do not usually cause focal neurologic deficits but instead cause seizures, disorientation, change in mental alertness, behavioral changes, and constant pacing. If the neurologic examination points to focal CNS deficits, metabolic disorders should be considered less likely. If the animal's problems are primarily indicative of a diffuse cerebral disorder, then metabolic disease should be a prime differential diagnosis in the older patient. Common metabolic disorders in the older dog include hypothyroidism, hypoglycemia owing to insulinoma, hepatic failure, hyperlipoproteinemia (in schnauzers), hyperviscosity syndromes (e.g., multiple myeloma, polycythemias), and diabetic ketoacidosis. A complete blood cell count, urinalysis, serum biochemistry panel, and/or fasting and 2-hour postprandial bile acid determinations often provide specific direction for establishing a definitive diagnosis.

Senile Degeneration

More older dogs are now being presented with signs relating to age-related mentation changes (Fenner, 1988; Luttgen, 1990a). These dogs are less mentally alert and responsive, tend to sleep a great deal, become forgetful in familiar environments, and lack a seizure history. Neurologic examination may reveal a slowing or decrease in some myotatic and cranial nerve reflexes but in general is usually normal. Metabolic or primary CNS diseases that cause dementia or mentation changes should be ruled out with a thorough neurologic work-up before the diagnosis of senile degeneration is rendered. Anecdotal reports have described treatment with nylidrin hydrochloride (Arlidin), which has produced improvement in mental alertness. The suggested dosage is 3 to 6 mg PO tid.

Cerebellar Disease

Cerebellar dysfunction is characterized by truncal ataxia, a broad-based stance, dysmetria in which the limbs either overstep (hypermetria) or understep (hypometria), and tremor that is most pronounced when the animal attempts a goal-oriented movement (i.e., intention tremor) (Kornegay, 1990b). Certainly, forebrain diseases may also localize to the cerebellum, but these will not be discussed in detail in this section. In addition, late-onset cerebellar degeneration has been reported in an adult male schnauzer-beagle mixed breed dog in which the signs of cerebellar disease were slowly progressive over 2 years (Chrisman et al, 1983). Cerebellar biopsy revealed active degeneration of Purkinje cells, gliosis, cytoplasmic granulation of glial cells, and pigment accumulation.

Brain Stem Disease

When cranial nerve dysfunction is associated with paresis/plegia of two limbs on one side (hemiparesis/plegia) or all four limbs (tetraparesis/plegia), focal brain stem disease or multifocal disease should be suspected. Common CNS diseases in older dogs that may localize to this neuroanatomic region include neoplasia, GME, and vascular disease (infarction).

Vestibular Disease

Vestibular dysfunction (ataxia, head tilt, nystagmus) results from diseases that affect either the central (brain stem, cerebellum) or peripheral (inner ear, vestibular nerve) parts of the vestibular system. If central vestibular signs (Table 19–4) are present, those disorders listed under brain stem disease should be considered. Otitis interna, neoplasia of the vestibular nerve (e.g., neurofibroma, lymphosarcoma), and geriatric vestibular syndrome are the three primary differential diagnoses for peripheral vestibular dysfunction (Table 19–4). Neoplasia of the vestibular nerve is extremely rare and consists mainly of primary nerve tumors (e.g., neurofibroma, neurofibrosarcoma, and lymphosarcoma) and tumors of the bullae or bony labyrinth that involve the vestibu-

TABLE 19–4. PERIPHERAL (INNER EAR) VERSUS CENTRAL (BRAIN STEM) VESTIBULAR SIGNS

SIGN	CENTRAL DISEASE	PERIPHERAL DISEASE
Head tilt	Present	Present
Falling, rolling	Present	Present
Nystagmus		
Horizontal	Present	Present
Rotary	Present	Present
Vertical	Present	Absent
May change with position of head	Yes	No
Cranial nerve deficits	Cranial nerves V, VI, VII	Cranial nerve VII may be involved
Horner's syndrome	No	May be present
Gait dysfunction	Severe ataxia, ipsilateral hemiparesis	Mild ataxia
Cerebellar signs	Possible	No

lar nerve. Likewise, tumors within the external ear canal (e.g., squamous cell carcinoma, ceruminous gland adenocarcinoma) may spread locally, extending into the inner ear resulting in vestibular nerve damage. If signs of facial nerve paralysis and Horner's syndrome are present, then coexisting middle ear disease should be suspected.

Geriatric vestibular syndrome is the most common cause of unilateral peripheral vestibular disease in old dogs (mean age at onset, 12.5 years) (Schunk and Averill, 1983). The disorder is characterized by sudden onset (usually appearing in less than 2 hours) of unilateral peripheral vestibular signs. Head tilt is toward the affected side, and the ataxia and falling may be severe enough that the dog is nonambulatory during the first 24 to 36 hours. The nystagmus is characterized as spontaneous and/or horizontal to rotary, with the fast phase opposite the head tilt. Proprioception and postural test reactions are normal, although during the first 24 to 36 hours, these may be difficult to assess because of the animal's disorientation. Approximately 30 per cent of dogs show transient nausea, vomiting, and anorexia. The diagnosis of geriatric vestibular syndrome is based on the elimination of other causes of peripheral vestibular dysfunction and/or with improvement in clinical signs over the 1 to 3 weeks after the onset of signs. The prognosis for recovery is excellent. Recurrent attacks are unusual but may occur on the same or opposite side.

Spinal Cord Disease

Spinal cord/column disorders seen more commonly in older dogs include cervical vertebral instability (wobbler disease), degenerative myelopathy (in German shepherd dogs), spondylosis deformans, and spinal cord tumors. Other disorders, such as inflammation (GME), infections (canine distemper and fungal, bacterial, or protozoal infections), trauma, and/or vascular disease (fibrocartilaginous embolic myelopathy) also occur.

Cervical Vertebral Instability (Wobbler Syndrome)

Canine wobbler syndrome is a major cause of cervical spinal cord compression in large breed dogs (e.g., Doberman pinscher) (Van Gundy, 1989). The spinal cord compression may be due to multiple anatomic changes and be either static or dynamic. Static compression can be secondary to (1) stenosis of the vertebral canal, (2) malformation of the articular processes and degenerative changes of the articular facets, (3) cervical disk protrusion (Hansen type II), or (4) hypertrophy of the ligamentum flavum and joint capsule. Dynamic compression produces intermittent pressure on the spinal cord that is dependent on neck posture. Causes of dynamic compression include (1) instability and excessive motion of the cervical vertebrae and (2) hypertrophy of the dorsal longitudinal ligament, which results in more spinal cord compression when the neck is extended.

The history is usually characterized by an insidious onset of paresis and/or ataxia of all four limbs, particularly of the hindquarters. When evaluating the gait, the thoracic limbs may appear normal at first, although the owner may report dragging of the toenails or a stiff gait in the forelimbs. On presentation, neurologic deficits related to a cervical lesion are evident. Deficits vary in severity from mild ataxia and hindlimb proprioceptive deficits to nonambulatory tetraparesis (Seim and Withrow, 1982). Additional thoracic limb abnormalities may include extensor spasticity and marked scapular muscle atrophy if the C_6–C_7 cord segments are involved. Sensory perception to the limbs is rarely, if ever, attenuated, and most dogs do not have overt pain.

Radiography, both plain radiography and myelography, provides the definitive diagnosis and facilitates exclusion of those conditions that have similar presenting signs. The changes recognized

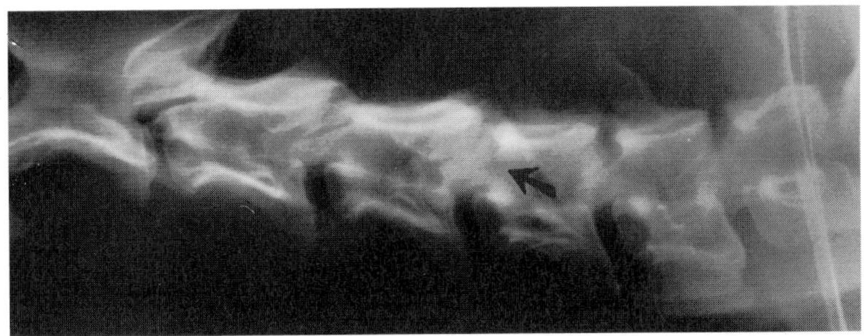

Figure 19–3. Lateral cervical spinal radiograph of a 10-year-old Doberman pinscher with wobbler syndrome. Note the degenerative changes in the articular facets (*arrow*) at the C_4–C_5 disk space and slight narrowing of the C_4–C_5 disk space.

with plain radiography (Figs. 19–3 and 19–4) include the following:

1. Tipping of the craniodorsal aspect of the vertebral body into the spinal canal (the site of vertebral tipping does not always correlate with the site of myelographic compression).
2. Stenosis of the vertebral canal, especially at the cranial aspect of the vertebrae.
3. Malformations of the vertebral bodies, with rounding of the cranioventral aspect.
4. Collapsed disk spaces or spondylosis.
5. Degenerative changes of the articular facets.

Despite these changes, myelography is always essential for accurate localization of spinal cord compression. Myelography (Figs. 19–5 and 19–6) visualizes extradural spinal cord compression by (1) dorsal cord compression resulting from hypertrophied ligamentum flavum (lateral view), (2) ventral cord compression resulting from hypertrophied dorsal annulus fibrosis (lateral view), (3) lateral cord compression resulting from articular facet malformation (ventrodorsal view), and (4) compression resulting from stenotic vertebral canal or instability manifested by vertebral tipping. In addition to routine myelography, stress myelography (flexion, extension, traction) (Fig. 19–7) may be useful in differentiating the nature of the compressive lesion (Seim and Withrow, 1982). Sites of compression vary in position and number. The highest incidence is at C_5–C_6. Incidence appears to decrease with increased distance from C_5–C_6. Approximately 70 per cent of the intervertebral disk–associated lesions are localized at C_6–C_7 (Seim and Withrow, 1982).

In addition to documenting wobbler syndrome in a clinically affected dog, radiographic studies may be helpful in identifying potential "wobblers." In a study of 115 mature dobermans that were clinically normal at presentation, 28 were considered to have radiographic changes similar to those identified in affected animals (Lewis, 1991). During the next five years, 20 (71.8 per cent) of these dogs developed clinical signs of cervical spondylomyelopathy. The remaining 87 dobermans during this 5-year period were considered normal by their owners. The author suggested that careful radiographic assessment may offer a real basis for the identification of potential wobblers and thereby may offer a means of identifying sound breeding stock as one method of reducing the increasing incidence of a serious multifactorial disease.

The clinical course of untreated wobbler syndrome is variable but usually is chronically progressive. Medical and/or surgical treatment attempts to relieve clinical signs temporarily or permanently. Medical therapy consists of glucocorticosteroids, rest, and/or a neck brace. Static compressive lesions, such as malarticulations,

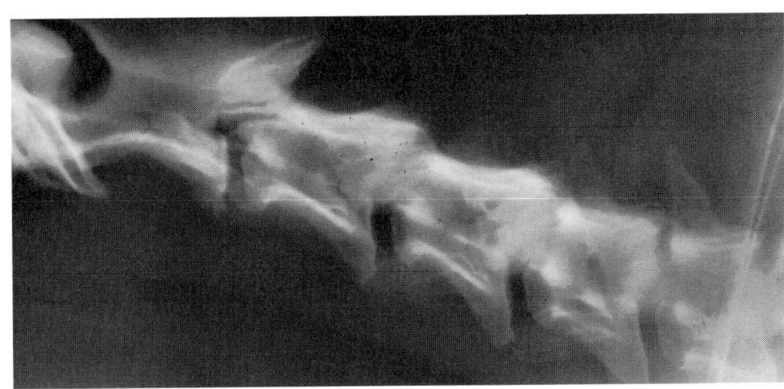

Figure 19–4. Lateral cervical spinal radiograph of an 8-year-old Doberman pinscher with wobbler syndrome. Note the degenerative changes of the articular facets at C_4 to C_5, narrowed disk space C_4–C_5, and rounding of the cranioventral aspect of the C_5 vertebral body.

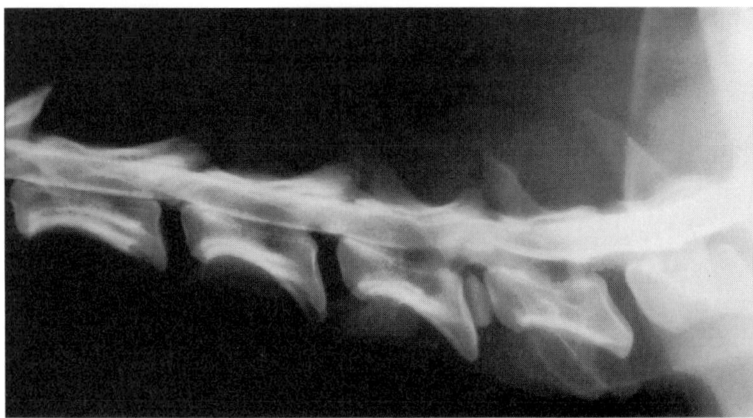

Figure 19–5. Lateral view of a cervical myelogram. Dorsal to the mineralized disk at C_5–C_6, note the dorsal deviation of the ventral dye column that is typical of compression seen secondary to hypertrophy of the dorsal annulus.

malformed vertebrae, and Hansen type II disks, cannot be alleviated with medical therapy alone. At best, dynamic lesions are ameliorated, but the underlying instability or malformation is still present. A neck brace, if used, should incorporate the cranial thorax as well as the entire cervical area to immobilize the caudal cervical region. Cage rest can also provide enough restriction to produce short-term relief, particularly when used in conjunction with glucocorticosteroids. Medical therapy can be used (1) to improve neurologic function before surgery, (2) for the old dog in which the risk of surgery negates the surgical option, and (3) for the dog whose owner cannot afford surgical treatment.

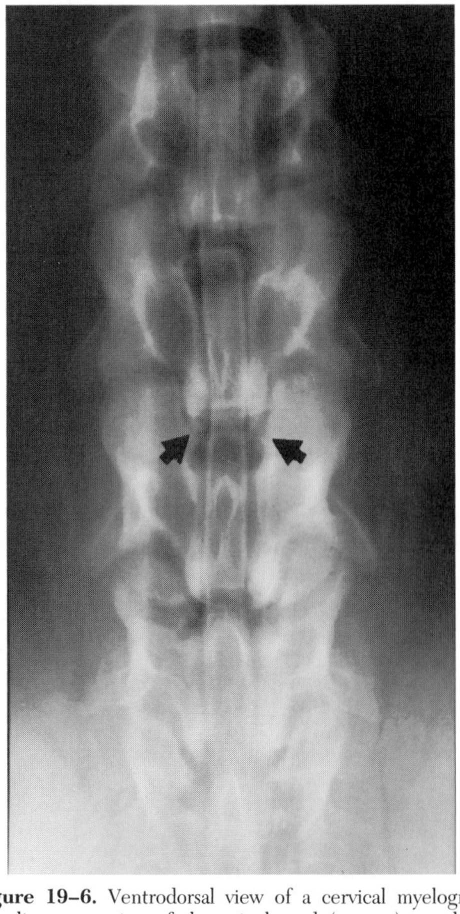

Figure 19–6. Ventrodorsal view of a cervical myelogram revealing narrowing of the spinal cord (*arrows*), resulting from articular facet malformation.

Surgical therapy is the only way to decompress an existing cervical lesion, whether static or dynamic. Two goals of neurosurgery are to decompress a compressive lesion and to stabilize an unstable patient. A static compressive lesion such as a Hansen type II disk protrusion will require a surgical approach different from that used for a dynamic lesion such as a hypertrophied dorsal longitudinal ligament and dorsal annulus fibrosis. In the former, a ventral decompressive surgery is needed, while in the latter, a distraction surgery at the site of instability is needed to keep the dorsal longitudinal ligament "stretched out" so that during neck movement (primarily neck extension), the redundant dorsal longitudinal ligament does not compress the spinal cord. Because of the different compressive lesions that may exist in the dog with wobbler syndrome, the importance of myelographic examination, including traction views, becomes apparent.

Degenerative Myelopathy

Degenerative myelopathy (DM), primarily a thoracolumbar spinal cord condition, has been recognized primarily in aged German shepherd dogs (age of onset, 5 to 14 years) (Averill, 1973). Other purebred and large mixed breed dogs of older age have been reported with this condition, but the incidence in the German shepherd dog far outnumbers that in other breeds. The patho-

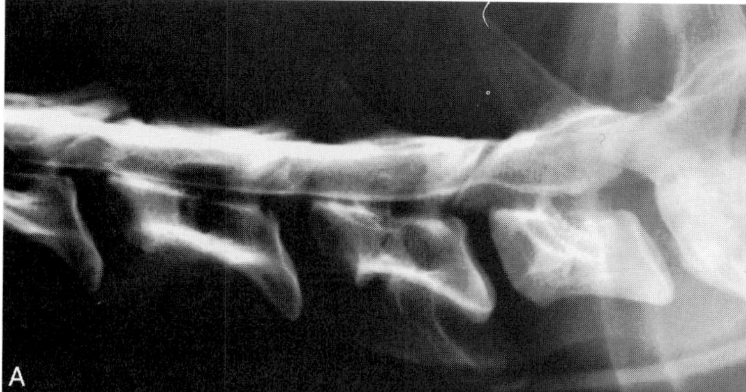

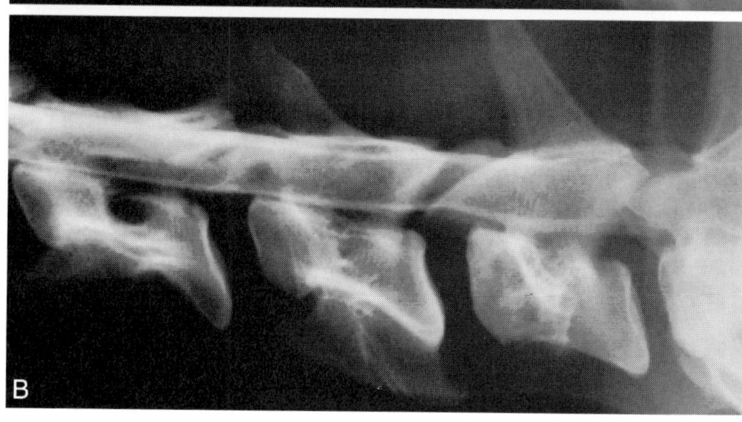

Figure 19–7. Lateral cervical myelography in an 8-year-old Doberman pinscher with wobbler syndrome. *A*, Note the dorsal deviation of the dye column at C_6 to C_7 in the lateral view (nontraction position). *B*, The lateral traction view reveals dissipation of the compressive lesion when forward traction was applied to the neck. This is most indicative of a dynamic compressive lesion from hypertrophy of the dorsal longitudinal ligament.

genesis of this disease is unknown. The history and clinical signs of affected dogs reveal a slowly progressive hindlimb dysfunction that begins with ataxia. This dysfunction is secondary to loss of proprioceptive function. The ataxia is initially characterized by knuckling of the toes, wearing of the nails of the inner digits of the rear paws, and stumbling. Later signs of hypermetria develop as the lateral funicular (spinocerebellar) pathways are affected. As the disease progresses, signs of upper motor neuronal dysfunction become evident and include (1) hyperreflexia of myotatic hindlimb reflexes, (2) presence of crossed extensor reflexes, and (3) development of Babinski's sign. Throughout this progression, weakness in the hindlimbs continues to develop. In the latter stages of the disease, urinary and fecal incontinence may develop.

Spinal myelography is the diagnostic test of choice to rule out Hansen type II intervertebral disk herniation and spinal neoplasia, which are the two primary differential diagnoses that may present similarly to degenerative myelopathy. The myelogram should be normal in dogs suffering only from DM. CSF analysis is also usually normal (Averill, 1973; Braund, 1986). Although no current therapy will resolve the lesions of DM, there is hope for control. Although nonsteroidal anti-inflammatory drugs appear to slow the progression of DM, the excessive levels required invariably lead to gastrointestinal irritation (Clemmons, 1989). The only treatment for DM that potentially alters the course of the disease is epsilon-aminocaproic acid (EACA) (Amicar) (Clemmons, 1989). The beneficial effect of EACA appears to occur secondary to its antiprotease activity, suggesting that blocking the final common pathway of tissue inflammation (i.e., reducing the activation of tissue enzymes) aids in preventing tissue damage. The suggested dosage for EACA is 500 mg PO every 8 hours. Side effects appear to be limited to gastrointestinal irritation. EACA does not cure DM but presumably controls the degenerative process.

Spondylosis Deformans

Spondylosis deformans (SD) is a degenerative disorder of the vertebral column in which vertebral osteophytes develop at intervertebral spaces independently of any inflammatory or traumatic processes, resulting in bony spurs or complete bony bridges on the ventral, lateral, and dorsolateral borders of the vertebral bodies (Fig. 19–8).

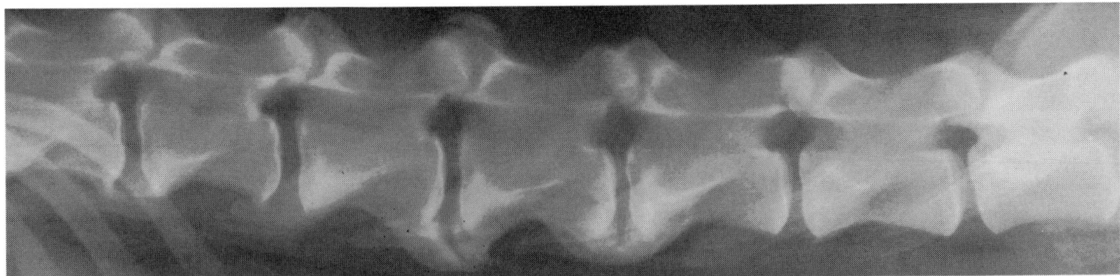

Figure 19–8. Lateral spinal thoracolumbar radiograph in an 12-year-old German shepherd dog showing bony spurs, ventral bridging at L_3 to L_4 and L_4 to L_5, and beginning of ventral bridging at L_1 to L_2.

Spondylosis deformans most often is an incidental finding on thoracolumbar spinal radiographs. Those dogs that do develop clinical signs often have a history of reluctance to rise, apparent spinal discomfort, and a straight back posture. These dogs usually have an insidious history, but if a bony bridge fractures, an acute history of localized spinal column hyperesthesia may be noticed by the owner. Hyperesthesia is the most common clinical sign, but ataxia and paresis in the rear limbs may occur secondary to cord compression. If the lumbosacral junction is affected, dogs may have difficulty rising and may show lower motor neuron dysfunction such as urinary and fecal incontinence or decreased hindlimb withdrawal reflexes. Treatment of spondylosis deformans is usually medical but at times surgical intervention may be needed. Those dogs displaying only hyperesthesia may be helped by analgesics or corticosteroids. Those not responding to medical management or displaying signs of spinal cord or nerve root compression probably need decompressive surgery.

Spinal Cord Tumors

Spinal cord tumors can be either primary or secondary (metastatic) (Table 19–5). The classic history is one of a slowly progressive loss of neurologic function in the limbs without periods of improvement. Occasionally, acute onset of signs may be seen when hemorrhage is associated with the tumor or when the spinal cord is affected by metastatic neoplasia. The signs of spinal cord dysfunction—spinal hyperesthesia, proprioceptive and motor deficits, and compromised deep pain sensation—vary in severity depending on the tumor location, extent of involvement, and type. Neck pain is a common sign of intradural-extramedullary and extradural tumors of the cervical spinal cord but is uncommon with intramedullary tumors (Gilmore, 1983). As with brain tumors, CSF analysis seldom provides specific information to diagnose a spinal tumor. Spinal cord lymphosarcoma is the only tumor type most likely to release malignant cells into the CSF.

Radiography remains the most valuable tool in the diagnosis of spinal cord tumors. Survey radiographs (Fig. 19–9) may show proliferation (e.g., with vertebral osteosarcoma); lysis of the bone (e.g., with multiple myeloma or nerve root/sheath tumors); or scalloped lamina, giving an expansible appearance to the spinal canal secondary to "pressure atrophy" (Fingeroth et al, 1987). Myelography (Fig. 19–10) is needed to clearly define the location of primary spinal cord neoplasia or other soft tissue neoplasms such as hemangiosarcoma or lymphosarcoma. CT and MRI can provide additional valuable information. Once the tumor has been localized with these techniques, surgical exploration and acquisition of tissue for histopathology are required for a definitive diagnosis.

TABLE 19–5. TUMORS OF THE SPINAL CORD AND VERTEBRAE

Extradural	Thyroid gland
Primary	Spindle cell
Osteosarcoma	Perianal gland
Fibrosarcoma	Hemangiosarcoma
Hemangioma	Malignant melanoma
Hemangiosarcoma	Fibrosarcoma
Reticulum cell sarcoma	Lymphosarcoma
Neurofibrosarcoma	Leiomyosarcoma
Meningioma	**Intradural-Extramedullary**
Lymphosarcoma	Meningioma
Neuroblastoma	Neurofibroma
Chondrosarcoma	Neurofibrosarcoma
Multiple myeloma	Medulloepithelioma
Metastatic	
Osteosarcoma	**Intramedullary**
Carcinoma	Astrocytoma
Mammary	Ependymoma
Squamous cell	Oligodendroglioma
Transitional cell	Primary sarcoma
Pancreatic	

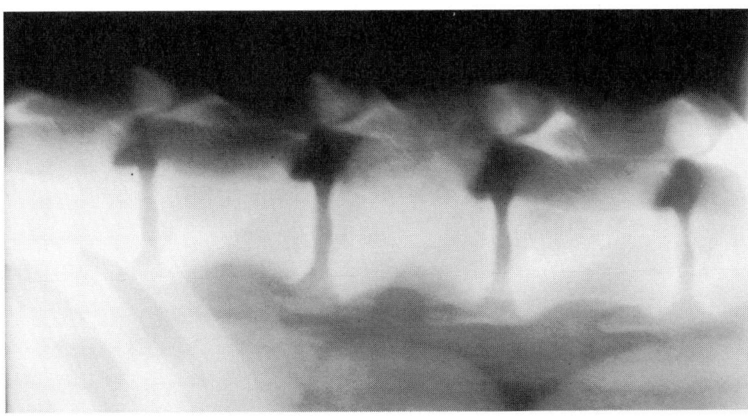

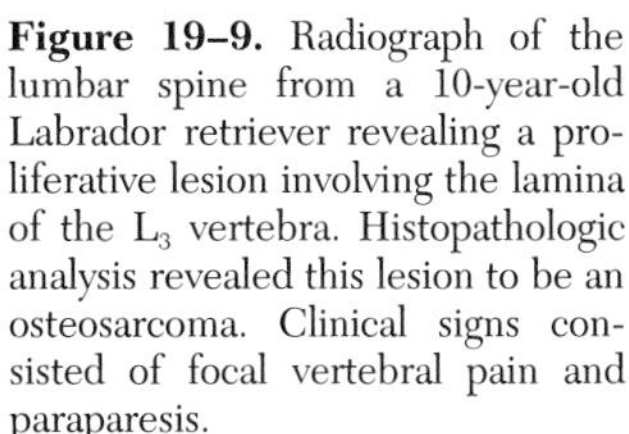

Figure 19–9. Radiograph of the lumbar spine from a 10-year-old Labrador retriever revealing a proliferative lesion involving the lamina of the L_3 vertebra. Histopathologic analysis revealed this lesion to be an osteosarcoma. Clinical signs consisted of focal vertebral pain and paraparesis.

Lumbosacral Disorders

Lumbosacral disorders display a characteristic clinical picture in dogs (i.e., urinary bladder, tail, or anal sphincter dysfunction) that is significantly different from that associated with other spinal lesions. Disorders affecting the lumbosacral junction include trauma, diskospondylitis or focal meningitis/neuritis, neoplasia, congenital vertebral malformations, intervertebral disk protrusion, and degenerative lumbosacral stenosis. Only neoplasia and degenerative lumbosacral stenosis are recognized more commonly in older dogs. Typically, larger working dogs (e.g., German shepherd dogs and Labrador retrievers) are most often affected. Historically, the most common signs associated with lumbosacral disorders are pain elicited in the lumbosacral area, unilateral or bilateral pelvic limb lameness or stilted gait, and weakness. Urinary or fecal incontinence is noted in approximately 25 per cent of dogs (Palmer and Chambers, 1991a). Ataxia, obvious proprioceptive abnormalities (knuckling), and biting or chewing at the limbs (paresthesias?) are occasionally part of the presenting history. Neurologic abnormalities include depressed tendon reflexes and/or postural test reactions; decreased muscle tone in the hindlimbs owing to involvement of the L_6, L_7, and S_1 nerve roots; and lumbosacral pain (Fig. 19–11).

Neoplasia

Neoplasia is a relatively rare cause of lumbosacral disease. Although primary extradural neoplasms are more common than tumors that metastasize to bone (Prata, 1977), prostatic and perianal gland adenocarcinomas often metastasize to the caudal lumbar and lumbosacral vertebrae (Lenehan, 1983). Neurofibrosarcoma and lymphosarcoma may also involve the lumbosacral nerve roots. The diagnosis of lumbosacral neoplasia may require one or all of the following tests: plain radiography, contrast radiography (myelography, epidurography), CSF analysis, electromyography, CT or MRI, and surgical exploration and biopsy (Palmer and Chambers, 1991b). Because lumbosacral neoplasia is relatively uncommon, objective prognostication is difficult. The prognosis is often poor to grave, because most tumors are primary neoplasms of bone or CNS.

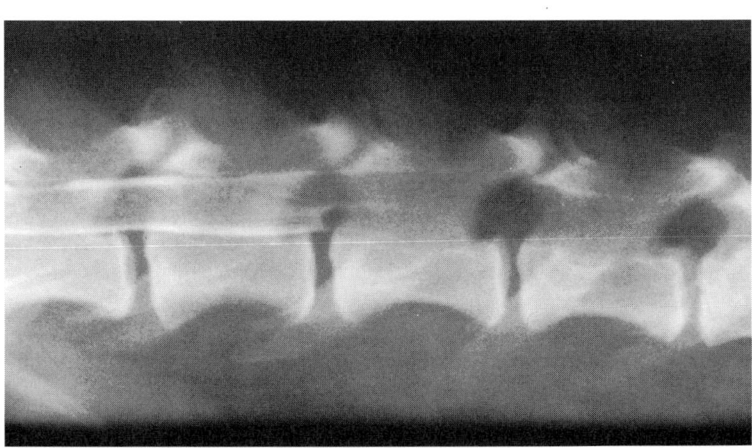

Figure 19–10. Lateral view from an iohexol myelogram showing obstruction to flow of contrast material at the L_2–L_3 vertebral level. Routine lumbar spinal radiographs were normal. At surgery a proliferative compressive soft tissue extradural mass was found, and histopathologic analysis revealed an anaplastic meningioma. Clinical signs consisted of a slowly progressive spastic paraparesis.

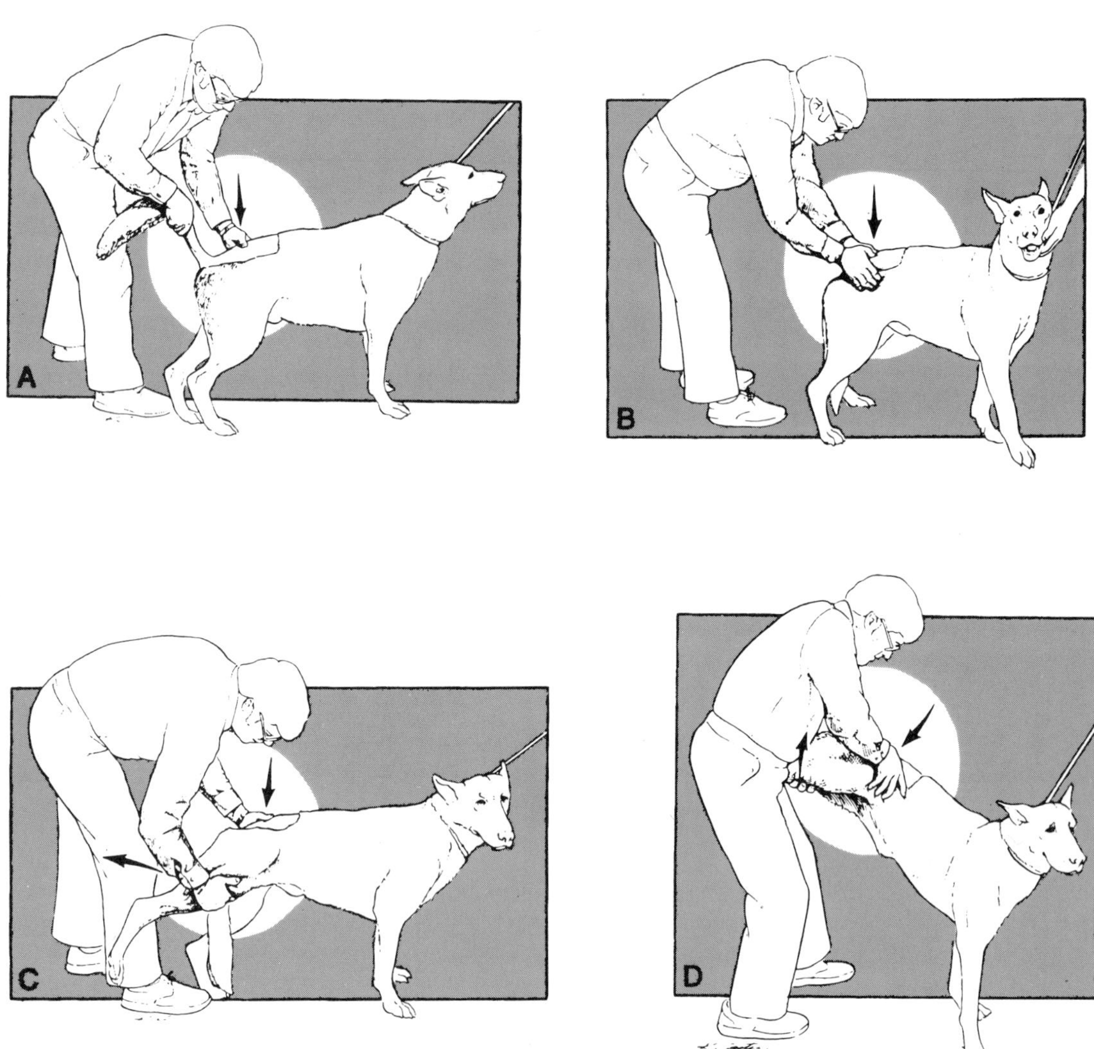

Figure 19–11. Physical examination to detect lumbosacral diseases. Arrows indicate the direction of pressure application. *A,* The tail is manipulated to check for tone and hyperesthesia. *B,* In the lumbosacral push test, pressure is applied at the lumbosacral junction. *C,* The hips are individually extended with and without pressure over the lumbosacral region. *D,* In the lordosis test, both hindlimbs are elevated and extended while pressure is applied at the lumbosacral junction. (From Chambers JN. Degenerative lumbosacral stenosis in dogs. Vet Med Rep 1:166, 1989. Reprinted with permission.)

Degenerative Lumbosacral Stenosis

Acquired stenosis of the lumbosacral canal is a disease that affects predominantly large dogs, with a higher incidence in German shepherd dogs, retrievers, and spaniels (Chambers, 1989). The techniques used to diagnose degenerative lumbosacral stenosis (DLSS) include electromyography; radiography, both plain and contrast, with both regular and stress views (epidurography, discography); and CT. The most frequent plain radiographic findings in DLSS include ventral and lateral spondylosis of the lumbosacral junction, sclerosis of the end plates of L_7 and S_1, ventral subluxation of the sacrum, and collapse of the L_7–S_1 intervertebral disk space (Figs. 19–12 and 19–13).

Early surgical intervention gives the best therapeutic results in cases of lumbosacral stenosis. In an animal that is displaying clinical signs for the first time or shows pain only, a conservative approach of cage rest, exercise restriction, and anti-inflammatory medications may be used, but this conservative management seldom provides good long-term results. Decompression by laminectomy and removal of encroaching tissue is the

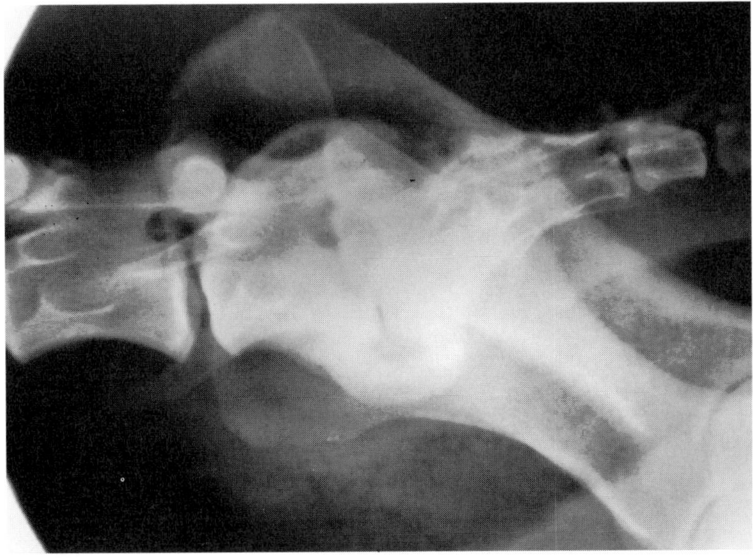

Figure 19–12. Lateral spinal radiograph in a dog with degenerative lumbosacral stenosis revealing collapse of the L_7–S_1 disk space and excessive ventral spondylosis. This dog was presented for evaluation of pain in the tailhead region.

preferred surgical approach. Dogs with DLSS often improve dramatically after surgery if pain is the only presenting sign (Chambers et al, 1988).

Peripheral Nerve Disease

Neoplasia

Tumors affecting the peripheral nervous system (PNS) may arise from neural tissue (neurofibroma) or from supporting structures (meningioma, osteosarcoma, fibrosarcoma) (Fig. 19–14). Neoplasia involving the PNS is generally localized, although multiple nerves may be affected at the same time. The brachial and lumbosacral intumescences are most commonly affected (Fenner, 1988), but cranial nerve involvement can also occur (Carpenter et al, 1987; Christopher et al, 1986; Hobbs and Cobb, 1990; Zachary et al, 1986). For these reasons the clinical signs associated with PNS tumors can be quite variable. The signs associated with peripheral nerve tumors generally have a gradual onset. The owner often notices a vague "lameness" in the affected limb

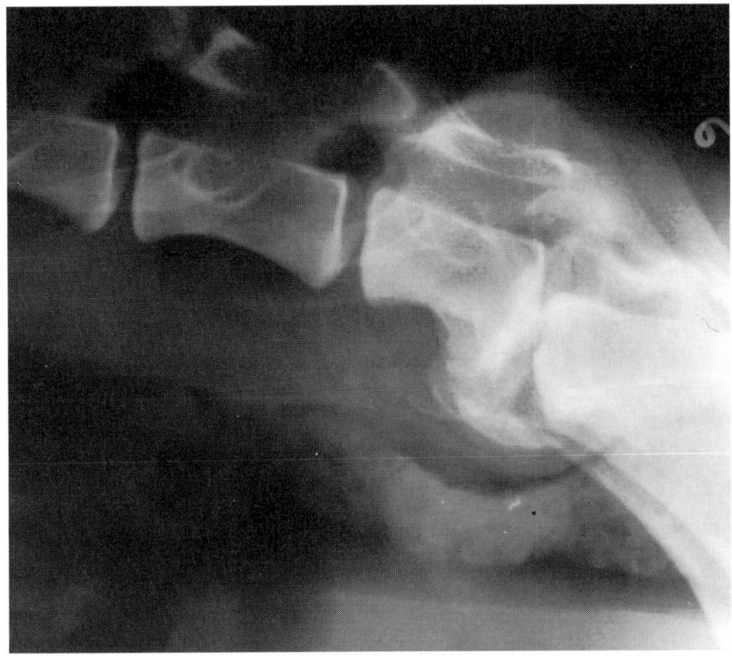

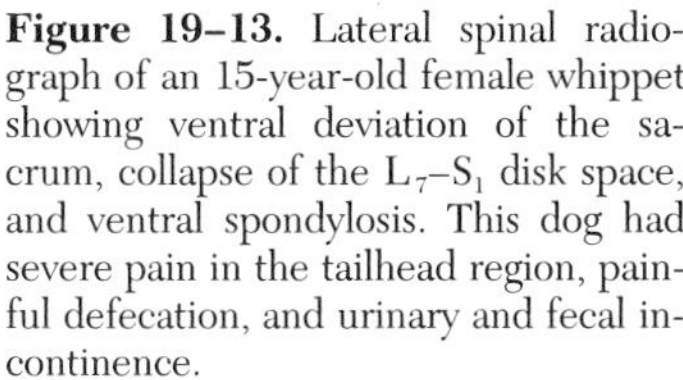

Figure 19–13. Lateral spinal radiograph of an 15-year-old female whippet showing ventral deviation of the sacrum, collapse of the L_7–S_1 disk space, and ventral spondylosis. This dog had severe pain in the tailhead region, painful defecation, and urinary and fecal incontinence.

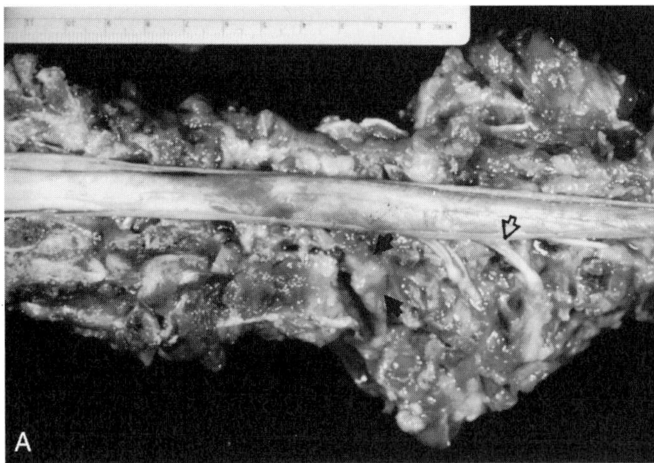
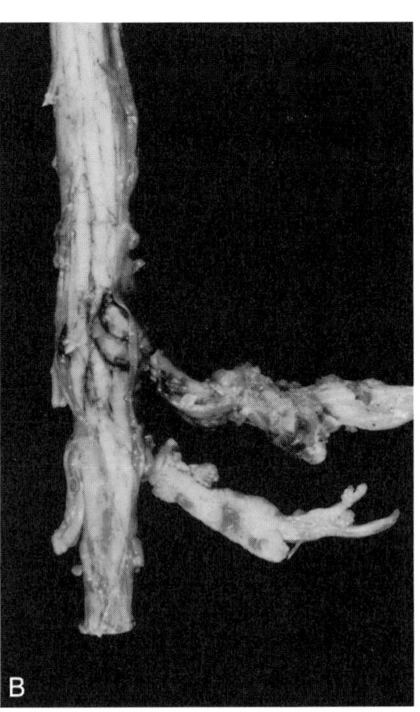

Figure 19–14. Examples of peripheral nerve root tumors in the dog. *A*, Neurofibrosarcoma (*solid arrow*) involving the C_5 nerve root on the left side. The unaffected C_7 nerve root and dorsal root ganglion are highlighted by the open arrow. *B*, Lymphosarcoma involving C_5 to C_6 nerve roots in a formalin-fixed specimen.

that progresses, over weeks to months, to loss of strength and muscle atrophy. The signs remain confined to the affected limb until late in the course of the illness. Occasionally the dog may self-mutilate the affected limb or cry out in pain when the limb is manipulated. Neurologic deficits will be noted in other limbs as the tumor grows into the spinal canal and causes spinal cord compression. If the tumor arises in the cauda equina, urinary and/or fecal incontinence may also be present.

Diagnosis. The diagnosis of PNS tumors is facilitated by the use of electrodiagnostic tests (e.g., electromyography and nerve conduction velocity tests), which help delineate the nerves involved. Plain spinal radiographs may reveal pressure-induced bone lysis if the tumor lies in the intervertebral foramen, resulting in enlargement of the foramen (Luttgen, 1990b). Myelography may help localize a compressive spinal cord lesion. CSF analysis does not generally contribute to the diagnosis. The definitive diagnostic test for PNS tumors is surgical exploration and biopsy of the affected nerves. As diagnostic methods such as CT and MRI become more widely available, they may come to be used to diagnose PNS tumors and, hopefully, aid in making a diagnosis at an earlier stage (McCarthy et al, 1993).

Treatment and Prognosis. Therapy for PNS tumors is very unrewarding (Carmichael and Griffiths, 1981; Fenner, 1988). If the tumor has not invaded the spinal cord, excision of the tumor may cure the disease but severely compromise the limb function. Secondary tumors (lymphosarcoma) may be amenable to chemotherapy or radiation therapy, but primary PNS tumors appear relatively resistant to these forms of therapy.

Miscellaneous Peripheral Neuropathies

Hypoglycemia, hyperglycemia, and hypothyroidism are metabolic/endocrine disorders with the potential to cause neuropathies. Currently there is no conclusive evidence that dogs that have beta cell tumors and associated hypoglycemia develop clinical peripheral neuropathy, although pathologic nerve changes occur in dogs with beta cell tumors (Braund et al, 1987). Clinical neuropathies in dogs with diabetes mellitus are uncommon, although pathologic neuropathies occur in diabetic dogs (Braund and Steiss, 1982; Johnson et al, 1983; Katherman and Braund, 1983; Steiss et al, 1981). Hypothyroidism may cause a neuropathy in affected dogs, but published studies unequivocally documenting this association are lacking. In humans, paraneoplastic neuropathy is a well-established clinical entity. In veterinary medicine, it has been suggested that dogs with neoplasms can demonstrate subclinical pathology (Braund et al, 1987) and clinical disease (Duncan and Griffiths, 1986). The pathogenesis of these neuropathies is still not fully understood in humans, and more complete studies are required to document their association in dogs and cats. In general, neuropathies associated with miscellaneous causes are more likely to affect multiple peripheral nerves, while single nerve involvement is more commonly seen with PNS neoplasia.

Tremors

An idiopathic tremor may occur in older dogs, primarily in wirehaired fox terriers, Airedale terriers, and other terrier breeds (Fenner, 1988). As affected dogs get older, a progressive tremor of the pelvic limbs begins and progresses to involve the thoracic limbs. These animals never display weakness and have normal neurologic examinations, and tremors are accentuated during the excitement that accompanies physical examination. They are primarily seen when the animal is standing and disappear when gaiting, making it unlikely that the tremors are of cerebellar origin. These tremors may be a form of benign essential tremor or an accentuation of physiologic tremor (Koller and Rubino, 1985). This benign condition must be differentiated from tremors caused by aflatoxicosis, "white dog shaker syndrome," cerebellar neoplasia, and hypocalcemia. The current recommendation is not to treat this condition, but rather to counsel the owner that the disorder is benign and rarely debilitating (Fenner, 1988).

Deafness

As in humans, dogs can be affected with progressive senile hearing loss. Senile deafness is probably caused by progressive degeneration of the cochlear receptor organ (sensory or nerve deafness) (Knowles, 1990) and/or progressive degeneration of the hair of ossicles in the middle ear (conduction deafness). Clinical signs of senile deafness relate to decreased or absence of hearing. The owner indicates that the dog is sleeping more soundly, is apparently inattentive, fails to respond to usual verbal commands, and fails to localize the source of a sound. The complaint may suggest acute hearing loss if the owner has missed the subtle signs of gradually developing deafness. Senile deafness can develop asymmetrically, thereby making it even more difficult for the owner to identify hearing loss in the early stages (Luttgen, 1990b). Otitis interna, neoplasia, and ototoxicity, in addition to senile deafness, are the primary differential diagnoses for hearing loss in the aged dog.

In addition to the neurologic and aural examination, evaluation with skull radiographs and brain stem auditory-evoked responses is indicated (Fig. 19–15). Radiographs should focus on the tympanic bullae and may reveal bony proliferation and sclerosis (chronic otitis media, bone neoplasia) or bony erosion (neoplasia). If the history rules out ototoxicity, aural examination and skull radiographs rule out otitis externa/media, and brain stem auditory-evoked responses con-

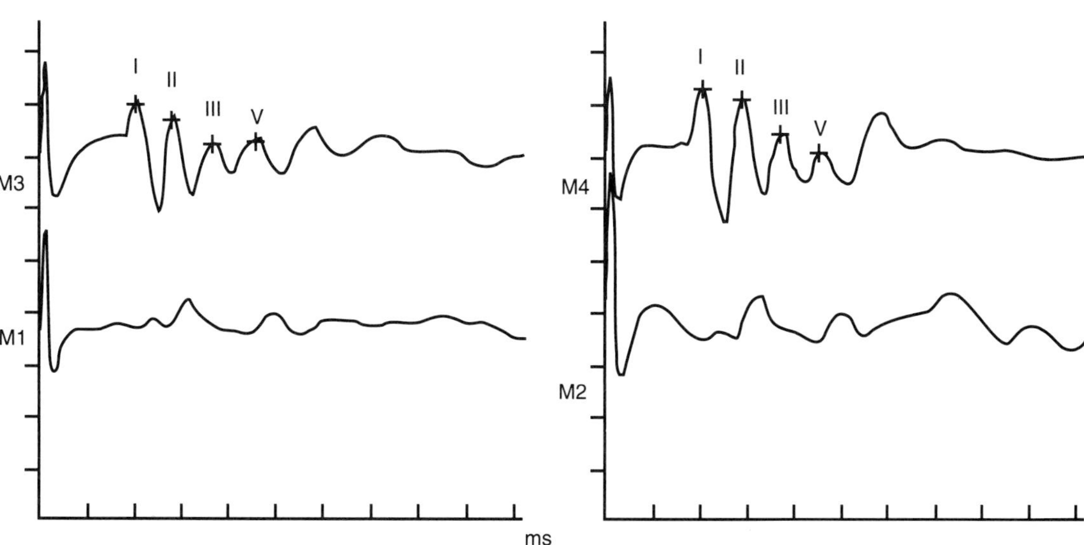

Figure 19–15. Brain stem auditory evoked potentials (BAEP) from an 11-year-old cocker spaniel with bilateral deafness. A normal BAEP is shown above the affected BAEP for comparison. Peak I represents cochlear nerve function. (Courtesy of George M. Strain, PhD, Louisiana State University.)

firm hearing loss, the veterinarian can be confident that the diagnosis of progressive senile hearing loss is correct (Luttgen, 1990b). The treatment of senile deafness in dogs is difficult because of the high likelihood that the dog will fail to adapt to hearing aids. The brain stem auditory-evoked response test is required before considering hearing aid therapy. This test helps determine (1) whether the dog has enough hearing function to make a hearing aid helpful and (2) which ear should be fitted (Marshall, 1990).

DISORDERS IN THE CAT

In general, the disorders affecting the nervous system of the older cat are not different from those affecting the nervous system of the older dog. Furthermore, the same general groups of diseases that affect older dogs also affect older cats, with a few exceptions.

Forebrain Disease

Neoplasia

Cats may develop primary brain tumors (e.g., astrocytoma, oligodendroglioma, ependymoma, meningioma) or secondary tumors (e.g., metastatic intracranial neoplasms, lymphosarcoma) (LeCouteur, 1989). Meningiomas are the most frequently reported intracranial neoplasm in the older cat (LeCouteur, 1990). In many cats the earliest sign of meningioma is altered behavior, manifested by lethargy, depression, dullness, inactivity, anorexia, and/or aggression (Lawson et al, 1984). Affected cats generally have an insidious, progressive onset of neurologic dysfunction, ultimately culminating in focal neurologic signs (e.g., circling, cortical blindness, postural test reaction deficits, positional nystagmus, various degrees of weakness, and seizures) (Nafe, 1979). Seizures rarely occur in these cats.

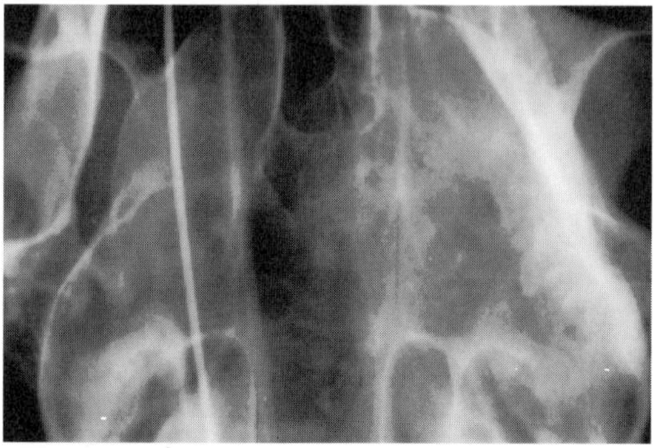

Figure 19–16. Ventrodorsal radiograph of the skull of a cat that reveals hyperostosis of the skull in association with a meningioma. (From Nafe LA. Topics in feline neurology. Vet Clin North Am [Small Anim Pract] 14:1292, 1984.)

Diagnosis and Treatment. The diagnostic approach to intracranial neoplasia in the cat is essentially the same as that in the dog. A major difference in the cat is that plain skull radiographs commonly show hyperostosis of the calvarium adjacent to the meningioma and/or partial calcification of the tumor (Fig. 19–16). Because meningiomas are commonly located on the surface of the cerebral hemispheres, surgical access is easier and more successful. Therefore, surgery should be encouraged, and owners can expect the cat to have extended quality of life.

Peripheral Nerve Disease

Diabetes mellitus in cats can cause a peripheral neuropathy, although the pathogenesis of the neuropathy is not understood (Keamek et al, 1984). The predominant pathologic change that occurs in peripheral nerves is axonal degeneration. The clinical signs relative to the neuropathy include a plantigrade stance, depressed patellar reflexes, hindlimb weakness, and diminished postural reactions. The diagnosis of feline diabetic neuropathy is based on history, clinical signs, presence of hyperglycemia, and electromyographic results. The treatment for the neuropathy is regulation of the diabetic state. In longstanding cases the neuropathy is less likely to respond to diabetic regulation than in cases of shorter duration.

References and Supplemental Reading

Ambrose J, Gooding MR, Richardson AE. An assessment of the accuracy of computerized transversed axial scanning (EMI scanner) in the diagnosis of intracranial tumor. A review of 366 patients. Brain 98:569, 1975.

Aronin PA, Mahaley MS, Rudnick SA, et al. Prediction of BCNU pulmonary toxicity in patients with malignant gliomas. N Engl J Med 303:183, 1980.

Averill DR. Degenerative myelopathy in the aging German shepherd dog: Clinical and pathologic findings. J Am Vet Med Assoc 162:1045, 1973.

Bailey CS, Higgins RJ. Characteristics of cisternal cerebrospinal fluid associated with primary brain tumors in the dog: A retrospective study. J Am Vet Med Assoc 188:414, 1986.

Braund KG. Clinical Syndromes in Veterinary Neurology. Baltimore, Williams & Wilkins, 1986, p 85.

Braund KG, Steiss JE. Distal neuropathy in spontaneous diabetes mellitus in the dog. Acta Neuropathol (Berl) 57:263, 1982.

Braund KG, Steiss JE, Amling KA, et al. Insulinoma and

subclinical peripheral neuropathy in two dogs. J Vet Intern Med 1:86, 1987.
Carmichael S, Griffiths IR. Tumors involving the brachial plexus in seven dogs. Vet Rec 108:435, 1981.
Carpenter JL, King NW Jr, Abrams KL. Bilateral trigeminal nerve paralysis and Horner's syndrome associated with myelomonocytic neoplasia in a dog. J Am Vet Med Assoc 191:1594, 1987.
Carrillo JM, Sarfatl D, Greenlee P. Intracranial neoplasm and associated inflammatory response from the central nervous system. J Am Anim Hosp Assoc 22:367, 1986.
Chambers JN. Degenerative lumbosacral stenosis in dogs. Vet Med Rep 1:166, 1989.
Chambers JN, Selcer JE, Oliver JE. Results of treatment of lumbosacral stenosis in dogs by exploration and excision. Vet Comp Orthop Trauma 3:130, 1988.
Chrisman CL, Spencer CP, Crane SW, et al. Late-onset cerebellar degeneration in a dog. J Am Vet Med Assoc 182:717, 1983.
Christopher MM, Metz AL, Klausner J, et al. Acute myelomonocytic leukemia with neurologic manifestations in the dog. Vet Pathol 23:140, 1986.
Clemmons RM. Degenerative myelopathy. In Kirk RW, Bonagura JD, eds. Current Veterinary Therapy X. Philadelphia, WB Saunders, 1989, p 830.
Cook JR. Chemotherapy for brain tumors. Vet Med Report 2:391, 1990.
Cordy DR, Holliday TA. A necrotizing meningoencephalitis of pug dogs. Vet Pathol 26:191, 1989.
Couto CG, Cullen J, Pedroia V, et al. Central nervous system lymphosarcoma in the dog. J Am Vet Med Assoc 184:809, 1984.
Cuddon PA, Smith-Maxie L. Reticulosis of the central nervous system in the dog. Compend Contin Educ Pract Vet 6:23, 1984.
Dimski DS, Cook JR. Carmustine-induced partial remission of an astrocytoma in a dog. J Am Anim Hosp Assoc 26:179, 1990.
Dow SW, LeCouteur RA, Rosychuk RW, et al. Response of dogs with functional pituitary macroadenomas and macrocarcinomas to radiation. J Small Anim Pract 31:287, 1990.
Duncan ID, Griffiths IR. Neuromuscular diseases. In Kornegay JN, ed. Neurologic Disorders. New York, Churchill Livingstone, 1986, p 169.
Fenner WR. Neurology of the geriatric patient. Vet Clin North Am [Small Anim Pract] 18:711, 1988.
Fenner WR. Metastatic neoplasms of the central nervous system. Semin Vet Med Surg [Small Anim] 5:253, 1990.
Fingeroth JM, Prata RG, Patnaik AK. Spinal meningiomas in dogs: 13 cases (1972–1987). J Am Vet Med Assoc 191:720, 1987.
Foster ES, Carrillo JM, Patnaik AK. Clinical signs of tumors affecting the rostral cerebrum in 43 dogs. J Vet Intern Med 2:71, 1988.
Gearhart MA, deLahunta A, Summers BA. Cerebellar mass in a dog due to granulomatous meningoencephalitis. J Am Anim Hosp Assoc 22:683, 1986.
Gilmore DR. Neoplasia of the cervical spinal cord and vertebrae in the dog. J Am Anim Hosp Assoc 19:1009, 1983.
Hammer AS, Couto CG, Getzy D, et al. Magnetic resonance imaging in a dog with a choroid plexus carcinoma. J Small Anim Pract 31:341, 1990.
Heidner GL, Kornegay JN, Page RL, et al. Analysis of survival in a retrospective study of 86 dogs with brain tumors. J Vet Intern Med 5:219, 1991.
Hobbs SL, Cobb MA. A cranial neuropathy associated with multicentric lymphosarcoma in a dog. Vet Rec 127:526, 1990.
Hoerlein BF, Redding RW, Hoff EJ, et al. Evaluation of naloxone, crocetin, thyrotropin releasing hormone, methylprednisolone, partial myelotomy, and hemilaminectomy in the treatment of acute spinal cord trauma. J Am Anim Hosp Assoc 21:67, 1985.
Holliday TA, Higgins RJ, Turrel JM. Tumors of the nervous system. In Theilen GH, Madewell BN, eds. Veterinary Cancer Medicine. 2nd ed. Philadelphia, Lea & Febiger, 1987, p 601.
Ingram M, Jacques DB, Freshwater DB, et al. Adaptive immunotherapy of brain tumors in dogs. Vet Med Report 2:398, 1990.
Johnson CA, Kittleson MD, Indrieri RJ. Peripheral neuropathy and hypotension in a diabetic dog. J Am Vet Med Assoc 183:1007, 1983.
Katherman AE, Braund KG. Polyneuropathy associated with diabetes mellitus in a dog. J Am Vet Med Assoc 182:522, 1983.
Keamek BA, Moise NS, Cooper B, et al. Neuropathy associated with diabetes mellitus in the cat. J Am Vet Med Assoc 184:42, 1984.
Knowles K. Reduction of spiral ganglion neurons in the aging canine with hearing loss. Proc Am Coll Vet Intern Med 8:105, 1990.
Koller WC, Rubino FA. Combined resting-postural tremors. Arch Neurol 42:683, 1985.
Kornegay JN. Central nervous system neoplasia. In Kornegay JN, ed. Contemporary Issues in Small Animal Practice: Neurologic Disorders. New York, Churchill Livingstone, 1986, p 78.
Kornegay JN. Imaging brain neoplasms. Computed tomography and magnetic resonance imaging. Vet Med Report 2:372, 1990a.
Kornegay JN. The nervous system. In Hoskins JD, ed. Veterinary Pediatrics: Dogs and Cats From Birth to Six Months. Philadelphia, WB Saunders, 1990b, p 106.
Lawson DC, Burk RL, Prata RG. Cerebral meningioma in the cat: Diagnosis and surgical treatment of ten cases. J Am Anim Hosp Assoc 20:333, 1984.
LeCouteur RA. Tumors of the nervous system. In Withrow SJ, MacEwen EG, eds. Clinical Veterinary Oncology. Philadelphia, JB Lippincott, 1989, p 325.
LeCouteur RA. Brain tumors of dogs and cats. Vet Med Report 2:332, 1990.
LeCouteur RA, Child G. Clinical management of epilepsy of dogs and cats. In Indeiri RJ, ed. Epilepsy: Problems in Veterinary Medicine. Philadelphia, JB Lippincott, 1989, p 578.
LeCouteur RA, Sisson AF, Dow SW, et al. Combined surgical debulking and irradiation for the treatment of a large frontal meningioma in 8 dogs. Presented at the 7th Annual Conference of the Veterinary Cancer Society, Madison, WI, 1987.
LeCouteur RA, Turrel JM. Brain tumors in dogs and cats. In Kirk RW, ed. Current Veterinary Therapy IX. Philadelphia, WB Saunders, 1986, p 820.
Lenehan TN. Canine cauda equina syndrome. Compend Contin Educ Pract Vet 5:941, 1983.
Lewis DG. Radiological assessment of the cervical spine of the doberman with reference to cervical spondylomyelopathy. J Small Anim Prac 32:75, 1991.
Luttgen PJ. Diseases of the nervous system in older dogs. Part 1. Central nervous system. Compend Contin Educ Pract Vet 12:933, 1990a.
Luttgen PJ. Diseases of the nervous system in older dogs. Part II. Peripheral nervous system. Compend Contin Educ Pract Vet 12:1077, 1990b.
Marshall AE. Hearing loss in aged dogs. Adv Small Anim Med Surg 2:6, 1990.
McCarthy RJ, Feeney DA, Lipowitz AJ. Preoperative diagno-

sis of tumors of the brachial plexus by use of computed tomography in three dogs. J Am Vet Med Assoc 202:291, 1993.

Meric SM. Seizures. In Nelson RW, Couto CG, eds. Essentials of Small Animal Internal Medicine. St. Louis, Mosby–Year Book, 1992, p 760.

Moore MP, Gavin PR, Kraft SL, et al. MR, CT, and clinical features from four dogs with nasal tumors involving the rostral cerebrum. Vet Radiol 32:19, 1991.

Moore MP, Gavin PR, Kraft S. Boron neutron capture therapy for management of canine tumors. Proc Am Coll Vet Intern Med 7:623, 1989.

Nafe LA. Meningiomas in cats: A retrospective clinical study of 36 cases. J Am Vet Med Assoc 174:1224, 1979.

Nafe LA. The clinical presentation and diagnosis of intracranial neoplasia. Semin Vet Med Surg [Small Anim] 5:223, 1990.

Palmer RH, Chambers JN. Canine lumbosacral diseases. Part I. Anatomy, pathophysiology, and clinical presentation. Compend Contin Educ Pract Vet 13:61, 1991a.

Palmer RH, Chambers JN. Canine lumbosacral diseases. Part II. Definitive diagnosis, treatment, and prognosis. Compend Contin Educ Pract Vet 13:213, 1991b.

Panciera DL, Duncan ID, Messing A, et al. Magnetic resonance imaging in two dogs with central nervous system disease. J Small Anim Pract 28:587, 1987.

Plummer SB, Wheeler SJ, Kornegay JN, et al. Computed tomography of non-neoplastic brain disorders. Proc Am Coll Vet Intern Med 9:891, 1991.

Prata RD. Diagnosis of spinal cord tumors in the dog. Vet Clin North Am [Small Anim Pract] 7:165, 1977.

Rosenthal RC. Chemotherapy. In Withrow SJ, MacEwen EG, eds. Clinical Veterinary Oncology. Philadelphia, JB Lippincott, 1989, p 63.

Sackman JE, Adams WH, McGavin MD. X-ray computed tomography-aided diagnosis of nasal adenocarcinoma, with extension to the skull and central nervous system, in a dog. J Am Vet Med Assoc 194:1073, 1989.

Sarfaty D, Carrillo JM, Greenlee PG. Differential diagnosis of granulomatous meningoencephalomyelitis, distemper, and suppurative meningoencephalitis in the dog. J Am Vet Med Assoc 188:387, 1986.

Schunk KL, Averill DR. Peripheral vestibular syndrome in the dog: A review of 83 cases. J Am Vet Med Assoc 182:1354, 1983.

Seim HB, Withrow SJ. Pathophysiology and diagnosis of caudal cervical spondylomyelopathy with emphasis on the Doberman pinscher. J Am Anim Hosp Assoc 18:241, 1982.

Sisson AF, LeCouteur RA, Dow SW, et al. Radiation therapy of granulomatous meningoencephalomyelitis. Proc Am Coll Vet Intern Med 7:1031, 1989.

Smedes SL. Geriatric ophthalmic disorders. In Kirk RW, Bonagura JD, eds. Current Veterinary Therapy XI. Philadelphia, WB Saunders, 1992, p 1077.

Smith MO, Turrel JM, Bailey CS, et al. Neurologic abnormalities as the predominant signs of neoplasia of the nasal cavity in dogs and cats: Seven cases (1973–1986). J Am Vet Med Assoc 195:242, 1989.

Sorjonen DC. Clinical and histopathological features of granulomatous meningoencephalomyelitis in dogs. J Am Anim Hosp Assoc 26:141, 1990.

Speciale J, VanWinkle TJ, Skinberg SA, et al. Computed tomography in the diagnosis of focal granulomatous meningoencephalitis: Retrospective evaluation of three cases. J Am Anim Hosp Assoc 28:327, 1992.

Steiss JE, Orsher AN, Bowen JM. Electrodiagnostic analysis of peripheral neuropathy in dogs with diabetes mellitus. Am J Vet Res 42:2061, 1981.

Stoffregen DA, Kallfelz FA, de Lahunta A. Cerebral hemorrhage in an old dog. J Am Anim Hosp Assoc 21:495, 1985.

Swanson JF, Morgan S, Green RA, et al. Cerebral thrombosis and hemorrhage in association with L-asparaginase administration. J Am Anim Hosp Assoc 22:749, 1986.

Swayne DE, Tyler DE, Batker J. Cerebral infarction with associated venous thrombosis in a dog. Vet Pathol 25:317, 1988.

Thomas JB, Eger C. Granulomatous meningoencephalomyelitis in 21 dogs. J Small Anim Pract 30:287, 1989.

Turrel JM, Fike JR, LeCouteur RA, et al. Radiotherapy of brain tumors in dogs. J Am Vet Med Assoc 184:82, 1984.

Turrel JM, Fike JR, LeCouteur RA, et al. Computed tomographic characteristics of primary brain tumors in 50 dogs. J Am Vet Med Assoc 188:851, 1986.

Van Gundy T. Canine wobbler syndrome. Part I. Pathophysiology and diagnosis. Compend Contin Educ Pract Vet 11:144, 1989.

Waters DJ, Hayden DW, Walter PA. Intracranial lesions in dogs with hemangiosarcoma. J Vet Intern Med 3:222, 1989.

Weiss RB, Issell BF. The nitrosureas: carmustine (BCNU) and lomustine (CCNU). Cancer Treat Rev 9:313, 1982.

Zachary JF, O'Brien DP, Ingles BW, et al. Multicentric nerve sheath fibrosarcomas of multiple cranial nerve roots in two dogs. J Am Vet Med Assoc 188:723, 1986.

Zaki FA, Nafe LA. Choroid plexus tumors in the dog. J Am Vet Med Assoc 176:328, 1980.

CHAPTER 20

The Reproductive System and Prostate Gland

JANICE L. CAIN
and AUTUMN P. DAVIDSON

Breeders often request veterinary services when deciding whether a particular dog or cat is too old for use in their breeding program. There is no set age after which breeding should be discontinued; however, the age of the dam or sire can affect reproductive efficiency. The general health of the potential dam or sire can determine its ability to produce offspring and may predict whether the breeding event or pregnancy could cause an adverse effect.

Bitch. The surface epithelium of the ovary remains proliferative throughout life in the bitch. Surface ovarian clefts develop and the ovary may become cauliflower-like in appearance after successive estrous cycles (Anderson, 1970b). As the bitch ages, the interestrous interval lengthens owing to an increased anestrus period. Beagle bitches averaged 1.65 estrous cycles per year at 18 months of age, whereas 7-year-old bitches averaged 1.40 estrous cycles per year (Anderson, 1970a). A lengthened interestrous interval may not affect fertility directly, but can frustrate the owner's attempt to predict when an estrous cycle will occur.

Hormonal influences of successive estrous cycles can cause uterine abnormalities. Cystic endometrial hyperplasia can adversely affect reproductive performance by causing infertility or decreased fecundity.

Advancing age can adversely affect reproductive efficiency by decreasing conception rate, decreasing litter sizes, and increasing puppy losses (Table 20–1). In colony-bred beagles peak fertility and the largest number of surviving puppies occurred when bitches were between 3 and 5 years of age; the second through fourth litters produced the largest number of healthy puppies (Anderson, 1970a). In one study of 10 colony beagle bitches bred on consecutive estrous periods, conception failures and/or puppy losses in-

TABLE 20–1. REPRODUCTIVE PARAMETERS AND DISEASES OF ADVANCING AGE IN THE BITCH

Increase in interestrous interval
Decreased conception rate
Decreased litter size
Increased puppy losses
Development of cystic endometrial hyperplasia
Development of ovarian cysts and neoplasia
Development of uterine neoplasia
Development of vaginal neoplasia

creased when bitches were between 4 and 6 years of age (Anderson, 1970a) (Table 20–2). Bitches older than 6 years of age had a marked increase in both conception failures and puppy losses.

Breeders often inquire whether parturition will have an adverse effect on an older bitch. In one clinical study of dystocia in 128 bitches, there was no significant difference in age between affected bitches (ages 8 months to 15 years) and the overall intact female hospital population (Gaudet, 1985). Also, 17 of 29 bitches had pregnancies with uncomplicated whelpings prior to development of dystocia. Some breeders believe that a primiparous bitch older than 5 years of age has a greater chance of whelping problems; however, prior whelpings do not preclude the need for veterinary assistance or cesarean section at later whelpings.

The general health of the bitch should be considered before breeding at any age, and only healthy individuals should be bred. Some metabolic illnesses have a greater tendency to occur with age. Before a bitch older than 6 years of age is bred, she should have a thorough physical examination, ideally including a screen for occult metabolic illness with a complete blood cell count, serum biochemistry profile, and urinalysis. A clinically nonapparent metabolic illness such as renal failure might not affect the outcome of pregnancy, but the physiologic changes resulting from pregnancy or dystocia could exacerbate the pre-existing disease condition.

Considering these factors of reproductive efficiency and general health, the question still persists: how old is too old for a bitch in excellent health to be bred? This question was asked of two breeders of each of 14 breeds, and responses indicate that 7 to 8 years is considered a common cutoff age for many dog breeds (Table 20–3). Some breeders also consider the total number of litters produced by an individual bitch, and some breed organizations evoke standards of age for breeding bitches and number of litters produced. If a breeder wants another litter from a bitch in good general health, most likely there is no harm in attempting the breeding as long as the potential for reduced rate of conception and high puppy losses are recognized. In addition to a thorough prebreeding evaluation, close monitoring of the bitch during and after gestation is recommended.

TABLE 20–2. REPRODUCTIVE RECORDS OF 10 BEAGLE BITCHES BRED ON CONSECUTIVE ESTROUS CYCLES

AGE RANGE (YR)	CONCEPTION FAILURE (%)	PUPPY LOSSES (%)
0.8–1.6	17	24
1.6–2.5	8	14
2.5–3.3	0	24
3.3–4.1	30	6
4.1–4.9	60	16
4.9–5.8	50	17
5.8–6.6	75	38
6.6–7.4	42	50
7.4–8.2	50	62
8.2–9.0	56	67

Adapted from Anderson AC. Reproduction. In Anderson AC, ed. The Beagle as an Experimental Dog. Ames, IA, Iowa State University Press, 1970, p 37.

TABLE 20–3. RESULTS OF A BREEDER SURVEY: THE OLDEST AGE TO CONSIDER BREEDING A MULTIPAROUS BITCH IN EXCELLENT GENERAL HEALTH*

BREED	AGE OF BITCH AT LAST LITTER (YR)
Bull mastiff	6
Corgi	8
Dalmatian	7
English setter	7–8
German shepherd dog	7–8
Golden retriever	7–8
Great dane	6–7
Irish setter	7
Irish wolfhound	7
Labrador retriever	7
Norwegian elkhound	7
Papillon	8
Rottweiler	7–8
Siberian husky	9

*Responses from at least two breeders in each breed. Age ranges represent a difference of opinion from the two respondents. All breeders consider the health and quality of previously produced litters, the ability of the bitch to recover from previous litters, and the total number of litters the bitch has produced. These ages represent an absolute maximum. Maiden bitches are generally not considered for breeding at these age ranges, but instead should have been bred at a younger age for the first litter.

Queen. As in the bitch, advancing age will affect the reproductive efficiency of the queen. Most queens will produce litters until approximately 5 years of age before an age-related reduction in litter size occurs (Schmidt, 1986). Litter size and kitten survival generally improve after the first litter, and most queens can produce a total of five to seven litters. There may be a relationship between age at first parity and kitten survivability. According to one report, if the first litter is obtained from a queen older than 3 years of age, higher kitten losses are expected (Lawler and Monti, 1984).

The relationship between age and dystocia has not been studied in the queen to our knowledge, but there appears to be a correlation between obesity and dystocia (Lawler and Monti, 1984). Obese cats are usually older, and therefore, it seems difficult to separate age and body weight in this regard.

Stud Dog. Advancing age may affect reproductive performance in the stud dog by altering semen quality and libido (Table 20–4). Semen quality and sperm quantity tend to decrease with advancing age (Amann, 1986), and the testes may become smaller and softer than normal. Consequently, the American Kennel Club will not register any puppies sired by a dog older than 12 years of age without veterinary certification of fertility. Systemic disease, drug therapy, and previous inflammation can contribute to bilateral testicular atrophy. Testicular asymmetry may be due to testicular neoplasms, inflammation, or unilateral atrophy (Fig. 20–1).

Systemic disease can alter semen characteristics in a dog of any age, but because some metabolic diseases are more common in older animals, a concurrent disease process should be considered if oligospermia or azoospermia is detected. Concurrent and previously used medications may also affect semen parameters. If abnormalities are detected during a semen evaluation, confirmation is recommended by repeating the sample collection and analysis at another time.

Older dogs can have decreased libido caused by otherwise occult prostatic disease (benign prostatic hyperplasia or prostatitis) and pain associated with ejaculation. Libido can also be decreased by orthopedic pain or a concurrent illness. In cases where semen quality is acceptable, artificial insemination may produce litters from stud dogs that are physically incapable of natural breeding. Some owners elect to have older stud dogs routinely breed by artificial insemination to prevent physical stress. In addition, artificial insemination allows semen evaluation at the time of breeding to ensure that fertility is adequate.

TABLE 20–4. REPRODUCTIVE PARAMETERS AND DISEASES OF ADVANCING AGE IN THE STUD DOG

Decreased sperm quantity
Decreased semen quality
Decreased libido
Decreased success of semen freezing
Development of testicular neoplasia
Development of benign prostatic hyperplasia
Development of bacterial prostatitis
Development of prostatic neoplasia

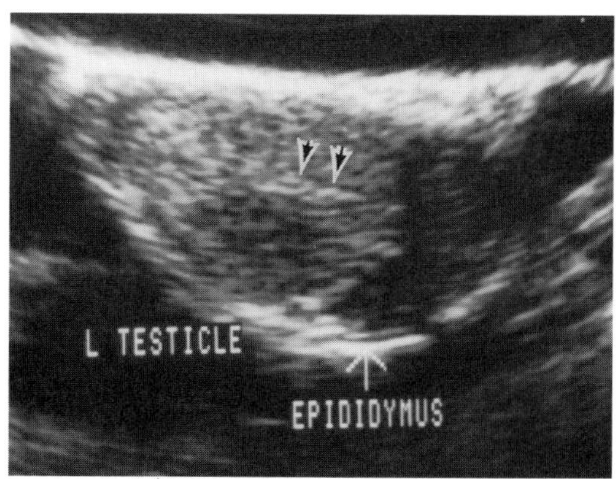

Figure 20–1. Ultrasonographic examination of a normal testicle. The normal testicle should have a very uniform echogenicity with a smooth, thin, hyperechoic capsule and central rete testis (*arrowheads*). The epididymis should be isoechoic or hypoechoic (as in this case) compared with the testicular parenchyma. Testicular atrophy may be identified by a testicular-to-epididymal measurement ratio of 3:1 or less (normal ratio, 4.5:1 to 3:1). This 11-year-old cocker spaniel has a testicular-to-epididymal ratio of 3.5:1. (Courtesy of Beth Partington, DVM, Louisiana State University, Baton Rouge, LA.)

To facilitate a breeding with an aged stud dog with oligospermia or poor semen quality, prediction of the time of ovulation in the bitch is recommended (Cain, 1992; Concannon and Lein, 1989). Ovulation timing is most accurate when serial evaluations of vaginal cytology, serum progesterone concentration, and vaginoscopic detection of vaginal mucosal crenelation are conducted during proestrus/estrus and prior to ovulation. This will allow the breeding, whether natural or by artificial insemination, to occur at a time the bitch is most likely to conceive. This technique was used by Cain to produce two litters sired by a 12-year-old Airedale terrier with oligospermia and 25 per cent motile sperm. Another possibility for producing litters from sires with poor semen quality is ovulation timing and surgical intrauterine insemination (Table 20–5). In a healthy bitch, surgical risk is minimal.

Age also can affect the success of semen cryopreservation. Sperm from some dogs older than 7 to 9 years of age are unable to withstand the stresses of freezing even when the fresh semen analysis appears normal (Goodman, personal communication, 1989). For this reason and because of the possible development of spontaneous infertility at any age, owners are encouraged to have their stud dog's semen frozen when the dog is between 2 and 6 years old.

Tom Cat. To our knowledge, information regarding the longevity of fertility for tom cats is not available. This may reflect the fact that tom cats are often neutered because of undesirable

TABLE 20–5. PROCEDURE FOR SURGICAL INTRAUTERINE INSEMINATION

Semen Preparation

Semen is collected by ejaculation and fractionated so that only the sperm-rich portion of the ejaculate is used. An extender is used to maintain sperm viability (Fresh Express-Semen Extender, International Canine Genetics, Inc., Malvern, PA). The maximal inseminant volume is 2 to 3 ml. If frozen semen is to be used, directions for thawing are followed to provide a maximal insemination volume of 2 to 3 ml. Using a syringe and a 22-gauge injection needle or a 22 × 2.5–inch spinal needle, semen is drawn into the syringe.

Surgical Procedure

The site is prepared as if for any ovariohysterectomy. A small incision is made 4 to 6 cm caudal to the umbilicus. The body of the uterus is exteriorized. The syringe containing the semen is held by the assistant, and the semen is transferred into a sterile syringe held by the surgeon. A new 22-gauge needle is attached to the sterile syringe and used to inject the semen into the uterus. A gentle finger clamp is formed caudal to the point of injection. The needle is directed into the lumen of the uterine body (through the uterine wall), and the semen is injected slowly toward the bifurcation. Each uterine horn will dilate as the semen is injected. Alternatively, each uterine horn can be injected individually with half of the inseminant. The finger clamp distal to the injection site is maintained for 30 to 60 sec. The uterus then is replaced into the abdomen, and abdominal closure is routinely done.

secondary sexual characteristics that often progress and may become intolerable as the cat ages.

DISORDERS OF THE FEMALE REPRODUCTIVE TRACT

Bitches and queens should undergo ovariohysterectomy after retirement from a breeding program. In addition to avoiding the behavioral and practical inconveniences of future estrous cycles, ovariohysterectomy will prevent the degenerative changes, hyperplasia, and neoplasia that occur with increased frequency in the reproductive organs of aged females.

Ovary

When faced with signs of possible ovarian disease in the aged bitch or queen, consideration must be given to all potential causes. Persistent estrus owing to functional follicular cysts has been documented in a wide age range of bitches. The age range for persistent estrus owing to ovarian neoplasia (especially granulosa cell tumors) overlaps that for estrus caused by ovarian cysts, but neoplasia is more common in the older bitch. A cystic neoplasm may be difficult to differentiate from an ovarian cyst without histopathologic examination. As with other cystic abdominal neoplasms, tumor seeding of the abdomen is possible if percutaneous fine needle aspiration is performed. Additional parameters, such as a complete blood cell count, serum biochemistry profile, and urinalysis, are part of the evaluation process. Exploratory laparotomy is both a diagnostic and a therapeutic procedure.

Ovarian Cysts

Ovarian cysts occur more commonly in aged bitches and queens and can be detected as incidental findings at elective ovariohysterectomy. Follicular cysts, also described as cystic follicles, result from incomplete resorption of fluid from an incompletely developed follicle. The cyst is lined by layers of granulosa cells, is thin walled, and contains watery fluid (Fig. 20–2). Luteinized follicular cysts, or luteal cysts, have a thicker layer of granulosa cells lining the cavity and may have a more opaque surface. Sixty-three of 400 2- to 5-year-old bitches (16 per cent) in one study had follicular cysts (Dow, 1960). Of the bitches with follicular cysts, 41 had solitary cysts, while 22 had multiple cysts involving one or both ovaries. Nearly 75 per cent of the bitches with follicular cysts were nulliparous (29 of 41 bitches with solitary cysts and 18 of 22 bitches with multiple cysts). In addition, nine bitches had luteal cysts, and of these, six were nulliparous. Cystic follicles are found most commonly in older, nulliparous queens and can cause persistent nonseasonal estrus and/or infertility (Stabenfeldt and Pedersen,

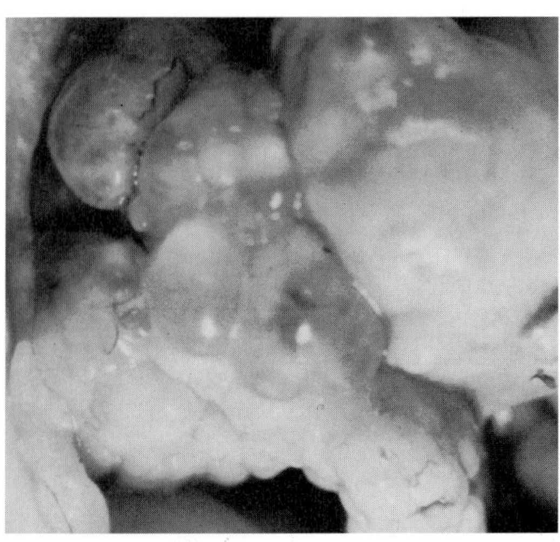

Figure 20–2. Ovarian cystadenoma in a dog.

1991). Queens are induced ovulators, and thus luteal cysts are rare (Carpenter et al, 1987).

Follicular and luteal cysts have the potential to produce reproductive steroid hormones, but when serum concentrations of these hormones are within normal limits, the cysts are considered nonfunctional. Functional follicular cysts have received the most attention in the veterinary literature because of the associated clinical signs. Increased estradiol production, similar to or exceeding that found in proestrus, causes signs of proestrus or estrus, and if levels are persistently elevated, bone marrow dyscrasias can result. Olson et al (1989) described 13 bitches with evidence of persistent estrus and functional ovarian cysts; 12 were 4 years of age or younger, and one was 9.5 years old. This age distribution may reflect the nature of bitches seen for treatment to preserve reproductive potential, rather than a true occurrence. Increased progesterone production has also been documented in bitches with follicular or luteal cysts.

Obstructed tubules on the ovarian surface epithelium cause epithelial tubular cysts. These can resemble follicular cysts but are differentiated histologically by a single layer of cuboidal epithelium lining the cyst. Cystic rete ovarii are the only cysts that occur in the hilar region of the ovary and generally are incidental findings (Dow, 1960; Gelberg et al, 1984).

Large ovarian cysts may be detected by abdominal palpation during a routine physical examination. Functional ovarian cysts are considered in the differential diagnosis for queens in persistent estrus and bitches with clinical or cytologic evidence of proestrus/estrus for more than 21 days. Conversely, functional ovarian cysts are also considered in the differential diagnosis for persistent anestrus. Masses can be detected by abdominal radiography but are better defined by ultrasonography. Cysts may be no larger than 1 cm but may range up to 10 cm in diameter. Serum estradiol concentrations may be elevated, but some bitches with functional follicular cysts have equivocally elevated serum estradiol concentrations. In Olson's description of bitches with persistent estrus and ovarian cysts, all had vaginal epithelial cornification, but only 6 of 11 bitches evaluated had serum estradiol concentrations consistent with or higher than that typical of proestrus (Olson et al, 1989). Neoplasia should also be considered in the differential diagnosis of any ovarian mass.

Ovariohysterectomy is the treatment of choice for functional or sizable ovarian cysts in an aged bitch with limited reproductive potential. Histopathologic evaluation of excised tissue can definitively differentiate a cyst from a cystic neoplasm. Suspected follicular cysts can be induced to luteinize by administration of either human chorionic gonadotropin (HCG) (500 to 1000 IU IM) or gonadotropin-releasing hormone (GnRH) (50 to 100 μg IM). Success is variable, and the need for repeated treatment is unknown. Increased estradiol and/or progesterone production can be associated with cystic endometrial hyperplasia. Subsequent increase in progesterone concentration associated with further luteinization of a cyst can create an increased risk for development of pyometra. Dow reported that 16 of 63 untreated bitches with follicular cysts also had cystic endometrial hyperplasia, and in the previously mentioned report by Olson et al (1989), pyometra occurred after medical treatment of ovarian cysts in two bitches (Dow, 1960).

Ovarian Neoplasia

With exception of teratomas, ovarian neoplasms are more common in older bitches and queens. The average age of bitches with ovarian tumors is 8 to 10 years (Heron, 1983; Withrow and Susaneck, 1986). The incidence of ovarian tumors is low (0.5 to 1.2 per cent) compared with that of other neoplasms. In another report evaluating a population of intact bitches, 6.25 per cent had ovarian tumors (Dow, 1960).

Ovarian tumors are generally classified as surface epithelial tumors, gonadal stomal tumors, germ cell line tumors, or metastatic neoplasia based on the origin of the neoplastic tissue (Susaneck and Barton, 1992).

Surface Epithelial Tumors. Papillary or cystic adenomas and adenocarcinomas have been described in bitches and queens. Cystadenomas are hyperplastic to adenomatous, poorly organized nodules of epithelial tubules seen commonly on ovaries of older bitches (Anderson and Simpson, 1973) and less commonly in queens (see Fig. 20–2). This may represent a continuum of the surface hyperplasia and cleft formation previously described in the aging bitch. Papillary adenocarcinomas extend beyond the neoplasm capsule and may be bilateral (Fig. 20–3). Ovarian adenocarcinomas may cause vaginal bleeding unassociated with the estrous cycle. Abdominal masses and ascites can result from metastasis. Persistent estrus resulting from ovarian adenocarcinoma has also been reported (Olson et al, 1989).

The treatment of choice for ovarian adenocarcinoma is surgical removal of the tumor, ovariohysterectomy, and exploratory laparotomy to

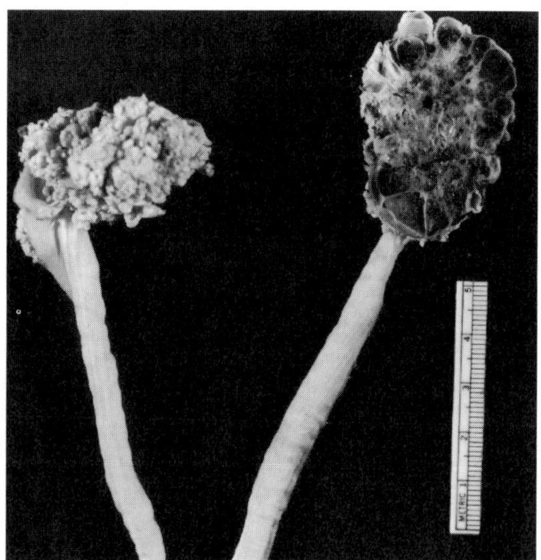

Figure 20–3. Bilateral ovarian cystadenocarcinoma in a 6-year-old dog. This figure shows neoplastic ovaries and normal uterine horns. This bitch had 6 L of serosanguineous ascitic fluid at necropsy and gross evidence of metastasis to the small intestine, colon, diaphragm, liver, urinary bladder, and vagina. Histologic evidence of metastasis was also detected in the spinal cord.

identify peritoneal metastatic lesions. Care should be taken during surgery to not disturb the tumor capsule. All metastatic lesions should be removed or debulked and subsequent systemic chemotherapy has been used (Withrow and Susaneck, 1986).

Gonadal Stomal or Sex-Cord Tumors. The most common neoplasms in this category are granulosa cell tumors, which represent approximately one half of the ovarian tumors reported in queens and bitches (Norris et al, 1969; Nielsen, 1983). Approximately 50 per cent of granulosa cell tumors are malignant in the queen, and 10 to 25 per cent are malignant in the bitch (Norris et al, 1969; Withrow and Susaneck, 1986). Thecomas and luteomas have been reported infrequently in bitches and queens.

Granulosa cell tumors can produce estradiol and/or progesterone and can be associated with irregular estrus, anestrus, persistent estrus, alopecia, gynecomastia, endometrial hyperplasia, and pyometra. Persistent estrus was documented in five bitches with ovarian tumors; four of these five bitches were older than 11 years of age (Olson et al, 1989).

A granulosa cell tumor should be suspected after discovery of an abdominal mass in an older intact female, especially if systemic endocrinologic effects are noted. Diagnostic confirmation relies on histopathologic examination. Surgical excision, as with ovarian adenocarcinoma, is the recommended treatment.

Germ Cell Line Tumors. Dysgerminomas and teratomas have been observed in bitches and queens. Dysgerminomas represent 15 per cent of ovarian tumors in queens (Carpenter et al, 1987). They resemble testicular seminomas and are usually benign. Ovarian teratomas are uncommonly reported and are found more frequently in younger animals.

Metastatic Neoplasia. The ovary can be the site of metastatic neoplasia such as lymphoma, squamous cell carcinoma, undifferentiated carcinoma, and mammary carcinoma (Withrow and Susaneck, 1986).

Uterus

Cystic Endometrial Hyperplasia-Pyometra Complex

Subsequent to ovulation the bitch has approximately a 2-month period of progesterone production from corpora lutea, even in the nonpregnant state. Progesterone stimulates endometrial hyperplasia and hypertrophy. Fluid accumulation within degenerated, cystic endometrial glands can lead to accumulation of fluid within the uterine lumen. The terms *hydrometra* and *mucometra* refer to the gross accumulation of sterile luminal fluid; the difference between the conditions depends on the mucin hydration of the accumulated fluid. Non-neoplastic, hyperplastic endometrial polyps that project into the uterine lumen can occur subsequent to cystic endometrial hyperplasia and may be confused with neoplasia (Barton, 1992).

Cystic endometrial hyperplasia (CEH) occurs more frequently in the aged bitch. Bitches with CEH may be infertile or have reduced fecundity, although the condition is often subclinical (Dow, 1957). Pyometra may occur as a sequela to CEH as a result of bacterial contamination of luminal fluid and occurs most commonly in aged bitches during diestrus (i.e., 4 to 10 weeks after estrus). During estrus, increased plasma estradiol concentrations cause the cervix to relax and allow ascent of cranial vaginal bacterial flora. Although other organisms have been implicated in pyometra, *Escherichia coli* is the most common bacterium in both the bitch and queen (Hardy and Osborne, 1974; Davidson et al, 1992). Ovarian progesterone production, in addition to inducing CEH, promotes pyometra by decreasing both the uterine luminal leukocyte response and myometrial contractility.

In queens pyometra may result from progesterone stimulation of the nonpregnant uterus. Because queens are induced ovulators, the uterus is not under the influence of progesterone between nonovulatory follicular cycles. The induction of pseudopregnancy in the queen either subsequent to an infertile breeding or as the result of stimulation to induce ovulation may result in the same circumstances for CEH production as occurs naturally in the bitch. In one study plasma progesterone concentration was increased in seven of nine queens at the time of pyometra diagnosis. The remaining two queens had basal plasma progesterone concentrations at diagnosis of pyometra, and thus it is possible that persistent plasma progesterone elevation is not required to induce or maintain pyometra in queens (see Davidson et al, 1992). It is also possible that these queens had transient plasma progesterone increases and concentrations were basal by the time pyometra was clinically recognized. Pyometra also occurs in unbred colony queens, implying a possible estradiol effect with recurring follicular cycles (Stabenfeldt and Pedersen, 1991). Whether the colony queens in that report could have been induced to ovulate unintentionally (i.e., communal grooming) and therefore could have been pseudopregnant prior to the development of pyometra is unknown, since plasma progesterone concentrations were not determined (Stabenfeldt, personal communication, 1991).

The clinical findings and treatment options for pyometra in the bitch and queen have been extensively reviewed (Barton, 1992; Johnson, 1989; Feldman and Nelson, 1987a; Davidson et al, 1992). To rule out a viable pregnancy and confirm the diagnosis, ultrasonography is recommended (Fig. 20–4). In the older animal, consideration of medical therapy (i.e., prostaglandin) versus surgical therapy (i.e., ovariohysterectomy) is based primarily on future reproductive potential. Prostaglandin therapy is not recommended for animals older than 8 years of age or in the presence of concurrent serious disease. A complete blood cell count, serum biochemistry profile, and urinalysis should be performed before surgical or medical therapy is begun. Care must be taken to avoid puncturing the distended uterus during cystocentesis, and therefore, ultrasound needle guidance is recommended. Alternatively, voided urine can be evaluated but will be unsuitable for bacterial culture if indicated. Ovariohysterectomy is recommended for any animal with a closed-cervix pyometra, especially if the bitch is older than 8 years of age.

Bacterial infection of the uterine stump in a neutered bitch or queen can occur at any age. Removal of the uterine body to just proximal to the cervix is recommended during ovariohysterectomy and may decrease subsequent stump pyometra. Ultrasonographic examination of the uterine stump is indicated if a purulent or sanguineous vulvar discharge occurs in a neutered female. Vaginoscopy is also recommended. The diagnosis may be more difficult in cases of a closed-cervix stump pyometra. Surgical excision of the stump is curative; concurrent systemic antimicrobial therapy is based on bacterial culture and sensitivity testing of the vulvar discharge.

Uterine Neoplasia

Uterine neoplasms are encountered more frequently in the aged bitch or queen but are relatively uncommon, accounting for less than 0.5 per cent of neoplasms detected (Brodey and Roszel, 1967). Leiomyoma is the most common

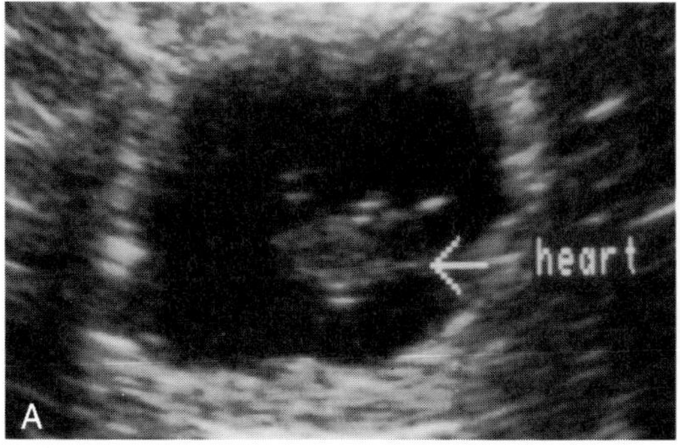

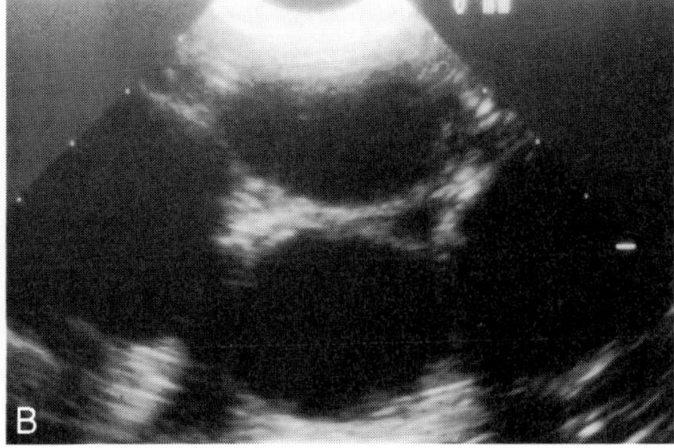

Figure 20–4. *A*, Ultrasonographic examination of a normal 16-day pregnancy in a cat. Circular to oval anechoic intrauterine fluid collections with fetal membranes, fetal poles with heartbeats, or moving fetuses are quickly distinguished from the thin-walled, tubular, anechoic fluid–filled uterus with a pyometra (*B*). (Courtesy of Beth Partington, DVM, Louisiana State University, Baton Rouge, LA.)

uterine neoplasm in the bitch, with an average age at diagnosis of 10 years, but is less common in queens (Loar, 1989). Leiomyomas can be incidental findings at ovariohysterectomy or necropsy and generally do not cause adverse clinical signs. Also, pyometra is occasionally evident at the time a benign uterine neoplasm is detected.

Endometrial adenocarcinoma is rarely described in bitches but is more frequent in queens. These neoplasms rapidly metastasize to regional lymph nodes, abdominal organs, lungs, and the central nervous system (Loar, 1989). Other less frequent uterine neoplasms include leiomyosarcoma, fibroma or fibrosarcoma, and choriocarcinoma.

Diagnosis of a uterine neoplasm may occur subsequent to detection of an abdominal mass during routine physical examination or as the result of investigation of abnormal vulvar discharge. Abdominal radiography and ultrasonography are useful in identifying a uterine neoplasm and differentiating other diagnoses (e.g., pregnancy or pyometra). Ovariohysterectomy and biopsy are useful diagnostic procedures. Metastatic lesions can be detected at primary tumor removal in queens with adenocarcinoma; thoracic radiography is indicated to detect radiographically discernible metastasis before surgery.

Uterine Torsion

Uterine torsion occurs in animals of any age but is more common in queens than bitches. Animals with uterine torsion usually have had large litters. Torsion of a single horn or of the entire uterus generally occurs near parturition. In addition, uterine neoplasms may predispose an animal to torsion (Barton, 1992). An abnormal vulvar discharge during gestation or prolonged nonproductive labor should prompt abdominal radiography and/or ultrasonography. The diagnosis of a uterine abnormality, with or without viable fetuses, necessitates surgical exploration. Torsion can result in uterine rupture and accumulation of fetal structures and/or serosanguineous fluid in the peritoneal cavity. Rupture of the uterine artery can result in hemorrhagic shock and sudden death.

Vagina

Congenital malformations of the vaginal canal and vaginal edema/hyperplasia are detected primarily in young bitches. Congenital vaginal lesions diagnosed in the older bitch are usually incidental findings. Extensive vaginal edema and hyperplasia during periods of estrogen stimulation (i.e., proestrus) are usually detected in young bitches but can recur with subsequent estrous cycles in an older bitch. Most owners elect ovariohysterectomy for a bitch with recurrent vaginal hyperplasia.

Vaginitis

Inflammation of the vaginal and/or vestibular mucosa can occur in a bitch of any age but rarely occurs in queens. Aerobic organisms, including (but not limited to) *E. coli*, *Streptococcus* spp., *Staphylococcus* spp., and *Pasturella* spp., are most often found in the normal vaginal flora (Olson et al, 1986). *Mycoplasma* and *Ureaplasma* organisms have been identified in the vaginal canal of reproductively normal, asymptomatic bitches; thus, they may be a constituent of the normal flora as well (Bjurstrom and Linde-Forsberg, 1992; Doig et al, 1981). Vaginitis attributable to overgrowth of normal vaginal flora occurs most likely secondary to an underlying condition. In many cases this predisposing condition is difficult to determine, but it can be obvious in some cases (i.e., vaginal foreign body, vaginal neoplasm, perineal dermatitis, vulvar skin fold redundancy, or congenital malformation). Less apparent causes of vaginitis include infection of the uterine stump and urinary tract abnormalities that lead to urine pooling in the vestibule (i.e., caudal to the urethral orifice). Urinary tract infection may be the cause or the result of a vaginitis.

Brucella canis and canine herpesvirus (CHV) should be considered as causative agents when evaluating vaginitis. Serologic testing for *B. canis* is readily available. Because agglutination tests for *B. canis* detection are sensitive but not very specific; negative screens are reliable, but positive titers require confirmation with a more specific assay system. Detection of *B. canis* in a blood or vaginal culture provides a definitive diagnosis, but a negative culture is less reliable. CHV may cause chronic recurrent vaginitis and infertility. Vaginal viral cultures for CHV may be attempted but, like those for brucellosis, are reliable only when positive. Serologic testing for CHV is less reliable than for *B. canis*, as antibody response is transient (Evermann, 1989).

In addition to a vulvar discharge, other clinical signs consistent with vaginitis include excessive vulvar grooming, scooting, and dysuria. Male dogs often exhibit sexual attraction to a neutered or intact bitch with vaginitis unrelated to hormonal fluctuations of estrous cycle activity. Diagnostic evaluation includes eliminating the possibility of pyometra as the source of vaginal discharge; thus, abdominal ultrasonography to evaluate the uterine lumen is indicated in an intact bitch. Vaginoscopy is also indicated, preferably by use of a rigid pediatric proctoscope on bitches of all breeds other than toy breeds. Vaginoscopy for small breeds may be accomplished with otoscopic or arthroscopic equipment. Thorough vaginoscopy is usually conducted without sedation in bitches free of any congenital vaginal malformations. Mucosal vesicles and ulcerations may be observed and biopsy specimens obtained. Vesicles may result from focal lymphoid response to inflammation, but CHV should also be considered and viral isolation from a vesicle attempted. Urine collected via cystocentesis is cultured for aerobic bacteria and mycoplasma.

Treatment is directed at eliminating the bacterial component of the inflammation with systemic antimicrobial therapy based on bacterial culture and sensitivity testing. Vaginal douching performed daily for 7 to 10 days using a very dilute povidone-iodine or chlorhexidine solution (e.g., human vaginal douche preparation) may expedite recovery. Correction of an underlying cause is attempted whenever possible. In cases of recurrent or persistent vaginitis, long-term appropriate antimicrobial therapy may be indicated.

Vaginal Neoplasia

Vaginal neoplasms are most common in older intact females and are usually incidental findings at necropsy. In both the bitch and the queen, fibromas and leiomyomas are most common (Loar, 1989). Malignant neoplasms (fibrosarcoma, leiomyosarcoma, mast cell tumors, squamous cell carcinoma, and transmissible venereal tumor) are less frequent. Extension of a transitional cell carcinoma from the urethra is uncommon but possible.

Vaginal neoplasms are detected either clinically, as a mass protruding from the vulva, or vaginoscopically during evaluation of infertility or investigation of vulvar discharge. Exfoliative cytologic examination may be nondiagnostic for encapsulated or submucosal neoplasms. Biopsy is indicated and can be obtained with vaginoscopy. Surgical removal and ovariohysterectomy should be considered concurrently in the intact bitch or queen.

DISORDERS OF THE MALE REPRODUCTIVE TRACT

Geriatric male dogs are often presented sexually intact. Stud dogs are used for breeding at an advanced age and are not commonly neutered after retirement from a breeding program. Tom cats are commonly neutered for development of behavioral disorders, and thus geriatric intact tom cats are rare. Disorders of the reproductive tract in the older male include infectious, inflammatory, neoplastic, and degenerative disorders. Each of these disorders can occur in the younger animal; however, neoplastic and degenerative disorders are more common in the aged male. Neutering at a young age will reduce or eliminate some diseases such as testicular neoplasia and benign prostatic hypertrophy.

Testes and Epididymides

The finding of an abnormal intrascrotal mass during physical examination of the older male warrants careful investigation as to its cause. Testicular neoplasia must be differentiated from chronic orchiepididymitis, testicular torsion, spermatocele, varicocele, hydrocele, or sperm granuloma (Johnson, 1986).

Testicular Neoplasia

Testicular neoplasia is rare in tom cats but very common in male dogs, ranking second in occurrence after cutaneous neoplasms (Susaneck and Withrow, 1986). Testicular neoplasms are more commonly reported in boxers, German shepherd dogs, Shetland sheepdogs, and weimaraners; thus, these breeds may be at an increased risk for developing testicular neoplasms (Daugherty, 1988). Testicular tumor types include Sertoli's cell tumor, seminoma, and interstitial cell tumor, and multiple testicular tumor types are commonly present in the same animal (Fig. 20–5).

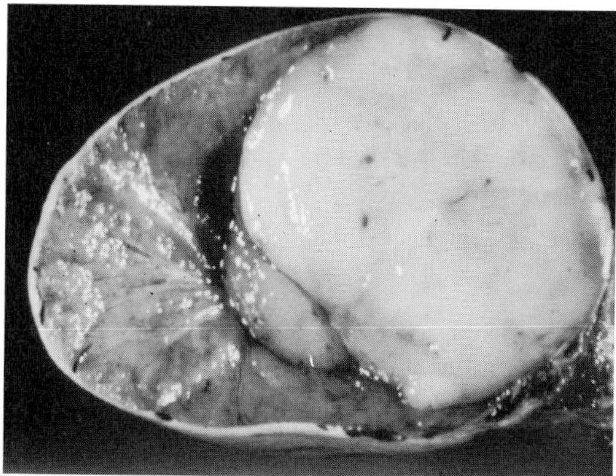

Figure 20–5. Seminoma within the testicle of a dog. Note the compression of the remaining testicular parenchyma to the left of the circumscribed neoplasm.

Cryptorchid testes were found to have a 13.6 per cent higher incidence of neoplasia, with the type varying with the location of the cryptorchid testis (Hayes and Pendergrass, 1976). The incidence of Sertoli's cell tumors and seminomas is higher in abdominal and inguinal cryptorchid testes, respectively, perhaps reflecting the temperature sensitivity of spermatogenic cells. Interstitial cell tumors are less frequent in extrascrotal testes (Feldman and Nelson, 1987b).

The majority of testicular neoplasms are benign, but 10 to 20 per cent of Sertoli's cell tumors and 5 to 10 per cent of seminomas are malignant (Loar, 1989). Most metastases are reported in regional lymph nodes, liver, and lungs. Adverse clinical signs of testicular neoplasms are usually related to their endocrine secreting capacity. Development of feminizing syndrome secondary to an absolute or relative excess of estrogenic compounds occurs most commonly with functional testicular neoplasms. Less commonly, excess androgen production occurs (Comharie et al, 1974). Sertoli's cell tumors are most commonly implicated in the male feminizing syndrome, with extrascrotal neoplastic testes having the highest association. Functional interstitial cell tumors and seminomas are more frequently associated with the production of androgens. Paraneoplastic disorders associated with excessive production of sex hormones include symmetric alopecia, cutaneous hyperpigmentation, gynecomastia, galactorrhea, prostatic squamous metaplasia, decreased libido, bone marrow dyscrasia, prostatic hyperplasia, perineal adenoma, and perineal hernias. Perineal hernias in otherwise healthy dogs without functional testicular tumors have not been found to be associated with abnormal estrogen or androgen levels (Mann et al., 1989). Testicular neoplasms can also cause clinical signs secondary to their size and location (e.g., abdominal distention or testicular torsion can result from the presence of an enlarged neoplastic intra-abdominal testis). Breakdown of the normally intact blood–testis barrier by neoplastic invasion can trigger an immune-mediated reaction against spermatogonia, with subsequent infertility (Feldman and Nelson, 1987b).

The diagnosis of testicular neoplasia is based on clinical signs and physical examination findings. Clinical signs vary depending on the tumor type, location, size, and functional status. Obvious clinical signs include testicular asymmetry and paraneoplastic endocrine abnormalities such as symmetric alopecia. Less obvious signs include hematologic or prostatic abnormalities and infertility. Testicular neoplasia should be suspected in an apparently neutered dog with an intra-abdominal mass unless a history of bilateral orchiectomy is known. Removing only the scrotal testes for sexual sterilization of a unilateral cryptorchid individual is unacceptable, because the retained testicle may become neoplastic. Cytologic evaluation of a fine needle aspirate of a testicular mass may be indicative of testicular neoplasia, but histologic evaluation is required for definitive diagnosis. Testicular ultrasonography may detect small neoplasms, differentiating intratesticular from extratesticular (epididymal) masses and determining the degree of local invasion or associated metastasis. The incidence of epididymal disease in the dog is low; most epididymal masses in humans are not neoplastic (Johnston et al., 1991).

Surgical removal of a neoplastic testicle is indicated and bilateral castration is advised if cryptorchidism is present. Presurgical evaluation for paraneoplastic disorders and evidence of thoracic and abdominal metastases should be performed. The prognosis after removal of benign testicular tumors is excellent, but the prognosis after removal of malignant or functional testicular tumors varies. In spite of supportive therapy, long-term prognosis for dogs with estrogen-induced bone marrow aplasia is grave. The use of hematopoietic colony-stimulating factors and bone marrow transplantation in pancytopenic dogs may be successful (Suess et al., 1992). Control of metastatic disease with adjunctive chemotherapy or external beam radiation can be attempted, but the prognosis is guarded (Crow, 1980; Loar, 1989). Return of fertility after removal of a functional testicular neoplasm depends on the recovery of the hypothalamic-pituitary-gonadal axis, reversal of atrophy in the remaining testis, and lack of other underlying testicular or reproductive disease. The prognosis for return to fertility after removal of a testicular neoplasm that has induced immunologic-mediated infertility is poor (Feldman and Nelson, 1987b). In general, bilateral orchiectomy is advised in a older dog with testicular neoplasia.

Testicular Torsion

Testicular neoplasms, when palpable, are usually nonpainful. The finding of a painful, warm, intrascrotal mass suggests the presence of an infectious or inflammatory disorder. Torsion occurs more frequently in an enlarged neoplastic intra-abdominal testicle and rarely occurs with scrotal testicles. Torsion results from rotation of the testicle along its horizontal axis, with resultant arterial and venous occlusion and tissue necrosis.

Acute onset of abdominal pain in a geriatric cryptorchid dog should prompt evaluation of the abdominal testicle for torsion. Orchiectomy is curative and is the preferred treatment.

Orchiepididymitis

Acute orchiepididymitis can result from trauma, septicemia, or extension of septic prostatitis or cystitis. There is an increased risk of orchiepididymitis in older dogs owing to the higher incidence of prostatic disease in the older dog (Krawiec and Heflin, 1992). Chronic, progressive, nonsuppurative orchiepididymitis can occur as a result of *B. canis*, canine distemper virus, or *E. coli* infection (Lein, 1977). Atrophy and fibrosis, sequelae of acute or chronic orchitis, can induce firm, irregular palpable changes in the testes. Inflammation may disrupt the blood–testis barrier leading to immune-mediated destruction of remaining spermatogenic cells.

Clinical signs of acute orchiepididymitis include localized pain, swelling, and heat within the scrotum, often making palpable differentiation of intrascrotal structures difficult. Abscess of the scrotum can occur, and signs of associated systemic illness (i.e., lethargy, fever, inappetence) may be present. Ultrasonography of the testes, prostate gland, and urinary bladder are indicated, as are urinalysis and bacterial urine culture. Cytologic examination and bacterial culture of both the sperm-rich (second) and prostatic (third) fractions of the ejaculate are indicated. Cytologic aspiration and bacterial culture of a testicular aspirate may be appropriate when collection of an ejaculate is not possible. Serologic screening for *B. canis* is indicated. A testicular biopsy is useful for diagnosing immune-mediated destruction of seminiferous tubules.

Supportive care, including fluid therapy and appropriate antimicrobial agents, should be initiated. Once adverse clinical signs are stabilized, orchiectomy is desirable if the dog is not a valued breeder. Unilateral orchiectomy is an option that may salvage the remaining testicle and the individual's fertility. Thermal and immunologic damage to spermatogenic cells can result from orchiepididymitis, and recovery of fertility depends on survival of spermatogonia and tubular patency (Feldman and Nelson, 1987b). Long-term appropriate antimicrobial therapy is indicated in chronic septic orchiepididymitis. Immunosuppressive therapy might be indicated in immune-mediated orchitis, but testicular degeneration and atrophy secondary to suppression of the hypothalamic-pituitary-gonadal axis are likely to occur with the use of corticosteroids. Therefore, the prognosis for return of fertility is guarded.

Prostate Gland

Prostatic disease is common in the older dog but rarely occurs in the cat. Such disease includes benign prostatic hyperplasia, parenchymal and paraprostatic cysts, calculi, acute and chronic infectious prostatitis, abscess, metaplasia, and neoplasia. Prostatic disease occurs in both intact and neutered dogs, with an increased incidence of infectious and inflammatory disorders in intact males. The incidence of prostatic disorders increases with advancing age for several reasons. As a dog ages, the prostate gland increases in size and develops an increased sensitivity to testosterone. Prostatic secretions, thought to have antibacterial properties, decline after 4 years of age. Communication with the urinary and reproductive tracts permits transfer of genitourinary pathogens to the prostate gland. Neoplastic transformation occurs with increased frequency in older dogs, and early neutering does not appear to be protective against prostatic malignancy (Obradovich et al, 1987).

Diagnosis of prostatic disease is based on the medical history, significant clinical signs (i.e., fecal tenesmus, dysuria, urethral discharge, systemic illness), and the results of specific diagnostic tests (i.e., prostate gland palpation, cytologic evaluation of urethral discharge, cytologic and bacterial/fungal evaluation of prostatic fluid, ultrasonography/radiography, prostatic gland aspirate, and biopsy). Different prostatic disorders can be present in the same dog, requiring a thorough diagnostic approach to the problem.

Benign Prostatic Hyperplasia and Cysts

Benign prostatic hyperplasia occurs in response to alteration of androgen-to-estrogen ratios in the older dog (Barsanti and Finco, 1989) (Fig. 20–6). Intraprostatic cystic hyperplasia occurs concurrently, sometimes producing large parenchymal masses. Benign hyperplasia becomes problematic when an enlarged prostate gland compresses the colon or urethra or bacterial or fungal infection compounds the condition (Krawiec and Heflin, 1992). Prostatomegaly secondary to benign hyperplasia has been implicated as a complication of perineal hernias (Mann et al, 1989). Although biopsy of the pros-

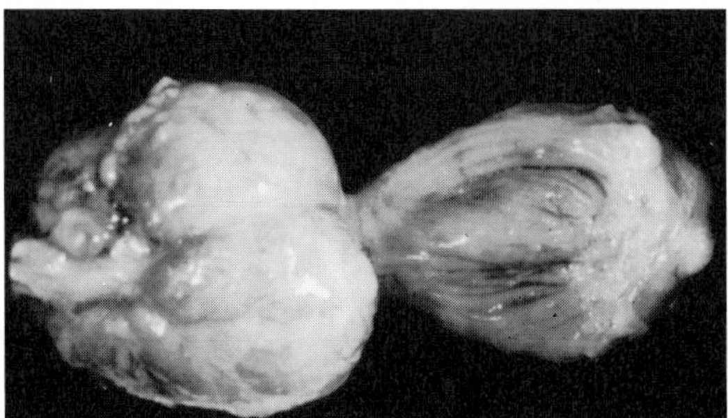

Figure 20–6. Benign prostatic hyperplasia in a dog. The circumscribed mass to the left is the enlarged prostate gland; the urinary bladder is to the right.

tate gland can confirm the diagnosis of benign hyperplasia, a presumptive diagnosis can be made from results of the physical examination and hematologic, cytologic, bacterial/fungal, and ultrasonographic evaluations (Fig. 20–7) (Feeney et al., 1987).

Orchiectomy is curative for uncomplicated benign hyperplasia, with a 70 per cent reduction in prostate gland size expected. Antiandrogenic medical therapy (ketoconazole, megestrol, and flutamide) is reportedly largely unsuccessful (Barsanti and Finco, 1989; Cartee et al, 1990). Treatment with estrogenic compounds is contraindicated because of their toxicity and the possible development of squamous metaplasia of the prostate gland.

Paraprostatic cysts can occur and can cause dysuria or tenesmus if the cyst is large. Ultrasonography confirms the diagnosis and allows guided fine needle aspiration of the cysts. Surgical drainage, excision, or marsupialization and concurrent orchiectomy are advised (Basinger and Rawlings, 1987).

Infectious Prostatitis

Acute and chronic infectious prostatitis are serious disorders of the intact dog. Bacteria ascending from normal urethral flora are most commonly implicated, with *E. coli* found most frequently. *B. canis* infection is also possible. Diagnosis is based on physical examination findings (i.e., painful prostatic palpation, hemorrhagic to purulent urethral discharge, signs of systemic illness) and clinical findings (i.e., microbiologic evaluation of an ejaculate, if obtainable, or an ultrasound-guided prostatic aspirate or biopsy) (Fig. 20–8). Appropriate antimicrobial therapy using bactericidal, lipid-soluble, basic antimicrobial agents for a minimum of 6 weeks is advised. A trimethoprim–sulfonamide combination, chloramphenicol, enrofloxacin, carbenicillin, and clindamycin are good antimicrobial choices (Barsanti and Finco, 1989). Orchiectomy is recommended. Studies have shown that orchiectomy early in the course of treatment of infectious prostatitis is of benefit, although concern about postoperative atrophy of prostate parenchyma around an infected nidus exists (Cowan et al, 1991). Prostatectomy may be complicated by surgical difficulty and postoperative urinary incontinence. Ineffectively treated infectious prostatitis can progress to chronic infection or abscess. Chronic prostatic infection is a potential cause of infertility in the older dog.

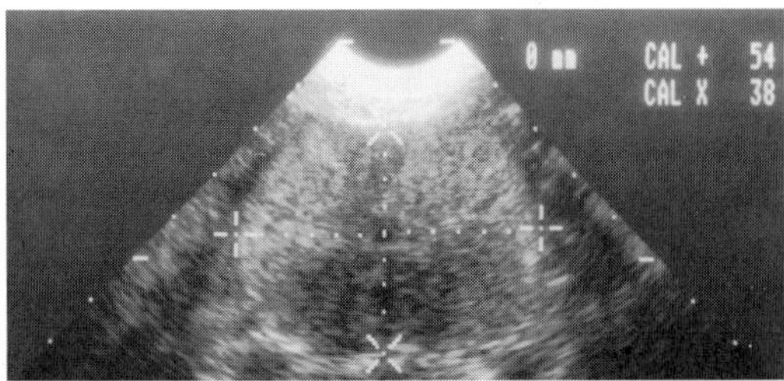

Figure 20–7. Cross-sectional ultrasonographic examination of an aged dog with benign prostatic hyperplasia. The prostate gland measures 5.4 × 3.0 cm in cross-sectional diameter and is uniformly hyperechoic and symmetric and contains no cavitations or mineralization. (Courtesy of Beth Partington, DVM, Louisiana State University, Baton Rouge, LA.)

Metaplasia and Neoplasia

Squamous metaplasia of the prostatic parenchyma occurs secondary to endogenous or exogenous hyperestrogenism. Squamous metaplasia

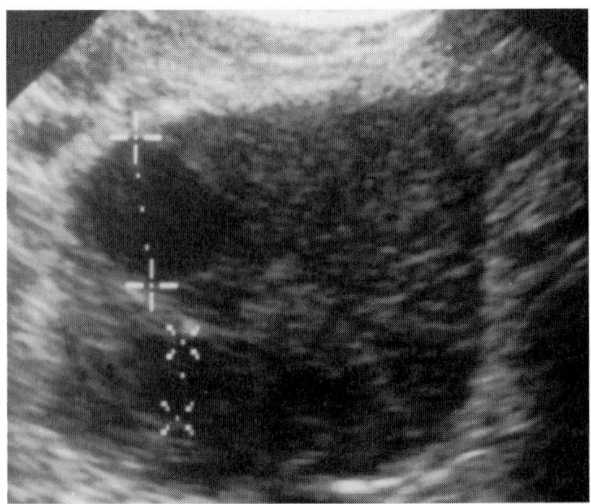

Figure 20–8. Cross-sectional ultrasonographic examination of a 5-year-old male dachshund with cavitating bacterial prostatitis. The prostate gland is enlarged, hypoechoic, and irregularly marginated and contains two anechoic circular cavitations identified with "t" and "x" measurement cursors. Ultrasound-guided fine needle aspiration of the cavitations for cytology and bacterial culture confirmed the diagnosis. (Courtesy of Beth Partington, DVM, Louisiana State University, Baton Rouge, LA.)

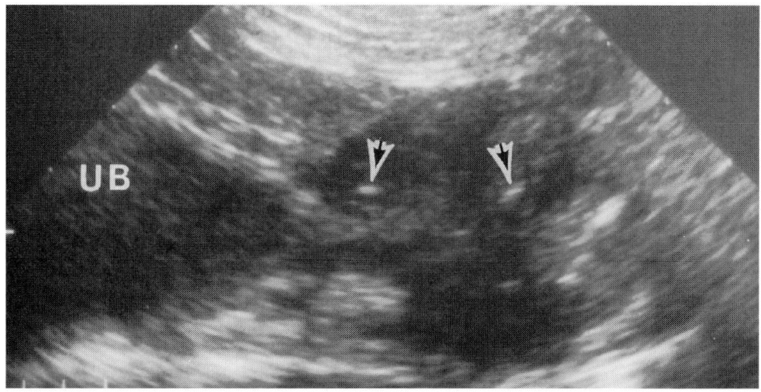

Figure 20–9. Longitudinal prostatic ultrasonographic examination of a 9-year-old castrated Airedale terrier with prostatic transitional cell carcinoma. The prostate gland is slightly enlarged, irregularly marginated, and complexly echogenic and contains several small mineralizations (*arrowheads*). UB, urinary bladder. (Courtesy of Beth Partington, DVM, Louisiana State University, Baton Rouge, LA.)

predisposes the prostate gland to cystic and infectious disorders. Identification and removal of the source of estrogen is recommended. Functional (estrogen-producing) Sertoli's cell tumors are most commonly responsible.

Malignant neoplastic conditions of the prostate gland occur with equal frequency in both intact and neutered geriatric dogs. Adenocarcinoma, transitional cell carcinoma, and squamous cell carcinoma occur most frequently (Figs. 20–9 and 20–10). Metastatic neoplasia of the prostate gland occurs as well. Common clinical signs include dysuria, tenesmus, irregular prostatomegaly, lumbar pain, cachexia, and posterior paresis. Definitive diagnosis by histopathologic analysis of biopsied tissue is advised because of the grave prognosis of the disease. Metastatic disease should be ruled out before therapy is undertaken. Radiation therapy and prostatectomy offer the best chance for palliation (Turrel, 1987).

Penile, Preputial, and Scrotal Disease

Neoplasia of the external genitalia may be observed in older dogs. Transmissible venereal tumors occur primarily in young dogs used for breeding. Other neoplasias of the external genitalia include squamous cell carcinomas, mast cell tumors, melanomas, fibromas, lymphosarcomas, hemangiosarcomas, adenomas, and papillomas (Feldman and Nelson, 1987b; Held and Prater, 1992). Clinical signs can include an abnormal preputial discharge, dysuria, and excessive self-grooming. Full extrusion of the penis from the prepuce permits thorough evaluation of its surfaces for a mass lesion. Therapeutic options vary with the tumor type, but complete surgical excision offers the best prognosis in most cases. Chemotherapy or adjunctive radiotherapy are other options that may be useful. To our knowledge, penile neoplasms have not been reported in the cat. Perianal gland adenomas are usually observed in the skin surrounding the anus but can be associated with the external genitalia. Perianal gland adenomas are hormone sensitive, and orchiectomy is indicated (Held and Prater, 1992).

Inflammatory conditions of the external genitalia, including scrotal dermatitis and balanoposthitis, can occur in the older male. Scrotal dermatitis can cause infertility as a result of the associated increase in scrotal and testicular temperature. Scrotal dermatitis can occur after exposure to traumatic kennel surfaces, excessively hot surfaces, or caustic chemicals such as disinfectants and may also be an extension of other dermatologic conditions. Balanoposthitis, an inflammation of the penile and preputial mucosa, is thought to arise from an overgrowth of bacteria normally present on the external genitalia. A purulent preputial discharge, accompanied by excessive self-grooming, can be present, although

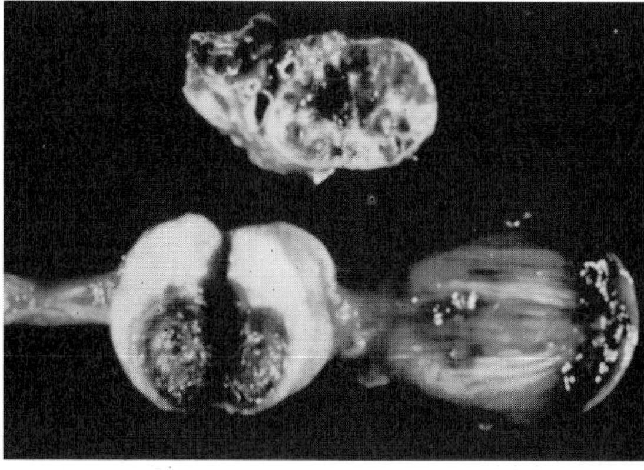

Figure 20–10. Prostatic adenocarcinoma in a dog. The prostate gland has been incised to expose the neoplasm; the urinary bladder is to the right of the prostate gland. Metastasis to a regional lymph node is included above.

many dogs are asymptomatic. The presence of a preputial foreign body or neoplasm should be considered in the differential diagnosis.

Therapy consists of antiseptic preputial lavage and inhibiting self-grooming. Systemic antimicrobial therapy may be beneficial (Johnston, 1989). Chronic balanoposthitis can result in paraphimosis (i.e., inability to reduce the penis within the prepuce). Chronic urethral obstruction in the tom cat can cause distal penile and preputial trauma and inflammation, resulting in partial paraphimosis. Spinal cord lesions in the older dog have been associated with priapism (persistent erection), and thromboembolism of the penile vasculature should also be considered.

References and Supplemental Reading

Amann RP. Reproductive physiology and endocrinology of the dog. In Morrow DA, ed. Current Therapy in Theriogenology 2. Philadelphia, WB Saunders, 1986, p 532.

Anderson AC. Reproduction. In Anderson AC, ed. The Beagle as an Experimental Dog. Ames, IA, Iowa State University Press, 1970a, p 31.

Anderson AC. Reproductive system-female. In Anderson AC, ed. The Beagle as an Experimental Dog. Ames, IA, Iowa State University Press, 1970b, p 312.

Anderson AC, Simpson ME. The Ovary and Reproductive Cycle of the Dog (Beagle). Los Altos, CA, Geron-X, 1973.

Barsanti JA, Finco DR. Canine prostatic diseases. In Ettinger SJ, ed. Textbook of Veterinary Internal Medicine. Philadelphia, WB Saunders, 1989, p 1859.

Barton CA. Diseases of the uterus. In Morgan RV, ed. Handbook of Small Animal Practice. New York, Churchill Livingstone, 1992, p 655.

Basinger RR, Rawlings CA. Surgical management of prostatic diseases. Compend Contin Educ Pract Vet 9:993, 1987.

Bjurstrom L, Linde-Forsberg C. Long-term study of aerobic bacteria of the genital tract in breeding bitches. Am J Vet Res 53:665, 1992.

Brodey RF, Roszel JR. Neoplasms of the canine uterus, vagina, and vulva: A clinical, pathologic study of 96 cases. J Am Vet Med Assoc 151:1294, 1967.

Cain JL. Introduction. In Morgan RV, ed. Handbook of Small Animal Practice. New York, Churchill Livingstone, 1992, p 637.

Carpenter JL, Andrews LK, Holzworth J, et al. Tumors and tumor-like lesions (female reproductive system). In Holzworth J, ed. Diseases of the Cat. Philadelphia, WB Saunders, 1987, p 520.

Cartee RE, Rumph PF, Kenter DC, et al. Evaluation of drug-induced prostatic involution in dogs by transabdominal B-mode ultrasonography. Am J Vet Res 51:1773, 1990.

Comharie F, Mattheeuws D, Vermeulen A. Testosterone and oestradiol in dogs with testicular tumors. Acta Endocrinol 77:408, 1974.

Concannon PW, Lein DH. Hormonal and clinical correlates of ovarian cycles, ovulation, pseudopregnancy, and pregnancy in dogs. In Kirk RW, ed. Current Veterinary Therapy X. Philadelphia, WB Saunders, 1989, p 1269.

Cowan LA, Barsanti JA, Crowell W, et al. Effects of castration on chronic bacterial prostatitis in dogs. J Am Vet Med Assoc 3:346, 1991.

Crow SE. Neoplasms of the reproductive organs and mammary glands of the dog. In Morrow DA, ed. Current Therapy in Theriogenology. Philadelphia, WB Saunders, 1980, p 640.

Daugherty SA. The geriatric dog: Understanding common manifestations of aging. In The Geriatric Dog Pedigree Forum, 1988, p 9.

Davidson AD, Feldman EC, Nelson RW. Treatment of pyometra in cats, using prostaglandin F2 alpha: 21 cases (1982–1990). J Am Vet Med Assoc 200:825, 1992.

Doig PA, Ruhnke HL, Bosu WTK. The genital *Mycoplasma* and *Ureaplasma* flora of healthy and diseased dogs. Can J Comp Med 45:233, 1981.

Dow C. Ovarian abnormalities in the bitch. J Comp Pathol 70:59, 1960.

Dow C. The cystic hyperplasia-pyometra complex in the bitch. Vet Rec 69:1409, 1957.

Evermann JF. Diagnosis of canine herpetic infections. In Kirk RW, ed. Current Veterinary Therapy X. Philadelphia, WB Saunders, 1989, p 1313.

Feeney DA, Johnston GR, Klausner JS, et al. Canine prostatic disease—comparison of ultrasonographic appearance with morphologic and microbiologic findings: 30 cases (1981–1985). J Am Vet Med Assoc 190:1027, 1987.

Feldman EC, Nelson RW. Canine female reproduction. In Feldman EC, Nelson RW, eds. Canine and Feline Endocrinology and Reproduction. Philadelphia, WB Saunders, 1987a, p 446.

Feldman EC, Nelson RW. Disorders of the canine male reproductive tract. In Feldman EC, Nelson RW, eds. Canine and Feline Endocrinology and Reproduction. Philadelphia, WB Saunders, 1987b, p 481.

Gaudet DA. Retrospective study of 128 cases of canine dystocia. J Am Anim Hosp Assoc 21:813, 1985.

Gelberg HB, McEntee K, Heath EH. Feline cystic rete ovarii. Vet Pathol 21:304, 1984.

Hardy RM, Osborne CA. Canine pyometra: Pathology, diagnosis, and treatment of uterine and extra-uterine lesions. J Am Anim Hosp Assoc 10:245, 1974.

Hayes HM, Pendergrass TW. Canine testicular tumors: Epidemiologic features of 410 dogs. Int J Cancer 18:482, 1976.

Held JP, Prater PE. Diseases of the external genitalia. In Morgan RV, ed. Handbook of Small Animal Practice. New York, Churchill Livingstone, 1992, p 667.

Heron MA. Tumors of the canine genital system. J Am Anim Hosp Assoc 19:981, 1983.

Johnson CA. Disorders of the canine testicles and epididymides. In Morrow DA, ed. Current Therapy in Theriogenology 2. Philadelphia, WB Saunders, 1986, p 551.

Johnson CA. Uterine diseases. In Ettinger SJ, ed. Textbook of Veterinary Internal Medicine. Philadelphia, WB Saunders, 1989, p 1797.

Johnson CA, Grace JA, Probst MR. The effect of maternal illness on perinatal health. Vet Clin North Am 16:435, 1986.

Johnston GR, Feeney CA, Johnston SD, et al. Ultrasonographic features of testicular neoplasia in dogs: 16 cases (1980–1988). J Am Vet Med Assoc 10:1779, 1991.

Johnston SD. Disorders the external genitalia of the male. In Ettinger SJ, ed. Textbook of Veterinary Internal Medicine. Philadelphia, WB Saunders, 1989, p 1881.

Krawiec DR, Heflin DH. Study of prostatic disease in dogs: 177 cases (1981–1986). J Am Vet Med Assoc 200:1119, 1992.

Lawler DF, Monti KL. Morbidity and mortality in neonatal kittens. Am J Vet Res 45:1455, 1984.

Lein DH. Canine orchitis. In Kirk RW, ed. Current Veterinary Therapy VI. Philadelphia, WB Saunders, 1977, p 1255.

Loar AS. Tumors of the genital system and mammary glands. In Ettinger SJ, ed. Textbook of Veterinary Internal Medicine. Philadelphia, WB Saunders, 1989, p 1814.

Mann FA, Boothe HW, Amoss MS, et al. Serum testosterone and estradiol 17-beta concentrations in 15 dogs with perineal hernia. J Am Vet Med Assoc 194:1578, 1989.

Nielsen SW. Classification of tumors in dogs and cats. J Am Anim Hosp Assoc 19:13, 1983.

Norris HJ, Garner FM, Taylor HB. Pathology of feline ovarian neoplasms. J Pathol 97:138, 1969.

Obradovich J, Walshaw R, Goullaud E. The influence of castration on the development of prostatic carcinoma in the dog: 43 cases (1978–1985). J Vet Intern Med 1:183, 1987.

Olson PN, Jones RL, Mather EC. The use and misuse of vaginal cultures in diagnosing reproductive diseases in the bitch. In Morrow DA, ed. Current Therapy in Theriogenology 2. Philadelphia, WB Saunders, 1986, p 469.

Olson PN, Wrigley RH, Husted PW, et al. Persistent estrus in the bitch. In Ettinger SJ, ed. Textbook of Veterinary Internal Medicine. Philadelphia, WB Saunders, 1989, p 1792.

Schmidt PM. Feline breeding management. Vet Clin North Am 16:435, 1986.

Stabenfeldt GH, Pedersen NC. Reproduction and reproductive disorders. In Pedersen NC, ed. Feline Husbandry. Goleta, CA, American Veterinary Publications, Inc., 1991, p 129.

Suess RP, Barr SC, Sacre BJ, et al. Bone marrow hypoplasia in a feminized dog with an interstitial cell tumor. J Am Vet Med Assoc 200:1346, 1992.

Susaneck SJ, Barton CA. Diseases of the ovaries. In Morgan RV, ed. Handbook of Small Animal Practice. New York, Churchill Livingstone, 1992, p 643.

Susaneck SJ, Withrow SJ. Tumors of the canine male reproductive tract. In Morrow DA, ed. Current Therapy in Theriogenology 2. Philadelphia, WB Saunders, 1986, p 561.

Turrel JM. Intraoperative radiotherapy of carcinoma of the prostate gland in 10 dogs. J Am Vet Med Assoc 190:48, 1987.

Withrow SJ, Susaneck SJ. Tumors of the canine female reproductive tract. In Morrow DA, ed. Current Therapy in Theriogenology 2. Philadelphia, WB Saunders, 1986, p 521.

CHAPTER 21

Anesthesia

ROBERT R. PADDLEFORD

The anesthetic management of the geriatric dog and cat can be challenging for the veterinarian. These animals are often suffering from multiple pathophysiologic conditions as well as decreased organ reserve capacity. Thus, the anesthetic episode may exacerbate a pre-existing subclinical organ dysfunction and produce overt organ failure. The primary goals in the anesthetic management of the geriatric dog or cat are to (1) keep anesthesia time to a minimum; (2) use anesthetic drugs that produce minimal cardiopulmonary depression; (3) use anesthetic drugs that can be antagonized, are readily metabolized, and/or require no metabolism; (4) maintain adequate renal function; and (5) closely monitor physiologic parameters.

PHYSIOLOGIC CHANGES ASSOCIATED WITH AGING

It is often difficult to define a geriatric dog or cat simply on the basis of chronologic age. Young dogs and cats may have organ system dysfunction more typical of a geriatric patient, and some geriatric dogs and cats have organ systems more typical of a younger patient. Some authors have suggested that patients be considered aged or geriatric when they have reached 75 to 80 per cent of their life expectancy; however, each patient must ultimately be evaluated as an individual and not simply as a "geriatric" patient.

There are some general considerations in regard to the physiologic changes associated with aging. The aged patient is likely to have more diseases and organ dysfunction than a young patient. In addition, the geriatric patient is more likely to have less functional organ reserve capacity than a young patient. This decreased organ reserve, termed *elderly normal*, may not become apparent until the patient is stressed by disease, hospitalization, anesthesia, or surgery, at which time overt organ failure may occur.

Much of the knowledge regarding the physiologic changes associated with aging has been derived from human studies. However, this information may be very applicable to the geriatric dog and cat.

Pulmonary System

Respiratory function progressively diminishes as a patient ages, resulting in a decreased functional reserve. There is a loss of strength in the muscles of respiration, chest wall compliance decreases, and there is a loss of elastic recoil (Knudson et al, 1977). The net effect of these changes is an increase in small airway closure, which produces a decrease in vital capacity and an increase in residual volume (Muiesan et al, 1971). In addition, there is a decrease in lung elasticity, respiratory rate, tidal volume, minute volume, oxygen consumption, carbon dioxide production, maximal diffusion capacity for oxygen, capillary blood volume, and protective airway reflexes in the aged patient (Muiesan et al, 1971). The decrease in protective airway reflexes (pharyngeal and laryngeal reflexes) puts the geriatric patient at a greater risk of aspiration in the perioperative period (Pontoppidan and Beecher, 1960). Finally, anatomic dead space and functional residual capacity increase (Muiesan et al, 1971).

Aging produces histologic changes in the lungs that include dilatation of alveolar ducts, loss of intra-alveolar septa, decreased numbers of alveoli, and a reduction in total lung surface area (Ryan et al, 1965). Human geriatric patients have a marked reduction in their ability to respond to induced hypercarbia and hypoxia (Kronenberg and Drage, 1973).

These changes in the respiratory system are significant in that even mild to moderate respiratory depression resulting from anesthesia may produce marked hypoxia and hypercarbia, and any pathologic disease of the respiratory system (e.g., pneumonia, edema, pulmonary fibrosis) will be greatly exacerbated in the geriatric patient. What is considered mild anesthetic depression in the young patient may be disaster in the aged patient.

Cardiovascular System

Geriatric patients have a decreased cardiac reserve compared with younger patients and may have difficulty compensating for the cardiovascular changes that occur during anesthesia. Geriatric patients have decreased baroreceptor activity, blood volume, cardiac output, blood pressure, circulation time, and vagotonia (Dodman et al, 1984). The conduction system of the heart is also affected by aging. In human patients it is not uncommon to see left bundle branch block, intraventricular conduction delay, ST segment and T wave changes, and atrial fibrillation (Fisch, 1981). This may make the geriatric patient more prone to anesthetic-induced dysrhythmias.

In addition, the geriatric patient may suffer from progressive and degenerative myocardial disease. This is usually associated with chronic valvular disease, which can lead to increased myocardial workload and oxygen consumption and demand and make the myocardium extremely sensitive to hypoxia. Geriatric patients often develop thickened elastic fibers and an increase in collagen and calcium in the walls of large arteries, which results in increased peripheral vascular resistance. The ability of the geriatric patient's cardiovascular system to adapt to hypotension is limited, and autoregulation is decreased (Owens, 1985).

The decreased cardiovascular function capabilities of geriatric patients make them very susceptible to anesthetic-induced cardiovascular depression, hypotension, and dysrhythmias.

Hepatic System

The aging process results in a reduction in the functional state of the microsomal enzyme systems in the liver. This reduction is present even when the standard biochemical function tests are normal (Green et al, 1982). Geriatric patients often have decreased hepatic blood flow, most likely as a result of their decreased cardiac output. Therefore, the plasma half-life of drugs dependent on hepatic excretion, metabolism, or conjugation are often increased in the geriatric patient. Altered hepatic function in the aged patient may lead to hypoproteinemia, delayed clotting function, and a greater susceptibility to hypoglycemia.

Renal System

The kidney is the major effective organ in fluid and electrolyte balance. Normal aging affects the kidneys in several ways (McLachlan, 1978). There is decreased renal blood flow, most likely as a result of the decreased cardiac output. There is a decrease in the total number of glomeruli to one half to two thirds that in young patients, and the nephron mass is reduced. Tubular changes occur, including atrophy, decreased tubular diameter, tubular disruption, and tubular hypertrophy. Glomerular filtration rate may be decreased by as much as 45 to 50 per cent in the aged patient, and there is a decreased ability to concentrate urine and excrete hydrogen ion because of decreased distal tubular function. The urine volume necessary for excretion of the obligatory solute load increases.

The result of these alterations is a diminished functional renal reserve, which makes the geriatric patient much less tolerant of body water deficits and excessive administration of fluids. Aged patients have a decreased capacity to excrete certain drugs and are more prone to acidosis, thus prolonging the plasma half-life of drugs dependent on renal excretion.

The effects of anesthesia and surgery on the kidney can be greatly exacerbated in the geriatric patient. Anesthesia and surgery generally cause increased activity of the sympathetic nervous system and the renin-angiotensin system, resulting in decreased total renal blood flow and a redistribution of intrarenal blood flow away from the renal cortex. General anesthesia may decrease renal blood flow and the glomerular filtration rate by up to 40 per cent. However, when the effects of the anesthetic agents terminate, renal function usually returns to normal. In addition, anesthesia and surgery may cause hypovolemia, hypotension, hypoxia, and hypercarbia, all of which will enhance pre-existing decreased renal function. All the foregoing factors make the geriatric patient much more susceptible to renal failure after anesthesia and surgery.

Central Nervous System

Aging produces changes in the central nervous system in human patients. There are alterations in cognitive, sensory, motor, and autonomic functions. Cerebral perfusion and oxygen consumption decline. Aging is also associated with a reduction in brain weight, which is most likely a result of individual neuron degeneration (Lorhan, 1971). The loss of brain weight is most evident in the cerebral cortex and the cerebellar cortex (Devaney and Johnson, 1980). Myelin sheaths also degenerate in the aged patient.

There is strong evidence that neurotransmitters change with age, with increased destruction and decreased production of neurotransmitters in the geriatric patient. The reduction in neurotransmitter function may be a result of the decreased quantity of neurotransmitters or a change in the receptors themselves.

The overall effects of these central nervous system alterations on the anesthetic management of the geriatric patient are not fully understood. The effects of local anesthetic agents seem to be enhanced in the aged patient, and the effects of neuromuscular blocking agents are prolonged. In addition, thermoregulatory center function is decreased, making the geriatric patient more susceptible to anesthesia-induced hypothermia.

Autonomic Nervous System

The autonomic nervous system loses some of its ability to respond to stress in the human geriatric patient. This appears to be most marked in the sympathetic nervous system. The aged patient has decreased vasoconstrictor responses and a decreased response to decreased cardiac preload (Collins et al, 1980). Despite this reduced response, there appears to be an enhanced response to iatrogenic epinephrine and norepinephrine, thus leading to the conclusion that perhaps the autonomic nervous system output is decreased but the receptors are more sensitive.

Endocrine System

Although aging does not appear to alter adrenocorticotropic hormone (ACTH)–stimulated plasma cortisol levels (Cherondache and Romanoff, 1967), there are reports that human geriatric patients may not have the adrenal gland reserves necessary to protect themselves adequately during stress from anesthesia and surgery (Lorhan, 1971). Renin and aldosterone hormones, which are necessary for water, sodium, and potassium balance as well as blood pressure control, are attenuated when the human geriatric patient is stressed (Weidman and DeMyttenoere-Buraztein, 1975).

Hyperadrenocorticism can be seen in middle-age and older dogs (Feldman, 1983). Clinical findings in hyperadrenocorticism patients include muscle weakness, reduced expiratory reserve volume, decreased chest wall compliance, expanded vascular volume leading to increased systolic and diastolic pressure, and pyelonephritis. The ability of these patients to ventilate adequately under anesthesia may be greatly attenuated.

Hypothyroidism is the most common endocrine disease in the dog (Rosychuk, 1983). Hypothyroid patients may have several clinical abnormalities that can be significant in anesthetic management. These patients are more prone to hypothermia as a result of thermoregulation abnormalities (Rosychuk, 1983). Cardiovascular problems may include sinus bradycardia, decreased myocardial contractility, cardiomyopathy, ischemic heart disease, and anemia (Rosychuk, 1983). These cardiovascular abnormalities make the hypothyroid patient more sensitive to the cardiovascular depressant effects of anesthetic agents. Hypothyroid patients also have a decreased ability to metabolize drugs (Rosychuk, 1983). This will prolong the effects of any preanesthetic and anesthetic agents that require metabolism and biodegradation to terminate their effects. Finally, many hypothyroid patients are obese, which can lead to a decrease in tidal volume and minute volume that in turn can be greatly exacerbated by hypoventilation during anesthesia.

Antidiuretic hormone increases with age owing

to an increased resistance of the distal renal tubules to its effects (Dodman et al, 1984). This can lead to impaired renal concentrating ability.

Pancreatic function may be altered in the geriatric patient. Glucose tolerance decreases with age, which may result from a decline in the ability of the insulin receptors to respond or from an actual decrease in the number of receptors (Davis and Davis, 1983). Diabetes mellitus is often encountered in the older patient and can be associated with osmotic diuresis, ketoacidosis, liver dysfunction due to fat deposition and cirrhosis, and concurrent infectious diseases. Hypoglycemia during and after anesthesia can be a problem in the aged patient because of altered pancreatic and liver function. The administration of fluids containing glucose may be warranted in the geriatric patient both during and after anesthesia.

PHARMACOKINETICS

Pharmacokinetics is the study of drug disposition in a patient. The most important age-related changes in the handling of anesthetic and preanesthetic drugs in the geriatric patient are in disposition (partitioning within the various distribution volumes) and clearance (excretion, metabolism, or conjugation of drugs). The slight reduction in plasma albumin concentrations in the aged patient is most likely not sufficient to produce clinically important changes in the amount of active or unbound drug in plasma after intravenous (IV) drug administration. Neither do data suggest that the aging process plays any significant role in altering the parenteral uptake of drugs (Ouslander, 1981).

The physical characteristics of drug molecules make them either lipophilic or hydrophilic and thus determine their ultimate partitioning between lipid tissues (brain, adipose tissue, and viscera) and aqueous body compartments (blood, extracellular fluid, and skeletal muscle). As a patient ages, there is a progressive decrease in the absolute volume of the aqueous fraction and an increase in the lipid compartments (Ritchel, 1983). Therefore, for hydrophilic drugs the decrease in the aqueous fraction of the body of an aged patient could produce higher than expected initial plasma levels after IV administration of recommended doses even when the dose has been adjusted for total body weight. The net pharmacokinetic effect is an enhancement of drug potency.

Because lipophilic drugs undergo some initial distribution to highly perfused nonadipose lipid tissues, the effects of the decreased aqueous fraction on the body is offset. However, because of the significant increase in total body lipid into which lipophilic drug molecules are ultimately distributed, the elimination process is markedly delayed, because the volume of the drug that must be cleared is increased in the geriatric patient (Richey and Bender, 1977).

Age also alters drug disposition or pharmacokinetics by significantly reducing both renal and hepatic function and thus decreasing the clearance of drugs eliminated through these pathways, regardless of whether a drug is lipophilic or hydrophilic.

PHARMACODYNAMICS

Pharmacodynamics, or the relationship between drug quantity and drug effect, is frequently altered in the geriatric patient. Geriatric patients have decreased circulating blood volume, which can produce high initial plasma concentrations of anesthetic drugs. However, the many observations of the need for reduced doses of anesthetic agents in geriatric patients cannot be solely explained by this (Berkowitz et al, 1975). Human studies involving tranquilizer and sedative drugs confirm that geriatric patients achieve a given drug effect at plasma concentrations that are significantly lower than those required for young adults (Giles et al, 1978). In addition, the minimum alveolar concentration (MAC) of volatile anesthetic agents is less in the aged patient than in young adults (Quasha et al, 1980). The mechanism by which age reduces the need for anesthetic agents is unclear, but the decreased anesthetic and analgesic requirements in the aged patient (Bellville et al, 1971; Muravchick, 1984) seem to correlate with the reduction in brain mass, the decrease in cerebral blood flow, and the decrease in the number and density of neurons and axons in both the central and peripheral nervous systems. These decreases and reductions occur in geriatric patients even in the absence of disease.

Other factors may play a significant role in reducing anesthetic requirements in the geriatric patient. Alterations in neurotransmitter activity have already been discussed, but other unknown factors may also play a role. It may be that this decreased anesthetic requirement is a result of decreased functional reserve of the nervous system rather than decreased nervous system function.

Regardless of the reasons for the pharmacokinetic and pharmacodynamic alterations of anesthetic agents observed in the geriatric patient, each patient must be examined on an individual basis, because no reliable universal guidelines are available. Some of the clinical consequences of these alterations are predictable, but they do not apply consistently to all the preanesthetic and anesthetic agents used.

ANESTHETIC CONSIDERATIONS

Any geriatric dog or cat presented for anesthesia should be considered on an individual basis. Each geriatric patient will have specific physiologic alterations or diseases unique to that individual. Thus, the anesthetic protocol needed for one aged patient may, out of necessity, change for the next patient.

As with any patient, a thorough and complete preanesthetic examination should be done. A complete history should be taken, with a special emphasis on present and past medical or surgical problems and any current medications the patient is receiving. Any previous anesthetic experience the patient has had should be noted, and close attention should be paid to any anesthetic complications or abnormal responses that occurred. A thorough preanesthetic physical examination should be performed to determine physiologic baseline values for future monitoring, as well as to ascertain any existing pathologic conditions within the patient. A complete blood cell count and serum biochemistry profile, with special emphasis on renal and hepatic function and electrolyte balance, should be obtained. Thoracic radiographs and a baseline electrocardiogram should be considered. Any abnormal preanesthetic findings should be thoroughly evaluated, and delaying the anesthesia and surgery should be considered.

Preanesthetic Drugs

The preanesthetic medications used in a particular geriatric patient will depend on that individual patient's physical condition, the amount of sedation or analgesia required, and the experience and preference of the veterinarian. Commonly used preanesthetic medications include anticholinergic agents, tranquilizers/sedatives, opioids, and neuroleptanalgesics (Table 21–1).

Anticholinergic Agents. Anticholinergic agents are used to decrease respiratory secretions and counteract sinus bradycardia. The two drugs available, atropine and glycopyrrolate, have simi-

TABLE 21–1. SUGGESTED DOSAGES FOR PREANESTHETIC MEDICATIONS IN THE GERIATRIC DOG AND CAT

DRUG	DOSE		DURATION OF ACTION (hr)
	Dog	Cat	
ANTICHOLINERGICS			
Atropine sulfate	0.022 mg/kg IM, SC	Same	1–1½
Glycopyrrolate (Robinul-V)	0.01 mg/kg IM, SC	Same	2–3
TRANQUILIZERS/SEDATIVES			
Acetylpromazine (Acepromazine)	0.1–0.2 mg/kg IM, IV to a maximum total dose of 2 mg	Same	3–6
Diazepam (Valium)	0.4 mg/kg IM, IV to a total dose of 10 mg	0.4 mg/kg IM, IV	½–3
Midazolam (Versed)	0.2–0.4 mg/kg IM, IV	Same	<2
Xylazine (Rompun)	0.1–0.2 mg/kg IM, IV	Same	1–2
Medetomidine	0.01–0.04 mg/kg IM	0.08–0.1 mg/kg IM	1
NARCOTIC ANALGESICS (AGONISTS-ANTAGONISTS)			
Pentazocine (Talwin)	1.0–3 mg/kg IM, IV	Same	1–2
Butorphanol (Torbugesic)	0.1–0.5 mg/kg IM, IV	Same	Up to 4
Buprenorphine	0.1–0.5 mg/kg IM, IV	Same	Up to 12
NARCOTIC ANALGESICS (AGONISTS)			
Morphine	0.05–1 mg/kg SC	0.002–0.1 mg/kg SC	3–6
Meperidine	0.5–3 mg/kg IM, IV	1.0–5.0 mg/kgIM, IV	2–4
Oxymorphone	0.1–0.2 mg/kg IM, IV to a maximal total dose of 4 mg	0.2 mg/kg IM, IV	2–4

IM, intramuscular; IV, intravenous; SC, subcutaneous.

lar actions except that glycopyrrolate does not cross the blood–brain barrier. Glycopyrrolate takes longer to exert its effects, but it lasts longer than atropine and is less likely to produce sinus tachycardia. However, glycopyrrolate does not seem to counteract severe sinus bradycardia as well as atropine.

The indiscriminant use of atropine or glycopyrrolate should be avoided in the geriatric patient to prevent an unwanted and potentially dangerous sinus tachycardia from occurring. The geriatric patient's heart may not be able to withstand the increased oxygen consumption and demand needed when sinus tachycardia occurs, and the sinus tachycardia may precipitate acute myocardial failure.

If sinus bradycardia occurs, atropine may be given IV to effect. If potent vagotonic drugs, such as the opioids, $alpha_2$ agonists (xylazine, medetomidine), or fentanyl-droperidol are to be used, an anticholinergic may be warranted. Half the normal dose of anticholinergic may be given intramuscularly (IM) as a premedicant, with additional anticholinergic given IV to effect if needed.

Tranquilizers/Sedatives. The primary tranquilizer/sedative preanesthetic agents available are the phenothiazine derivatives, butyrophenone derivatives, benzodiazepine derivatives, and thiazine derivatives.

Acetylpromazine is the most common phenothiazine-derivative tranquilizer in use. For the healthy geriatric patient, the use of *low*-dose acetylpromazine is a reasonable choice for a preanesthetic. Acetylpromazine causes general CNS depression without producing analgesia. However, it lowers the seizure threshold, so it should not be used in epileptics. Acetylpromazine can produce hypotension because of a peripheral vasodilating effect rather than a direct myocardial depressive effect. It does possess antidysrhythmic activity owing to either a quinidine-like effect or a local anesthetic effect on the myocardium, and it does inhibit myocardial sensitization to catecholamines. At low doses the effect of acetylpromazine on the respiratory system is usually negligible. There may be a slight decrease in respiratory rate, but this is usually compensated for by an increase in tidal volume, resulting in a normal minute ventilation. Acetylpromazine does not delay the respiratory center response (threshold) to increases in partial arterial carbon dioxide pressure ($Paco_2$), although the maximum ventilatory response (sensitivity) may be decreased. Acetylpromazine undergoes extensive biodegradation in the liver, and thus patients with hepatic dysfunction may have extremely long recovery times. This may explain why aged patients may have prolonged recovery times after receiving acetylpromazine.

The three butyrophenone derivatives used in veterinary anesthesia are droperidol (Inapsine), azaperone (Stresnil), and lenperone (Elanone-V). All three drugs have similar physiologic effects. They have little or no direct effect on cardiac output, but they do decrease arterial blood pressure, total peripheral resistance, and heart rate; respiratory depression can also occur. The butyrophenones are biodegraded by the liver. Lenperone has been approved for dogs and cats, azaperone is primarily used in swine, and droperidol is mainly used in combination with the narcotic fentanyl.

The main benzodiazepine-derivative tranquilizer used in small animal anesthesia is diazepam. Diazepam is dissolved in propylene glycol, and thus its absorption from IM injection sites may be unpredictable and erratic. In addition, propylene glycol is a cardiopulmonary depressant, and rapid IV administration may cause hypotension, bradycardia, and apnea. Benzodiazepine tranquilizers are considered "minor" tranquilizers, meaning they have minimal CNS depressant activity. They produce a calming or taming effect and reduce fear and anxiety without marked sedation. They are good muscle relaxants. The benzodiazepines have broad-spectrum anticonvulsant activity and usually produce minimal cardiopulmonary depression. Because of the minimal cardiopulmonary depression, they are often used as a preanesthetic in the aged patient. When combined with an opioid, they can be very effective. These drugs are highly protein bound and are metabolized in the liver.

Midazolam (Versed) is a water-soluble benzodiazepine. It is highly lipid soluble and has a short duration of action, with a rapid elimination half-life and total body clearance. Midazolam has been used at a dose of 0.1 to 0.2 mg/kg IV or IM as a preanesthetic tranquilizer. It has been used in combination with opioids, barbiturates, dissociative agents, and inhalant agents. The cardiopulmonary effects of midazolam are similar to those of the other benzodiazepines. Higher doses of midazolam have produced dysphoria in dogs. Behavioral effects, including restlessness, pacing, vocalization, and difficulty in handling, have been reported in cats after midazolam administration. If midazolam is used in combination with an opioid, the behavioral effects can be attenuated.

A specific antagonist has been developed for the benzodiazepine tranquilizers. Flumazenil (Mazicon) is a benzodiazepine antagonist that competitively and reversibly binds with the benzodiazepine central nervous system receptor sites. It reverses the sedative, muscle relaxant, amnesic, and anxiolytic effects of the benzodiazepine tranquilizers while having minimal intrinsic pharmacologic activity itself. Flumazenil does have weak agonistic effects with high doses. A dose of 0.1 mg/kg IV of flumazenil will antagonize the effects of diazepam or midazolam in the dog and cat.

There are two $alpha_2$ agonists that are being used in small animal practice, xylazine and medetomidine. Xylazine (Rompun) is a thiazine derivative that has sedative, analgesic, and muscle relaxant properties. However, its marked cardiovascular effects and its unpredictable respiratory effects may limit its use in the geriatric patient. Xylazine can produce significant bradycardia as well as second-degree atrioventricular heart block. It also appears to sensitize the myocardium to catecholamines, thus making dysrhythmias more likely. The bradycardia and heart block are vagally induced; atropine can counteract these effects. Xylazine's effect on respiration is extremely variable and may range from minimal to marked depression of respiration rate and tidal volume, leading to hypoxemia and hypercarbia. Xylazine should be used with extreme caution in geriatric patients and/or debilitated patients with cardiovascular or pulmonary dysfunction.

Medetomidine differs from xylazine in that it has more potency and efficacy at $alpha_2$ receptors, is more lipophilic, and is eliminated faster (Tranquilli and Benson, 1992). The physiologic effects of medetomidine are very similar to those of xylazine, and the precautions for its use in the geriatric patient are the same as those for xylazine.

One advantage to the use of xylazine and medetomidine is that specific antagonists are available to counteract their effects (Table 21–2). Yohimbine, tolazoline, idazoxan, and atipamezole are all $alpha_2$ antagonists. Yohimbine and tolazoline are commercially available and will completely and rapidly antagonize the CNS and cardiopulmonary depressant effects of xylazine and medetomidine.

Opioids. Opioids and narcotic analgesics are often used alone or in combination with tranquilizers in the geriatric patient as preanesthetic medications. Various opioid agonists have been used, including morphine, meperidine, oxymorphone, and fentanyl. The opioid agonist-antagonists (e.g., butorphanol, buprenorphine, pentazocine, and nalbuphine) have also been used.

There are at least four major opioid receptor sites. The mu receptors are associated with respiratory depression, supraspinal analgesia, euphoria, and physical dependence; the kappa receptors are associated with spinal analgesia, sedation, and miosis; the sigma receptors are associated with dysphoria, hallucinations, and respiratory and vasomotor stimulation; and the delta receptors are associated with dependency and behavioral alterations. Opioids such as morphine, meperidine, oxymorphone, and fentanyl act as agonists at all four receptors. Butorphanol, buprenorphine, pentazocine, and nalbuphine are agonists at the kappa and sigma receptors but are antagonists or partial antagonists at the mu and

TABLE 21–2. VARIOUS ANTAGONISTS, THEIR DOSAGES, AND DURATION OF ACTION

ANTAGONIST	DOSE	ANTAGONIZES THE EFFECTS OF	DURATION OF ACTION
Levallorphan (Lorfan)	0.02–0.2 mg/kg IV	Narcotic agonist-antagonist	1.5–3 hr
Nalorphine (Nalline)	1.0 mg/kg IV, IM, SC	Narcotic agonist-antagonist	1.5–3 hr
Naloxone (Narcan)	20–100 μg/kg IV, IM, SC	Pure narcotic antagonist (only antagonist for pentazocine)	15–45 min
4-Aminopyridine	0.3 mg/kg IV	Partial antagonist for xylazine, ketamine, and barbiturates	
Yohimbine (Yobine)	0.15 mg/kg IV	$Alpha_2$ agonists (xylazine, medetomidine)	
Tolazoline (Priscoline)	0.4–2 mg/kg IV	$Alpha_2$ agonists (xylazine, medetomidine)	
Flumazenil (Mazicon)	0.1 mg/kg IV	Benzodiazepine derivatives	1 hr

IM, intramuscular; IV, intravenous; SC, subcutaneous.

delta receptors. Thus, they are less likely to produce the degree of respiratory depression and addiction that pure opioid agonists do.

The advantages of the opioids are that they produce analgesia and sedation, they produce minimal direct myocardial depression, and their effects can be readily antagonized (see Table 21–2). However, they can produce mild to significant depression of minute ventilation; and therefore, respiratory rate and depth should be closely monitored. Opioids often slow the heart rate, but this may be advantageous in the geriatric patient, as the slow heart rate may lead to decreased myocardial oxygen consumption and demand and more forceful contractions. Because this bradycardia is vagally induced, an anticholinergic agent may be used to counteract it if necessary.

Butorphanol (Torbugesic, Torbutrol, Stadol) has been used as an effective pre- and postanesthetic analgesic in the dog and cat. However, currently it has only been approved for use as a cough suppressant in small animals. Butorphanol is an uncontrolled synthetic opioid agonist-antagonist of the nalophane-cyclazocine class, with a chemical structure similar to that of morphine but with pharmacologic activity similar to that of pentazocine. Its analgesic potency is five times that of morphine, 15 to 30 times that of pentazocine, and one third to one half that of oxymorphone. Butorphanol can produce a dose-related respiratory depression similar to that produced by morphine; however, butorphanol seems to reach a "ceiling" beyond which higher doses do not cause significantly more depression. Butorphanol can produce decreases in heart rate, cardiac output, and blood pressure, but the depression is less than that produced by morphine and oxymorphone. It is rapidly absorbed after IM injection, with peak blood levels occurring in 15 to 30 minutes. Butorphanol is extensively metabolized in the liver, with its analgesic activity lasting 2 to 4 hours. It is rapidly and completely absorbed from the gastrointestinal tract; however, because of significant first-pass hepatic metabolism, only about 17 per cent of the administered dose is available systemically. Its effects are readily antagonized with naloxone.

Butorphanol has good analgesic properties and fair sedation properties. When it is combined with a tranquilizer such as diazepam or acetylpromazine, a very acceptable neuroleptanalgesic is produced. Butorphanol's main advantages in the geriatric patient are that it produces minimal respiratory depression and minimal to moderate cardiovascular depression, it provides good analgesia, and it is an uncontrolled opioid.

Neuroleptanalgesic Agents. A neuroleptanalgesic agent is a combination of a tranquilizer (neuroleptic) and an opioid (analgesic). The use of such agents may be very beneficial in the geriatric patient. Various neuroleptanalgesic combinations are available (Table 21–3). The pharmacologic effects of a neuroleptanalgesic agent will depend on the tranquilizer and opioid used. Neuroleptanalgesic agents, used alone or in combination with local anesthetic agents, may be all that is needed for minor diagnostic or surgical procedures in the geriatric patient. As with any patient, cardiopulmonary function should be closely monitored when neuroleptanalgesic agents are used, as these drugs may produce respiratory depression ranging from slight to significant.

Injectable General Anesthetic Agents

Injectable general anesthetic agents can be used in the geriatric patient, but they should be used with care because of the often altered hemodynamics, the decreased plasma protein binding, and the decreased ability of the liver in the aged patient to biodegrade drugs. The two major types of injectable agents used in the dog and cat are the ultra–short-acting thiobarbiturates and the dissociative agents. In addition, two new injectable agents, propofol and etomidate, are also being evaluated for use in the small animal patient.

Ultra–Short-Acting Barbiturates. Ultra–

TABLE 21–3. NEUROLEPTANALGESIC COMBINATIONS FOR THE GERIATRIC DOG AND CAT

NEUROLEPTIC (TRANQUILIZER)	ANALGESIC (NARCOTIC)
Acetylpromazine 0.1 mg/kg IM or IV, not to exceed a maximum total dose of 1.5 mg	Oxymorphone 0.2 mg/kg IM or IV not to exceed a maximum total dose of 3 mg
Diazepam 0.25 to 0.45 mg/kg IM or IV to a maximum total dose of 10 mg	Oxymorphone (as above)
Acetylpromazine (as above)	Meperidine 1 to 4.5 mg/kg IM or IV
Acetylpromazine (as above)	Butorphanol 0.2–0.45 mg/kg IM or IV
Diazepam (as above)	Butorphanol (as above)

IM, intramuscular; IV, intravenous.

short-acting thiobarbiturates (methohexital, thiopental) can be used to induce anesthesia and for short surgical procedures; however, the lowest possible dose necessary for the procedure should be used. These drugs are highly protein bound, and their effects will be greatly exacerbated in any patient that is hypoproteinemic. Acidosis in a patient will also greatly enhance their effects by causing more nonionized barbiturate to be available and by decreasing the amount of protein-bound barbiturate. Both factors increase the amount of active barbiturate available.

The effects of the ultra–short-acting barbiturates on the cardiovascular system are variable and depend on the species, specific barbiturate, and dose given. In general there is usually an increase in heart rate as a result of depression of the vagal center and/or arterial pressoreceptor reflexes; a decrease in stroke volume and myocardial contractility related to calcium-dependent mechanisms; an initial increase in cardiac output, followed by a decrease; and an initial decrease in total peripheral resistance, followed by a return to normal. The ultra–short-acting thiobarbiturates may produce transitory cardiac dysrhythmias, which are usually premature ventricular contractions and of a bigeminal nature.

The ultra–short-acting barbiturates are potent respiratory depressants, depressing both rate and tidal volume and, thus, minute ventilation. The respiratory center response to increases in $PaCO_2$ is delayed, and the maximum ventilatory response is decreased. The carotid-aortic chemoreceptors are also depressed. Although initial arousal from an ultra–short-acting thiobarbiturate is dependent on redistribution of the drug into the various body tissue compartments, ultimately the drug must be metabolized in the liver to be excreted. If a patient receives an overdose of a thiobarbiturate or redistribution is hindered because of a lack of body fat, hepatic biodegradation then becomes the main pathway for arousal and awakening. Because dogs and cats do not readily metabolize the thiobarbiturates, very prolonged recovery times (6 to 24 hours) may be observed. If hepatic dysfunction is also evident in the patient, the recovery from a thiobarbiturate may be even longer if tissue redistribution is altered.

Because of the ability of the ultra–short-acting thiobarbiturates to depress the cardiovascular system and, especially, the respiratory system, such agents should be used with extreme care in geriatric patients that may already have cardiopulmonary compromise. In addition, the geriatric patient may have decreased plasma protein binding capabilities, hepatic dysfunction, and an increase in the total body lipid into which the thiobarbiturates are ultimately distributed. These three factors may cause a marked increase in the physiologic effect and duration of action of a given dose of ultra–short-acting thiobarbiturate.

Dissociative Anesthetic Agents. Dissociative anesthetic agents are cyclohexanone derivatives that produce a cataleptic state characterized by CNS excitement rather than depression, analgesia, immobility, dissociation from one's environment, and amnesia. The two drugs in this group available for veterinary anesthesia are ketamine and tiletamine.

Ketamine and tiletamine have the same basic pharmacologic effects. They appear to selectively depress the thalamocortical system (i.e., the association region of the cerebral cortex) while stimulating the reticular-activating and limbic systems. Ketamine and tiletamine appear to potently inhibit gamma-aminobutyric acid (GABA) binding in the CNS, enhance inhibitory mechanisms through the action of the GABA systems, and block neuronal transport processes for the monamine transmitters such as 5-hydroxytryptamine (serotonin), dopamine, and norepinephrine.

These drugs tend to stimulate the cardiovascular system, but the mechanism by which this occurs is not completely understood. Ketamine and tiletamine exert a selective positive inotropic effect on heart muscle that is independent of heart rate and/or the autonomic nervous system. They tend to cause an increase in heart rate, cardiac output, mean arterial blood pressure, pulmonary arterial blood pressure, and central venous pressure either by directly stimulating the central adrenergic centers or by indirectly preventing the uptake of the catecholamines. Both dissociative agents seem to have antidysrhythmic activity. An increase in heart rate can produce a marked increase in myocardial oxygen consumption and demand. Large doses of ketamine and tiletamine, especially when administered IV, can have a marked depressant effect on the cardiovascular system.

Both drugs can produce apneustic ventilation—that is, a ventilatory pattern characterized by a prolonged pause after inspiration. Although the respiratory rate may decrease, the tidal volume usually remains normal. In general, these respiratory alterations do not affect the blood gases; however, in some patients the dissociative agents can produce marked hypoxia and hypercarbia, especially when additional CNS depressant drugs, such as tranquilizers, sedatives, or opioids, are used in combination with them. Dissociative agents do not depress the pharyngeal or laryngeal reflexes, although they may be activated only with stimulation; therefore, a patient may be more prone to laryngospasm, bronchospasm, and coughing because of these agents' activity. The dissociative agents increase salivation and respiratory secretions, sometimes to the point of aspiration and respiratory obstruction. For this reason, the use of an anticholinergic agent in combination with these drugs may be indicated.

The dissociative agents produce muscle tonus and increased limb rigidity, often necessitating the additional use of a tranquilizer/sedative to produce better muscle relaxation. Patients under the effects of these drugs may have spontaneous, random limb movements unassociated with pain. Eyelid and corneal reflexes remain intact, and the eyes remain open; therefore, eye ointment should be used to prevent corneal drying. Because coughing, swallowing, corneal, and pedal reflexes are maintained, these reflexes cannot be used to adequately judge the depth of anesthesia.

In the dog ketamine and tiletamine undergo extensive hepatic biodegradation, with the water-soluble metabolites being excreted in the urine. Because both drugs are rapidly metabolized by the dog, the duration of anesthesia from an IM dose is approximately 20 to 30 minutes, with full recovery in 2 to 4 hours. In the cat, the majority of the injected dissociative agent is eliminated intact by the kidneys, with only 25 to 35 per cent of the dose metabolized by the liver. Therefore, even though anesthesia time from a single IM dose of one of these drugs may last 20 to 40 minutes in the cat, full recovery may take 5 hours or more. Both drugs are highly lipid soluble, which accounts for the rapid induction of anesthesia following IM administration.

Ketamine has been used IV in the dog and cat at a dose of 2 to 4 mg/kg to induce general anesthesia and for short surgical procedures lasting less than 10 minutes. Ketamine may produce seizures, especially in the dog, and for this reason diazepam, at a dose of 0.4 mg/kg IV is often administered with it. Acetylpromazine may also be used with ketamine at a dose of 0.1 mg/kg IV or IM, to a maximum total dose of 2 mg. Acetylpromazine aids in providing better muscle relaxation and will help prevent ketamine-induced seizures because of its dopamine-blocking capabilities.

At present, tiletamine is available only as Telazol, which is a combination of equal parts by weight of tiletamine and zolazepam (a nonphenothiazine diazepinone tranquilizer). It is supplied in sterile vials containing 500 mg of active drug (250 mg of tiletamine and 250 mg of zolazepam). Five milliliters of sterile diluent are added to produce 100 mg/ml of active drug. Telazol is a Class III controlled substance approved only for IM use in the dog and cat.

In the dog Telazol is recommended as an anesthetic for diagnostic examinations, restraint, treatment of lacerations and wounds, castrations, and any procedure requiring mild to moderate analgesia. The dose range is 6 to 12 mg/kg IM. Supplemental doses may be given, but any supplemental dose should be less than the initial dose, and the total dose given (initial dose plus supplemental doses) should not exceed 20 mg/kg in the dog. Telazol is not recommended as the sole agent for use in the dog for procedures requiring major analgesia (e.g., abdominal or thoracic procedures).

In the cat Telazol is recommended as an anesthetic for procedures ranging from diagnostic examinations and restraint to declawing and ovariohysterectomies. The dose range is 9 to 15 mg/kg IM. As with the dog, supplemental doses may be given, but any supplemental dose should be less than the initial dose and the total dose given should not exceed 50 mg/kg. Telazol has a wider margin of safety in cats than in dogs.

Repeated doses of Telazol increase the duration of effect of the drug but may not further diminish muscle tone; recovery is extended with multiple doses. The quality of anesthesia varies with repeated doses, because the ratio between tiletamine and zolazepam within the patient changes with each injection. Therefore, giving repeated doses of Telazol to prolong anesthesia time should be avoided if possible.

In the dog both tiletamine and zolazepam undergo extensive biodegradation in the liver, with less than 4 per cent of the injected dose excreted unchanged. In the cat both drugs are excreted virtually intact by the kidneys. After IM injection, patients lose the righting reflex in 3 to 4 minutes, with onset of surgical anesthesia in 6 to 7 minutes. The duration of surgical anesthesia ranges from 20 to 30 minutes. Righting reflexes return in 2 to 3 hours, with full recovery in 4 to 6 hours. Supplemental doses will prolong the recovery period.

Ketamine and Telazol should be used with caution in geriatric patients with pre-existing cardiovascular or pulmonary dysfunction. The sinus tachycardia produced by both drugs may be disadvantageous in the geriatric patient because of the marked increase in oxygen consumption and demand. The geriatric patient may not have the cardiac reserve to withstand this increased heart rate. The dissociative agents may also exacerbate any pre-existing pulmonary dysfunction and further compromise the patient. Patients with renal or hepatic dysfunction may be expected to have prolonged recovery times.

Propofol (Diprivan). Propofol is a new injectable anesthetic agent that has found widespread use in human anesthesia and will most likely be approved for use in veterinary anesthesia. Propofol is a highly lipid soluble alkylphenol that is a rapid-acting IV anesthetic agent. It is insoluble in water and must be solubilized in a lecithin-containing emulsion. Propofol is formulated as a 1 per cent emulsion containing 10 per cent soybean oil, 1.2 per cent egg lecithin, and 2.25 per cent glycerol. Propofol can be used for short periods of anesthesia (5 to 10 minutes) after a single bolus. More prolonged anesthesia can be maintained with repeated bolus injections or continuous infusion.

Propofol's rapid onset time is similar to that of methohexital and thiopental. A single bolus injection of propofol produces a rapid onset of anesthesia (less than 60 seconds), lasting 5 to 10 minutes (Table 21–4). The induction is smooth and excitement free; however, transient local pain may occur as a result of venoirritation during induction. Propofol-induced excitatory activity, such as movements, myoclonic twitching, and muscle tremors, have been reported in some patients.

Recovery is very rapid, even after repeated doses of propofol. It is rapidly redistributed and rapidly metabolized by glucuronidation and sulfonation. After 30 minutes, less than 20 per cent of the dose can be recovered as unchanged compound. Total body clearance exceeds hepatic blood flow, and although hepatic metabolism plays a major role in clearance, other tissues (e.g., lung) are also involved. Ninety percent of propofol is excreted in the urine as water-soluble glucuronide and sulfate conjugates, and there are no known active metabolites. Cats have a deficiency in their ability to conjugate phenols, and although the reported recovery times after single or repeated doses of propofol are similar in dogs and cats, continuous infusion may produce more prolonged recoveries in cats.

The total calculated dose used for anesthetic induction in the dog and cat is 6 mg/kg IV. The drug is administered to effect in much the same way as methohexital and thiopental. Approximately one fourth to one third of the dose is administered every 30 to 45 seconds until the desired level of anesthesia is produced. The total dose given will depend on the preanesthetic sedatives used, the degree of patient sedation, and the physical status of the patient. After propofol induction, anesthesia can be maintained with inhalation agents or with repeated bolus injections or continuous infusions of propofol. Propofol can be used at a maintenance infusion of 0.2 to 0.4 mg/kg/min, which is increased or decreased depending on the desired anesthetic level of the patient.

The cardiopulmonary effects of propofol are similar to those of barbiturates (Table 21–5). Propofol causes a decrease in cerebral blood flow and oxygen consumption, as well as direct myocardial depression, peripheral vasodilation, venodilation, and hypotension. Propofol can also produce respiratory depression. The incidence of apnea with propofol is comparable to that with barbiturates, but the duration of apneic episodes may be slightly longer. The cardiopulmonary effects of propofol are dose dependent.

Propofol's pharmacokinetics in patients with renal and hepatic dysfunction is similar to that in nondiseased patients, suggesting that it would be suitable for patients with renal and/or hepatic impairment. Propofol has been safely used in sighthound dog breeds.

Propofol seems ideally suited for use as a continuous infusion for the maintenance of anesthesia. Recovery is rapid, with minimal "drug hangover." There does not appear to be a problem of drug buildup with propofol when compared with barbiturates or the dissociative agents. Myoclonic

TABLE 21–4. PHARMACOKINETICS OF INTRAVENOUS GENERAL ANESTHETIC AGENTS

DRUG GROUP	DRUG NAME	DISTRIBUTION HALF-LIFE (min)	ELIMINATION HALF-LIFE (hr)
Barbiturates	Thiopental	2–4	10–12
	Methohexital	5–6	3–5
Imidazoles	Etomidate	2–4	2–5
Arylcyclohexylamines	Telazol	11–17	2–3
Alkylphenols	Propofol	2–4	1–3

TABLE 21–5. SUMMARY OF COMPARATIVE PHARMACOLOGIC PROPERTIES OF IV INDUCTION AGENTS

PROPERTIES	THIOPENTAL	ETOMIDATE	TELAZOL	PROPOFOL
Solubility	Water	Propylene glycol	Water	Egg lecithin
Dose (mg/kg)	8–12 (IV)	1.5–3.0 (IV)	4–16 (IM) 1–2 (IV)	2–6 (IV)
Onset	Rapid	Rapid	Rapid	Rapid
Induction	Smooth	Pain/myoclonus	Excitatory/smooth	Smooth/pain
Cardiovascular effects	Depression	Minimal	Stimulation	Depression
Respiratory effect	Depression	Minimal	Minimal/moderate depression	Depression
Analgesia	None	None	Superficial—yes Deep visceral—?	None
Amnesia	Minimal	Minimal	Minimal	Minimal
Recovery	Rapid	Rapid	Intermediate	Rapid

IM, intramuscular; IV, intravenous.

twitching, muscle tremors, and muscle movements have been reported in humans and dogs during maintenance of anesthesia with propofol. During these episodes, anesthetic depth appeared adequate, and arterial blood gases and pH were normal. Diazepam, 2.5 to 5.0 mg given slowly IV, has been used to control the myoclonus when necessary.

Propofol may be suitable for use in the geriatric patient, as recovery times do not seem to be prolonged in patients with renal or hepatic dysfunction. However, because its cardiopulmonary depressant effects are very similar to those of the thiobarbiturates, it should be used with caution in any patient with pre-existing cardiopulmonary disease or dysfunction.

Etomidate (Amidate). Etomidate is another new injectable anesthetic finding use in human anesthesia. Etomidate is a carboxylated imidazole-containing compound that is structurally unrelated to any other IV anesthetic. It is a sedative-hypnotic agent with a rapid onset of action and a rapid recovery. It is a weak base dissolved in propylene glycol; therefore, IV infusion can be associated with pain and venoirritation.

Etomidate has been used in veterinary anesthesia, although it has not yet been approved for use. The induction dose of etomidate in the dog and cat is 1.5 to 3.0 mg/kg IV. This dose is given to effect and will depend on the preanesthetic sedatives given to the patient and the physical status of the patient. A single bolus injection produces a rapid loss of consciousness with a duration of action of 5 to 10 minutes. Etomidate undergoes rapid hepatic hydrolysis to inactive metabolites. This results in rapid recovery and a lack of accumulation when used in repeated boluses or as an infusion.

At doses used to produce general anesthesia (3.0 mg/kg IV), etomidate produces no change in heart rate, cardiac output, or mean arterial blood pressure. Cardiovascular stability may be better with etomidate, because it better maintains baroreceptor-mediated responses. Etomidate can produce a mild to moderate dose-dependent respiratory depression (see Table 21–5).

Several adverse side effects have been reported with etomidate. Pain and phlebitis have been associated with IV injections, possibly because of the carrier agent propylene glycol. Excitement during induction and recovery have been reported, but this can be partially or completely eliminated by using preanesthetic sedatives. Retching, myoclonus, and apnea have been reported in humans and dogs during induction. Etomidate has been demonstrated to temporarily inhibit adrenal steroidogenesis in humans and dogs, but whether this inhibition is significant to the patient is controversial.

Etomidate's minimal cardiopulmonary depressant effects and its rapid metabolism and recovery would make it seem ideally suited for the geriatric patient. However, the adverse side effects during induction may limit its use, at least at present.

Inhalant General Anesthetic Agents

Inhalant general anesthetic agents are probably the anesthetic agents of choice in the geriatric patient, especially for procedures lasting longer than 10 to 15 minutes and in very debilitated patients. Methoxyflurane, halothane, or isoflurane can all be used either with or without nitrous oxide.

Methoxyflurane. Methoxyflurane is a methyl

ethyl ether that is the most potent (lowest MAC requirement) of the volatile inhalant anesthetic agents. Because of its high blood and rubber solubility, induction and recovery from methoxyflurane is slow when compared with the other inhalant agents. Methoxyflurane depresses heart rate, stroke volume, and cardiac output in a dose-dependent fashion. Spontaneous cardiac dysrhythmias are not common during methoxyflurane anesthesia.

Methoxyflurane can produce hypotension primarily because of the decreased cardiac output. At normal anesthetic concentrations, peripheral resistance is usually maintained; therefore, large decreases in arterial blood pressure may not be observed. However, with high doses of methoxyflurane, peripheral resistance will decrease, and significant drops in arterial blood pressure may occur. Methoxyflurane also produces a dose-dependent respiratory depression by decreasing the respiratory rate and tidal volume. It can produce a transitory hepatic depression, but it does not appear to be directly hepatotoxic. Methoxyflurane may alter renal function by decreasing renal blood flow, and it has also been shown to produce direct renal toxicity in humans through its metabolic by-products, primarily oxalic acid and inorganic fluoride ion. The renal toxicity produced by methoxyflurane is characterized by proximal renal tubular necrosis with high-output renal failure, hypernatremia, elevated blood urea nitrogen levels, and dehydration. As much as 80 per cent of the inspired methoxyflurane is metabolized by the liver. Although there are no specific contraindications to the use of methoxyflurane, it should be used with caution in the presence of renal or hepatic dysfunction.

Halothane. Halothane is a halogenated hydrocarbon that produces a fairly rapid induction and recovery from anesthesia. Halothane can cause significant cardiovascular depression that is directly related to the administered concentration. Myocardial contractility, heart rate, and cardiac output are decreased in a dose-dependent manner. Halothane can also produce marked arterial hypotension owing to direct myocardial depression, decreased peripheral resistance, and direct depression of the vasomotor center. Spontaneous cardiac dysrhythmias are more common with halothane than with methoxyflurane, because halothane sensitizes the myocardium to catecholamines and also slows the conduction impulses through the His-Purkinje system, allowing for reentry of impulses. Halothane, like most inhalant and injectable anesthetic agents, has an additive effect on sinoarterial or atrioventricular conduction disturbances. Halothane has the lowest cardiac index of the volatile anesthetic agents. (A low cardiac index equates to more myocardial depression.) It produces the same amount of respiratory depression as methoxyflurane at equipotent doses. Halothane does not have direct nephrotoxic effects, although it can produce a transitory decrease in renal function by decreasing blood flow. Up to 50 per cent of inspired halothane can be metabolized by the liver.

Halothane has been implicated as a possible cause of postanesthetic hepatitis in human patients. The phenomenon is extremely rare and is most likely related to the metabolites of halothane biodegradation. Halothane can be metabolized via an oxidative hepatic microsomal enzyme pathway (the major pathway), which produces relatively harmless metabolites, or via a reductive pathway (the non–oxygen-dependent, minor pathway), which produces potentially harmful metabolites. The reactive intermediate metabolites produced by the reductive pathway can covalently bind to hepatic proteins, lipoproteins, and lipids, altering their function and resulting in hepatic necrosis. Certain factors seem to increase the risk of "halothane hepatitis" in human patients, including intraoperative hepatic hypoxia, reductive metabolism of halothane by the liver, and genetics of the patient. Repeated halothane exposure seems to be less important.

Halothane should be used with extreme caution in patients with cardiac conduction problems or other dysrhythmias and in patients with myocardial disease. Halothane is contraindicated in patients that have previously developed an unexplained postanesthetic hepatitis after its use or in patients with active hepatitis. Chronic liver dysfunction should also preclude the use of halothane.

Isoflurane (AErrane). Isoflurane, a halogenated ether, is the newest of the volatile inhalant agents. It is the least soluble of the volatile inhalation anesthetic agents in blood, body tissues, and conductive rubber components of the anesthetic circuit. This accounts for its very rapid induction time (3 to 5 minutes) and its very rapid recovery time (often less than 5 minutes). The MAC for isoflurane is 1.3 and 1.6 in the dog and cat, respectively, and thus it is less potent than methoxyflurane or halothane. In normal patients the isoflurane concentrations needed to provide clinical surgical anesthesia will have minimal depressant effects on the cardiovascular system. Its cardiovascular margin of safety seems to be greater than that for halothane or methoxyflurane; in fact, it has the highest cardiac index of the volatile inhalant anesthetic agents. Although isoflurane does decrease the stroke volume, the heart rate remains the same or increases slightly and compensates for the decreased stroke volume; therefore, cardiac output does not fall significantly. Isoflurane does decrease arterial blood pressure in a dose-related fashion, owing primarily to a decreased vascular resistance (vasodilation) and not to a decreased cardiac output. Peripheral perfusion is adequately maintained at normal anesthetic concentrations. Isoflurane decreases myocardial oxygen consumption and coronary vascular resistance without decreasing coronary blood flow. It produces an extremely stable heart rhythm because it does not seem to sensitize the myocardium to catecholamines, and it does not slow the conduction of impulses through the His-Purkinje system. Isoflurane depresses respiration in a dose-related fashion and is a slightly more potent depressant than methoxyflurane and halothane. It does not appear to produce any liver damage, even when used for long procedures or during hypoxia. Isoflurane, like other inhalant anesthetic agents, produces a transitory decrease in renal blood flow, glomerular filtration rate, and urine flow. No direct renal toxicity has been reported. Only about 0.2 per cent of the inhaled isoflurane undergoes hepatic biodegradation. There are no major precautions or contraindications to the use of isoflurane, and it is probably the volatile inhalant anesthetic of choice in the geriatric patient.

Nitrous Oxide. Nitrous oxide is an inorganic gas that can be used in combination with any of the volatile anesthetic agents. The minimum alveolar concentrations in the dog and cat are 200 and 250 per cent, respectively. Thus, it is a very weak CNS depressant and is not capable of producing general anesthesia by itself; to obtain surgical anesthesia, hypnotics, narcotics, or other inhalation anesthetic agents must be used in combination with it. Nitrous oxide has minimal effects on cardiopulmonary function unless hypoxia occurs and has no appreciable effects on other organ systems. Nitrous oxide can be used with the more potent inhalant anesthetic agents during mask induction to induce anesthesia more rapidly in the patient owing to a concentrating or "second gas" effect of the nitrous oxide.

Nitrous oxide must be combined with other CNS depressant drugs or anesthetic agents for maintenance of anesthesia. For maintenance, it is recommended that 50 to 66 per cent nitrous oxide be used in combination with 50 to 33 per cent oxygen. At least 30 per cent oxygen should always be administered with the nitrous oxide. The concentration of the other more potent inhalation anesthetic agents can be decreased by one third to one half when nitrous oxide is used in combination with them. Nitrous oxide and oxygen can be used in combination with hypnotics, narcotics, or local anesthetic agents for minor procedures in the geriatric patient.

The veterinarian must be aware of several precautions with nitrous oxide. General anesthesia cannot be produced with nitrous oxide alone. Nitrous oxide may cause increased tension in the gas pockets of the body, and therefore, it may compound problems when used in the presence of a pneumothorax or intestinal obstruction. Diffusion hypoxia may occur when nitrous oxide is discontinued and the patient is allowed to breathe room air immediately. For this reason the patient should be allowed to breathe 100 per cent oxygen for a minimum of 5 minutes after discontinuation of nitrous oxide. Hypoxia is always a danger with nitrous oxide unless at least 30 per cent oxygen is administered with it. If the patient develops cyanosis while receiving nitrous oxide, nitrous oxide should be discontinued immediately and 100 per cent oxygen administered.

MISCELLANEOUS CONSIDERATIONS

Regardless of the anesthetic techniques used in a particular geriatric patient, certain protocols should be incorporated. Geriatric patients should be preoxygenated for 2 to 5 minutes before anesthetic induction to help prevent hypoxia from developing during induction. When a general anesthetic is used, the patient should be intubated to provide a patent airway. Close monitoring of cardiovascular and respiratory parameters are essential, and if necessary, the geriatric patient's ventilation should be assisted or controlled.

Adequate fluid replacement should be given to prevent a renal crisis and to help maintain a proper hemodynamic state in the geriatric patient. The specific fluid used will be dictated by the particular patient's needs; however, in most situations, a balanced electrolyte solution, such as lactated Ringer's or Normosol-R solution, is a reasonable choice. Because hypoglycemia can be a problem during and after anesthesia in the geriatric patient, administering fluids containing glucose may be warranted. The rate of IV fluid administration will depend on the particular patient's needs but will most likely be in the range of 10 to 20 ml/kg/hr. This rate will be decreased in a geriatric patient where the risk of cardiovascular overload, with the subsequent development of pulmonary edema, is a concern. Fluid therapy may have to be continued for several hours to several days after anesthesia and surgery.

Methods should be used to prevent or decrease hypothermia during and after the surgical procedure. Intraoperative monitoring should be continued into the postoperative period or until the geriatric patient has returned to the preanesthetized state.

References and Supplemental Reading

Bellville JW, Forrest WH, Miller E. Influence of age on pain and relief from analgesics: A study of postoperative patients. JAMA 217:1835–1841, 1971.

Berkowitz BA, Ngai SH, Yang JC, et al. The disposition of morphine in surgical patients. Clin Pharmacol Ther 17:629–635, 1975.

Cherondache CN, Romanoff LP. Hormones in aging men. In Gitman L, ed. Endocrines and Aging. Springfield, IL, Charles C Thomas, 1967, p 76.

Collins KJ, Exton-Smith AN, James MH, et al. Functional changes in autonomic nervous responses with aging. Age Ageing 9:17–24, 1980.

Davis PJ, Davis FB. Endocrinology and aging. In Reichel W, ed. Clinical Aspects of Aging. Baltimore, Williams & Wilkins, 1983, pp 396–410.

Devaney KO, Johnson HA. Neuron loss in the aging visual cortex of man. J Gerontol 35:836–841, 1980.

Dodman NH, Seeler DC, Court MH. Aging changes in the geriatric dog and their impact on anesthesia. Compend Contin Educ Pract Vet 6:1106–1112, 1984.

Feldman EC. The adrenal cortex. In Ettinger SJ, ed. Textbook of Veterinary Internal Medicine, Diseases of the Dog and Cat. Philadelphia, WB Saunders, 1983, pp 1650–1696.

Fisch C. Electrocardiogram in the aged—an independent marker of heart disease? Am J Med 70:4–6, 1981.

Giles HG, MacLoed SM, Wright JR, et al. Influence of age and previous use on diazepam dosage required for endoscopy. Can Med Assoc J 118:513–514, 1978.

Green DJ, Sellers EM, Shader RJ. Drug disposition in old age. N Engl J Med 306:1981–1988, 1982.

Knudson RJ, Clark DF, Kennedy TC, et al. Effect of aging alone on mechanical properties of the normal adult lung. J Appl Physiol 43:1054–1062, 1977.

Kronenberg RS, Drage CW. Attenuation of the ventilatory and heart rate responses to hypoxia and hypercapnia with aging in normal men. J Clin Invest 52:1812–1819, 1973.

Lorhan PH. Physiological considerations. In Lorhan PH, ed. Anesthesia for the Aged. Springfield, IL, Charles C Thomas, 1971, pp 31–33.

Lytle LD, Altar A. Diet, central nervous system and aging. Fed Proc 38:2017–2022, 1979.

McLachlan MSF. The aging kidney. Lancet 2:143–146, 1978.

Muiesan G, Sorbini CA, Grassi V. Respiratory function in the aged. Bull Physiopathol Respir 7:973–1009, 1971.

Muravchick S. Effect of age and premedication on thiopental sleep dose. Anesthesiology 61:333–336, 1984.

Ouslander JG. Drug therapy in the elderly. Ann Intern Med 95:711–722, 1981.

Owens W. The geriatric patient—physiology of aging. Proc Am Soc Anesthesiol 275A:1–4, 1985.

Pontoppidan H, Beecher HK. Progressive loss of protective reflexes in the airway with the advance of age. JAMA 174:2209–2213, 1960.

Quasha AL, Eger EI III, Tinker JH. Determination and application of MAC. Anesthesiology 53:315–334, 1980.

Richey DP, Bender AD. Pharmacokinetic consequences of aging. Ann Rev Pharmacol Toxicol 17:49–65, 1977.

Ritchel WA. Pharmacokinetics in the aged. In Pagliaro LA, Pagliaro AM, eds. Pharmacologic Aspects of Aging. St. Louis, CV Mosby, 1983, pp 219–256.

Rosychuk R. Management of hypothyroidism. In Kirk RW, ed. Current Veterinary Therapy VIII. Philadelphia, WB Saunders, 1983, pp 869–876.

Ryan SF, Vericent TN, Mitchell RS, et al. Ductasia—an asymptomatic pulmonary change related to age. Med Thorac 22:181–187, 1965.

Tranquilli WJ, Benson GJ. Advantages and guidelines for using alpha-2 agonists as anesthetic adjuvants. Vet Clin North Am 22(2):289–293, 1992.

Weidman P, DeMyttenoere-Buraztein S. Effect of aging on plasma renin and aldosterone in normal man. Kidney Int 8:325–333, 1975.

CHAPTER 22

Surgical Protocol

GISELLE HOSGOOD

Aging is a complex biologic process that reduces the individual's ability to maintain homeostasis during internal physiologic and external environmental stresses. Thus, the older animal is more vulnerable to disease and less able to handle its consequences (Allen and Roudebush, 1990).

Age does not prohibit surgery. However, the geriatric dog or cat often has multiple problems. These problems can significantly affect the animal's ability to tolerate anesthesia and surgery and hence warrant careful consideration during surgical planning (Table 22–1). It is important to evaluate the animal as a whole and avoid focusing only on the surgical problem. This enables the veterinary surgeon to offer the owner and the animal the most rational plan.

PHYSIOLOGIC CHANGES OF AGING AND THEIR POTENTIAL IMPACT ON SURGERY

Metabolic System

Multiple organ systems undergo change during aging (Table 22–2). Metabolic changes include a decreased basal metabolic rate, diminished ability to withstand stress, decreased capacity for thermoregulation, decreased function of the thyrotropin-thyroid system, altered sleep patterns, and reduced sensitivity to thirst (Mosier, 1989). Thermoregulatory control is less efficient owing to decreased heat production and slower peripheral vasomotor reactions. Hence, it is important to keep animals warm during surgery and recovery. In addition, reduced sensitivity to thirst in the older animal makes monitoring of hydration crucial (Mosier, 1989).

The percentage of body weight composed of fat increases with age (Mosier, 1990), and this, accompanied by decreased muscle mass, can alter parenteral drug absorption and distribution (Aucoin, 1989).

TABLE 22–1. CONSIDERATIONS WHEN PERFORMING SURGERY IN GERIATRIC DOGS AND CATS

- Physiologic changes of aging with potential impact on surgery
  - Metabolic system
  - Hepatorenal system
  - Cardiovascular system
  - Respiratory system
  - Integument
- Preoperative considerations
  - History and physical examination
  - Preoperative evaluation
  - Preoperative care
  - Surgical planning
- Intraoperative considerations
  - Body system support
  - Tissue handling
  - Suture selection and stapling devices
- Postoperative considerations
  - Monitoring and body system support
  - Analgesia
  - Nutritional support

TABLE 22–2. PHYSIOLOGIC CHANGES OF AGING WITH A POTENTIAL IMPACT ON SURGERY

ORGAN SYSTEM	PHYSIOLOGIC CHANGES WITH AGING
Metabolic system	Decreased basal metabolic rate
	Decreased thermoregulation
	Reduced sensitivity to thirst
	Reduced ability to withstand stress
	Loss of muscle mass and increased body fat
Hepatorenal system	Glomerular sclerosis
	Reduced adaptability to changes in fluid intake
	Decreased number of hepatocytes
	Increased intra- and extracellular hepatic fat
Cardiovascular system	Reduced response to catecholamines
	Reduced blood vessel wall compliance
Respiratory system	Increased pulmonary dead space
	Increased lung compliance
Integument	Atrophy of epidermis, dermis, and appendages

Immunologic competence decreases with age, as evidenced by decreased phagocytosis and chemotactic functions, despite the presence of normal numbers of lymphocytes (Tizard and Warner, 1987). This may increase the susceptibility of the geriatric animal to infection (Mosier, 1989).

Hepatorenal System

Age-related changes in the kidney have been observed in both humans and rodents (Brown et al, 1986). These changes are characterized by glomerular sclerosis, although the renal tubules and interstitium are also affected (Brown et al, 1986). Similar lesions have been observed in dogs (Guttman and Andersen, 1986), but their effect on renal function and their clinical significance are unknown. These changes may be significant in reducing the rate of drug excretion (Polzin, 1989). In addition, the aging kidney is less able to adapt to fluctuations in fluid intake, and the geriatric animal is more likely to develop dehydration and prerenal azotemia (Brown et al, 1986). Overt chronic renal failure caused by aging alone is uncommon, but the effects of age and the presence of certain risk factors associated with surgery (Table 22–3) may predispose the geriatric animal to develop acute renal failure (Polzin, 1989). These factors are additive and should be prevented or at least controlled. Prophylactic therapy such as parenteral fluid administration or diuretics should be considered. Preoperative and postoperative diuresis is required in the renally compromised animal.

Liver function declines with age as the number of hepatocytes decreases, the amount of interstitial fibrous tissue increases, and the intracellular and overall fat content of the liver increases (Mosier, 1989).

Cardiovascular System

The heart of the healthy geriatric animal maintains normal contractile elements; however, its ability to respond to catecholamines is reduced. This contributes to the geriatric animal's inability to increase the heart rate and force of contraction to levels attained by the young adult animal. In addition, less compliant blood vessels increase the afterload and reduce the baroreceptor reflexes. This affects the ability of the geriatric animal to maintain blood pressure during periods of stress (Hamlin, 1990; Shimada et al, 1985; Vestal et al, 1979).

Respiratory System

The lungs become more compliant with age, requiring less work on inspiration but making

TABLE 22–3. RISK FACTORS FOR ACUTE RENAL FAILURE IN THE GERIATRIC ANIMAL UNDERGOING SURGERY

Pre-existing or active renal disease
Volume depletion
Nephrotoxic drugs
Chronic administration of NSAIDs
Fever
Sepsis
Metabolic acidosis
Hypokalemia

NSAIDs, Nonsteroidal anti-inflammatory drugs.

expiration more difficult. This contributes to more air remaining in the lungs of the geriatric animal after expiration compared with a young adult animal (Robinson and Gillespie, 1973). The percentage of lung occupied by conducting airways (dead space) increases in the geriatric animal, and hence the surface area available for gaseous exchange decreases (Hamlin, 1990).

Integument

The effect of aging on skin is well documented in humans (Grove, 1989; Lavker et al, 1989). Senile changes in the skin of dogs, characterized by atrophy of the epidermis, appendages, and dermis with a decrease in hair number, have been reported. These changes are far more subtle than those observed in humans, and the senile elastosis and dermal basophilia described in humans does not occur (Baker, 1967).

Wound healing is delayed in geriatric rats (Quirinia and Viidik, 1991; Sussman, 1973) and humans (Holt et al, 1992; Mann and Bednar, 1977). Whether age has a critical effect on wound healing in geriatric dogs and cats is uncertain; however, the effect of concurrent disease is likely to have an impact on wound healing (Quirinia and Viidik, 1991).

PREOPERATIVE CONSIDERATIONS

History and Physical Examination

A complete history and physical examination are essential, as they provide information on concurrent drug administration and past and current medical problems that may have an impact on the selection of anesthetic and surgical protocols. Prolonged corticosteroid and antimicrobial administration for dermatologic disease or nonsteroidal anti-inflammatory drug (NSAID) administration for degenerative joint disease is not uncommon. These agents may affect wound healing, renal function, microbial resistance, and blood clotting.

A drug history is important, as drug interactions are more likely to occur in the geriatric animal. Reasons for this include increased incidence of major illness, presence of undiagnosed illness, simultaneous use of multiple drugs, changes in the pharmacokinetics and pharmacodynamics of drugs owing to reduced renal excretion and diminished hepatic metabolism, altered drug distribution owing to a lower total body water content and higher body fat content, and decreased protein binding of drugs. In addition, the possibility of drug–drug interactions or drug–organ interactions must be considered (Aucoin, 1989; Polzin, 1989). For example, the administration of an NSAID for degenerative joint disease and the presence of cardiac failure may impair renal function in the geriatric animal (Polzin, 1989).

Clinical signs evident on physical examination may indicate undiagnosed conditions that warrant specific evaluation before surgery is scheduled. For example, an undiagnosed cough, lameness, mass, or behavioral change may point to a serious problem that requires attention before surgery can progress.

Preoperative Evaluation

The preoperative evaluation is generally dictated by the primary surgical problem and any pre-existing disease. In elective procedures, a minimum data base for the geriatric animal should include a complete blood cell count, serum chemistry panel, urinalysis, and a lead II electrocardiogram. Most cases warrant thoracic radiographs to assess cardiac and pulmonary status, and if neoplasia is suspected, both left and right lateral recumbent projections and a ventrodorsal projection should be included to rule out visible metastatic disease. A history of prolonged NSAID administration may indicate the need for blood coagulation screening using buccal mucosal bleeding time and activated clotting time tests. A history of prolonged, indiscriminate administration of corticosteroids may indicate the need for adrenal function testing.

Any unidentified lesion on the animal, whether it is the primary problem or a concurrent finding, can be preliminarily (and sometimes definitively) assessed by fine needle aspirate biopsy and subsequent cytologic examination. This can generally be performed without anesthesia; sedation is required only in a minority of animals. Invasive biopsies using a biopsy punch or Tru-Cut needle (Travenol Laboratories, Inc., Deerfield, IL), can be performed under local anesthesia and sedation. Information obtained from biopsy specimens may be vital to constructing a rational surgical plan.

Ultrasonography and endoscopy are useful, noninvasive tools for evaluation, particularly in the geriatric animal. Ultrasonography rarely requires anesthesia and only occasionally requires

TABLE 22–4. CONCEPTS TO IMPROVE OPERATIVE EFFICIENCY IN THE GERIATRIC ANIMAL

CONCEPT	COMMENTS
Clip the surgical site immediately before anesthetic induction	Applicable in the cooperative or premedicated animal Do not clip the day before surgery, as this allows microlacerations of the skin to become infected and may increase the chance of surgical site contamination
Be familiar with the procedure	Know the anatomy Select the best approach (i.e., one that allows good exposure and uninhibited progress) Have the appropriate equipment Be prepared for problems; have contingency plans formalized
Crossmatch before surgery if blood loss is likely	Have blood collected before surgery Have personnel available to collect blood if needed

sedation of the animal. Although endoscopy does require general anesthesia, the procedure time is often shorter than surgery, and essential information can be obtained from biopsy samples taken during the procedure.

Preoperative Care

The older animal, especially one with chronic disease, may be undernourished. Provision of preoperative nutrition may be indicated to improve the overall health of the animal and its candidacy for surgery. The stress of surgery can increase the basal metabolic rate 50 to 100 per cent (Crowe, 1986). Hence, good nutrition before and after surgery is extremely important. Providing a high-energy, high-protein diet may be all that is required for the animal that is eating. Nasogastric tube feeding offers a noninvasive route of hyperalimentation that does not require general anesthesia for tube placement (Abood and Buffington, 1991). Percutaneous gastrostomy tube placement may be indicated in some animals, and although it does require general anesthesia, the procedure is short and has few complications (Armstrong and Hardie, 1991; Bright et al, 1991).

Depriving the geriatric animal of water during the fasting period before surgery is contraindicated, and free-choice water should always be available. In fact, because the older animal has less control of body fluid homeostasis, preoperative fluid therapy may be necessary. This applies not only to the animal with renal compromise, but also to any animal whose hydration status is questionable. Monitoring of urine output, at least qualitatively, may provide useful information during this period. Quantitative urine output may be indicated in the renally compromised animal.

Surgical Planning

The most critical periods of any surgical procedure for a geriatric animal are probably the time of anesthesia induction, the period when the animal is under general anesthesia, and the early postoperative period. The surgeon should attempt to minimize stress on the animal preoperatively. Often an elective surgery patient can be examined and evaluated as an outpatient, then presented the morning of surgery after being fasted with access to free-choice water only (Waldron and Budsberg, 1989). It has been said that "the art of surgery in the aged patient is to be swift and gentle" and "to keep it simple" (Cohen, 1990). The surgeon should attempt to maximize the efficiency of the surgical procedure so that anesthesia time and stress on the animal are reduced (Table 22–4).

Age is not an indication for perioperative antimicrobial therapy. The need for such therapy is based on the type of procedure and likelihood of contamination, the presence of host defense impairment, and the duration of the surgical procedure. Surgical procedures lasting longer than 90 minutes are associated with a higher risk of bacterial contamination and wound complications than are shorter procedures (Hosgood, 1992; Vasseur et al, 1988). Antimicrobial drug selection, dosage, and administration intervals should be based on the primary route of drug excretion, the function of the organ system involved in excretion (i.e., hepatic or renal), and the pharmacokinetics of the drug (half-life, metabolism, and apparent volume of distribution) (Brown et al,

1986). Perioperative antimicrobials should be given immediately prior to surgery, intraoperatively if the procedure extends for more than 90 minutes, and for one or two doses postoperatively (Cohen, 1990; Dispiro et al, 1983; Kasier, 1986). Antimicrobials administered later than 6 hours after surgery show limited benefit in preventing surgical infection (Dispiro et al, 1983; Kasier, 1986).

INTRAOPERATIVE CONSIDERATIONS

Body System Support

Anesthetic needs have been discussed previously. It is important that close monitoring of the animal be done at all times. Monitoring blood pressure, either with noninvasive Doppler equipment or oscillometric monitoring (Dinamap or Critikon, Johnson and Johnson, Tampa, FL) using a pneumatic cuff or with invasive techniques using an arterial catheter, provides a sensitive indicator of the animal's cardiovascular status (Figs. 22–1 and 22–2). Intraoperative fluid therapy (normal rate, 10 to 20 ml/kg/hr) is required to prevent a renal crisis and provide cardiovascular support (Paddleford, 1988). The type of fluid used will be dictated by the specific needs of the animal; however, for the otherwise healthy animal, a balanced electrolyte solution such as lactated Ringer's solution is suitable.

Keeping the animal warm during surgery is important, as the older animal has less efficient thermoregulatory control. Warm water circulating blankets and the use of warm lavage solutions are indicated. Intraoperative monitoring of the animal using a rectal or esophageal thermometer or intermittent manual methods can be useful.

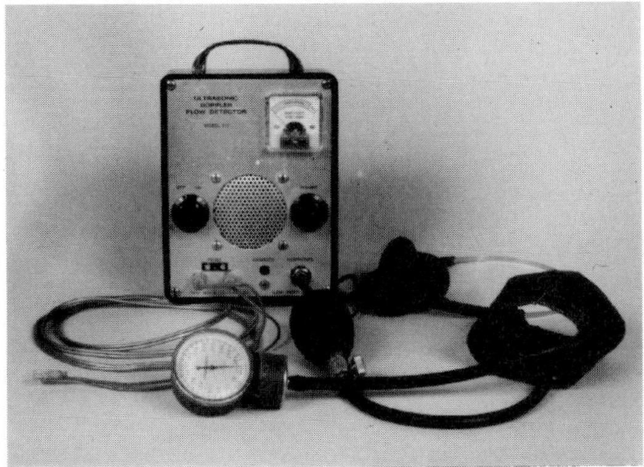

Figure 22–1. An electronically activated Doppler crystal that senses blood flow and is audibly broadcast can be used to monitor blood pressure.

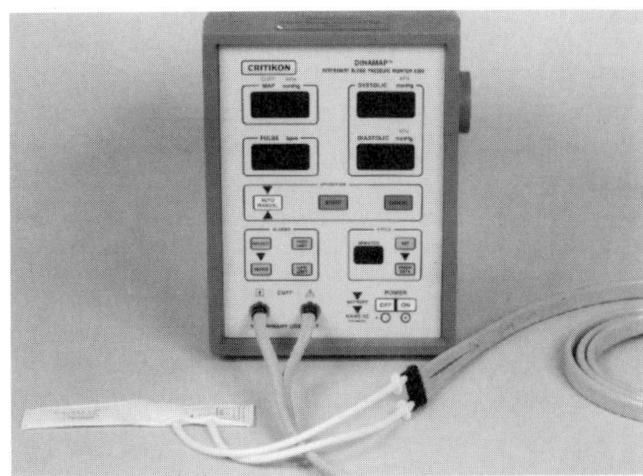

Figure 22–2. An oscillometric peripheral pulse monitor can be used to monitor pulse rate and blood pressure.

Tissue Handling

Tissue handling should be gentle and meticulous to minimize trauma and hemorrhage and maximize healing without complication. Electrocautery may facilitate hemostasis but should be used judiciously because of its deleterious effect on healing (Fucci and Elkins, 1991). Because time is important, using the correct instruments facilitates the efficiency of the surgical procedure.

Minimizing traction on viscera (which causes vagal stimulation) and avoiding compression of large veins such as the caudal vena cava help avoid fluctuations in blood pressure during surgery. Inadvertent leaning on the animal and hindering respiration should be avoided.

Suture Selection and Stapling Devices

Wound healing in older animals is retarded; however, concurrent disease probably has a greater impact on healing than age (Cohen, 1990). Animals with diabetes mellitus, hyperadrenocorticism, and other debilitating diseases have delayed wound healing (Swaim, 1980). Before selecting a suture material, the strength of the tissue, the rate of tissue healing, and the condition of the animal should be considered (Table 22–5). In the otherwise healthy animal, a rapid gain in wound strength is observed 7 to 10 days after surgery. Most absorbable suture materials pro-

TABLE 22–5. SUTURES SUITABLE FOR USE IN THE GERIATRIC ANIMAL UNDERGOING SURGERY

SUTURE DESCRIPTION	SUTURE TYPE
A. Multifilament absorbable without prolonged absorption	Polyglactin 910 Polyglycolic acid
B. Monofilament absorbable with prolonged absorption	Polydioxanone Polyglyconate
C. Monofilament nonabsorbable	Polypropylene Nylon Polybutester Stainless steel
D. Skin staples	

SUITABLE SUTURE

Patient Status	Linea Alba	Soft Tissue	Skin
Healthy	A or B; avoid catgut owing to unpredictable absorption	A	C or D, caprolactam
Concurrent disease that delays wound healing	B	A or B	C or D, caprolactam
Severely debilitated	B or C	A or B	C or D, caprolactam

vide adequate tensile strength for this period. Catgut should be avoided because of its unpredictable rate of absorption. Soft, nonirritating absorbable suture such as polyglactin 910 (Vicryl, Ethicon, NJ) and polyglycolic acid (Dexon, Davis and Geck, Puerto Rico) are suitable. Polydioxanone (PDS II, Ethicon, NJ) and polyglyconate (Maxon, Ethicon, NJ) have a prolonged rate of absorption and, although suitable in any animal, may be preferred for animals with diseases causing delayed wound healing or for debilitated animals. Inert, nonabsorbable, monofilament suture material such as polypropylene (Prolene, Ethicon, NJ), nylon (Ethilon, Ethicon, NJ), polybutester (Novofil, Ethicon, NJ), and stainless steel (Surgical Steel, Ethicon, NJ) may also be indicated in these animals. However, buried nonabsorbable monofilament suture has an increased likelihood for development of suture sinuses than absorbable suture (Hosgood et al, 1992). Burying multifilament and/or coated nonabsorbable suture materials such as polyester and caprolactam (Braunamid, B. Braun, Melsungen AG, Germany) is contraindicated; however, caprolactam is suitable for use in the skin.

Use of continuous suture patterns in the linea alba (Rosin, 1985) and skin are safe and help to decrease operative time. Stapling offers considerable time savings to the surgeon and in some instances provides a more secure method of closure than suturing (Pavletic, 1990). The thoracoabdominal (TA) instruments (United States Surgical Corporation, Norwalk, CT) are available in three sizes, producing staple lines of 90, 55, and 30 mm. The TA 30-V3, designed for cardiovascular use, creates three staggered rows of staples rather than two. The TA can be used for complete and partial lung lobectomy, partial hepatectomy and splenectomy, and intestinal anastomosis (Fig. 22–3). The gastrointestinal anastomosis (GIA) and end-to-end anastomosis (EEA) instruments (United States Surgical Corporation, Norwalk, CT) are used in gastrointestinal surgery. The GIA is available in two sizes producing staple lines of 50 and 90 mm (Pavletic, 1990). The EEA is available in three sizes, with outer diameter cartridges of 31, 28, and 25 mm producing anastomoses with an internal diameter of 21, 18, and 15 mm, respectively (Pavletic, 1990). Ligate-and-divide staplers (LDS, United States Surgical Corporation, Norwalk, CT) produce a double staple ligation and automatically cut between the two staples. They are useful during procedures that require many ligatures. Vascular staple units (Surgiclips, United States Surgical Corporation, Norwalk, CT) that fire a single vascular staple are also available (Fig. 22–4). Although disposable units for all staplers are available, reusable stapling equipment can be used on loan from the manufacturer, with only the cost of the staple cartridges incurred. For skin, disposable staples (Precise Vista Skin Stapler, 3M, St Paul, MN) are preferred, and are quick, convenient, and effective. Partially used skin staplers can

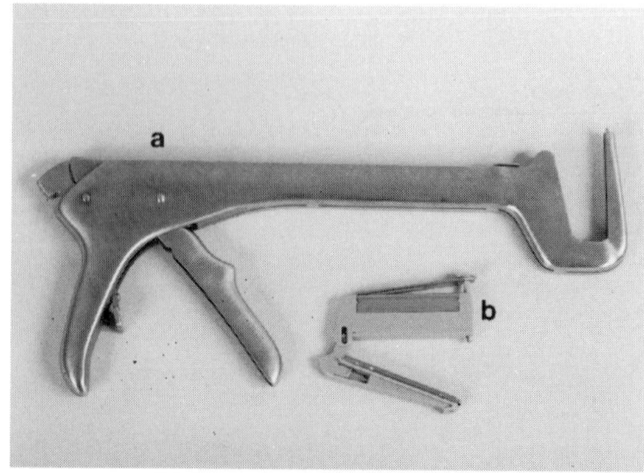

Figure 22–3. A reusable thoracic-abdominal (TA) surgical instrument (a) and cartridge (b). Staple sizes available in color-coded cartridges are: blue = 90-mm-long staple line, 4.8-mm staples; green = 55-mm-long staple line, 3.5-mm staples; white = 30-mm-long staple line; 3.0-mm staples.

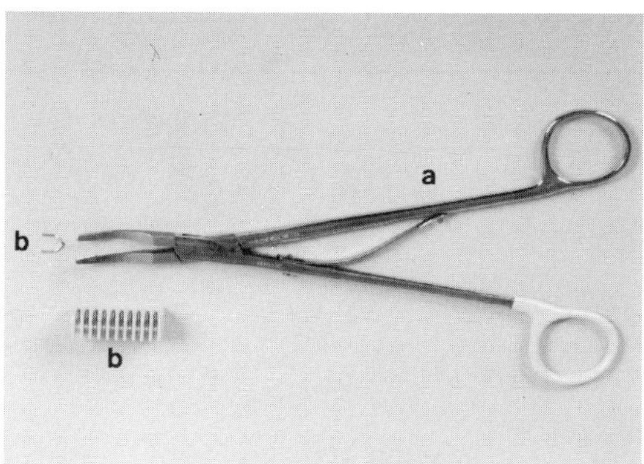

Figure 22–4. A reusable vascular staple applicator (a) and staples (b).

be resterilized with ethylene oxide (Pavletic, 1990). Based on time savings, the cost of stapling is not prohibitive.

POSTOPERATIVE CONSIDERATIONS

Monitoring and Body System Support

Continuous monitoring of vital signs (body temperature, pulse, capillary refill time, and respiration) is important in the early postoperative period (Table 22–6). Thoracic auscultation is indicated, especially if aggressive fluid therapy is instituted. Blood pressure, central venous pressure (through a jugular catheter), urine output, and electrocardiographic monitoring is necessary in the critical patient. Fluid therapy should be continued for at least 12 hours (Waldron and Budsberg, 1989); however, the duration depends on the needs of the animal. Unless diuresis is indicated, maintenance fluid rates (approximately 40 to 60 ml/kg/day) are adequate. Normal urine output of at least 1 to 2 ml/kg/hr should be maintained at this rate. If not, fluid rates should be increased, and diuretic therapy may be indicated. Monitoring the packed cell volume and total solids concentration can provide information regarding the effects of intraoperative or ongoing hemorrhage and is a good indicator of changes in hydration.

Oxygen should be available. A nasal oxygen tube can be easily placed at the end of the surgical procedure if the animal is predicted to need one. It can be removed later if not required. Oxygen masks should also be available.

Careful, slow rewarming of the animal is required to reverse hypothermia. This is accomplished most effectively by wrapping the animal in a circulating warm water blanket (Haskins, 1981). Care must be taken if heat lamps or hot water bottles are used, as thermal injury can occur (Dunlop et al, 1981).

The animal should be turned frequently to prevent hypostatic pulmonary congestion and atelectasis, enhance the removal of inhalant anesthetics, and prevent accumulation of airway secretions (Brown, 1985). Soft bedding and frequent turning are especially important in the animal that is recumbent for prolonged periods to prevent decubital ulcers. This is a serious postoperative complication that can significantly stress the already debilitated animal.

Analgesia

Careful attention to the analgesic needs of the animal is required. Geriatric animals are equally sensitive to pain, and analgesic treatment can remove undue stress and distress caused by pain (Cohen, 1990). Opioids do not depress myocardial contractility, are well tolerated, and provide excellent analgesia (Table 22–7). They will produce sinus bradycardia, which may require administration of an anticholinergic drug (e.g., atropine or glycopyrrolate). However, indiscriminate use of anticholinergic drugs can produce a potentially dangerous sinus tachycardia, and therefore, such agents should be used to effect only (Paddleford, 1988). Opioids may produce respiratory depression, especially with intravenous administration. The use of naloxone to reverse the action of opioids should be considered in the animal

TABLE 22–6. POSTOPERATIVE CONSIDERATIONS IN THE GERIATRIC ANIMAL

CONSIDERATION	COMMENT
Monitoring and body system support	Continuous monitoring of vital signs until normal Blood pressure assessment in the critical patient Fluid support for at least 12 hours Nasal oxygen if required Slow rewarming of animal Frequent turning
Analgesia	Important to reduce stress and distress of animal
Nutritional support	Necessary in debilitated animals and those unable to eat

TABLE 22–7. OPIOID ANALGESICS FOR USE IN THE GERIATRIC DOG AND CAT

ANALGESIC	POTENCY COMPARED WITH MORPHINE	DOSAGE	DURATION (hr)
Morphine	1	Dog: 0.1 to 2 mg/kg SC Cat: 0.01 mg/kg SC	3–6
Meperidine	0.2	Dog: 1 to 4.5 mg/kg IM, IV Cat: Same	2–4
Oxymorphone	10	0.2 mg/kg IM, IV, with maximum total dose of 3 mg Cat: Same	2–4
Butorphanol	5	Dog: 0.2 to 0.45 mg/kg IM, IV Cat: Same	Up to 4
Buprenorphine	25	Dog: 0.01 to 0.02 mg/kg SC Cat: 0.0025 to 0.005 mg SC	8–12

IM, intramuscular; IV, intravenous; SC, subcutaneous.

that is nonresponsive to ventilatory support. Morphine is used less often owing to its severe respiratory depressant side effects. Meperidine has limited use because of its minimal analgesic effects and short duration of action (Sackman, 1991). Oxymorphone provides excellent analgesia but will cause respiratory depression, auditory hypersensitivity, and altered thermoregulation (Sackman, 1991). Butorphanol is particularly useful, as it produces good analgesia without severe cardiopulmonary suppression; it can be reversed with naloxone (Paddleford, 1988). Buprenorphine is not yet approved for use in animals but has been used by the author. It provides excellent analgesia for 8 to 12 hours without sedation (Jenkins, 1987; Raffe 1988). However, respiratory depression may occur that is not easily reversed by naloxone, possibly because of high receptor affinity of buprenorphine (Jenkins, 1987; Raffe 1988).

Nutritional Support

Maintaining a positive nitrogen balance and good nutritional support of the animal is important in the recovery period. Those animals that require preoperative nutrition will usually require postoperative support. Animals with questionable nitrogen balance or those undergoing a procedure likely to impair eating should have a feeding tube placed at the end of the surgical procedure. It is imperative that nutritional therapy be instituted early, before the animal has gone several days without eating. The obese animal should not be neglected, as the animal will be in negative nitrogen balance if it is not eating.

Suture removal in the healthy animal can be performed 7 to 10 days after surgery. In debilitated animals, those with disease known to delay wound healing, or those in which electrocautery was used, suture removal should be delayed until 10 to 14 days (Fucci and Elkins, 1991).

References and Supplemental Reading

Abood SK, Buffington CA. Improved nasogastric intubation technique for administration of nutritional support in dogs. J Am Vet Med Assoc 199:577–579, 1991.

Allen TA, Roudebush P. Canine geriatric nephrology. Compend Contin Educ Pract Vet 12:909–917, 946, 1990.

Armstrong PJ, Hardie EM. Percutaneous endoscopic gastrostomy: A retrospective study of 54 clinical cases in dogs and cats. J Vet Intern Med 4:202–206, 1991.

Aucoin DP. Drug therapy in the geriatric animal: The effect of aging on drug disposition. Vet Clin North Am [Small Anim Pract] 19:41–47, 1989.

Baker KD. Senile changes of dog skin. J Small Anim Pract 8:49–54, 1967.

Bright RM, Okrasinski EB, Pardo A, et al. Percutaneous tube gastrostomy for enteral alimentation in small animals. Compend Contin Educ Pract Vet 13:15–23, 1991.

Brown NO. Patient aftercare. In Slatter DH, ed. Textbook of Small Animal Surgery. Philadelphia, WB Saunders, pp 373–389, 1985.

Brown WW, Davis BB, Spry LA, et al. Aging and the kidney. Arch Intern Med 146:1790–1796, 1986.

Cohen MM. Perioperative responsibilities of the surgeon. Clin Geriatr Med 6:469–480, 1990.

Crowe DT. Enteral nutrition for critically ill or injured patients—part I. Compend Contin Educ Pract Vet 8:603–613, 1986.

Dispiro JT, Bivins BA, Record KE, et al. The prophylactic use of antimicrobials in surgery. Curr Probl Surg 2:70–73, 1983.

Dunlop CE, Daunt DA, Haskins SC. Thermal burns in four dogs during anesthesia. Vet Surg 8:242–246, 1981.

Fucci V, Elkins AD. Electrosurgery: Principles and guidelines in veterinary medicine. Compend Contin Educ Pract Vet 13:407–415, 1991.

Grove GL. Physiologic changes in older skin. Clin Geriatr Med 5:115–125, 1989.

Guttman PH, Andersen AC. Progressive intercapillary glomerulosclerosis in aging and irradiated Beagles. Radiat Res 35:45–60, 1986.

Hamlin RL. Identifying the cardiovascular and pulmonary diseases that affect old dogs. Vet Med 85:483–497, 1990.
Haskins SC. Hypothermia and its prevention during general anesthesia in cats. Am J Vet Res 42:56–61, 1981.
Holt DR, Kirk SJ, Regan MC, et al. Effect of age on wound healing in healthy human beings. Surgery 112:293–298, 1992.
Hosgood G. Pharmacologic features of butorphanol in dogs and cats. J Am Vet Med Assoc 196:135–136, 1990.
Hosgood G. Wound complications following thoracolumbar laminectomy in the dog: A retrospective study of 264 procedures. J Am Anim Hosp Assoc 2:47–52, 1992.
Hosgood G, Pechman RD, Casey HW. Suture sinus in the linea alba of two dogs. J Small Anim Pract 33:285–288, 1992.
Jenkins WL. Pharmacologic aspects of analgesic drugs in animals: An overview. J Am Vet Med Assoc 191:1231–1240, 1987.
Kasier AB. Antimicrobial prophylaxis in surgery. N Engl J Med 315:1129–1138, 1986.
Lavker RM, Zheng P, Don G. Morphology of aged skin. Clin Geriatr Med 5:53–67, 1989.
Mann M, Bednar B. Influence of aging and different drugs on the healing process in human skin wounds. Gerontology 23:277–289, 1977.
Mosier JE. Effect of aging on body systems of the dog. Vet Clin North Am [Small Anim Pract] 19:1–12, 1989.
Mosier JE. Caring for the aging dog in today's practice. Vet Med 85:463–471, 1990.
Paddleford RR. Anesthetic management in the critical geriatric patient. Semin Vet Med Surg [Small Anim] 3:22–29, 1988.
Pavletic MM. Surgical stapling devices in small animal surgery. Compend Contin Educ Pract Vet 12:1724–1740, 1990.
Polzin DJ. The effects of aging on the canine urinary tract. Vet Med 85:472–482, 1990.
Quirinia A, Viidik A. The influence of age on the healing of normal and ischemic skin wounds. Mech Aging Dev 5:221–232, 1991.
Raffe MR. Management of pain in the traumatized animal. Semin Vet Med Surg 3:210–215, 1988.
Robinson NE, Gillespie JR. Lung volumes in aging beagles. J Appl Physiol 35:317–321, 1973.
Rosin E. Single layer, simple continuous suture pattern for closure of abdominal incisions. J Am Anim Hosp Assoc 21:751–756, 1985.
Sackman JE. Pain. Part II. Control of pain in animals. Compend Contin Educ Pract Vet 13:181–193, 1991.
Shimada K, Kitazumi T, Sadakane N, et al. Age-related changes in baroreflex function, plasma norepinephrine, and blood pressure. Hypertension 7:113–117, 1985.
Sussman MD. Aging of connective tissue: Physical properties of healing wounds in young and old rats. Am J Physiol 224:1167–1171, 1973.
Swaim SF. Wound healing. In Surgery of Traumatized Skin: Management and Reconstruction in the Dog and Cat. Philadelphia, WB Saunders, 1980, pp 70–115.
Tizard I, Warner D. State of animal's immune system key to longevity. DVM 1987; 1:27–28, 1987.
Vasseur PB, Levy J, Dowd E, et al. Surgical wound infection rates in dogs and cats. Data from a teaching hospital. Vet Surg 1:60–64, 1988.
Vestal RE, Wood AJ, Shand DG, et al. Reduced beta-adrenoreceptor sensitivity in the elderly. Clin Pharmacol Ther 26:11–16, 1979.
Waldron DR, Budsberg SC. Surgery of the geriatric patient. Vet Clin North Am [Small Anim Pract] 19:33–40, 1989.

CHAPTER 23

Client Services

C. GUY HANCOCK

Geriatric dogs and cats are at much greater risk of life-threatening illness and are reaching the end of their natural lives. In recent years veterinarians have shown more interest in helping owners cope with the emotions caused by pet loss. This discussion will include the topics of pet loss, services for the owners of geriatric pets, memorialization, and hospice concepts that are applicable to veterinary medicine. As veterinarians learn more about the significance of the human–animal bond, they are more obligated to address the grief that occurs when that bond is broken by death.

PET DEATH AND THE GRIEF REACTION

The grief reaction may occur any time there is a perceived loss. The reaction to pet loss has been noted for its intensity and duration. Studies point out the similarity between people's relations to children and to pets, and how people tend to prefer child-like physical features in pets, such as proportionally larger heads and eyes. In addition, people's emotional relationships with pets are more like their relationships with children than with adults. The death of a child is widely recognized as being extremely stressful because of the perceived innocence and purity of the adult–child relationship. It follows that because of the similarities in relationships with children and pets, pet death could be expected to induce strong feelings.

After a loss, people experience many emotions such as denial, anger, guilt, depression, and others. These emotions continue to recur with gradually less intensity until resolution is complete. People progress toward resolution by talking about their feelings. It is important for sympathetic, active listeners to be available so that people feel safe enough to express their feelings.

However, the resolution of pet loss grief is complicated by two special difficulties not associated with other losses. First, people lack widely accepted social customs such as funerals and burials to provide opportunities for expression of grief. Second, it is difficult to identify people who have an understanding of pet loss and can listen sympathetically. Rather than risk derision or unhelpful comments such as, "It was only a dog," people keep their emotions bottled up inside. They avoid the immediate hurt by being silent, with the consequence that grief is prolonged because they are unable to deal with or express their feelings.

Many veterinary hospital staff may not realize that they, too, often suffer a loss and experience grief when a patient dies. Their first reaction may be denial ("I can't believe [—] is dead!") followed by anger over losing a patient. If this anger is directed at the owner, it may relieve the staff at the expense of serving the owner. This is followed by guilt and depression ("If I had only noticed this or done that, he might still be with us."). The significance of the loss and, therefore, the intensity of the grief will vary from case to case, of course. The average veterinarian may lose as many as six patients a week, based on a caseload of 3000 patients with average life spans of 10 years. However, veterinarians are spared somewhat because not all of them die in the hospital or during veterinary care. Despite this, the fact remains that veterinarians face a significant amount of pet loss owing to the shorter natural lives of their animal patients when compared with people.

USEFUL TECHNIQUES FOR VETERINARIANS AND HOSPITAL STAFF

Advance Preparation of Owners for Pet Loss

American society has been described as worshiping youth and denying death. There are some widely accepted rituals that help people to cope with the death of a loved one, but there are no generally accepted traditions, customs, or rituals for dealing with animal deaths. The person coping with a pet's death does not attend a memorial service, a funeral home, or, usually, a cemetery internment. Without these rituals, there is little opportunity to express one's feelings and share them with sympathetic friends. The support group of friends, relatives, and others is mostly lacking in reference to pet loss.

It is important for veterinarians to become proactive in preparing owners for a pet's death, beginning several years in advance. A mention of realistic life expectancy for the species presented for examination on the first visit is appropriate. If owners work through the process of planning some of the details of their pet's last days and disposition of the body, they can avoid making poor decisions during the most emotional time of their grief. Poor decisions made under emotional strain may prolong the recovery from grief of one or more members of the pet's household.

One technique that may be borrowed from human medicine, with appropriate modifications, is the concept of advance directives. These directives were part of the Federal Omnibus Budget Reconciliation Act of 1990 and went into effect on December 1, 1991. The Act requires hospitals and other health care providers to give information to patients about their right to make personal health care decisions, including accepting or refusing medical treatment. Advance directives allow the patient to specify in advance whether he or she wants, or wishes to avoid, resuscitation, maintenance on feeding tubes, and other procedures.

Modified veterinary advance directives offer the potential to help owners make decisions and prepare for the inevitable death of their pet (Fig. 23–1). By asking owners to complete an advance directive questionnaire, the veterinarian can help everyone in the household begin to consider the elements of their pet's quality of life, how to decide on euthanasia if it should be needed, and what should be done with the pet's remains. Some questions that can be asked in an advance directive are as follows:

- Where would you wish to have your pet spend its last hours: at home or in the veterinary hospital?
- What criteria would you use to evaluate your pet's quality of life (e.g., appetite, mobility, interest in surroundings)?
- Would you consider euthanasia of a very ill pet?
- How would you decide when euthanasia is indicated?
- What would you do if your pet was diagnosed with a progressive incurable illness?

These questions must be worded carefully so as not to unnecessarily frighten owners or lead them to think that owning a pet is not a pleasurable experience. They can be presented as one way for owners to provide optimal care for their pet by thinking ahead about how they can best meet their pet's needs.

Opportunities to Provide Service

Acknowledging Grief. Astute veterinarians and practice management consultants have recommended a variety of ways to provide better service to grieving owners. The first is attempting to schedule euthanasia conferences or euthanasia appointments at the beginning or end of the day to avoid the busy times. This allows the veterinarian to spend more time with the owners at this critical time in their pet's life and spares them the embarrassment of having a waiting room full of strangers witnessing their grief. A second step is preparing owners by explaining the process and what to expect at each step. It is helpful to answer questions about what the animal will experience as well as any other questions. The further this can be done in advance, the better, as it preconditions owners for the approach of the end of their pet's life. Finally, a sensitive way to han-

1. Who will participate in discussions and decisions about the patient's care?

Name	Relation	Phone	Scale of attachment
____________	________	________	Low 1 2 3 4 High
____________	________	________	Low 1 2 3 4 High
____________	________	________	Low 1 2 3 4 High

Who will not participate?

____________	________	________	Low 1 2 3 4 High
____________	________	________	Low 1 2 3 4 High

2. Who, if anyone, is the primary caregiver of the patient?

3. If the patient's condition becomes terminal, who wants to be sure to visit and have a last opportunity to say goodbye?

4. How important are the following factors in causing you to consider euthanasia?

Scale: Euthanasia is not a consideration	1	2	3	4	5	Euthanasia highly desirable
Reduced mobility..........................	____	____	____	____	____	
Poor appetite	____	____	____	____	____	
Weight loss.................................	____	____	____	____	____	
Need medication 3 times daily........	____	____	____	____	____	
Need increasing nursing care.........	____	____	____	____	____	
Chronic pain	____	____	____	____	____	
Loss of eyesight	____	____	____	____	____	
Loss of bowel control	____	____	____	____	____	
Loss of urinary control	____	____	____	____	____	

Note: these items should be discussed among all the caregivers in the household, or separate forms should be completed by each member.

5. If you could choose where your pet will die, would it be at home or at the hospital? ____________

6. If you were forced to choose euthanasia, who among the family would want to be present?

____ All caregivers ____ Only the primary caregiver
____ None of the caregivers ____ Other (list) ____________

7. What is your preference in caring for the remains?

____ Burial in a common grave ____ Burial at home
____ Burial in a marked grave ____ Freeze drying
____ Cremation and mass burial ____ Cremation, return ashes
____ Other ____________

8. Which of the following, if any, would you consider doing in memory of your special relationship with this pet?

____ Pet cemetery memorial service
____ Memorial service at home
____ Hang a special picture
____ Plant a tree or living memorial
____ Make a donation to an animal organization
____ Make a donation to a veterinary/veterinary technology college

9. How would you direct close friends to acknowledge their sympathy?

____ Cards ____ Flowers
____ Telephone call ____ Donation to ____________

Figure 23–1. Sample of veterinary advance directives form.

dle billing is to meet with the owner beforehand or to mail a bill afterward.

For a number of years it has been recommended to send a card, sympathy note, or some remembrance to the family soon after a pet's death. Some veterinarians have a personal preference for handwritten sympathy notes; veterinarians often write personal notes to reassure owners that they (the owners) are not responsible for their pet's death. Staff members should sign the letter if they had much interaction with the pet or the family. These expressions of sympathy are greatly appreciated.

Another well-received follow-up is a donation to a charity that then sends a letter stating that a donation was received from the veterinarian in the name of the deceased pet. This is a good idea, but the processing of the donation and the follow-up letter is not under the veterinarian's control and may not be as timely as the veterinarian would like. A note from the veterinary facility is worthwhile even when a donation is made.

Caring for the Remains. The disposition of the remains is an important issue that is best decided far in advance of the necessity. The veterinarian should use terminology that implies that the body of the deceased pet is an object worthy of respect in proportion to the respect accorded the pet during its life. The phrase "dispose of the body" implies that the body is a waste object and not of value. Such words as "care," "treat," "prepare," or even "handle" do not have the negative connotation of "dispose."

It is important to be both knowledgeable and helpful to the owner, as well as nonjudgmental about the owner's wishes or choice in the matter. Products such as urns and cardboard pet caskets are available and should be considered as a way to add dignity to the handling of a pet's remains. Veterinarians who are proactive in helping families to face the issue of what to do with the remains will obtain information about pet cemeteries, cremations, and local laws to give to owners. Owners can be encouraged to consider the options long before the actual need occurs through the use of advance directives. Some human cemeteries allow burial of pets with people, some have a special pet area, and others refuse pets. Some pet cemeteries accept human remains so that family members can be interred with their pets.

Memorialization. In the foreword to *Rituals for Living and Dying*, Stanley Kippner states, "Mary Chadwick, a psychoanalyst, has described the fear of death as the western individual's most fundamental anxiety." Kippner further quotes Dr. Chadwick: "Rituals build community, creating a meeting ground where people can share deep feelings, positive and negative. Rituals and rites of passage are traditionally among the most powerful culturally sanctioned vehicles available for exerting this influence. They are social inventions for instructing the human spirit on its journey into the world" (Feinstein and Mayo, 1990). People use rituals to deal with significant events in their lives.

In *Rituals for Living and Dying*, Feinstein and Mayo (1990) state the following:

> Rituals, like myths, address
>
> - our urge to comprehend our existence in a meaningful way,
> - our search for a marked pathway as we move from one stage of our lives to the next,
> - our need to establish secure and fulfilling relationships within a human community, and
> - our longing to know our part in the vast wonder and mystery of the cosmos.
>
> The guidance the culture's mythology has to offer is etched into the mind and body of every person participating in the ritual. In this manner, rituals—family ceremonies, community celebrations, church liturgies, the sacraments of baptism, marriage, and burial—help to form the individual's personal mythology and continue to shape it with each life passage.

Memorialization is a technique for creating personal rituals, where none exist, to add meaning to the life shock of a pet's death. Memorialization is a way to recognize the significance of the pet's role in an owner's life and the uniqueness of that pet. It is also a way to create opportunities in which it is permissible to express grief. Because memorialization is very important, both in affirming the value of an individual pet and in helping resolve grief over the loss, it must not be left to chance. Veterinarians must take the initiative to be proactive in helping the owners consider ways to memorialize the pets they have lost.

Bereavement Services. Bereavement services can be characterized as crisis intervention, support groups, and counseling. Pet loss crisis intervention hotlines are available at the University of California at Davis, University of Florida, and perhaps other colleges of veterinary medicine. The first hotline was founded by Mader and Hart (Human-Animal Bond Program, University of California at Davis), who solicited volunteers from the veterinary students. The students undergo crisis intervention training and then answer calls on a rotating basis under the supervision of Mader. The service is modeled after community crisis intervention hotlines that deal with suicide prevention and similar problems.

Pet loss support groups offer a complementary service to crisis intervention. The support group is a safe place for self-disclosure of grief. Talking about the strong feelings accompanying a loss is therapeutic. Hearing others who are at different stages in the process talk about their grief is reassuring. It shows that progress toward resolution is possible, and that a person is not alone in having very strong feelings about a pet's death. These groups are usually provided free or for a minimal fee. However, they should be facilitated or led by an experienced bereavement counselor with the proper credentials to provide mental health counseling. Veterinary associations or individual practices may sponsor pet loss support groups, but one of the greatest difficulties is maintaining steady attendance, as many people attend only once. It may be necessary to put regular notices in the newspaper, send cards to owners who lose pets, and distribute brochures in veterinary facilities and pet cemeteries to keep reaching people currently in need. Even though many people attend the group only one time, receiving enough benefit that further visits seem unnecessary to them, others attend regularly for many months.

Hospice Philosophy

It is important to examine human hospice care, because so much about hospice is applicable to helping families faced with the approaching death of a pet. The term *hospice* is derived from the same root word used for hospital, hotel, hostel, and hospitality. In more ancient times it referred to a place where a traveler could find rest, refreshment, and safety. A Greek hospital in 1134 B.C. is described as having hot and cold baths; gymnasiotherapy; an amphitheater for entertainment; sunshine and fresh air, combined with pleasant vistas; libraries; and rooms for visitors (Stoddard, 1991).

The modern hospice movement in the United States began in the early 1970s and has gained considerable momentum. A National Hospice Organization survey in 1991 indicated that approximately 2000 hospices are operating in the United States. The development of these hospices was precipitated by the belief that dying patients and their families were not being served very well by the medical care system. "There is a difference between prolonging life and prolonging the act of dying until the patient lives a travesty of life." says Stoddard (1991) in her book, *The Hospice Movement*. Although modern hospitals are capable of amazing accomplishments in curing and saving patients, their focus is on treating and curing illness. When the patient is not curable, however, to persist in applying inappropriate care as if a cure was possible is pointless. It subjects patients to many indignities and discomforts and isolates them from many things that are important. Dame Cicely Saunders, a physician and the founder of St. Christopher's Hospice in England, said that "a patient should no more undergo aggressive treatment, which not only offers no hope of being effective, but which may isolate him from all true contact with those around him, than he should merely be relieved of symptoms when the underlying cause is still treatable—or has once again become so" (Stoddard, 1991).

The National Hospice Organization defines hospice as ". . . a medically directed, nurse coordinated program providing a continuum of home and inpatient care for the terminally ill patient and family. (It provides) . . . palliative and supportive care to meet the special needs arising out of the physical, emotional and spiritual, and social and economic stresses experienced during the final stages of illness, and during dying and bereavement. This care is available 24 hours per day, 7 days per week and is provided on the basis of need, not ability to pay" (Cohen, 1979). Hospice is characterized by palliation of symptoms, a caring environment, sustained expert care, and the pledge that families and patients will not be abandoned.

In the hospital environment, the patient and immediate family are often helpless to stop procedures and practices that none of them desire. Life may be prolonged, but so is suffering, and there is no quality of life. Use of the hospice concept maximizes the quality of life for terminal patients by supporting them with psychosocial services, providing respite care to relieve primary caregivers, and maintaining most patients in their homes. More than 90 per cent of hospice patients die at home, unlike nonhospice patients, 75 per cent of whom die in hospitals.

Hospice care is administered by a team that includes an administrator, medical director, nurse, home health aide, social worker, pastor, and volunteers. It combines skilled medical care with social, psychological, and spiritual support for the patient and family group. After the patient's death the survivors receive bereavement assistance through support groups and volunteers.

Hospice Practices. Patients are frequently referred to hospice by their primary physician when the physician recognizes that the life expectancy is less than 6 months. The hospice philosophy involves assisting the patient and family to acknowledge the imminence of death. The patient and family then begin to make realistic plans for maintaining the highest quality of life for whatever time remains.

Other key concepts of hospice philosophy are very important. The first is expert medical care. The physician and nurse use every resource to keep the patient free of pain and to minimize symptoms. Another concept is that the unit of care is the family. Psychosocial counseling and support are an important element of hospice care, and this care for the family continues for up to 1 year after the patient's death. A hospice may include a physical building with inpatient beds, but many hospices have only an office building. Patients are served primarily in their homes and in nursing homes and hospitals as needed. Most hospices are nonprofit organizations and serve everyone, regardless of ability to pay. Medicare and Medicaid reimbursement are the most important source of funds for patient care.

The patients served by hospices are under care for an average of 60 days. By diagnosis, 78 per cent have cancer, 8 per cent have heart disease, 5 per cent have respiratory disease, 4 per cent have acquired immunodeficiency syndrome, and 5 per cent have other conditions.

The Hospice Concept for Pets. There are many parts of the hospice concept that are applicable to veterinary medicine, yet some major differences from human medicine deserve discussion. In pets it may be even more difficult than it is in people to know when the pet has 6 months or less to live, as fewer statistics are available regarding animal life spans after any particular diagnosis. Also, 6 months is a much larger proportion of life in dogs and cats than in humans.

Another difference is that a pet's primary caregiver makes the decisions regarding treatment, not the pet. This corresponds more closely to pediatric hospice care.

The third difference is that in human medicine, a patient's physician refers him or her to hospice where physicians more experienced in palliative care may consult or participate in treatment. However, for veterinarians there is no hospice to which to make a referral. The veterinarian must make the transition from the "cure" state of mind to the "care" approach. This is not an easy transition, because the veterinarian must face a loss just as the members of the pet's household.

One physician said (Rossman, 1977):

> The basic aim in this hospital is to get people cured and out of the hospital as soon as possible. We are not running a luxury hotel devoted to making patients happy, but we are organized for efficiency to mobilize all possible resources for cure. The dying person who lingers in such a hospital is seen by the medical staff as one of their failures. And scientists do not wish to fail—even when there is no further chance of sustaining a meaningful and happy life, the tempo of efficiency is maintained or even increased with more discomfort, pain, machines, more needles stuck in veins, more impossible expense—and all for nothing in so many cases. As the clergy and psychiatrists seek to relieve anxieties, they are being increasingly frustrated as to how to help families that are caught up in the misery of such prolonged deaths.

Veterinarians want to use all their talents, knowledge, and technology to save patients. However, there are many cases in which a cure cannot be achieved; the reasons vary from lack of understanding of illness to the owner's lack of funds. In every case and for whatever reason, a crossroad will be reached where it is imperative to reassess what is best for the patient: continued attempts to cure or a new primary emphasis on care.

It is not easy to recognize when a patient's prognosis has become certain, nor is it easy to face the owner with this news and recommend a change of goals from cure to care. Yet in serving the patient and the family, veterinarians must make this difficult transition and help those last days to be counted among the best. The benefits to patients are to prolong quality of life and reduce suffering and pain (Max, 1990; Short and Van Poznak, 1991). The benefits to owners include more time to adjust to the impending death of the pet and possibly the ability to avoid facing the euthanasia decision.

Applications in Veterinary Medicine

Presuming both a desire to offer hospice care and the ability to make the philosophical transition, examining the human hospice helps to identify services and techniques adaptable to veterinary medicine. In presentations given at Delta Society Annual Conferences, Harris, Hancock, and Mader have conveyed many insights and experiences regarding the concept of hospice care for animals (Harris et al, 1991).

As a first step the veterinary staff can inform owners that hospice care exists as an alternative to either prolonged suffering or immediate euthanasia. This means providing continuous relief of pain—not relief after pain is evident, but prevention of pain through the regular use of analgesic agents. Second, many of the services comparable to those provided in human hospice care can be provided by using veterinary hospital staff. Skilled nursing care in the patient's home can be arranged by having veterinary technicians and other staff make house calls on the way to work, during the lunch hour, or after work, as needed.

The third component of hospice care is psychosocial services for the patient's family. The resources to provide this support are not part of the typical veterinary hospital and must be found elsewhere. Current and former human hospice employees may be willing to serve in a part-time or volunteer role. Local psychologists and social workers in private practice may be willing to take these cases on a fee basis or as volunteers. Hospital bereavement counselors may also be prospects. If these people have not had hospice experience or training, it will be valuable for them to obtain such training. The local hospice is the best resource to obtain guidance, training, or educational materials.

The fourth component is volunteers, which most veterinary hospitals seldom use. Perhaps there is an untapped opportunity to better use volunteers in many areas of the veterinary hospital, including in hospice care. Hospice volunteers provide support to the family and patient by running errands, allowing caregivers to take a break from patient care, and spending time with the family. They continue this support for up to a year after the patient has died. Most of the hospice volunteers are friends, relatives, and family served by the hospice during the death of a loved one.

The volunteers must be well trained before they have patient contact and are part of the hospice team. The greatest difficulties anticipated for veterinary hospitals are providing volunteer training and operating as a team. Perhaps the local hospice can include veterinary volunteers in their training classes. The team concept requires meetings and communication among team members. Being a human hospice volunteer may be the best way to understand the concepts and learn techniques that can be applied in the veterinary setting. Specifics tasks and assignments of various team members are presented in Table 23–1.

A final area of concern in hospice care is record keeping or charting. This is a consistent, well-structured, and closely monitored process in human medicine. Veterinary records do not usually contain any significant information about the human–animal bonds and relationships within the household. Unless this information is recorded routinely, it will not be there when needed by the hospital or hospice team.

Dr. Al Marshall of Largo, FL, suggested a simple way to record this information in the patient record. He envisioned a chart with pets in one column and household members across the top (Fig. 23–2). In each box can be recorded the significant activities in which each person participates with a particular animal. He believes this will be useful for managing medical cases and obtaining accurate histories, as well as for managing bereavement and hospice issues.

An approach like that in Figure 23–2 will help all of the veterinary staff keep in mind how various members of the household may be affected by the terminal illness or loss of a particular patient. It serves as a basis for discussion and further record keeping by the hospice team. It is also recommended that information about owners—any illnesses, losses of pets, friends, family, job, whether they live alone, and whether they appear to be extremely attached to the pet—be kept in the records. All of these factors can predispose owners to increased loneliness, more dependence on the relationship with the pet, and

Name	James					Doris					Heather					Richard					Arthur				
Relationship	Spouse					Spouse					Daughter, 8 yrs					Son, 10 yrs					Father-in-law				
	P	F	W	I	B	P	F	W	I	B	P	F	W	I	B	P	F	W	I	B	P	F	W	I	B
Snoopy	X				X		X			X				X	X				X	X			X		X
Garfield						X	X			X						X			X	X				X	X

Figure 23–2. Human–animal interactions and relationships. P, Primary (pet "belongs" to this person); F, feeds pet daily; W, walks pet daily; I, interacts regularly (plays with, talks to, trains); B, highly bonded.

TABLE 23–1. TIMELINE PHASES OF TERMINAL CARE*

	SIX MONTHS BEFORE DEATH	LAST MONTH BEFORE DEATH	AFTER DEATH
Patient signs	Ambulatory; coherent; some side effects from medication; initial stages of grief, anger, and denial	End-stage pronounced withdrawal; requires total care; intensive management of symptoms and pain; no appetite	
Medical director	Initial examination of patient; develops plan of care	Monitors/assesses plan of care; increased need for medication changes to manage symptoms and control pain	May have further communications with the family
Nurse case manager	Assessment of hospice conference with family; confers with physician; develops plan of care; orders medications; orders durable medical equipment; trains/instructs primary caregivers	Daily monitoring of end-stage process, side effects of medication, symptoms manifested, and pain management; coordinates preparation for death with other team members, increasing support for both family and patient	Calls and/or visits family; assesses special bereavement needs; may attend funeral; completes discharge charting
Social services	Assesses patient/family psychosocial/bereavement needs to develop plan of care; establishes trusting relationships with patient/family	Continued monitoring of approved plan of care; assists patient/family in resolution and closure; ensures final arrangements; facilitates support systems	Calls and/or visits family; may attend funeral; begins bereavement follow-up, identifies dysfunctional grieving, and initiates appropriate intervention
Volunteers	Confer with hospice team for direction; learn interest of patient; make initial visitations	Provide respite periods for family; provide patient with emotional support	Provide bereavement support to family/significant others; maintain regular contact for up to 12 months

*This table is excerpted from a National Hospice Organization publication. The original has columns for each month from 6 months before death up to the last month, and rows for additional personnel. Some of the items that are more applicable to veterinary medicine are shown.

From Timeline Phases of Terminal Care. Progressive Changes in Physical and Psychologic Conditions: Six-month Hospice Plan of Care. A publication of National Hospice Organization, 1901 N. Moore St., Suite 901, Arlington, VA 22209.

increased grief should the pet die. These are risk factors, not guarantees that the grief will be more intense or last longer. Having the information simply makes veterinarians more aware of the grief potential and more sensitive to the needs of the owners. This information should be recorded and updated by the staff as it is volunteered by the owner. It will then be available to everyone as needed.

SUMMARY

Veterinarians can apply knowledge about the grief response, advance directives, memorialization, and hospice care concepts to assist owners with geriatric pets through the inevitable loss they will endure. The results will be a more satisfactory closure to special human–animal relationships, quicker resolution of grief, and a greater appreciation of the human–animal bond.

References and Supplemental Reading

Cohen K. Hospice: Prescription for Terminal Care. Germantown, MD, Aspen Systems Corporation, 1979.

Feinstein D, Mayo PE. Rituals for Living and Dying, How We Can Turn Loss and the Fear of Death into an Affirmation of Life. San Francisco, Harper San Francisco, 1990.

Harris JM, Hancock G, Mader B. 10th Annual Delta Society Conference, Portland, OR, Oct. 10–12, 1991.

Max MB. Improving outcomes of analgesic treatment: Is education enough? Ann Intern Med 113:885–889, 1990.

Rossman P. Hospice: Creating New Models of Care for the Terminally Ill. New York, Association Press, 1977.

Short CE, Van Poznak A. Animal Pain. New York, Churchill Livingstone, 1991.

Stoddard S. The Hospice Movement. A Better Way of Caring for the Dying. New York, Vintage Books, 1991.

Index

Note: Page numbers in *italics* indicate illustrations; page numbers followed by t indicate tables.

ISBN 0-7216-4584-4